DIXON *AND* STEIN'S
Encounters With
CHILDREN
PEDIATRIC BEHAVIOR AND DEVELOPMENT

FIFTH EDITION

DIXON *AND* STEIN'S
Encounters With
CHILDREN
PEDIATRIC BEHAVIOR AND DEVELOPMENT

JENNY S. RADESKY, MD
Division Director, Developmental Behavioral Pediatrics
Associate Professor
Department of Pediatrics
University of Michigan Medical School
Ann Arbor, Michigan

CAROLINE J. KISTIN, MD, MSC
Associate Professor
Hassenfeld Child Health Innovation Institute
Department of Health Services, Policy, and Practice
Brown University School of Public Health
Providence, Rhode Island

ELSEVIER

Elsevier
1600 John F. Kennedy Blvd.
Ste 1800
Philadelphia, PA 19103-2899

DIXON AND STEIN'S ENCOUNTERS WITH CHILDREN: PEDIATRIC BEHAVIOR AND DEVELOPMENT, FIFTH EDITION

ISBN: 978-0-443-10704-7

Notice

Previous editions copyrighted 2006, 2000, 1992, 1987 by Mosby Inc.

Publisher: Sarah Barth
Senior Content Development Specialist: Ranjana Sharma
Publishing Services Manager: Deepthi Unni
Senior Project Manager: Beula Christopher
Senior Book Designer: Renee Duenow

Printed in India

Last digit is the print number: 9 8 7 6 5 4 3 2 1

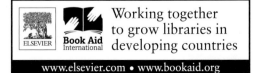

LIST OF CONTRIBUTORS

Shaquita Bell, MD, FAAP
Clinical Professor
Department of Pediatrics
University of Washington School of
    Medicine;
Senior Medical Director
Odessa Brown Children's Clinic
Seattle Children's Hospital
Seattle, Washington

Caitlin Camfield, MD
Fellow
Department of Pediatrics, Division of
    Adolescent Medicine
Seattle Children's Hospital
University of Washington
Seattle, Washington

**Erika Gabriela Cordova Ramos,
MD**
Assistant Professor
Department of Pediatrics
Boston Medical Center
Boston, Massachusetts

Kelsey A. Egan, MD, MSc
Assistant Professor
Department of Pediatrics, Division of
    Health Services Research
Boston University Chobanian and
    Avedisian School of Medicine,
    Boston Medical Center
Boston, Massachusetts

Yolanda N. Evans, MD, MPH
Division Director, Adolescent Medicine
Associate Professor of Pediatrics
Department of Pediatrics
University of Washington
Seattle, Washington

Yuan He, MD, MPH, FAAP
Assistant Professor
Department of Pediatrics
Perelman School of Medicine at the
    University of Pennsylvania
Philadelphia, Pennsylvania

Caroline J. Kistin, MD, MSc
Associate Professor
Hassenfeld Child Health Innovation
    Institute
Department of Health Services, Policy,
    and Practice
Brown University School of Public Health
Providence, Rhode Island

Anna Klunk, MPH, BS
Osteopathic Manipulative Medicine
    Clinical Scholar
Philadelphia College of Osteopathic
    Medicine
Philadelphia, Pennsylvania

Alana K. Otto, MD, MPH
Assistant Professor
Department of Pediatrics
University of Michigan
Ann Arbor, Michigan

**Lauren K. O'Connell, MD, MSc,
FAAP**
Assistant Professor
Department of Pediatrics
University of Michigan
Ann Arbor, Michigan

Jenny S. Radesky, MD
Division Director, Developmental
    Behavioral Pediatrics
Associate Professor
Department of Pediatrics
University of Michigan Medical School
Ann Arbor, Michigan

Cassie N. Ross, PsyD
Psychiatry and Behavioral Health
Nationwide Children's Hospital –
    Toledo;
Clinical Assistant Professor of
    Pediatrics
The Ohio State University
Columbus, Ohio

Destiny G. Tolliver, MD, MHS
Assistant Professor
Department of Pediatrics
Boston University Chobanian and
    Avedisian School of Medicine
Boston, Massachusetts

FOREWORD

Where do you go when you need help? Many of us turn to our own healthcare providers, our trusted partners in times of great stress and of great joy. These practitioners are the ones we turn to for answers, for reassurance, and for support. We trust our most precious gifts, our children, to our pediatrician. In turn, pediatricians turn to compendiums and tools to help them balance the competing demands of a busy office visit and stay up to date with best practices.

Over 20 years ago, when the first edition of *Encounters With Children* was published, the landscape of pediatric practice was somewhat simpler. Social media and other technologies were in the beginning stages of development, there were no global pandemics like COVID-19 wreaking havoc on the very framework of medicine, and the rates of mental health disorders in youth were far less. Now, practicing providers must balance medicine with rapidly evolving technology interfaces, social drivers of health, media consumption, and the increasing likelihood that the youth and adolescents they encounter have been or will be diagnosed with a mental, emotional, developmental, or behavioral health disorder.

As best practices have evolved, so has the actual role of a pediatrician. A doctor was once the person you visited when you were due for a physical or were feeling sick, but their role has evolved into one of advocacy across clinical, community, organizational, and political settings. In the last 5 years, organizations like the American Academy of Pediatrics have stepped into the national spotlight, providing expertise on topics ranging from racism to firearm violence prevention. Our duty to children does not start and stop in an examination room. Because of the wide range of drivers impacting child health, the role of a pediatrician extends far beyond shaping policy, legislation, and even societal dialogue. The adage, with great power comes great responsibility, has never been truer. The evolution of our role will come more easily for some clinicians than for others, but nonetheless, it is a mindset shift that must happen.

Drs. Radesky and Kistin approached the fifth edition of *Encounters With Children* with a determination to update clinicians on current issues. They partnered with pediatricians, medical students, and residents to understand the ever-evolving concept of clinical care that is rooted in justice and social advocacy, with the intent of moving the text to a more antiracist, inclusive collection. There is a focus on how to meet patients and their families where they are. Similarly, there is an emphasis on thinking about the child in the context of their community and how all our communities are linked. Drs. Radesky and Kistin demonstrate a clear intention to use language that promotes the dignity of children, adolescents, and families from all walks of life. This information will help guide pediatricians on what skills are needed to approach their practice from a holistic lens of health and well-being. It is then up to us to find ways to learn, practice, and implement those skills into our daily practice. I realize that growth and change surrounding the role of the advocate can be uncomfortable sometimes, as learning often is. Addressing trauma is a heavy load to bear. However, as pediatricians we are committed to the idea that our learning never stops and that ultimately this is about protecting and helping children and adolescents.

As clinicians caring for children and adolescents, we are uniquely positioned to share space with youth who are brave enough to share their hopes, dreams, and visions for the future … as well as their questions and concerns. Using techniques in this textbook, we can work toward creating safe spaces for youth and adolescents to explore their identity, their communities, and the world around them. One small practice change that has been used in our clinic in Seattle, Washington, is leveraging the electronic medical record for screening housing, transportation, and food security. This practice has led to more effective screenings, interventions, and the ability to measure needs over time.

It brings me immense joy to see our profession on the front lines of advocating for future generations. With tools like *Encounters With Children*, fifth edition, we have a framework for equity and excellence in our clinical practice. Most importantly, we have the tools to help all children be their healthiest and most productive.

Shaquita Bell, MD, FAAP

This book allows the professional to set the stage to allow children to tell us what they are about, to prompt families to bring forward the issues and concerns they have, to get at the things that really matter to them.

Dixon and Stein, Encounters With Children, Preface to the fourth edition

It has been a great responsibility updating this edition of *Dixon and Stein's Encounters With Children*. In our own training as pediatricians, we have found this textbook to be an essential guide to understanding how to connect with children, understand their behavior, and support parents through the surprises, joys, and frustrations of child-rearing. Constant through all the previous editions of *Encounters With Children* is a child-centered approach to understanding developmental stages, a focus on practical strategies for child health clinicians interacting with children and families, and the alignment of the content with the well-child visit schedule, making it highly relevant to new and experienced clinicians alike. *Encounters With Children* is well known for bringing the child's perspective into medical training through the use of children's drawings, which we have preserved throughout the book.

When we were asked to edit this new edition, we were in the middle of the first wave of the COVID-19 pandemic in 2020. The world was in various stages of social distancing, children were attending school over video from their bedrooms, grocery store aisles were empty, a national emergency in youth mental health was about to be declared, and healthcare systems were overwhelmed. Existing inequities in access to basic needs and services were both illuminated and exacerbated, and it became starkly clear that our systems were failing children's health and well-being. We accepted the task of updating this textbook to its fifth edition with the goal of updating the scientific content and recommendations about child development and behavior to reflect the environment that children are growing up in now, as well as ensuring that the text reflects diverse family experiences.

To that end, we have collaborated with pediatric scholars, clinicians, and experts across the country to identify opportunities to add additional content and perspectives to the text. With over half of the US child population living in poverty, we aimed to write and edit this book to explicitly incorporate psychosocial context into care. Each chapter attempts to call attention to the social, educational, cultural, and technological structures that shape children's opportunities, as well as the enormous impact trauma, racism, and marginalization exert on parent-child relationships and brain development. We aimed to use a strengths-based approach and teach child behavior and development in a way that would support clinicians in humble partnering with families rather than assuming an "expert" stance.

Similar to previous *Encounters With Children* editions, we foreground how relationships are central to a child's life course well-being. We added descriptions of contemporary theories of the drivers of child development, including attachment theory, infant mental health, strengths-based socioecological frameworks, adverse childhood experiences, toxic stress, and racism, in Chapter 2. In infancy chapters, we focus on supporting caregiver-child attachment through helping caregivers understand and mentalize about their child's experience. Toddler and preschool-aged chapters have been updated to include more information about autism screening, digital media, and taking a trauma-informed perspective with difficult behaviors and preschool expulsion. The school-aged chapters contextualize the child's entry into school within families' trust of the educational system, ability to navigate it, and advocacy opportunities. Finally, the preadolescent, adolescent, and emerging adulthood chapters take a strengths-based approach to the development of identity, reproductive health, positive relationships, and mental health.

Our sincere hope is that the fifth edition of *Dixon and Stein's Encounters With Children*, like the editions that came before it, provides child health clinicians in training and in practice with a useful guide to child development that increases knowledge, supports meaningful engagement with patients and families, and deepens the enjoyment of clinical medicine.

Jenny S. Radesky and Caroline J. Kistin

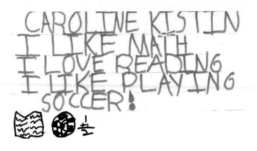

Caroline J. Kistin, early artwork (a very clear sense of self!)

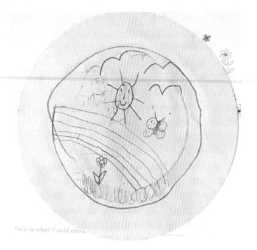

Jenny S. Radesky, early artwork on a paper plate (with prior drawing erased that I must have been unhappy with!)

ACKNOWLEDGMENTS

We are thankful for the many people who have made this work possible. We want to recognize the leadership of Drs. Suzanne Dixon and Martin (Marty) Stein and their dedication to *Encounters With Children* over the prior four editions. We are thrilled to present the fifth edition, renamed in their honor as *Dixon and Stein's Encounters With Children*. This edition also builds on the work of prior contributors, whose names are mentioned in each relevant chapter. To our many colleagues who provided in-depth reviews and authored novel content: it has been a joy to collaborate with you to craft this updated text, and we are thankful for your expertise and commitment to equitable, excellent care for children and teens. We are grateful as well for the guidance of the skilled editorial team; without you, this undertaking would not have been possible. On a personal note, we want to recognize the mentors and mentees who instruct and inspire us, the families with whom we have had the privilege to work over the years, our own partners and children, and the many people in our lives who make it possible for us to do the work we love.

Jenny S. Radesky
Caroline J. Kistin

CONTENTS

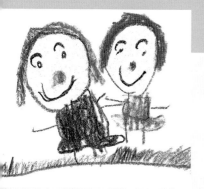

The Importance of Child Behavior and Development in Life Course Health

Caroline J. Kistin and Jenny S. Radesky

This is a book about child development for clinicians who care for children. The importance of evaluating development at different stages, as well as the growth and changes in a child's abilities over time, distinguishes pediatric medicine from other specialties. We believe that professionals delivering child health care should have knowledge in this area on a par with other sciences that touch their work. This book seeks to lay the foundation for knowledge of child development in the course of practice, clinical encounter by clinical encounter, preparing the clinician to effectively engage with caregivers, provide guidance, and advocate for the support families deserve.

In this book, the chapters are organized by child age and aligned with the typical visit schedule of well-child preventive clinical care. Although a child's development evolves along several dimensions at any one time, we have found that some strands of development are particularly prominent at predictable times. We have included topics in chapters based on the age of the child when a particular developmental or behavioral theme is prominent, important to the family, and easy to observe in the child. The immediate clinical relevance of a topic allows the clinician to review the full range of a specific developmental theme across the ages.

Within each chapter's specific developmental themes, the foundations of the developmental processes that have occurred earlier and the anticipated rollout of these processes in the future are also reviewed. This expanded discussion of a topic allows the clinician to see the matter in context and how it changes over time. It also allows for a review of the theoretical and research background relevant to the topic. As one goes through the entire book, a full course in child development is presented in a way that is relevant to the child health care clinician. The presentations

of developmental skills and behavior at each age are necessarily short; each chapter is a condensation of the large body of material that exists in the worlds of developmental psychology, psychiatry, developmental and behavioral pediatrics, neurology, and public health and counseling. In the type, length, format, and relevance of the material, we have kept the child health care professional in mind.

The material in this book is designed to provide clinicians with a map of typical child development, with its multiple themes and overlapping processes. The mental map is built on the learning that can occur at each health care visit, as the everyday encounters with children and parents in pediatric medicine offer a remarkable course in child development. All of us, young and old, experienced or on our first clinical rotation, can learn from each patient who comes in the door. Through careful listening, discussion, and observations, a child and family will teach us what we need to know. By reading a chapter before an office visit and then seeing a child and family at a particular age, the clinician builds a full picture of the developmental processes over time. Each encounter can then be met with an in-depth understanding of how development is progressing in a particular child.

There are developmental milestones we need to be aware of to ensure children who have developmental delays or need additional support have timely assessment and intervention. There are multiple validated screening instruments that help identify delays on a population level, which are referenced in this text, but this book will focus more on the interactions that occur during clinical encounters that help build the clinician's understanding of the child and family. While it is beyond the scope of this book to include a detailed discussion of the diagnosis or treatment of every developmental condition, we hope to provide the reader with skills that can be applied to each of their patient's specific circumstances, including guidance around supporting caregivers, observing child behavior,

---

Original chapter by Suzanne D. Dixon and Martin T. Stein.

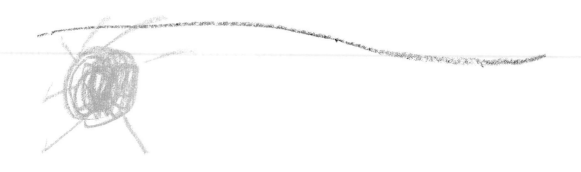

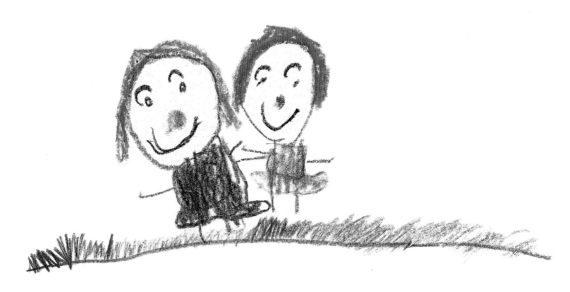

"Me and my sister." By Meike Messick, age 6.

and understanding what resources are available to families. For readers interested in pursuing more in-depth knowledge of child development, we provide resources at the end of each chapter, in Chapter 27, and in the Appendix. There are additional prompts in each chapter, under the "Heads Up" feature, that describe clinical findings that may be early signs of developmental delays or other issues that should be considered.

In most child health care settings, practice has become increasingly digitized and automated—from scheduling systems to treatment guidelines. There are many aspects of assessment, however, that cannot and should not be passed off to an automated system. We do not think it sufficient or even advisable to work only from checklists of milestones, to counsel families from rote lists of anticipatory guidance topics, or to see children in a "normal"/"not normal" developmental dichotomy that adds stigma and overly simplifies strengths and challenges. A broader perspective sets the clinician up for a more enlightened approach to the work of everyday practice. In this book, most chapters include a brief list of milestones that we expect to see at a given age, the "Quick Check" feature. We intend this to be used not as the focus of the visit but rather as a quick refresher of specific elements of developmental issues at each age.

The following perspectives inform the content of this book and underpin our recommendations for clinicians in their work with children and families.

1. **Caregiver-child relationships are the bedrock of life course well-being.** Ample research has demonstrated that a child's parents and caregivers are not only their first teachers but also their most influential guides through the stages of growth and development throughout childhood. A child's individual abilities and developmental trajectory both reflect this critical relationship and also shape it, as children change and influence their caregivers and families as well. This book takes the mindset that it is a privilege for us to be given access to this relationship. Clinicians and caregivers are partners in the process of discovering who a child is and how to support their individual strengths and challenges. Clinicians should center on and learn from the family's expertise with their child, and care should be taken to ensure that anticipatory guidance and any recommended interventions empower rather than disempower a child's family members. Often the best way to support children is to support their caregivers, which we discuss in relevant chapters.

2. In addition to examining development and behavior in the context of the caregiver-child relationship, **children and families need to be understood and supported within their home and neighborhood context, school and childcare context, and larger societal and cultural context.** The old models of the child marching along in a preset course of development, unaffected by environmental conditions, have been completely debunked. New models see the child's development intricately evolving through the interaction between the child and the whole of the environment. Summarizing the complexities of the developmental processes as we know them in the 21st century, Shonkoff and Phillips present us with the scope of our work as clinicians "from neurons to neighborhoods" and beyond. Assessment, guidance, and support will not be effective unless they incorporate an understanding of the factors at play in a child's experience across this whole gamut. Moreover, if we ignore the contextual factors that shape a child's access to health-promoting resources (e.g., nutritious food, high-quality educational instruction, positive family interactions) and pursue a one-size-fits-all approach to pediatric care, we run the risk of increasing inequities in child health and developmental outcomes.

3. Previous approaches to child development and pediatric practice relied on research and assumptions that were largely based on the experiences of White, heterosexual, and cisgendered middle-class or upper-middle-class families. Other ways of being or supporting children were often viewed as "other" or pathologized, and these views contributed to **conscious and unconscious bias and racism in clinical practice that reinforce and worsen inequities in child and family outcomes.** In addition to interpersonal bias and racism (which includes the discriminatory beliefs and actions of individuals), historical and present-day institutional and structural bias and racism (which includes unjust policies, laws, and practices) have profoundly shaped family circumstances and experiences with the health care system, education system, and social services—all of which impact child development. This text highlights historical and present-day inequities and calls on clinicians to reflect on their personal assumptions and blind spots, as well as the policies and practices of the family-facing institutions that influence child and family well-being. Approaching each clinical encounter with curiosity and open-mindedness, with the aim of working with families in a way that fosters mutual understanding and trust, is a common thread in these chapters. We also include recommendations for providing families with help meeting their material needs and connecting to community-based supports, as well as offering opportunities for advocacy that take into account the root causes of inequities and unmet needs that are present in clinical practice.

In addition to the key perspectives above, the following **guiding tenets** about children and child development, which are endorsed by experts in the field, shape the content of the book:

- **Children are active participants in their own development.** Children have an inherent agency to explore and master the world, the challenges of life, and the barriers that come up. Children inherently self-regulate and respond to change, the demands of the environment, and their own maturation by achieving a new balance. They can be observed learning new skills, handling emotions, and altering their course if required. They can be expected to work at resolving discrepancies and crises in their views of the world, minimizing emotional pain, and getting what they need from the environment by drawing on internal and external resources. A deeper understanding of these processes can spark both respect for and trust in the child from clinicians and caregivers.

- **Child behavior is understandable.** Virtually all behavior is both explainable and adaptive if one sees beyond the behavior to the core issues confronting a child and to the context in which such behavior occurs. This tenet is based on the premise that *behavior has meaning*. Even the most unusual behavior usually has some adaptive worth or explanation, and clinicians and family members should be intrigued to discover those adaptive forces that merge with developmental processes in a given circumstance. A solid grounding in child development will help clinicians understand what they and the family observe.

- **Families love their children, have expertise in their strengths and challenges, and want to support their growth and development.** In the vast majority of cases, parents want their children to do well, and they apply whatever resources they have to forward that agenda. These include not only physical resources but also knowledge, their individual life experiences, the support systems available to them, and the cultural understanding of what a good parent is and what good child rearing is. Child priorities are lined up with other family and personal demands on attention and energy. The clinician can be a source of information, an interpreter of the child's needs and behavior, and an observer of the child's strengths. With a shared goal of what is best for the child, a therapeutic alliance is set in place.

- **Development is not an even process.** Developmental progress is one of gains and plateaus in one area. Then another area becomes a prominent issue. Forward progression in one area may be accompanied by a seemingly short-term decline in another. Periods of plateau are times of consolidation and refinement of skills and should not be interpreted as a lack of developmental progress. The big shifts seem to be triggered by predictable neurological maturation, which sets the child up to act on the environment in a new and exciting way. Child development is more like climbing a series of peaks rather than ascending one big mountain. Some skills seem to fall into place overnight, whereas other gains are made one baby step at a time. A linear mentality will confuse the clinician over the expected ups and downs in watching children mature. An undulating, interweaving model is more appropriate and, in fact, more interesting.

- **Children will do their own developmental assessment if you give them a chance.** Children always practice the leading edge of their developmental competency, work at an emerging or newly acquired skill, and delight in a toy or activity that is just a little new and challenging. Through knowledge of developmental sequences, a wise clinician will set up toys or ask questions aimed at that developmental edge. The office visit should be orchestrated so that the assessment occurs automatically, seemingly incidentally, through the process of checking in, weighing, measuring, playing in the waiting room, and being observed in the examination room. The clinician should lay the agenda, set the stage, and then let the drama unfold. With this proactive, playful, and easy approach, rich information is gathered with little extra time or effort. However, this process depends on the clinician knowing what to look for, what to ask, and what simple maneuvers can be done quickly with a child and family.

- **Child health care should be fun.** Our day-to-day encounters can be particularly enjoyable if we continually marvel at the exciting development of children and the incredible adaptability of children and families. Watching these processes and seeing children grow and develop in individual ways should add delight to one's practice. By setting the agenda for each visit, setting up an office with a developmental focus, and really connecting with families, the clinician can claim back some of the excitement of pediatric practice.

This book aims to provide a professional perspective on the overall well-being of the patients seen and the families met. We hope that those in training and practice will take this opportunity to keep a broad perspective on the developmental forces that move children forward. This perspective should make practice not only more effective but also more intellectually satisfying. Being less bound by checklists and guided more by an understanding of child development and family needs, one can have the freedom to determine the agenda of each encounter and set the stage to evaluate the important issues affecting a child and family.

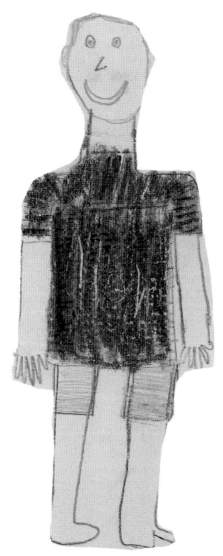

"A self-portrait." By Neil Hennessy, age 8.

This book, then, is a guide for learning child development and a guide for clinical practice. It is meant to be useful for learning one of the vital basic sciences of pediatric health care and to be a guide for adding behavioral and developmental depth of knowledge to pediatric medicine. It is a roadmap to allow one, from personal experience, to learn the principles of pediatric behavioral medicine, build a matrix of developmental expectation, and understand the patients and families one encounters each day in child health care.

RECOMMENDED READINGS

Berk L. *Child development*. Pearson Higher Education AU; 2015.

Cole M, Cole S. *The development of the child*. ed 4. New York: Worth Publishers; 2001.

Shonkoff JP, Phillips D, eds. *From neurons to neighborhoods: the science of early child development*. Washington, DC: National Academy Press; 2000.

Zuckerman BS, Augustyn M. *Zuckerman Parker handbook of developmental and behavioral pediatrics for primary care*. Wolters Kluwer; 2019.

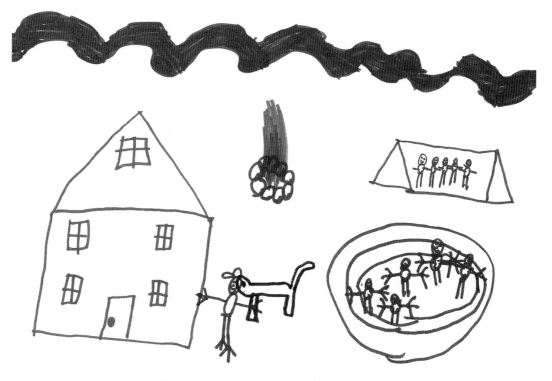

"My family outside." By David Betts, age 11.

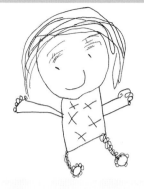

2

Understanding Children: Theories, Concepts, and Insights

Jenny S. Radesky and Caroline J. Kistin

This chapter presents the major theoretical perspectives on child development that have arisen over the last 150 years and contribute to our understanding of children. The major points of each theory, their enduring features and areas where each is most applicable, and their limitations, are presented. The thinkers, experimenters, and clinicians who have shaped our understanding are named within their own schools of thought. This chapter aims to inform the healthcare provider on the basic lines of thinking that give us established and emerging insights into the development of children.

KEYWORDS

- Developmental theories
- Attachment
- Scaffolding
- Mentalization
- Infant mental health
- Adverse childhood experiences
- Toxic stress

WHY LEARN THEORIES?

Like children themselves, theoretical frameworks of child psychology are always changing and developing. Child development theories are naturally shaped by the norms, cultures, scientific approaches, and sociopolitical context of the time. Although most cultures have folk theories and traditions for children's unique abilities, developmental processes, and place in the family, many early Western theories were dominated by perspectives of white European patriarchal societies. Over time, more diverse theoretical approaches have shed light on the blind spots in prior theories, while scientific advances have allowed more rigorous, empirical, and reproducible testing of child development concepts. Despite improvements over time, no theory is perfect or all-encompassing. So why learn about theories at all?

Theoretical perspectives provide insights for our everyday encounters with children and caregivers. Theories allow us to think about behavior, family interactions and developmental achievements and to then make sense of them. They allow us to demystify challenging child behaviors to parents, anchor their concerns in evidence about how children develop, and help them recognize the unrealistic pressures they feel from popular culture.

Theoretical insights also allow us to **organize observations**. With theoretical perspectives, we are helped to organize the seemingly random or chance behavior of a child into recognizable patterns. Without this lens, children's behavior—whether in the exam room or through a parent's narrative—makes less sense, and is more likely to elicit feelings of anger or guilt in parents. When we have a view of what a child is up to broadly from a developmental perspective, small behaviors, incidental observations and expected and unexpected responses all become recognizable units of data that help us in our understanding of a child and their family. Rather than be overwhelmed by the behavior and development of children, or react to behavior with punitive or harsh responses, a theoretical framework will add some explanatory foundation, as well as some interest and delight to our work lives and the experiences of caregivers. With a strong theoretical framework, a clinician can make use of every behavior, every action and every interaction with a child to gather and use data. Even a tantrum in your exam room is "data"—and the more we explain this to parents, the more they will hopefully feel understood rather than judged.

Based on prior edition chapter by Suzanne D. Dixon.

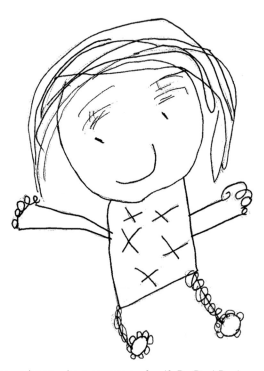

A girl shows her exuberant sense of self. By Dori Dedmom, age 6.

Anticipatory guidance becomes easy when we understand what will come next and why. Developmental surveillance becomes a professional matter of monitoring the progression of expected events rather than the technical job of just checking off items on a list. With limited time provided for well child encounters, it helps to have a big picture of what development is all about, so that we can maintain a high level of awareness of the core issues of our patients. When we encounter an unusual or troublesome behavior, we can be intrigued by what it means and model curiosity to caregivers. *Theories make us better observers and better thinkers.*

However, thinkers need help to put ideas and observations together. Theories on the development of children support our thinking processes by grouping behavior into manageable stages to remember and to guide further observations. Accordingly, if we observe a child having a tantrum, we can see that as part of the greater process of acquiring independence, so it is logical that other behavior may reflect this process, such as food refusal and sleep resistance. We can ask the right questions, provide guidance that anticipates these bumps in parenting and frame it as normative and not pathological. We can also generate additional observations based on what we see as the organizing theme of the child's behavior. We can contextualize our observations about a child and help give their actions meaning for our own thinking and that of families.

Second, new theories evolve not so much by building on the past but by challenging the old through highlighting their discrepancies and deficiencies and then proposing alternatives. In this chapter, we have tried to distill the enduring aspects of each school of thought, even if orthodox adherence to that theory is no longer common. They have left us a legacy of understanding some aspect or characteristic of the child. Finally, few theories claim to give us *all the answers on all aspects of development* or claim to explain all types of behavior. Typically, theories focus on one area and spend only passing reference to other areas.

As clinicians, we should not subscribe wholly to any one theoretical perspective. We can pick and choose what seems to fit for a given child at a given time and in a given area. This eclectic approach, however, requires that we have a solid grounding in the science so that our application is neither random nor glib. Throughout this textbook, we have tried to highlight the perspectives that seem salient to the age and event before us as examples of this flexible approach.

We can draw on all the rich insights available to us from developmental theory to give our work professionalism, perspective, focus, interest and amazement as children become at once predictable and totally surprising as individuals.

HISTORICAL THEORIES

MATURATIONAL THEORY–NORMATIVE APPROACH

Maturational theory was one of the earliest attempts to describe child development, starting in the 18th century but becoming more prominent under **G. Stanley Hall** and his student **Arnold Gesell** working at Yale University in the early to mid-20th century. This theory regards development as the inevitable unfolding of events determined internally by the forces of genetics and the neuromaturational processes that the genes direct. This perspective runs parallel to health professionals' understanding of embryology, developmental physiology and physical growth. In this model, development depends entirely on neurological and physical maturation, and it proceeds in fixed sequences—in fact, it underlies the idea of developmental "milestones" that compares the rate of attainment of different competencies. The concept of cephalocaudal progression of development originated here; for example, control of the head comes before control of the legs. These theorists gave us extensive data on the normative course of specific developmental gains and provided the earliest standards for expectations of typical development—which allows comparison of children as developmentally delayed, typical, or accelerated.

Limitations of the maturational perspective are that the child's environment is seen as having an impact only in that it can *impede* the developmental sequence. Temperament and individuality are acknowledged, but not specified. Gesell's concept of internal readiness for a task has endured in the childcare advice that began with Gesell but has influenced **Benjamin Spock's, T. Berry Brazelton's** and others' perspectives to the present. Gesell saw babies as inherently self-regulating and self-righting, progressing from periods of imbalance and instability to new levels of organization as they acquired new abilities. Very little depended on parents; they were supposed to step back, marvel and follow the child's lead. Although this was an improvement from prior, overly controlling parenting practices, it did not acknowledge the important role of the environment and secure relationships in shaping infants' brain architecture, development and sense of self (see "Attachment" section below). Furthermore, the discontinuities in developmental processes, abrupt shifts in competencies and new abilities that seem to appear without an antecedent basis are all at odds with orthodox maturational models. Much of the complexity and variability in development is left unexplained by this model.

Gesell's norms were based on upper-middle-class US children and did not capture the richness of cognitive or emotional development in infants and toddlers. The major contribution of maturational theory stems from the valuable norms that it has provided for the systematic observation of development in children. We still need and use these norms today. We will see this application most clearly in the chapters on motor development (see Chapters 11 and 13). Gesell's own perspective that babies are inherently "wise," being the depository of millions of years of evolutionary adaptations, is an important perspective for the clinician and parent alike (Box 2.1).

FREUD AND THE PSYCHOANALYTIC APPROACH

Sigmund Freud's work influenced several theories that continue to be relevant to pediatric clinical practice, although his perspective on human psychology had significant biases that limit its direct applicability. We outline here the contributions of his theories, including the ideas of conscious/unconscious processes, stages of development throughout childhood, and tensions between drives and impulse control—while recognizing that they are not empirically based.

Freud drew attention to the consequences of early childhood experience in later life and the centrality of emotional life in shaping personality. This model (Box 2.2) emphasizes the importance of both unconscious and conscious mental processes that shape development and influence behavior. A person's self-concept results from the interface of the child's inner needs (*biological drives and instincts*) with the demands of the external world around them (*social expectations*), which are viewed as conflicting. The drives and instincts revolved around "psychosexual tensions" centered on specific body areas listed in Table 2.1.

The three parts of personality were described as the *id* (housing the basic drives and instincts), the *ego* (the aware and rational self), which develops in late infancy and toddlerhood, and the *superego* (the conscience), which emerges from ages 3 to 6. The way these components are integrated and function in concert in early childhood are theorized to determine the individual's ability to function over the long term.

Successful *resolution of specific inner conflicts* at each stage leaves the child ready for a new level of emotional and social maturity. Freud was the first to introduce the concept of distinct stages in development. His model is like a staircase, not linear. He viewed the source of mental illness as

---

BOX 2.1   Key Insights—Maturational Theories

- Children develop along fixed sequences, a continuum of developmental gains controlled by genes.
- Individual children's development can be categorized as typical, accelerated or delayed when compared with large population norms.
- Rates of development vary by individual but the sequence does not.
- Behavioral change is linked to physical maturation.
- Children must have an inner readiness to perform a task for teaching to be effective.
- Children have inherent abilities to self-regulate in terms of sleeping, eating, activity and engagement.
- Children are "wise" because they carry thousands of years of evolutionary adaptiveness.
- Appropriate child rearing is responsive to the individual child, not as predetermined by adult care providers.

BOX 2.2   Key Insights—Freudian Theories

- Development occurs in distinct stages that vary by the drives and interests to be mastered in the service of meeting social expectations.
- Emotional life has a powerful influence on behavior and development.
- Emotions, dreams, disappointment, feelings, and frustrations matter.
- Unconscious processes shape behavior, concurrent and ongoing.
- Interactions between parent and child influence personality, resiliency, adjustment, and behavior into adulthood.
- Children do have an active mental life even before the emergence of speech.
- This mental life contributes to the child's adjustment both during childhood and later in life.
- Unconscious wishes and thoughts influence both present and future behavior, thus making it imperative when assessing behavior to look at the child's history, particularly their emotional past.
- Psychological growth is prompted by a moderate degree of frustration.
- The child's interpersonal experience with loved ones, most often their parents, is central to overall adjustment and functioning.

TABLE 2.1　Theoretical Perspectives of Human Behavior

Age	THEORIES OF DEVELOPMENT			SKILL AREAS		
	Freud	Erikson	Piaget	Language	Motor	Possible Psychopathology
Birth–18 months	Oral	Basic trust vs. mistrust	Sensorimotor	Body actions; crying; naming; pointing; shared social communication	Reflex; sitting; reaching; grasping; walking; mouthing	Autism; colic; disorders of attachment; feeding and sleeping problems
18 months–3 years	Anal	Autonomy vs shame, doubt	Symbolic preoperational	Sentences; telegraph; unique utterances; sharing of events	Climbing; running; jumping; use of tools; using toilet; early self-care	Separation issues; negativism; fearfulness; feeding and toileting problems; shyness; withdrawal; aggressiveness
3–6 year	Oedipal	Initiative vs. guilt	Intuition, preoperational	Connective words; can be readily understood; tells and follows stories, questions	Increased coordination; tricycle; jumping; writing	Toileting problems (enuresis, encopresis); anxiety; aggressive acting out; phobias
6–12 year	Latency	Industry vs. inferiority	Concrete operational	Communicating in sentences; reading and writing; language reasoning	Increased skills; sports; recreational cooperative games	School phobias; obsessive reactions; psychosomatic reactions; depressive equivalents; anxiety; attention deficit/ hyperactivity disorder; aggression
12–17 year	Adolescence (genital)	Identity vs. role confusion	Formal operational	Reason abstract; using language; abstract mental manipulation	Refinement of skills	Antisocial or illegal behavior; mood disorders; anorexia nervosa; suicide
17–30 year	Young adulthood	Intimacy vs. isolation	Formal operational	Reason abstract; using language; abstract mental manipulation	Refinement of specialized skills; sports skills peak	Depression; anxiety; schizophrenia; adjustment disorders; development of intimate relationships; difficulties with relationships
30–60 year	Adulthood	Generativity vs. stagnation	Formal operational	Reason abstract; using language; abstract mental manipulation	Refinement of skills	Depression; self-doubts; career development issues; family social network; neuroses
>60 year	Old age	Ego integration vs. despair	Formal operational	Some loss of skills; decreased memory focus	Loss of functions	Involutional depression; anxiety; anger; increased dependency

an outgrowth of developmental failure, not moving along satisfactorily to the next stage. Disruptions or abnormalities at a specific stage (e.g., anal) are seen as the basis for psychological conflict (e.g., obsessive behavior) that continues into adult life, when it results in unresolved anxiety (*neuroses*) or major psychological disturbances (*psychoses*).

Following Freud, other important thinkers emerged and provided additional insights. **Margaret Mahler** and her colleagues taught us that a child's mental and physical relationship with their mother gradually moves from one of total *symbiosis* (as in pregnancy) to independence through a series of stages in the first 3 years of life. These predictable landmarks of emotional development allow for the child's increasingly solid sense of self as an individual. These processes of *separation and individuation* become increasingly complex with time. Chapters 15 and 16 on the toddler years draw on this construct. Freud's daughter, **Anna Freud**, extended psychoanalytic thinking to specific observations of young children. Using individual play therapy and studies of orphan children, she conceptualized *lines of development* based on psychosexual theory.

ERIKSON AND STAGE-BASED APPROACHES

Erik Erikson broadened and extended Freudian theory to include the whole life cycle. He brought in the influence of society beyond the family in determining the outcome of each developmental stage. His *psychosocial stages* are shown in Table 2.2. Each stage is characterized by negotiation of one central issue that is necessary for emotional advancement to the next stage. Variation in these stage-locked tasks through the forces of culture, family, individual differences and the changing demands of society makes it widely applicable. Erikson's theory extends through adulthood and highlights some of the generic issues confronting parents as part of their own development. Erikson believed that "the child can be trusted to obey the inner laws of development." Under this umbrella, child rearing calls for child responsiveness rather than a proscriptive process. These Ericksonian broad themes can help us step back from specific issues or types of behavior that are brought to our attention clinically. If we see what the child's "big job" is at that stage, we can often find a way out of an immediate dilemma.

In the Ericksonian formulation, life is a journey to establish a *personal identity* that is built over time. Inherent factors such as physical maturation pose a series of crises; how each is resolved is influenced by one's place in a culture, in history and even in the political dimensions that surround us.

Erikson's language in labeling the core developmental task at any given time is helpful in organizing our own thoughts, especially those regarding atypical behavior, and in communicating issues with families (Box 2.3). The infancy chapters, particularly Chapters 10 and 12, use this framework to look at affective development, and the school-age years, as developed in Chapter 20, highlight this construct.

BEHAVIORISM AND SOCIAL LEARNING THEORY

This group of theorists, dominant in American thinking for most of the 20th century, shares the perspective that only behavior that is observable can be studied (i.e., not motives, beliefs, unconscious forces) and that the environment is the primary source of behavioral change. The environment supplies *patterns of reinforcement* or rewards that shape the child's behavior. The child becomes *conditioned* to respond in a certain way based on the environment's shaping of their behavior. The child's association of certain stimuli with responses (i.e., the *stimulus-response model)* influences behavior in increasingly complex patterns over time. Types of behavior that are rewarded stay; those ignored or punished disappear or are *extinguished* with predictable regularity. These theorists sought to make the study of child behavior an objective science and applied their efforts

TABLE 2.2	Erikson's Stages of Development	
Stage	**Age**	**Issue**
1	Birth–18 months	Trust vs. mistrust
2	18 months–3 year	Autonomy vs. shame and doubt
3	3–6 year	Initiative vs. guilt
4	6–11 year	Industry vs. inferiority
5	Adolescence	Identity vs. role confusion
6	Young adulthood	Intimacy vs. isolation
7	Adulthood	Generativity vs. stagnation
8	Old age	Ego integrity vs. despair

BOX 2.3   Key Insights—Erikson and Followers

- Development continues across the life span. We all have a developmental dimension, young and old alike.
- The process of development is the building of a personal identity.
- Biological maturation creates a series of crises that have to be resolved by each person, dependent in part on the wider social milieu.
- Society as a whole and historical and sociopolitical factors, as well as cultural ones, have a powerful

influence on how these developmental hurdles are negotiated. Explanations for variations in human behavior and development must take these factors into account.

- The social context of a person strongly influences behavior. Look at the context.
- Each person's unique life history shapes his individuality.

BOX 2.4   Key Insights—Learning and Behavioral Theories

- The environment, especially the social environment, has a powerful influence on behavior. Look at the environment when you evaluate behavior.
- Behavior is shaped (at least in part) by reinforcers in the environment. This concept can be used to change specific behavior.
- Children learn from the models, adults and children, around them, particularly in such matters as aggression, sex roles, social consciousness and action, and social norms of behavior. Evaluate the models when you evaluate behavior.
- Children learn from seeing and experiencing the consequences of their own behavior and adjust accordingly.

- Behavioral change is promoted by an ever-advancing sense of self-efficacy. Without a sense of efficacy and the experience of success, children will withdraw either physically or psychologically.
- Behavior modification programs do work to change behavior, but not to address the basis of that behavior.
- The closer the reinforcer to the action, the more likely one is to link the two.
- Positive reinforcers work better than negative ones.
- Social reinforcers work the best of all.

---

in laboratory settings. In traditional behaviorism, internal factors such as biology and temperament were minimized. Children are seen as lumps of clay to be shaped through experiencing positive and negative consequences of their actions. Behavioral problems and solutions come from patterns of reinforcement in the environment. Child rearing was seen in the earliest days (1930s–40s) as *child engineering*. Much of the early work was a transposition of animal studies to children. Indeed, the behaviorists were the first to apply a theory to rigorous laboratory studies. **Ivan Pavlov, J.B. Watson** and **B.F. Skinner** are names associated with the earliest behaviorist perspective.

Social learning theory, with **Albert Bandura** as a major figure in this school, evolved from behaviorism. It highlighted the importance of modeling in the processes of development. Children learn within a specific social context that provides feedback on behavior. This theory has now evolved to account for the child's internal processes of organizing, regrouping and drawing on memory to shape a behavior in a new environment or situation. Although a lot

of learning is still derived from observation, other types of behavior emerge from a child's ability to combine patterns and learn from imaginings of their own and through processes of self-evaluation. Children become more selective in what and whom they use as models, in line with an increasing sense of self and self-efficacy in their own worlds. This model presents development as a series of upward spirals, with forward progress fueled by the experience of successes or failures in the past. The model is one of a steady uphill progression, shaped by what you encounter on the journey.

Behavioral theories (Box 2.4) have prompted a great deal of applied research, as well as clinical intervention strategies, including conditioning children to consequences (*reinforcers*), positive and negative, associated with problem behavior. Programs targeted to get rid of negative early childhood behavior through withdrawal of privileges or positive reinforcement of desired behaviors rely on these *behavior modification* techniques (see Chapters 14 and 16). Therapies designed to foster learning to deal with fears and phobias are also based on these principles. Programs for treatment of autism spectrum disorder, for eliminating fears of medical treatments and for managing bedwetting are examples of interventions founded on this theoretical base.

Strict behaviorism does not take into account a child's inner life, emotions, motivations, and style in adapting to new circumstances and demands, and it is now used in combination with other interventional approaches (e.g., relational support, self-regulation strategies) in modern therapies. Other limitations of strict behaviorism include the fact that the environment in which children develop is much more complex than a series of reinforcers or even a series of models.

Behaviorist techniques are attractive to clinicians because they can be prescribed for almost any condition or situation presented by a troubled parent. Moreover, in many circumstances the techniques work, provided that one has typical children and typical circumstances. Caution should be exercised, however, because these techniques are directed at changing behavior alone and not at addressing the basis for that behavior. Children's behavior has meaning, no matter how seemingly maladaptive or disruptive, and addressing the underlying driver of the behavior is most important. This may include addressing a language delay that is leading to aggression when the child is frustrated, addressing insecure attachment that is leading to toddler dysregulation, or addressing an attention deficit that is leading to disruptive classroom behavior.

PIAGETIAN PERSPECTIVES

Jean Piaget revolutionized our "thinking about thinking" in children by proposing a new idea: children think differently than adults do. He posited that children learn through active interaction with the environment. Piaget developed his view of the active role of the child through detailed observations of children; he attended as much to their errors in problem solving and the patterns of exploration as to their successes. These "mistakes" told him how children reason about and understand their world. The funny things little kids say often reveal their beliefs about the world, beliefs that they have constructed through perceptions mulled over in a very active mental life.

His observations led to a *stage theory of development*. A child's way of acting on the world, physically and mentally, shifts radically between these stages. Table 2.3 shows these stages. This sequence is invariant, although the rate of progression may vary. The world is understood by the child with increasingly complicated mental structures. The model here, again, is a staircase, but one that a child actively climbs, dancing a bit on each step.

Piaget's insights dramatically changed the dominant behaviorist schools in America through his premise that the child is an active learner rather than a passive recipient or target of environmental forces. Such concepts as the importance of discovery and exploration to the child, now the foundation of early education, come from his

TABLE 2.3 Piagetian Stages of Development

Stage	Approximate Age (Years)	Ways of Understanding the World	Basic Concepts to Be Mastered
1. Sensorimotor	Birth–2	Through direct sensations and motor actions	Object permanence, causality, spatial relationships, use of instruments, etc.
2. Preoperational	2–6	Mental processes that are governed by the child's own perceptions and linkage of events; no separation of internal and external realities	Sense of animism; egocentrism, idiosyncratic associations, transductive reasoning
3. Concrete operational	6–11	Can reason through real and mental actions on real objects; can reverse changes in the world mentally to gain understanding; can reason with a stable rule system; understands some patterns	Mass, number, volume, linear time deductive reasoning conservation tasks; objective causality; decentering—can see another's perspective
4. Formal operations	12 and older (variable)	Abstract thought; can reason about ideas, impossibilities, and probabilities; broad abstract concepts	Mastery of abstract ideas and concepts; possibilities, inductive reasoning, complex deductive reasoning

work. Much work in developmental psychology today has Piagetian ideas as the explicit or implicit foundation.

Children develop, in this view, by a process of *assimilation* (taking in information through any and all the senses), *accommodation* (taking one's current abilities/understandings and modifying them to adjust to the new circumstance or challenge) and organization of this into a new mental structure or physical action, a *schema*. Such development creates a new level of mental *equilibrium* that lasts until there is something new experienced in the environment. Novel, surprising events that are discordant with previous experiences then challenge the child to develop newer schema. The social and physical environments are important parts of this learning.

Piaget theorized that in infancy, children are in the *sensory motor period*, in which infants learn through their own senses and actions on objects. These baby "experiments" begin with reflexes and the infant's spontaneous actions. The infant observes the results of such behavior and repeats it. Then they modify their actions slightly and observe this outcome. These are called *circular reactions*. Through increasingly complex interactions, the infant constructs their own world view. This world is eventually found to contain objects and people that exist even when you do not see them, a concept called *object permanence*. It also has consistent connections between actions and results (*causality*) and is mapped in three dimensional space (*spatial perception*). An infant banging a rattle in more and more complex ways, a baby playing peek-a-boo and a young child winding up a toy or finding a hidden toy are examples of this infant scientist at work. More specifics of these observations are covered in the infancy chapters (see Chapters 10–13).

The *preoperational period* (preschoolers) is cognitively egocentric. Children at this age believe that the world is organized around them and their wishes; events depend on their actions. Objects are viewed as having a life (*animism*), including toys and technology. They reason *transductively*, assuming a causal link or a permanent association when two events are experienced in close proximity (e.g., I had a temper tantrum in the clinic, so now I get a shot; the nurse blows up my mom's arm every time she gets checked because she is having a baby—that is why her belly just keeps getting bigger). Their logic is faulty, although they are mentally active in creating linkages and associations. Fantasy, imagination and their own desires influence thinking at this age. The world is a magical place, and they see themselves pulling the strings. Chapter 16 in particular uses these themes.

The *concrete operational child* (grade-schooler) becomes more logical and can reason about objects in front of them. They can imagine that changing the shape of an object or the distribution of an array of objects does not change their essence such as mass or number. They can imagine changes in real objects in their head. This mind-set is called *conservation* and is the mental basis for much of school work, games and sports (mental aspects) and social interactions. Deductive reasoning becomes possible. They can *decenter* enough to understand that others may have ideas, feelings, and desires different from their own. They can look for the order of things beyond their own idiosyncratic groupings. The tasks of school and learning call up these perspectives and are applied in Chapters 18 through 20.

With the *formal operational* person, an adolescent or adult, abstract, theoretical, inductive thinking becomes possible. Hypothetical situations, multifaceted causality, and consequence networks can be imagined. This is discussed in the adolescent chapters (see Chapters 21–23).

The chapters on illness (see Chapter 25) and on stress and loss (see Chapter 26) use this framework to explain childhood thinking in these circumstances. Our clinical approach changes when we know children experience the world qualitatively different than we do.

Despite Piaget's influential theories, they have limitations. Piaget may have underestimated the capabilities of infants and toddlers, or what any child can learn with help or practice. Cross-cultural observations support Piaget's ideas about the universals of cognitive development in young children, but the mental structures of older children and adults seem to vary across the globe, seemingly in response to the particular cognitive demands placed by a specific environment. Finally, the Piagetian stage-based theory has been modified by many in favor of a more continuous and heterogeneous view of mental development in children. Children roll along rather than bounce from one stage to another in these revisionist views. However, Piaget's work contains a rich legacy of important insights and probably inspires more current research in child development than any other view (Box 2.5).

MORAL DEVELOPMENT

Piaget applied his theories to moral development with the description of two stages, divided at about age 10. At the younger stage, children see rules as immutable, handed down by an authority and requiring obedience to the letter. The seriousness of a crime is judged by the damage done or the extent of the violation, not by motivation. After age 10, children appreciate that people have different perspectives on what the rules that guide conduct are or should be and that these rules might be changed. **Lawrence Kohlberg's** work evolved from Piaget; he also used stages to describe the generic characteristics of children's moral problem solving, the way in which they reason about moral situations. Children and adults all over the world seem to solve moral dilemmas along this continuum, although the

---

BOX 2.5 Key Insights—Piaget and Followers

- Learning is an active process for children. They build their own mental constructs from environmental input.
- Children understand, reason about and act on their world in qualitatively different ways than adults do.
- Cognitive development proceeds in stages that are distinct and invariant in sequence.
- The child is self-regulating in what they take in and how it is organized.
- Readiness to learn a specific task is necessary if it is to be achieved.
- Supports, prompts and interaction with objects and people can move a child up the next level but cannot advance them beyond their ability to assimilate that input.
- Shifts in cognitive development are associated with changes in social interaction and competence, moral judgments, and emotional regulation.

---

context and values may vary by context, culture, religion, and even sociopolitical influences.

Kohlberg's view of the progression of moral judgment has been challenged by several investigators, prominently **Carol Gilligan**, in whose view this schema is inherently male, Western and falsely hierarchical. Values placed on cooperation, caring and compassion are more characteristic of the way females and indigenous cultures make moral judgments, and these factors are not accounted for in Kohlberg's scheme. Experimental work supports these differences but still shows that young children see rules as rigid and absolute, that guilt depends on the damage done rather than motivation and that the likelihood of punishment has strong sway. Lecturing a preschooler on the broad social order, the perspectives of others or even empathy is unlikely to have much salience or effectiveness. In contrast, many adolescents will love to discuss the complexity of moral decision-making and will broaden their own perspective when exposed to others who base judgments on the values of adherence to human rights, human dignity, and other broad values.

SOCIOCULTURAL THEORIES

The current era has seen a rediscovery of this school as initiated by the work of the Russian psychologist **L.S. Vygotsky**. With an eclectic background, an Eastern approach to life and living in a Marxist regime, Vygotsky provided an entirely new view of the child. He saw a child as embedded in the whole of the cultural, historical and social milieus; no behavior or developmental gain can be explained without taking these influences into account. The culture defines what skills are needed for functioning and then gives the child tools in the form of language, numbers, writing, technologies, ideas, and patterns of behavior. With these they solve their own social problems, seen broadly as how to get along and succeed. The *child-in-context* is the only observable unit—a given child is inherently different in different contexts. A change in a child's routine, physical attributes, and skills changes everything. Newer research in psychological anthropology, sociology, and developmental psychology has incorporated these ideas with greater specification of the context of each child's behavior and evaluation of a child in an activity or within a specific surrounding. Cross-cultural work has changed significantly with this perspective and greater inclusion of diverse children and families.

Perhaps a greater contribution of the sociocultural model is Vygotsky's framework of *zone of proximal development* that has influenced education and childrearing. He proposed that a child on their own will function at the bottom of that zone, the *functional level*. However, with good teaching, parenting, coaching, motivation and modeling, the child will function at a much higher level, their *potential level*. This higher level is achieved through a process of *scaffolding*, where the mentor assesses what the child can do and then builds on that, step by step, by guiding, modeling, and suggesting strategies or approaches. This entails presenting activities just above the child's current level of functioning and helping them reach for that new level. If the level of input is too low, the child gets bored and disengages or makes things more lively. (Envision the child throwing spitballs instead of doing spelling words.) If it is too hard or presents unattainable tasks, the child simplifies the task, does part of it or disengages. (See the child daydreaming, doodling and asking to go to the restroom at math time.) An environment that prompts healthy development is one that keeps the child at the top margins of their zone, with adjustments made for advancing skills and backtracking if the child becomes overwhelmed. Scaffolding remains a very important clinical concept as discussed in the early childhood Chapters 14 through 17.

IMPORTANT CONTEMPORARY THEORIES FOR CLINICAL PRACTICE

TEMPERAMENT

The unique way a child behaves, develops, and respond to their world is called *temperament*. *Temperament can be defined as stable, individual modes of responding to the environment based on differences in emotional reactivity, activity level, attention, and self-regulation that appear consistently across situations and are relatively stable over time.* The concept of temperament as an important characteristic of a child and a strong predictor of behavioral concerns and problems began with the seminal work of **Stella Chess** and **Alexander Thomas**. Their longitudinal studies clearly showed remarkable stability of the characteristics of temperament and how they elicit caretaking responses.

The dimensions of child temperament often used in clinical practice and research are shown in Table 2.4. Clinical appraisal of these dimensions can be done informally in a primary care setting over time, but was standardized by **William Carey** and **Sean McDevitt** with the use of questionnaires. Other researchers such as **Mary Rothbart** use slightly different language and clustering, but there is considerable overlap in all schemas.

Substantial evidence indicates that these characteristics are "hard-wired" in any individual and cluster in families. Twin studies show that identical twins are more alike temperamentally than fraternal twins are, even when raised apart. When characteristics group in families—such as shyness, poor adaptability and irregularity in biological functions—this can lead to caregivers really understanding their children, or being very frustrated by them. Additional evidence shows that resting heart rates, cortisol levels, and even frontal lobe electroencephalographic activity vary by temperament in infancy and beyond. Children with specific genetic conditions (e.g., Williams syndrome, Lesch-Nyhan syndrome, Angelman syndrome) may have their own unique temperamental profiles.

Longitudinal studies show that infant temperament predicts the occurrence of later behavioral challenges. Infants with "difficult" temperament (i.e., low adaptability and self-soothing, high emotional intensity, and physical activity)

are four times as likely as easy infants to have preschool and school difficulties. Children with inhibited temperament (i.e., low adaptability, slow to warm up to new experiences, easily overstimulated with sensory input) are more likely to have shyness, anxiety, social withdrawal, or difficulty adjusting to new school or social settings. These links are particularly strong for children who are at the extremes, such as a very fearful infant or a very active toddler. Because temperament traits track from childhood into adulthood, it can help if clinicians reframe for caregivers that some temperament characteristics feel challenging to parent in early childhood, but are beneficial traits later in life. Active, gregarious, talkative school-age children may spend a lot of time in the principal's office in elementary school but be very successful entrepreneurs and activists as adults. Children labeled slow to warm up may find a niche in a profession that requires precision and caution.

Characterizing a child's individuality on dimensions of temperament allows the clinician to assist parents in seeing the child's unique needs and in developing behavior management strategies that are likely to be successful. For example, a child with low adaptability will need help in anticipating and coping with change. A high-activity child will need more help to wind down before bed. Good advice follows from a clear understanding of these individual characteristics. The concept of temperamental match or *goodness of fit* between parent and child predicts adaptability and resilience in the face of stress; poor alignment is often the source of interactional difficulties and behavioral complaints. For example, a quiet, low-intensity child who withdraws in new situations may be a source of worry to an anxious parent who responds with overprotection or avoidance of new challenges. A high-intensity, persistent, child with a negative mood may be regarded by parents as angry, ungrateful and generally difficult, particularly if

TABLE 2.4 Temperament Dimensions

Dimension	Description
Activity level	Amount of physical movement during sleep and awake periods
Rhythmicity	Regularity of physiological functions, such as sleep, hunger, elimination
Approach-withdrawal	Nature of the initial response to new stimuli
Adaptability	Ease or difficulty with which reactions can be modified
Persistence-attention span	Length of time that an activity is pursued
Intensity of reaction	Energy level of the responses regardless of quality or direction
Distractibility	Effectiveness of extraneous environmental stimuli in interfering with ongoing behavior
Threshold of responsiveness	Amount of stimulation (e.g., light, sound, touch) necessary to draw a discernible response from the child
Quality of mood	General emotional tone of the child's response and interactions

the parents tend to be inflexible or emotionally reactive themselves. In these circumstances, the clinician must help families see these differences as hard-wired and part of the individuality of the child. If caregivers respond with altered expectations and a child-rearing style that is supportive and does not reinforce negative behaviors, the child is likely to do well and show more adaptive functioning.

A child with a negative mood, poor adaptability, irregularity in habits and a highly intense reaction presents a challenge to any parent and may elicit a punitive, controlling parenting style unless such behavior is seen in the context of an individual style and responded to positively and consistently. Temperament will enter into many chapters of this textbook because it is an important concept.

Other longitudinal work done in Hawaii by **Emmy Elizabeth Werner** and colleagues, though not strictly of temperament, shows the role of these individual factors in development. The concept of the effect of *resiliency* in the face of overwhelming stress on the processes of development was evaluated over the life span. This work showed that children with a positive demeanor, a ready approach to what life brought and an ability to inspire passionate devotion in at least one adult care provider were more likely to succeed in all aspects of their lives despite a myriad of risk factors. These individual features were more predictive than other biological (except direct insults to the central nervous system such as meningitis) or even sociological variables when examining the outcomes of children monitored into adult life. Such is the power of temperament and positive relationships to influence development. Without a strong understanding of how temperament influences behavioral and developmental issues, the clinician will have a hard time evaluating behavior, behavior problems and difficulties that children and families face in all the systems that change their lives.

ATTACHMENT AND EARLY RELATIONAL HEALTH

Attachment theory was first introduced in the 1960s by John Bowlby, who considered the formation of attachment relationships to be the dominant organizing force of infant and early childhood social development. Infants are thought to be drawn to closeness and interactions with caregivers to promote survival; over time, based on these interactions, infants and children start to conceptualize their caregivers as available and responsive. The daily serve-and-return interactions that act as the context for development of attachment, and how clinicians can support them are described in greater detail in Chapters 8 and 10. As the infant develops the ability to walk and move independently, they are increasingly able to use their caregiver as a *secure base* from which they can explore the environment and then return for comfort. Several factors

influence attachment development, from child and caregiver individual differences to household and structural factors (see Box 12.1).

Attachment has been researched empirically in several ways. **Mary Ainsworth** developed the Strange Situation Experiment to examine the separations and reunification of young children and their caregivers, including response of the child to an unfamiliar adult. The patterns of attachment observed during this experiment are described in Chapter 12. Secure child-caregiver attachment is a strong predictor of social-emotional outcomes later in childhood and adulthood, while insecure or disorganized attachment patterns predict more dysregulated behavior, hostile and untrusting relationship, lower empathy, and weaker sense of self.

Another approach for measuring attachment that is relevant to pediatric clinical practice is the Working Model of the Child Interview. Created by **Charles Zeanah** and further developed by **Kate Rosenblum and Maria Muzik**, this caregiver interview explores what types of adjectives they use to describe their child, the narratives they tell about their parenting experience, and how they **mentalize** about the motivations and feeling states underlying their child's behavior. Caregivers with secure attachment describe their child in sensitive ways that understand the child's unique abilities and challenges, reflect on their experience as a parent and how their behavior influences their child. In contrast, insecurely attached caregivers may describe their child in emotionally distanced, disorganized, simplistic, or negative ways, or may be preoccupied with other factors (e.g., their own relationship with their parents) that dominate the interview. Pediatric clinicians may notice similar elements of narratives when taking a clinical history. When a caregiver is being overly harsh or negative about a child, it can help to wonder out loud about what the child might be thinking, feeling, and trying to master—to help the caregiver mentalize about the child's perspective.

Other research methods examine moment-to-moment changes in how caregivers and young children interact, and how this influences attachment formation. In **Ed Tronick's** famous Still Face Experiment, parents and infants are asked to play together for several minutes, and then the parent is instructed to make a flat facial expression for several minutes (which is upsetting to most infants; this acts as a relational "disruption"), and then the child and parent "repair" (usually the parent calming down the distressed infant and helping them play again.). An important takeaway from this research is that the process of *disruption and repair* is common and is an important part of the developmental process for infants. In other words, caregivers do not have to be perfectly attuned to their child's emotions all the time; but, if they can respond to moments of distress with sensitivity and warmth that help the child recover, the child will learn something in the process. Mutual regulation is believed to help children develop awareness of their own self and emotions—to recognize and regulate them—through caregiver mirroring and labeling of child emotional and mental states.

The interventional field of **infant mental health** (now often referred to as Early Relational Health) applies attachment principles to clinical care and grew out of **Selma Fraiberg's** work with caregiver-infant dyads. Her approach emphasized: (1) importance of direct observation of caregiver-child interactions, (2) identifying caregiver and child strengths to be built on, as well as challenges and risks to be targeted with intervention, and (3) creating a *parallel process* in which the clinician *understands and responds to the caregiver's needs* with the goal of *strengthening the caregiver's capacity to understand and respond to child needs*. This approach is inherently strengths-based and adapts to the needs of families, regardless of their mental health, resources, or structural barriers. It is often carried out through home visiting, pediatrics, early education, and early intervention and as such is an interdisciplinary field.

Important concepts in infant mental health/early relational health include:

- Caregiver and child emotion regulation and coregulation
- Safe, stable, and nurturing caregiver-child relationships
- Sensitive and responsive caregiver-child interactions and play (see Chapter 10)
- Caregiver reflective functioning and mentalization about the child's emotional experiences
- Multigenerational and culturally embedded models in which the health of the child depends on the well-being of the caregivers and may be impacted by the family history of stress and trauma, and resilience of the community

Therefore early relational health has been identified by the American Academy of Pediatrics as an important approach to supporting child social competence and emotional well-being, while also buffering children from the impact of toxic stress and adverse childhood experiences. "Serve-and-return interactions occur within the context of simple daily routines such as feeding, dressing and bedtime, and are enhanced by safe and nurturing environments that support exploration and learning. Throughout each day, relational health is promoted by simple moments of positive parenting/caregiving activities such as reading aloud, interactive play, talking, singing and participating" (Council on Early Childhood, 2014). Early relational health is inherently a trauma-informed practice because it aims to understand families within their unique psychological lived experience and social context, and therefore is an important concept for current pediatric practice.

SOCIOECOLOGICAL SYSTEMS MODEL

Closely allied with the sociocultural views are those with *ecological* perspectives as influences on child development. In this view, a broad and interlocking set of systems influence the developmental processes. Table 2.5 describes these systems. No longer is the child viewed as being influenced by the interface with family, peers and school alone. Rather, the whole sociopolitical and cultural environment has a profound impact on the one hand and incredible potential for intervention on the other. Beginning in

TABLE 2.5 Ecological Systems That Influence and Determine Child Development

System	Description	Examples
Microsystem	Direct, reciprocal interactions between adults and children; also includes others who influence those directly acting on the child	Parents, siblings, care providers, teachers
Mesosystem	Environments that serve as connections between individuals in the microsystem	Home, school, daycare
Exosystem	Social settings that affect children, but do not contain them; community-based organizations, services and forces that influence the child-family microsystem; and informal community support systems for families	Health and welfare services, workplace policies and programs, social networks/social media, financial aid, jobs, recreational opportunities for families
Macrosystem	Cultural values, laws, customs, resources and the priorities that children and children's issues have in the community	Daycare standards, educational standards and expectations, policies/laws such as paid parental leave or federal antipoverty programs

infancy and increasing dramatically as they age, children are influenced by—and in turn shape—their environments. **Uri Bronfenbrenner** is a key proponent of this perspective, which was inspired by his work on daycare. In related work, **Michael Rutter** and colleagues have called attention to the tremendous impact of the school milieu on children (Box 2.6).

The essence of this theory is that the child is nested in concentric circles of influence, which include their family, community, and larger policies and systems. The outer systems mediate their effects through alteration of the microsystem that surrounds the child. For example, the structural components of a healthcare system will change when, how and where a child gets care and even what elements will be included in that care. Increases in societal isolation and dependence on social media during the COVID-19 pandemic influenced levels of trust in neighbors and institutions, which impacted child well-being through alterations in the parent-child interface. The impact of each factor varies, depending on the developmental status of the child and all the other factors in this system (Box 2.7). The child is enveloped by the family; however, this is not an impervious cocoon, but an ever-changing environment. It is also a two-way street—the child's own needs, personality and developmental level prompt change in the interface between them and their family, which in turn prompts changes in the family's interface with their community.

Within the socioecological framework, there are factors at each level of influence that support optimal child health and development. The Strengthening Families Protective Factors framework, from the **Center for the Study of Social Policy**, highlights five interrelated areas of focus for child and family well-being. First, at the policy and system level, is the family's ability to access necessary services and support when needed. This may include access to medical or educational resources, assistance with food or housing programs, or the ability to obtain other types of support as necessary. Second, at the level of the community, is the formation of meaningful social connections with others. The third and fourth factors operate at the level of the family and include parental resilience, or the ability to cope with daily challenges or stressors, and the parent's knowledge of child development and parenting practices that foster child growth, communication, self-regulation, and curiosity. The fifth protective factor, at the level of the child, is impacted by all of the others and is the child's own social and emotional skills and behaviors. For the child health clinician, an ecological systems approach therefore mandates a broad perspective on pediatric care and wellness. Sometimes we can act at one level and sometimes at another in the course of taking care of patients. These spheres of advocacy are seen in Fig. 2.1. One cannot care for children without taking these systems into account.

BOX 2.6   Key Insights—Sociocultural Theories

- The child's development is enmeshed in a social, cultural fabric from which they cannot be separated.
- Behavior can be understood only as a child-in-context.
- Children learn only in social contexts. They solve social problems presented by the real world in which they live. They learn the skills and acquire the tools that allow them to survive and thrive.
- Children learn within a certain range of environmental input, at the lowest level when left to their own devices, at the highest level when given appropriate support. If the environment is overwhelming, they will do something to lower the input or alter the task downward. If too low, they will add some spice to the situation.
- Development is better characterized by what children can accomplish with support and how they evolve over time in an environment of social support. Assessment should be interactive and dynamic over time.
- Teaching, coaching or parenting at its best teaches strategies to learn, not specific skills or information.

BOX 2.7   Key Insights—Ecological Systems

- Development is determined by a child's interaction with their family.
- The interface between the child and the family is in a state of constant change in response to intrafamilial and extrafamilial forces.
- Societal forces have a powerful influence on the child, primarily through the medium of alterations in the interactions in the family.
- The child's own behavior alters the caretaking milieu.
- To support a child's optimal development, one may need a family systems approach or community advocacy.
- Trauma, racism, and other significant stressors can interfere with healthy child development, particularly during critical developmental windows or in the absence of robust support.

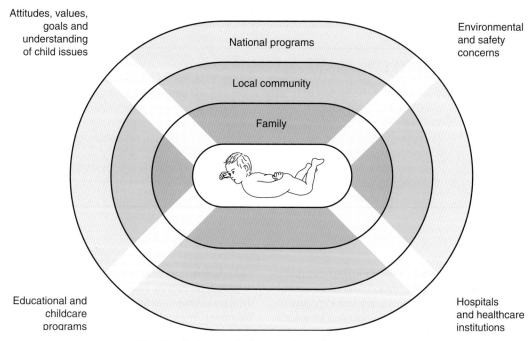

Fig. 2.1 Spheres of advocacy in pediatric practice.

INDIVIDUAL DIFFERENCES

Akin to the concept of temperament, **neurodiversity** describes the spectrum of different abilities that vary between individuals. Children and adults with autism spectrum disorder, attention deficit hyperactivity disorder, dyslexia, and other learning disabilities may identify as neurodiverse. This framing, rather than deficit or "disorder" based, respects the unique strengths of people with different abilities and reduces stigma. For example, children with autism may have strong visual-spatial skills or memory, which can help them compensate for the skills that do not come as easy to them. It also raises awareness of the fact that children respond differently to the same environments, and therefore may need accommodations to help them function best in environments such as home or school.

Howard Gardner's idea of multiple intelligences aligns to some degree with the neurodiversity ideas just described. In his view, some individuals are particularly primed to be responsive to certain kinds of information and skill acquisition. They are innately set up to process information in specific ways, to learn in specific ways more easily than in others. These clearly varying differences in a child's "hard wiring" identify strengths and vulnerabilities that influence how a person functions. Each type is neurologically based

with its own developmental course (Table 2.6). Gardner dismisses the notion of general intelligence entirely. Schools base their teaching and assessment on linguistic intelligence, but a child with strengths in other areas may not be successful in that particular milieu. As above, Gardner's theories allow the framing of many difficulties with learning as *learning differences* rather than learning "disorders." His view is that we miss a lot of human potential when we fail to allow these other mental abilities to blossom.

THREATS TO CHILD DEVELOPMENT AND EXPANSION OF THE SOCIOECOLOGICAL MODEL

Just as there are conditions that support healthy child development, there are also threats that should be understood by the child health clinician. A number of theories have expanded on the socioecological systems model to further explain how exposure to major stressors, including trauma and racism, impact child development and short and long-term health outcomes.

The ecobiodevelopmental model, toxic stress, and adverse childhood experiences

The ecobiodevelopmental model, developed by **Jack Shonkoff** and colleagues, describes the interplay between a child's biology, or genetic predisposition to certain

TABLE 2.6   Multiple Intelligences

Intelligence	Description
Linguistic	Sensitivity to language; language-based functions
Logicomathematical	Abstract reasoning, manipulation of symbols, detection of patterns, logical reasoning
Musical	Detection and production of musical structures and patterns; appreciation of pitch, rhythm, musical expressiveness
Spatial	Visual memory, visual-spatial skills, visualization
Body—kinesthetic	Representation of ideas, feelings in movement; use of body, coordination, goal-directed activities
Naturalistic	Classification and recognition of animals, plants
Social	Sensitivity and responsiveness to moods, motives, intentions and feelings of others
Personal	Sensitivity to self, feelings, strengths, desires, weaknesses and understanding of intention and motivation of others

conditions, and the stressors in their family, community, and societal environments. The model identifies critical periods of development, such as infancy, when exposure to adversity may have a particularly significant and long-lasting impact. In this model, close attachment to a responsive caregiver is a protective factor, which can buffer the impact of a stressor on the child's developing brain and nervous system and allow the child to successfully adapt to the situation. When that supportive relationship is absent, or when the stressful exposure is too persistent or overwhelming to be buffered, the child experiences "toxic stress" which dysregulates the autonomic nervous system and can lead to physiologic changes and future challenges with emotional regulation, cognition, language development, and behavior. Research on the impact of adverse childhood experiences (ACEs) on adult health, conducted by **Vincent J. Felitti** and colleagues, found associations between childhood experiences of abuse, neglect, and other household stressors and an increased incidence of poor mental and physical health in adulthood.

Racism and Child Development

The original studies on toxic stress and ACEs did not include the specific impact of racism, a significant contributor to disparate health outcomes. The theoretical model of the levels of racism by **Camara P. Jones** describes how institutional, interpersonal, and internalized racism operate and impact health and well-being. *Institutional racism* includes historical and present-day discriminatory laws, practices, and norms that impact access to education, employment, healthcare, housing, and other needs, as well as the power and influence that an individual can wield. *Interpersonal racism* includes conscious and unconscious bias and discrimination that upholds institutional racism and can manifest as lack of respect, dehumanization, exclusion from opportunities, and harsh judgment. *Internalized racism* refers to one's own belief in the harmful stereotypes about one's worth and abilities, based on race, which can impact self-esteem and the ability to form supportive social ties.

Newer models of child development, such as the Social Determinants of Early Learning (SDoEL) model and the Racism + Resilience + Resistance Integrative Study of Childhood Ecosystem (R³ISE) model by **Iheoma U. Iruka** and colleagues, incorporate the ways in which racism impacts child development, with an eye towards identifying and developing interventions to improve equitable outcomes. The SDoEL model examines early learning and development outcomes in the context of three areas of influence: the structural socioeconomic and political context, a family's own socioeconomic position, including social class, income, experience, and power, and the resources available to the individual child. Historical and present-day racism and discrimination act at every level in this model and influence a child and family's opportunities and challenges, with direct impact on early learning. The R³ISE model examines the ways in which cultural racism (ideologic beliefs that position non-White culture and people as inferior), institutional racism, interpersonal racism, and internalized racism impact child development through the influence on family assets, including material resources but also strengths such as strong community ties, social capital, efficacy, adaptability, and others. The model is focused on identifying interventions that mitigate the impact of racism and increase family assets, with the aim of promoting child development and wellness.

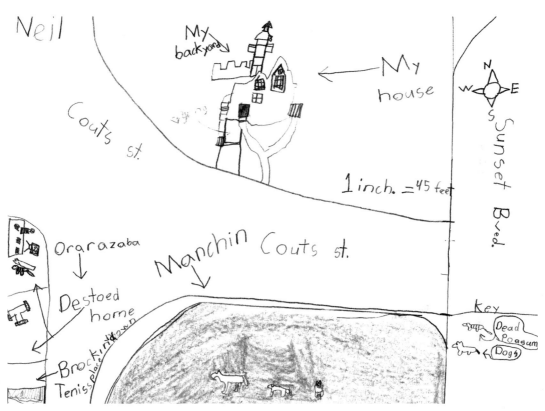

The child in context, in the neighborhood. Note the size and centrality of the child's house and the animals, including a dead possum, which are features most adult inhabitants would miss.

SUMMARY

There is a wealth of information on the development and behavior of children that is waiting to be applied to the clinical encounters we have every day. A comparison of the major historical theories is presented in Table 2.1. These perspectives, together with the modern theories described in this chapter, help us organize our observations and our thinking, they assist us in becoming efficient in data collection, and they give us insight into many behavioral tools at our disposal to assist families in supporting their own child's development.

RECOMMENDED READINGS

Blair C, Raver CC. School readiness and self-regulation: A developmental psychobiological approach. *Annual review of psychology*. 2015 Jan 3;66:711–731.

Crain W. *Theories of Development: Concepts and Applications*. 4th ed. Upper Saddle River, NJ: Prentice-Hall; 2000.

Felitti VJ, Anda RF, Nordenberg D, et al. Relationship of childhood abuse and household dysfunction to many of the leading causes of death in adults. The adverse childhood experiences (ACE) study. *Am J Prev Med*. 1998;14(4):245–258. https://doi.org/10.1016/S0749-3797(98)00017-8.

Hornor G, Davis C, Sherfield J, Wilkinson K. Trauma-informed care: Essential elements for pediatric health care. *Journal of Pediatric Health Care*. 2019 Mar 1;33(2):214–221.

Iruka IU. Using a social determinants of early learning framework to eliminate educational disparities and opportunity gaps. *Getting It Right: Using Implementation Research to Improve Outcomes in Early Care and Education*. 2020:63–86. New York: Found. Child Dev.

Iruka Iheoma U, Gardner-Neblett Nicole, Telfer Nicole A, Ibekwe-Okafor Nneka, Curenton Stephanie M, Sims Jacqueline, Sansbury Amber B, Neblett Enrique W. Effects of racism on child development: Advancing antiracist developmental science. *Annual Review of Developmental Psychology*. 2022;4:109–132.

Jones CP. Levels of racism: a theoretic framework and a gardener's tale. *Am J Public Health*. 2000 Aug;90(8):1212–1215. https://doi.org/10.2105/ajph.90.8.1212. PMID: 10936998; PMCID: PMC1446334.

Kagan J. *The Nature of the Child*. New York: Basic Books; 1984.

Miller PH. *Theories of Developmental Psychology*. 4th ed. New York: Worth Publishers; 2002.

Rosenblum KL, Dayton CJ, Muzik M. Infant social and emotional development: The emergence of self in a relational context. In: Zeanah CH, ed. *Handbook of infant mental health*. 3rd ed. NY: Guilford Press; 2009:80–103. Available at. http://digitalcommons.wayne.edu/soc_work_pubs/43.

Shonkoff JP, Garner AS, Committee on Psychosocial Aspects of Child and Family Health; Committee on Early Childhood, Adoption, and Dependent Care; Section on Developmental and Behavioral Pediatrics The lifelong effects of early childhood adversity and toxic stress. *Pediatrics*. 2012 Jan;129(1):e232–e246. https://doi.org/10.1542/peds.2011-2663. Epub 2011 Dec 26. PMID: 22201156.

Thomas RM. *Comparing Theories of Child Development*. 5th ed. Belmont, CA: Wadsworth/Thompson Learning; 2000.

The Center for the Study of Social Policy – Protective Factors Framework https://cssp.org/our-work/projects/protective-factors-framework/

Willis DW, Eddy JM. Early relational health: Innovations in child health for promotion, screening, and research. *Infant Mental Health Journal*. 2022 May;43(3):361–372.

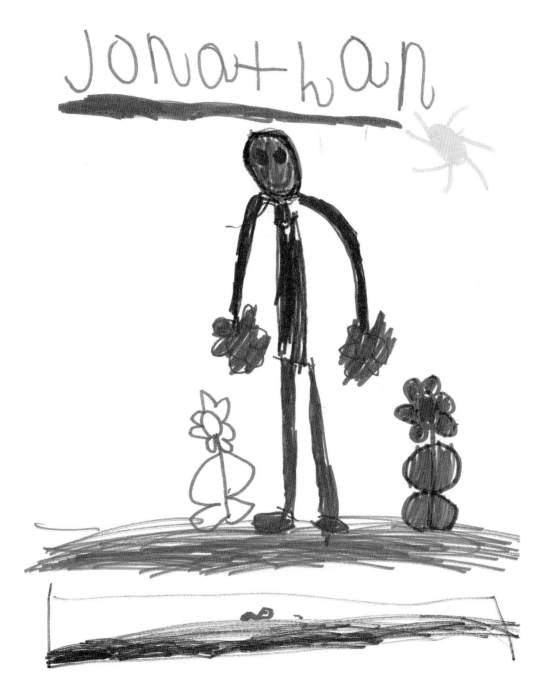

Developmental Parallels. "Jonathan," a 6-year-old sets himself amidst the growing flowers. By JM.

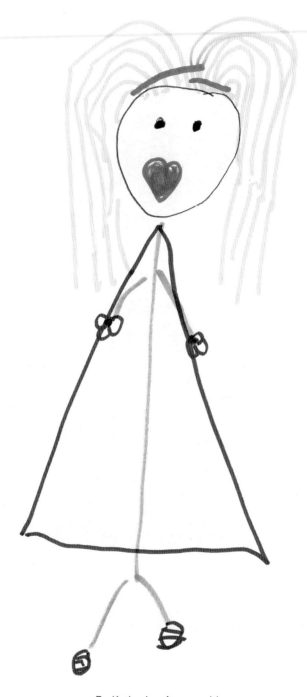

By Katherine Auerswald

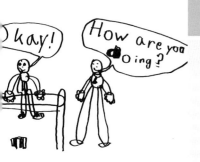

3

Preparing Your Practice for Socially and Emotionally Responsive Care

Yuan He

This chapter describes a focus on building relationships with children and parents in the context of the clinical encounter, which can make each visit more effective and responsive. Specific components and methods of interviewing are illustrated to show how different approaches can be used to make the most of each encounter. The physical layout of the office and the structural elements of the practice can enhance the quality and efficiency of care for the child and the whole family as well.

KEYWORDS

- Interview
- Clinician-family partnership
- Verbal and nonverbal communication
- Process and content
- Explanatory model
- Active listening
- Transference
- Reflection and self-awareness

Families are the primary context in which life is experienced, especially for children. Pediatricians tend to focus on the child's symptoms, developmental skills, and behavior and spend less time assessing family strengths, stressors, and life event changes. By incorporating the caregiver(s) and the child as equal partners during the clinical interview, the clinician discovers important information about a family's strengths, the child's relationship with others in the family and community, and about potential stressors, such as caregiver discord, mental health concerns, exposure to violence or other trauma, and economic and social uncertainties.

The family-directed interview model supports the notion, confirmed by research and clinical experience, that the developmental potential of children is affected

Original chapter by Martin T. Stein.

by the environment in which they live. Family-directed interviewing also encourages the generation of data about the child's home and neighborhood environment, which has been shown to have an important impact on a child's development. Recognition that trauma is not only common, but that certain populations are at a higher risk for trauma exposure (e.g., those with minoritized racial, ethnic, gender, and sexual identities, who have developmental or behavioral problems, have prior contact with the child welfare and/or criminal legal systems, or are immigrants) can help ensure that clinicians approach families with sensitivity and a trauma-informed approach.

THE ENCOUNTER AS A RELATIONAL EVENT

The clinical practice of preventive pediatric care is built on an educational model. When the clinical encounter is orchestrated in a manner that provides an educational experience for the caregivers, child, and clinician, expanded gains emerge from the encounter. By *planned orchestration* of the style and content of the interview, a new dimension is added to the practice of pediatrics that makes it both more effective and more rewarding than simply adhering to an impersonal checklist of tasks at each encounter. The manner in which questions are asked, the types of questions asked, the direction of the questioning (to the parent and to the child), and the actual interaction with the child are critical components of the interview. They influence not only the information gathered but also what caregivers and

29

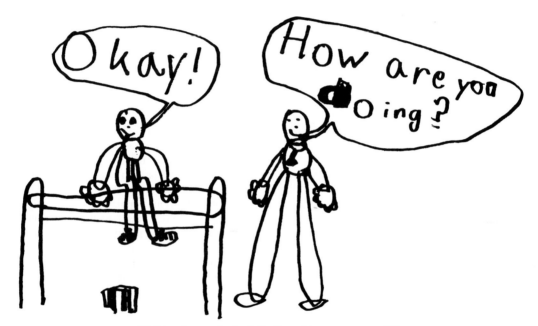

"Talking to my doctor." By Ryan Hennessy, age 7½.

children learn about growth and development during times of illness and health.

THE PHYSICAL LAYOUT

The potential for an "educational experience" during a pediatric office visit begins before the actual visit. The physical and social ecology of a medical office that serves the needs of children requires forethought in planning and continuous modification and would benefit from the solicitation and inclusion of perspectives and opinions of patients, families, and staff alike. An appreciation that personnel, space, color, and design can interact to create a positive, health-promoting atmosphere may generate interesting ideas that allow the office environment to enhance child development, parent-child-clinician interactions, and assessments of health and development. The pictures or children's drawings selected for the walls, the availability of crawl and walk spaces, the toys in the reception area, and the educational material made available to parents and children are at first seemingly unrelated decisions, but they may come together to create a cohesive theme in each office. While there may be stress and/or big emotions related to the medical visit, families may appreciate that the practice has been designed to be a safe and welcoming place where children are expected to explore, developmental considerations are front and center, and caregivers will be supported by the clinicians, staff, and other expertise available.

Whether a new office or clinic facility is being planned or modification to an established office seems possible, two questions should be asked:

"How can we plan to use the available space in a manner that is consistent with the developmental needs of the children and parents who will come to the facility?"

"Can the design promote comfort, relieve anxiety, nurture the parent-child relationship, and maintain a learning and educational environment?"

Priorities, budgets, and available space will vary among settings, but a core group of developmental principles are applicable to most pediatric offices, including the following:

- *A busy waiting room is like a neighborhood park.* Caregivers can observe their children learning to play and interact with other children. Toys, books, or a wall board equipped for drawing can make these interactions more interesting and entertaining for caregivers and children. The waiting room might also serve as an after-hours meeting place or informal classroom. It can be used for educational events, group care visits, or places for families of children with special needs.
- *The waiting area should allow for movement and play of children.* The choices of flooring, wall covering, and furniture should take into account the developmental requirements of children in various age groups. Safety, clean lines, and cheerfulness are key elements. Avoid overstimulating, noisy, or trendy décor. Doors should shut off main traffic areas.
- *Furniture and play objects can be safe but still engaging and instructive.* A concern for a safe environment should not create a sterile office. Providing a space for the containment of busy toddlers and a separate area for older youth and teens is ideal. Smaller, semicontained areas set a quieter and more contained tone for families.
- *Pictures of children and their families or drawings created by children* in the practice invite children to feel comfortable in the office and encourage conversation about the pictures' content among caregivers and other children.
- *A fish tank in the waiting room* may help alleviate the boredom, anxiety, and/or fears that children may experience when visiting a physician's office. Many children enjoy the visual sensory experience of watching fish swim.
- *Tables and chairs designed for toddlers and young children* and placed in the reception area may encourage a child to separate from the parent and independently open a book or play with a puzzle. Anxiety may be momentarily decreased as the child learns to manage a fear independent of the parent.
- *The availability of paper and marking pens or a chalkboard* will encourage children to draw pictures that may help them redirect fears about their symptoms, an illness, or the concern observed in a parent.
- *Observation of children and caregivers together by office personnel* allows staff to note when a child may be having a hard time, which can be communicated to the clinical team. It may be possible to alter the child's rooming process and measurement of vital signs and to help anticipate that additional support might be needed.
- *Televisions in the waiting room* may send the unintended message that TV is a good strategy to entertain children during downtime. Consider getting rid of the TV or using it to show prosocial, calm, and educational programs that will benefit both the child and the parent.

POSITIONING THE PARTICIPANTS

Certain aspects of the interview environment controlled by the clinician determine the quality and quantity of data that will be obtained. Planning the clinical space in an examination room may be guided by knowledge that the word *interview* is derived from *between* and *seeing*. By implication, the process of interviewing is a mutual communication of thoughts that can be influenced by the nature of the space between the clinician and patient. The clinician can and should actively determine that spacing. The following are issues to consider to create the best interview environment possible:

- The clinician should be positioned at the same or lower level to ensure eye contact and to prevent the caregiver from having to look up at the clinician, exacerbating unequal power dynamics. If the caregiver is sitting, the clinician should also sit or position themselves to be at or around eye level.
- The decision to conduct the interview in a sitting or standing position will change with the type of visit.
- For a new patient or a new problem that requires an extensive history, sitting down with the parent and child may encourage greater information exchange as well as allow the clinician to pay more attention to nonverbal cues.
- For an established patient with an acute illness, the history may be taken while the parent and clinician are standing.
- A young child who is ill may remain in the arms of the parent or in close physical contact.
- The placement of chairs in an examination room and the proximity of the clinician and patient influence the style and content of the interview.
- A computer between a practitioner and the caregiver/child can be a barrier to optimal communication but can also be used to share information if the monitor is positioned for both the clinician and the family to view. This behavior can be used to signal transparency and can turn the screen into a teaching tool, rather than a barrier. If using the electronic health record during the encounter, continue to frequently physically turn to the parent and child and give full attention when the parent or child shares information.
- Picking up a chair and moving it closer to a parent may facilitate the exchange of information; the act itself may enhance a therapeutic relationship.
- When interviewing a child or a teen, apply the same principles of spacing and eye contact.

To maximize the quality of the interview of a child at any age, the clinician should be at the same level as the child. For a tall clinician, positioning is especially important when interviewing young children and caregivers. A younger child should be allowed to scan the physician at a distance first and become familiar with her. Eye-to-eye contact may feel threatening to a child younger than 2 years or to a child of any age if the contact is initiated early in an interview. A friendly interchange with the caregivers first allows the child to size up the clinician before the interaction.

AN INTERACTIVE MODEL

As the clinician acquires information from the family, a broad social and medical database is generated. The caregiver and older child receive information from the clinician that focuses on diagnosis, treatment, and education. During the interview, caregiver-child interactions provide the clinician an opportunity to assess developmental skills of the child, as well as parenting skills and the dynamics of family interaction. The interview is an opportunity to observe the interaction between child and parent—how the baby is undressed/dressed, fed, spoken to, spoken for, and disciplined, and how the child looks for comfort and receives it—and provide strength-based affirmations and reflections where appropriate. The rewards of the clinical interview can be a shared learning experience, long-term gains in understanding the family, and a clearer focus for care and guidance going forward.

If parent and child are using mobile devices when the interview starts, the clinician can prompt more focused engagement in the interview by saying something like "it's OK for [child] to be occupied with a device right now, because I'm going to talk to you first, so I only need your attention" or "they can keep playing with the phone, I just need to talk to you right now." Remember that parent mobile device use during clinical encounters can be a sign of stress, avoidance, or sheer habit, so it helps to respond in a pragmatic, nonjudgmental way. One study showed that clinicians actually had a *better* understanding of their patient's developmental issues when children were allowed to use devices during well-child visits, likely because the parent was able to provide a more coherent or in-depth history, compared to children who were not allowed to use a device. While this single study is not an argument for *recommending* child device use during visits, it does suggest that keeping the child occupied, for example, with drawing (Chapter 4) or a book, may allow for richer clinician-caregiver communication.

THE CLINICIAN-FAMILY PARTNERSHIP

The pediatric interview encompasses the notion of the clinician-family partnership as an essential relationship in the care of the child. The caregiver and child are treated both as individuals and as an interactional unit, and the parent's expertise and experience are centered. Although most of the historical facts during an interview will come from the caregiver, the child also provides important clues through verbal and nonverbal interactions. Two frequent shortcomings of the pediatric interview are that the clinician spends most of the visit telling the caregiver information, rather than asking questions or listening, and that the clinician communicates exclusively with the caregiver, rather than actively involving the child. In a visit with a 3-year-old patient, for example, expressive and receptive language skills provide the child with the ability to communicate symptoms and concerns to the clinician. If you find yourself talking more than half the time, it usually means that you may not be getting all the information *you* need from the interview. As a rule, family members should talk more than the clinician.

The interview should provide information and supportive care to the child and the family unit, through direct questioning of the participants and sensitive, strengths-based observations of their interactions. It is useful to think about the process as involving a story or stories from the family members, and the work of the clinician is to hear the story and its personal meaning for each participant. The "therapeutic triangle" (Fig. 3.1) illustrates the influence of caregivers (and the extended family) on the relationship between the clinician and child; simultaneously, the child's clinician supports the relationship between the child and family because this is the vehicle of intervention, care, and support for the child. However, it is important to note that this "therapeutic triangle" is influenced by many factors, and any observations made about the caregiver and patient should be interpreted within the specific context of that clinical encounter. Patients and families have varying and sometimes negative experiences and impressions of clinicians and the healthcare system due to social and structural determinants of health, including racism, sexism, other forms of bias and discrimination, and other systemic influences that shape each encounter. Clinicians should approach each visit with cultural humility, compassion, and a trauma-informed approach that prioritizes emotional safety, trust building, and partnership with the family.

Questions should be directed to children with age-appropriate words and eye contact that will encourage the child's participation. Direct interaction with a child of any age acknowledges the important contribution that any individual child has on his own rearing, health, and development. An appreciation of the clinician-family partnership directs the clinician's attention to concerns of both the caregiver and the child and to the important role that the interaction between them really plays. This approach enhances traditional pediatric advocacy for the needs of the child. (See Chapter 17, the 4-year-old health supervision visit, and subsequent chapters for examples of a coordinated parent-child interview.) One way of emphasizing the child's importance is to ask a child familiar to the office to state their reason for the visit first and to give them the last word as well.

OBSERVING FAMILY INTERACTIONS

Information from the clinical interview is derived from two major sources: **verbal and nonverbal communication** (Box 3.1). Interactional behavior—how the baby is held, fed, stroked, spoken to, looked at, and so on—is also part of the nonverbal database. Similarly, the relationship between an older child and parent should be observed and assessed during the interview. Observations about communication style and content regarding discipline and self-help skills (e.g., undressing and getting on the examination table) can provide important clues about caregiver-child relationships, as well as developmental capacities. Children who are delayed or whom the caregivers perceive to need care appropriate for a younger age will show this behavior during the interaction. In fact, motor, social, adaptive, and individual temperament skills can be assessed in a young child by observing the child's activity while the parent is providing the medical history, provided that the room and your focus are set in that direction.

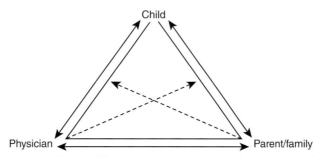

Fig. 3.1 The therapeutic triangle in pediatrics. The educational model for the clinical pediatric interview should follow a pattern in which information exchange is dynamic for the three participants. (Adapted from Doherty WJ, Baird MA: *Family therapy and medicine: toward the primary care of families*, New York, 1983, Guilford Press, p 13.)

Nonverbal data are as important as verbal statements and should be incorporated into the medical evaluation, again within the cultural and social context. Due to discomfort, fear, or mistrust, families may vary in how much they share with the clinician, both verbally and nonverbally. Similarly, cultural and language barriers may prevent accurate interpretation of verbal and nonverbal communication, sometimes even with the aid of a language interpreter. However, when appropriate, certain observations may be included in the medical record and incorporated into the assessment (e.g., a child with a flat affect—rule out depression; a caregiver who seems easily upset throughout the visit, which may indicate increased stress that warrants connections to community based services and other supports; an active child who is running around the room, with concern for inattention and hyperactivity). If needed, they should be incorporated into the problem list to ensure appropriate attention during follow-up care. In practices that use a child behavior checklist or a parent-family psychosocial screening instrument completed before the office visit (see Appendix), nonverbal observations can be compared with the parent's written observations. Confirmations and discrepancies may provide useful clinical information.

Nonverbal cues given by caregivers and children are a component of the process portion of the interview as opposed to the content portion. Although the process of an interview is interwoven with the content, it is helpful for the clinician to be aware of the two components as separate. In that way, verbal data can be understood within the context of the nonverbal information that was generated simultaneously by the parent or the child and monitored by a sensitive clinician. For example, a mother of a 2-month-old infant reporting her anxiety as she describes several concerns related to the baby may raise suspicion in the clinician regarding postpartum depression and/or anxiety, if accompanied by relevant nonverbal clues.

TALKING WITH CHILDREN: WORDS AND FEELINGS GO BACK AND FORTH

When interviewing a child who has achieved interactive language skills at about 3 to 4 years of age, the clinician can speak directly to the child, ask questions, and listen carefully to responses. It is helpful to remember that receptive language development is often ahead of expressive language. A 2-year-old may understand as many as 300 words, but expression may be limited to 50 to 100 words, for example. Children may reveal information of which the parent is either unaware or has suppressed. In addition, allowing the child to participate in the interview provides an opportunity to assess language development and auditory functioning. Furthermore, it provides the child with an experience of actively participating in the visit to the physician, which may encourage a sense of responsibility and participation in personal health and medical care. It may also provide a model for caregivers in listening to and respecting the opinions of the child. Beginning with the health supervision visit for a 4-year-old (see Chapter 17), the clinician has the opportunity to conduct the interview with the child and parent in a parallel fashion. This rich clinical experience does not take much additional time but requires a knowledge of age-appropriate developmental skills and a comfort level in communicating simultaneously with an adult and child. This book describes what to observe at each encounter and say at that age. Like other clinical skills, the ability to effectively interact with families during the clinical encounter will improve with practice.

EVERY VISIT AS A TEACHING ENCOUNTER

The clinician's interactions with the child during the interview and physical examination provide multiple opportunities to affirm positive interactions and behaviors that can increase caregivers' self-esteem while continually engaging both the patient and caregiver. There may also be opportunities to model certain types of behavior in the visit, incorporating developmentally appropriate language that also helps provide guidance and reassurance regarding different milestones. For example, a physician holding, rocking, and stroking the infant while talking to the parent can help model effective soothing techniques, while normalizing the stress and anxiety that can be associated with a fussy infant. Providing firm behavioral boundaries to a toddler with a calm, concise, and authoritative statement may help the parent experience the effect of appropriate limit setting and discipline.

A note of caution—there can be a fine line between supportive modeling of discipline and implied criticism of the caregiver for doing it differently. When a child is showing negative behaviors, it can be helpful to ask the caregiver: "how do you manage it when he [hits/runs around/etc.]?" If a caregiver does not have an answer, it is an opportunity to offer new behavioral management strategies. If the caregiver provides a response that effectively handles the child behavior, this allows the clinician to support the caregiver's agency and status as an "expert" on their own child. It is also an opportunity to ask whether the child's behavior has been a problem at home. These chance events, when a behavioral or developmental issue naturally comes up, open up "teachable moments" that become part of the real output or gain of the encounter itself. When a caregiver realizes that their approach to their child's challenging behavior is met with support, rather than judgment, this also increases trust in the clinician.

Asking a 5-year-old whether she'd prefer the left or right arm for an immunization may illustrate to the caregiver the value of providing choices for a child facing something that is really nonnegotiable. In addition, the clinician may demonstrate the powerful effect of reflecting on a child's feelings when an emotional response is intense. For example, to a tearful youngster about to undergo a painful procedure, the clinician might say, "Are you worried that it will hurt?" The child's altered emotional response to these "feedback" statements is often dramatic and encourages further communication about the child's feelings. In engaging in these interactions during the clinical encounter, clinicians should be mindful of using this approach to demonstrate new or additional ways to interact with the child, rather than to criticize the caregiver's behavior and style of child rearing. Any concerns about caregiver discipline style or parenting approach should be addressed directly, rather than implied through demonstration.

STRUCTURING THE INTERVIEW

The clinician sets up an effective and efficient practice by structuring the well-child medical interview. Such orchestration of these visits is helpful in ensuring complete data collection as well as providing a framework for controlled digressions. An opening statement should include an introduction by name if this is the first visit. A concerned, friendly, and empathetic demeanor is most effective in child healthcare practice. It can be established by a warm introduction and immediate eye contact with the caregiver. The language and nonverbal approach may need to be modified according to the cultural context. A brief statement about the goals for the visit may be helpful at the beginning of the interview. This can be followed by asking, "What concerns about your child's health would you like to discuss during this visit?" A similar question might be directed to an older child. This approach, early in the visit, ensures that the patient or family member has an opportunity to state the agenda for the visit; it allows the clinician an opportunity to structure and address that agenda and to partner with the family to develop shared goals for the visit.

The content of an interview depends on the child's age and significant developmental themes. Specific chapters in this book provide directions for each age so that the themes or issues most likely to emerge can be targeted at that time. To encourage a developmental perspective for the well-child visit, questions and educational information should be organized around the major issues at a particular age. In this manner, specific goals can be established for each visit. For example, at the visit when the infant is 6 months of age, the encounter highlights the emerging motor skills of grasping and reaching out. Advice about solids (especially finger foods), toys, and poison prevention should be provided to caregivers in the context of specific current and anticipated developmental skills. Knowing this theme means that the clinician can use a block, pen, or stethoscope to extend to the child as she enters the room. The key observation is made in 3 seconds, and conversation, advice, and teaching follow easily. *Choosing a central concern or theme gives the visit more cohesiveness* and less of a feeling of an assembly line or check-off list, both for the clinician and the parent. The chapters in this book on each health supervision visit prepare clinicians for this task. The contents of the clinical interview, both data gathering and instruction, for each age will be outlined in subsequent chapters.

FINE-TUNING THE INTERVIEW

Open and Closed Questions

The interview should start with open-ended questions, such as "How is your baby doing?"; "What's new with the baby's development?"; or "What do you like about your baby?" Such questions generate more spontaneous, less structured responses. They allow the caregivers to bring up problems of greatest concern to them and acknowledge the caregivers' responsibility in establishing priorities in the interview. The interview should start with these types of questions. Open-ended questions allow the child's or the caregivers' "explanatory model" of the illness or problem to come out. The explanatory model is the culturally dependent perspective of an illness that the family brings to the medical encounter. This is the first step in meeting the family's needs for addressing an issue.

When open-ended questions lead to confusing answers, the clinician may want to get some clarity and focus. This should be done carefully and should always start with "I," for example, "I'm not clear about when this problem started; help me understand that part better."

Open-ended questions can be followed by closed-ended questions that are focused, specific, and more concrete (e.g., "Is the baby sitting up without support?," "How is breastfeeding going?," "Are you getting any help with child care?"). Such questions provide important concrete data and shift control of the interview to the interviewer. The clinician's explanatory model and agenda for the interview can be brought out by the careful use of these questions. It can be helpful for the clinician to put the questions into context, such as saying, "I like to hear a parent's concerns first" or "I always ask children their understanding of why they came here today." Planned, thoughtful use of these types of questions allows the clinician to get the information needed and build a relationship.

When emotionally difficult issues are discussed, the clinician should use their best judgment to gauge whether gentle reassurance or periods of silence may be more helpful. In some cases, time spent in silence may allow the patient to collect thoughts and express feelings. It carries with it the message that you care enough about the patient to take the time to listen to concerns about the child and family. If families are not yet ready to open up or disclose emotionally difficult or sensitive issues, the clinician should take additional time to build trust and foster the relationship and may elect to set up a follow-up appointment to discuss at a future visit.

Repetition of Important Phrases

When a patient makes a statement that appears significant from either verbal or nonverbal cues but stops the communication abruptly, the clinician may choose to repeat or interpret an important phrase that was just mentioned. This approach encourages further exploration, clarification, or modification by the patient.

Dealing With Surprise

When caregivers say surprising things, the clinician can start by repeating their comment back in an even voice without comment. For example, "You give him Coca-Cola every night at bedtime." The ball is then passed to the caregiver to explain, clarify, or expand the startling comment. With some statements, we can make a supportive connection with a parent by acknowledging their intent (e.g., the intent of corporal punishment is to help the child understand that a behavior is unacceptable) and then listening to the parent's response before offering a preferred alternative. At other times, the use of an "I" phrase may be the best way

to respond to a concerning statement (e.g., "I worry that …" or "I think that's a pretty powerful statement"). Keep your tone and body language even, to maintain a nonjudgmental and empathic approach.

Active Listening

Active listening refers to the process of giving undivided attention to what a person is saying through words and body language. It requires, above all, the ability to concentrate. The assumption underlying active listening is that the patient will provide most of the important information spontaneously, verbally or nonverbally, if given an opportunity, and that the encounter is set up correctly. A clinician who listens actively uses open-ended questions, pauses, silences, and repetitions of important phrases. Such an empathetic listener can discover, through a unique, interpersonal style, a way that brings about a succinct and accurate acceptance of the patient's feelings, concerns, and perceptions. This understanding of the patient is communicated through facial expressions, posture, hand movements, and head nodding. Active and empathetic listening can decrease a patient's anxiety, increase trust in the clinician, encourage greater patient participation in the interview process, yield more information, and increase the clinician's satisfaction in the relationship. It is a skill that can be learned and is one of the most effective and efficient ways to build a complete database. Most mistakes have to do with too much talking. If one finds that one is doing more talking than listening, a great deal of needed information will probably be missed.

Transference

Primary pediatric care is based on the development of a long-term relationship with families. When continuity of health care is provided in this framework, a special relationship develops between the caregiver and the patient and family. In pediatric practice, caregivers often have respect and admiration for their child's physician; it is the foundation for a trusting, long-term relationship. This relationship is a powerful tool in effecting change for the child. It is also one of the rewards of primary care. At the same time and to a variable degree as a result of this close and special relationship, a caregiver may respond to the pediatrician as someone who is symbolically and psychologically identified with another important person in their own life, past or present. This **"transference"** phenomenon may surface only at times of deep emotional expression, such as joy, relief, and/or admiration after a successful therapeutic intervention. It may also be the unconscious source of hostility directed toward the clinician by the parent of a child with a chronic, functionally disabling illness. An appreciation of parental reactions mediated by transference may assist the clinician in providing more appropriate and helpful responses during medical interviews and in understanding some aspects of the interaction.

Clinicians should be aware that transference can go both ways and should be mindful of their own strong positive and negative reactions to patients and families. The American Academy of Pediatrics Committee on Bioethics calls on clinicians to set and maintain professional boundaries with families. When pediatricians and parents already know each other or have contact outside of the office setting, either in person or online, patients will benefit from explicit discussions about how their privacy and confidentiality will be protected.

Reflection and Self-awareness

Effective clinicians monitor their work with patients through reflection and self-awareness to examine their own belief systems and values, manage strong feelings about patients, and make difficult decisions. This critical self-reflection enables physicians to listen attentively to patients' distress, recognize their own errors, refine their technical skills, make evidence-based decisions, and clarify their values so that they can act with compassion, technical competence, presence, and insight. Reflection and self-awareness during an interview can be achieved by conscious use of your own response to a child, parent, and other family members to help you develop skills in regulating strong emotions in the clinical setting and identifying personal biases, triggers, or situations that are personally stressful.

Pay attention to your own feelings in an encounter and your own responses to a child. If you feel your shoulders slumped, your face dropped, and your movement slowed, you may just have had an emotional visit with a family in a challenging situation and may be experiencing secondary trauma. If you find a child particularly challenging, demanding, or obstructive, reflect on what you personally found difficult and what additional skills may make a similar encounter go well the next time. If you find yourself handling a baby overcautiously or lowering your voice, look at what the source of that reaction is. Better understanding and managing our own stress responses can improve our ability to provide support for children and parents during difficult times.

Set for Success

Analyses of pediatric interviews through videotape records have documented the clinical skills to which caregivers are most responsive. Process and outcome measures, such as parental understanding of a diagnostic label and compliance with a medical regimen, have been evaluated and correlated with specific traits of clinicians that yield optimal results. Effective interviewing skills go a long way toward optimal results. Dr. Barbara Korsch, a pioneer in pediatric interview research, suggests that the following traits produce the most effective medical encounters:

- Pay attention to the *concerns of patients*. Three open-ended questions will elicit *most* concerns for a child with a problem:
  1. Why did you bring your child to the clinic today?
  2. What worries you most?
  3. Why did that worry you?
- *Acknowledge the parent's expectation* for the medical visit and the parent's explanation of the child's problem, or the explanatory model. Caregivers may bring to the visit their own explanatory models of illness and health. It is important to bring those models to the surface and show the caregivers that you understand their perception, whether it is similar to or different from your own.
- Caregivers need an *explanation of the diagnosis and cause*. If the medical explanation is inconsistent with the caregivers' own understanding, the clinician should try to reconcile the difference. For example, a parent who believes that the child acquired a cold from rain exposure may be assisted by the statement, "While many believe that colds are caused by being cold in the rain, we have learned that common colds are actually caused by viruses."
- Nurture the *doctor-patient relationship*. Be relaxed, friendly, positive, and warm in manner.
- *Limit medical jargon*. This is often a protective barrier for yourself. Jargon can be used to establish power over another or to hide ignorance when you feel threatened. Rather than hide behind words, try to deal with the situation directly.
- Most caregivers prefer a *friendly, professional attitude* rather than an authoritative, businesslike stature or an overly casual or familiar manner.
- *Attend to parental anxieties* as manifested by nervousness and tension during the interview. Examples of responses are the following: "You look nervous to me today … is there something you want to bring up?" or "My explanation for his symptoms don't seem to be resonating with you—can you share what you're thinking?"

These skills can be acquired during medical training or in pediatric practice. As with most aspects of learning, supervision is extremely helpful in gaining insight into interviewing techniques. A video of a patient encounter can be played back in front of the student and teacher. Videotaping has the advantage of allowing comments periodically when the tape is stopped and replayed.

Communication during the medical interview remains a powerful and effective way to gather data, teach, and develop the specifically human way of connecting with another human being empathetically and therapeutically.

We owe it to ourselves and to our patients to develop these skills optimally.

Identifying Other Concerns

Caregivers who bring children to a physician for an illness visit are frequently motivated to come to the office because of a concern that is not immediately apparent. The "secondary diagnosis" often originates from a behavioral, psychosocial, or developmental uncertainty that the parent may be unaware of at the time of the visit or one that seems inappropriate to bring to the attention of the child's clinician. The real concern must be uncovered or it can prompt additional, preventable office or emergency room visits.

These concerns reflect fears and anxieties about the child's health and provide insight into family functioning and caregiver perceptions that are critical to growth and development of the child. In one study, caregivers in 10% of visits saw their child as "vulnerable" because of a previous illness or event in the life of the child, a family member, or a close friend. Providing the parent with a brief opportunity to express any additional concerns may be therapeutic in itself. The clinician then has a window of opportunity to place the symptom in perspective and, when appropriate, reassure the parent about the health of the child and the limited duration of the current illness. When these fears have created significant or chronic parental anxiety, a future visit may be necessary. Caregivers may not even be aware of these underlying concerns themselves. Like a hidden infection, they need to be identified or they will continue to fester.

These explorations in causality are the rewards of sensitive interviewing. For the child and family, the therapeutic value may be as important as discovery of the pathophysiology of a cardiac murmur. The long-term benefit comes from the relationship that begins to be built when clinicians give caregivers the message that their concerns are important and worthy of the physician's time.

Cultural Sensitivity and Humility

Although most of the general principles of effective medical interviewing reviewed in this chapter are applicable when there are cultural differences between a clinician and patient, such differences may pervade the encounter at many levels. Patcher has defined culturally sensitive pediatrics as "care [that] *respects the beliefs, attitudes and cultural life-styles of patients*. It acknowledges that concepts of health and illness are influenced by patients' ethnic values, religious beliefs, linguistic considerations and cultural orientations." A culturally sensitive pediatric clinician discovers ways to blend ethnomedical interpretations of a child's developmental skills and behavior with a biomedical understanding. Cultural humility goes further to include the practice of self-reflection and interrogation of how our own backgrounds and identities impact our clinical practice.

Some clinicians may be frustrated by the false impression that to accomplish an effective medical interview that also nurtures a therapeutic relationship, a clinician must possess specific information about a family's cultural beliefs and practices. Instead, clinicians should be aware that differing customs regarding deference and respect (e.g., how much or how long to sustain eye contact, or how much the parent/caregiver speaks for the patient), privacy (e.g., how much personal/family information to share with an "outsider"), and even engagement with preventive healthcare (as opposed to seeking health care only when urgently or emergently ill) may shape clinicians' interactions and ability to build trusting relationships with families. In addition, two strategies may guide and assist medical encounters across cultures without an extensive knowledge of specific customs and beliefs.

Explanatory Model for Symptoms

All patients have a culturally based model for understanding health status at times of health and disease. Their interpretation and explanation of symptoms may be different from the assumptions of the clinician. Through a process of specific questions, the family's explanatory model of health and illness will emerge (Box 3.2).

Mini-ethnography

In the process of an empathetic, respectful interview with the caregivers and a child, the pediatric clinician should strive to understand cultural and personal meanings and interpretations of the child's development and behavior. When the patient is seen in the context of continuity of care, defining a mini-ethnography for a child and family over time is a clinically and personally rewarding exercise. Other family members and interpreters may be essential in the development of a meaningful history. Box 3.3 gives guidelines for a bilingual medical interview.

Finally, understanding and addressing our own biases and assumptions, and how they play out in the clinical setting, is a key component of practicing effective, equitable medicine.

Eliciting Information

The clinic visit offers an opportunity to learn more about a child's growth and development, understand parental concerns, and identify household needs or stressors. While in the past, parent and child questionnaires for health supervision visits focused primarily on child development, there are now widely available screening tools for behavioral health, health-related social needs, and family history of adverse events that may provide additional important information (see Appendix).

BOX 3.2   **Questions for a Health Beliefs History**

- What would you call this problem?
- Why do youm think your child has developed it?
- What do you think caused it?
- Why do you think it started when it did?
- What do you think is happening inside the body?
- What are the symptoms that make you know your child has this illness?
- What are you most worried about with this illness?
- What problems does this illness cause your child?
- How do you treat it?
- Is the treatment helpful?
- What will happen if this problem is not treated?
- What do you expect from the treatments?

Modified from Patcher LM: Practicing culturally sensitive pediatrics, *Contemp Pediatr* 14:139, 1997; Kleinman A: *Patients and healers in the context of culture*, Berkeley, 1980, University of California Press, p 106.

BOX 3.3   **Guidelines for A Bilingual Medical Interview**

Always use an interpreter (ideally a trained professional rather than an ad hoc interpreter), unless you are fluent in the family's language.
- Try to match the individual interpreter to the individual patient and clinical setting.
- Reassure the parent or child regarding confidentiality.
- Avoid technical terms, jargon, lengthy explanations without breaks, ambiguity, idioms, abstractions, figures of speech, and indefinite phrases.
- Use clear statements planned in advance with language appropriate for the interpreter and expect to spend twice the usual time.
- Be prepared to obtain information via narrative or conversational modes.
- Ask the interpreter to comment on nonverbal elements, the fullness of the parent's or child's understanding, and any culturally sensitive issues.
- Learn the basic language and common health-related beliefs and practices of patient groups regularly encountered.

Modified from Putsch RW III: Cross-cultural contamination: the special case of interpreters in health care. *JAMA* 254:3334–3338, 1985.

Epidemiological studies indicate that an increasing number of school-age children have a disorder in psychosocial function and that pediatricians identify only a small percentage of these disorders during most office visits. Some clinicians may find that behavior screening instruments, such as the Pediatric Symptom Checklist (see Appendix), are helpful in setting the agenda for health supervision by giving the parent (and child) the message that behavioral concerns are appropriate and that discussion is encouraged during the visit. A behavioral screening test can be used as a springboard to initiate the dialogs and therapeutic alliance necessary to explore behavioral concerns.

In its 2016 policy statement on poverty and child health, the American Academy of Pediatrics (AAP) recommended universal screening for social determinants of health (SDOH)–related basic needs, with the goal of identifying and addressing identified needs to improve child and family well-being. Since then, many practices have implemented different screeners to identify social needs, with mixed results regarding acceptability by caregivers and enrollment in community resources to address identified needs. Recent qualitative work has found that caregivers are more receptive and likely to discuss SDOH with clinicians who can successfully build rapport with families, explain the connections between the topic and child health, and had knowledge and could provide assistance around how to address identified needs and risk factors. Screening for social needs without providing the appropriate support or connections to services should be avoided.

Similarly, there have been robust discussions around the merits and potential harms of screening for adverse childhood events (ACEs), which have been shown to have strong associations with negative physical and mental health. While there may be opportunities to address downstream effects of ACEs, such as physical, mental, and/or behavioral manifestations of trauma, there is little evidence to show that trauma-directed therapy and treatments are effective in mitigating ACE exposure if there are no symptoms or manifestations of trauma. There are also potential unintended consequences of ACE screening, as answering personal questions about ACEs may potentially retraumatize caregivers and/or raise concerns around child maltreatment that require mandated reporting to child protective services. Instead, clinicians can consider screening for traumatic stress symptoms using validated tools, such as the Pediatric Traumatic Stress Screening Tool. Clinicians who ask about ACEs and other trauma exposures should be trained in trauma-informed, person-centered approaches to sensitive questions and have knowledge regarding available resources and support to address concerns that arise.

COMMUNITY RESOURCES

Developmentally based pediatric practice also means that a clinician has comprehensive knowledge about resources in the community that enhance preventive and therapeutic goals for patients. Community resources serve as an extension of the pediatric clinician for consultation, referral, and intervention. An effective "medical home" means that the primary care staff can direct children and families to preventive and therapeutic services in the community. Knowing who your allies are in the community and in what situations they can be accessed is a critical element of effective primary care.

Community resources go beyond knowing about medical subspecialty referrals (Table 3.1). They include early intervention programs, effective ways to access school programs for children with special needs, services for children with language delays (including instances when the pediatrician has a concern about autism spectrum disorder), programs that assist with accessing public benefits, and mental health professionals for both children and caregivers. Knowledge about recreational community resources is also useful, especially when that knowledge can be tailored to specific communities—for example, after-school programs and recreation programs (including supervised sports activities) where a child can be safe from community violence, and summer programs that are accessible to families experiencing low income. In some communities, a social service agency may accumulate this information; in other communities, pediatricians have the responsibility to organize the resources available for their practice. Assigning the organizing role to an individual office staff person who maintains an up-to-date binder on a broad range of community resources is an effective strategy.

TABLE 3.1   Community Resources for Prevention, Evaluation, and Treatment of Children and Their Families With Problems in Development and Behavior

Early intervention services (0–3 years old)
Public school services for children with special needs
Home visiting networks
Mental health services
Recreation services
Nutrition services
Speech and hearing
Occupational and physical therapy
Programs for students with learning disabilities
Preschools/daycare—child care resource and referral agency
Early Head Start and Head Start programs
Parent support/respite care

WRAPPING IT UP

Clinicians should provide a summary statement after the history and physical examination. When the child's health and development are satisfactory, the clinician should report that finding positively, emphatically, and with enthusiasm. The caregiver should be congratulated on the care and health of the child. These supportive statements encourage a high level of self-esteem with regard to parenting skills and strengthen the relationship between the caregiver and clinician. Parents may feel that the visit is a checkup of them as parents and may appreciate affirmation of their parenting and their child's well-being. Give it honestly and enthusiastically.

If a problem has been uncovered and discussed during the visit, review the problem briefly during the summary statement. This should include an assessment of how serious the clinician judges the problem to be and the advised plan to address it. Provide a time frame for decisions, assessments, or future reevaluations and clearly state potential options. Caregivers may raise an important question or concern when their options are reflected back to them and after they have digested the information presented to them. Do not be surprised if this summary prompts a whole set of questions, a new level of awareness, and raw emotions. That is what such a summary is designed to do.

Each well-child visit should terminate with a *closing question* that allows the parent and older child to express an uncovered problem or concern. "Was there anything else you wanted to bring up?" may encourage the caregiver or child to mention a sensitive problem that they are able to express only after a sense of trust has been established at the end of a visit. These *out-the-door questions* as the visit is about to end frequently reflect significant issues that have previously been hidden.

If the concern is nonemergent and time for an adequate response is not available, a statement such as "It sounds like something we should talk about when we both have more time together" may be followed by arranging the next available appointment. Although the clinician should not feel obligated to answer all out-the-door questions, interest and concern can be expressed by making an immediate, appropriate follow-up arrangement as part of a new contractual agreement, thereby acknowledging that the concern was heard.

The same response can be made to families who are late for their appointments or who bring up big issues on visits for acute illnesses. The clinician can say, for example, "This issue is too important for the very little time we have together today. Let's set a time when we can really work on this together." Then get specific and set up a time. Do not let the family leave without a specific appointment to address the issue. This practice helps clinicians feel as though they are in better control and able to do better work. Obviously, emergency concerns have to fit in, but others can usually wait. Most families appreciate a little longer time slot when the clinician can sit down and really listen. Wise clinicians do not let out-the-door comments derail their day, but they do recognize them as entrees to important information.

Each clinician develops a personal style for interviewing that optimally encourages the establishment of a helpful and healthy therapeutic relationship with children and caregivers. If education, guidance, and developmental monitoring are the objectives of a visit, a flexible, empathetic, and compassionate approach is helpful to ensure optimal communication between the clinician and the family. Awareness of the tools available to the clinician in constructing the interview will create a form and foundation for the art of medicine.

Innovations in Pediatric Primary Care

Focus on Early Relational Health

The concept of early relational health recognizes the relationship between parent and child as the foundation for social and emotional development and growth and a key driver of future child well-being. Many innovations in pediatric care, including those described here, have been developed with the aim of supporting positive parent-child emotional interactions, centering the parent and family experience, and fostering connections between families at the individual and community levels.

Group Well-Child Care

In this practice model, children are seen for health supervision visits in the first 2 to 3 years of life in small groups of parents and infants. Beginning with the first well-child visit after birth, a group of five to six infants and parents meet (usually 45 minutes) to discuss the contents included in the *Guidelines for Health Supervision IV* or *Bright Futures*. Parent concerns guide the discussion. The clinician is in the role of both an educator and facilitator. With children of similar age, parents often have shared concerns. They learn from each other, as well as from the clinician facilitator. After the group discussion, each child is examined; the physical and developmental assessments can occur within the group or individually. Group well-child care is cost-effective, efficient, and satisfying to parents and includes all the content found in traditional individual care. It has the added advantage of creating a supportive group of parents who can share their parenting experiences while observing a range of developmental and behavioral characteristics.

Parent Cafes and Group Discussions

Parents are invited to come together with other caregivers for support and educational talks by clinicians in the practice, followed by a group discussion. The focus may be on a developmental stage (e.g., toddlers, school-age children, adolescents), a particular topic (e.g., nutrition, tantrums and discipline, home safety, school underachievement, substance abuse), or a condition (e.g., asthma/allergies, recurrent ear infections, attention-deficit/hyperactivity disorder, eating disorders). Parent cafes and support groups often have a community-building component as well so that parents can socialize with others and often normalize common issues that they may be facing at the same time. Parent group discussions focused on a specific age group may also be organized before selected health supervision visits in the first 3 to 5 years of life, with the discussion being followed by an examination.

Healthy Steps

Healthy Steps is an approach to primary care for children from birth to 3 years of age, which aims to increase a clinician's ability to address behavioral, emotional, and cognitive development. To achieve this goal and create a strong bond between clinicians and parents, a Healthy Steps specialist (trained in pediatric nursing, early childhood education, or social work) is available to the practice to ensure enhanced well-child care, home visits, child development/family health checkups, availability of written materials, access to a child development telephone information line, links to community resources, and parent groups. The Healthy Steps specialist performs a standardized developmental screening test at targeted times and meets with parents during well-child visits to discuss behavioral and developmental issues. Teachable moments in the office encounter are emphasized. Research has demonstrated that parents in the program acquire more knowledge about child development/behavior and are better able to use community recourses than parents exposed to traditional pediatric care.

Reach Out and Read

Developed to promote literacy, language skills, and a close parent-child attachment through reading to children at an early age, the Reach Out and Read program offers a developmentally appropriate book to a family at each health supervision visit in the first 5 years. The books may be taken home, and office clinicians and staff emphasize the importance of reading aloud to young children. In the waiting room, volunteers read to children, thereby modeling techniques for parents. Reach Out and Read has been shown to increase parental attitudes and activities that encourage early literacy and to improve language scores on standardized tests at 2 years.

Video Interaction Project

The Video Interaction Project integrates coaching and feedback for parents of children ages 0 to 3 into the primary care encounter and aims to support parent strengths and encourage positive parent-child interactions. As a part of each session, parents and children are filmed playing with a toy or reading a book together. The video is then watched by the parent and a coach to identify strengths in the interaction and plan for age-appropriate interactions at home to support development. The model has been shown to increase positive parent-child interactions.

Medical-Legal Partnership

In recognition of the complex issues that impact the health of many families, the medical-legal partnership model includes lawyers as an integrated part of the healthcare team to help address structural and policy-related barriers to wellness. Lawyers in this model provide training to clinical practices on the best approaches to meeting family needs, as well as guidance to clinicians and families on specific issues, such as how to combat a housing eviction, advocate for a child with special educational needs, or where to access longer term legal services.

Home Visiting Partnerships

Given strong evidence that home visiting programs improve both maternal and child health, a number of primary care clinics have developed partnerships and even integrated home visitors into the pediatric primary care setting to enhance communication, collaboration, and coordination of care between home visitors and pediatric providers.

Embedded Maternal Mental Health Care

Perinatal and maternal depression are underdiagnosed and undertreated, leading to the AAP recommendation that mothers be screened for postpartum depression in pediatric primary care visits. In recognition that there are many barriers to accessing treatment, some clinics have gone beyond mere screening and identification to embed psychiatrists in pediatric clinics such that mothers who are identified to be at risk for perinatal or maternal depression can be seen on the same day for psychiatric intake and continue longitudinal treatment within the pediatric setting, if indicated and desired.

SUMMARY

- The child and the parent are both key members of the clinician-family partnership.
- The "therapeutic triangle" illustrates the influence of parents (and the extended family) on the relationship between the clinician and the child.
- Between 6 months and 2 to 3 years of age, stranger anxiety often guides the examination, and the child may be more secure in the lap of a parent.

- By 3 years old, a child begins to contribute to oral history; by 4 years, she is a major player.
- Adolescents should be interviewed separately from their parents to encourage autonomy and promote communication.
- Methods to enhance the clinical interview include the following:
    Open-ended and closed-ended/focused questions
    Pauses and silent periods
    Repetition of important phrases
    Active listening
  Transference and countertransference
- The processes of "reflection" and "self-awareness" by clinicians are associated with improved listening to patients in a nonjudgmental way, recognition of clinician errors, and refinement of technical interviewing skills.
- Knowledge about and respect for the beliefs, attitudes, and cultural lifestyle of children and their families yield important clinical information and enhance the therapeutic alliance.

! HEADS UP DEVELOPMENTALLY BASED OFFICE

- Periodically review the content and quality of information in your waiting room about development and behavior for parents and children.
- Clinical data are generated from verbal and nonverbal clues. Both are important.
- When entering the exam room, address the child with a comment before opening communication with a parent.
- Look for "teachable moments" and the opportunity to model a behavioral response and/or provide verbal/written information.
- Do not neglect an "out-the-door" question from a parent. It may be the main concern for the visit.
- Have paper and a marker (or crayon) available for drawing while waiting to be seen.
- The "explanatory model" of a parent or child for either health or illness may be different from the assumptions of a Western-trained clinician.
- A parent may have additional concerns that reveal behavioral or developmental uncertainty. Through active listening and focused questions, these concerns often come to the surface.
- Have an up-to-date, comprehensive list of community resources available for referrals.

RECOMMENDED READINGS

Allmond BS Jr, Tanner JL, Gofman HF. *The family is the patient.* ed 2. Baltimore: Williams & Wilkins; 1999.

American Academy of Pediatrics. *Guidelines for health supervision III.* Elk Grove Village: American Academy of Pediatrics; 2002.

American Academy of Pediatrics. Family pediatrics. *Pediatrics.* 2003;111(Suppl):1539.

Conn A-M, Szilagyi MA, Jee SH, Manly JT, Briggs R, Szilagyi PG. Parental perspectives of screening for adverse childhood experiences in pediatric primary care. *Families Syst Health.* 2018;36(1):62–72. https://doi.org/10.1037/fsh0000311.

Doyle S, Chavez S, Cohen S, Morrison S. *Fostering social and emotional health through pediatric primary care: common threads to transform practice and systems.* Center for the Study of Social Policy; 2019. Available at: https://cssp.org/wp-content/uploads/2019/10/Fostering-Social-Emotional-Health-Full-Report.pdf.

Duffee J, Szilagyi M, Forkey H, Kelly ET, Council on Community Pediatrics Council on Foster Care Adoption, and Kinship Care Council on Child Abuse and Neglect, and committee on Psychosocial Aspects of Child and Family Health Trauma-informed care in child health systems. *Pediatrics.* 2021;148(2): e2021052579.

Epstein RM. Mindful practice. *JAMA.* 1999;282:833–839.

Green M, ed. *Bright futures: guidelines for health supervision of infants, children, and adolescents.* ed 2. Arlington: National Center for Education in Maternal and Child Health; 2002.

Jee S, Forkey H. Maximizing the Benefit of Screening for Adverse Childhood Experiences. *Pediatrics.* 2022;149(2): e2021054624.

Liu YH, Stein MT. Talking with children. In: Parker S, Zuckerman B, eds. *Developmental and behavioral pediatrics: a handbook for primary care.* ed 2. Boston: Little, Brown; 2004.

Mendelsohn AL, Huberman HS, Berkule SB, Brockmeyer CA, Morrow LM, Dreyer BP. Primary care strategies for promoting parent-child interactions and school readiness in at-risk families: the Bellevue Project for Early Language, Literacy, and Education Success. *Arch Pediatr Adolesc Med.* 2011;165(1):33–41. https://doi.org/10.1001/archpediatrics.2010.254. PMID: 21199978; PMCID: PMC3095489.

National Center for Medical Legal Partnership: Available from: https://medical-legalpartnership.org/.

Penumalee L, Lambert JO, Gonzalez M, Gray M, Partani E, Wilson C, Etz R, Nelson B. "Why do they want to know?": a qualitative assessment of caregiver perspectives on social drivers of health screening in pediatric primary care. *Acad Pediatr.* 2023;23(3):329–335.

Roby E, Miller EB, Shaw DS, Morris P, Gill A, Bogen DL, Mendelsohn AL. Improving parent-child interactions in pediatric health care: a two-site randomized controlled trial. *Pediatrics.* 2021;147(3).

Stein MT, Jellinek M, Wells RD. The difficult parent: a reflective pediatrician's response. *J Dev Behav Pediatr.* 2003;24.

Utah Pediatric Integrated Post-Trauma Services: *Child traumatic stress care process model.* https://utahpips.org/cpm/

Willis DW, Eddy JM. Early relational health: Innovations in child health for promotion, screening, and research. *Infant Mental Health J.* 2022;43(3):361–372.

Young CA, Burnett H, Ballinger A, et al. Embedded maternal mental health care in a pediatric primary care clinic: a qualitative exploration of mothers' experiences. *Acad Pediatr.* 2019;19(8):934–941. https://doi.org/10.1016/j.acap.2019.08.004.

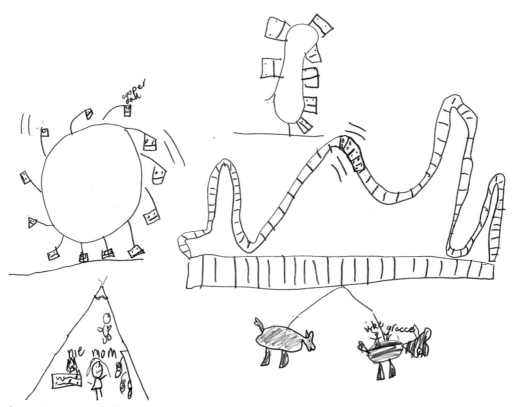

Some days in the office seem as busy and frenetic as a day at an amusement park, depicted here by a girl on an excursion with her family. The movement lines make it all seem to be whirling around. By, EB, aged 9.

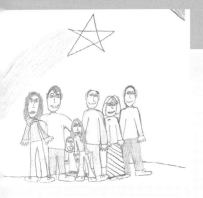

4

Use of Drawing by Children at Health Encounters

Jenny S. Radesky

This chapter describes approaches for understanding children's perspectives during clinical encounters, focusing on the use of children's drawings. The use of books and other playful ways of engaging with children are also briefly presented. Insights into child temperament, strengths, and challenges gleaned from artwork and reading-related behaviors—and caregivers' responses to the child's abilities—are presented from early childhood through adolescence. Ways to look at drawings as revealing of a child's inner life and social context are described.

KEYWORDS

- Fine motor skills
- Visual-motor integration
- Mentalization
- Early literacy promotion
- Shared book reading
- Digital media

Children are often anxious when attending pediatric visits. They may associate their pediatric primary care provider's office with vaccinations, blood draws, blood pressure cuffs that squeeze their arms, and black plastic cones that adults try to fit into their ear canals. Caregivers are also often stressed in pediatric offices, worried about the child's health, how their family's health behaviors will be judged by a physician, or how their child will behave—and children will pick up on this stress. Therefore children can often be overly inhibited or dysregulated, or even aggressive, during clinical encounters. Smartphones and tablets are commonly employed by caregivers to regulate their young child's behavior—or by preteens and adolescents who relieve boredom or stress associated with doctors' visits by turning to their phones.

Previous chapter authors: John B. Welsh, Susan L. Instone, and Martin T. Stein.

Therefore it can be helpful for clinicians to develop an array of drawing or reading activities to help children feel at ease. At the least, this provides children a distraction to facilitate collecting a detailed history from the caregiver; at best, it provides important insight into the child's emotions and challenges. While it is not feasible to have toys for each child to use—particularly in light of infection control—offices can encourage caregivers to bring a few of the child's favorite small toys from home. Blank paper and crayons or a sanitized pen can be available in examination rooms. Pediatric practices engaging in literacy promotion programs such as *Reach Out and Read* can provide a book to facilitate assessment of the child's early literacy and language skills. Each of these approaches provides an observable moment related to child development and opportunities for a child-centered discussion among caregivers, children, and clinicians.

DRAWING

Developmental Aspects of Drawing

Most children naturally like to draw or scribble. By 18 to 24 months, typically developing toddlers understand symbolically what pens and pencils are used for and therefore will try to write with these objects when they pick them up. A definite sequence, beginning with basic scribbles that progress to more complex diagrams and designs, is seen early in the drawings of toddlers and young preschool children.

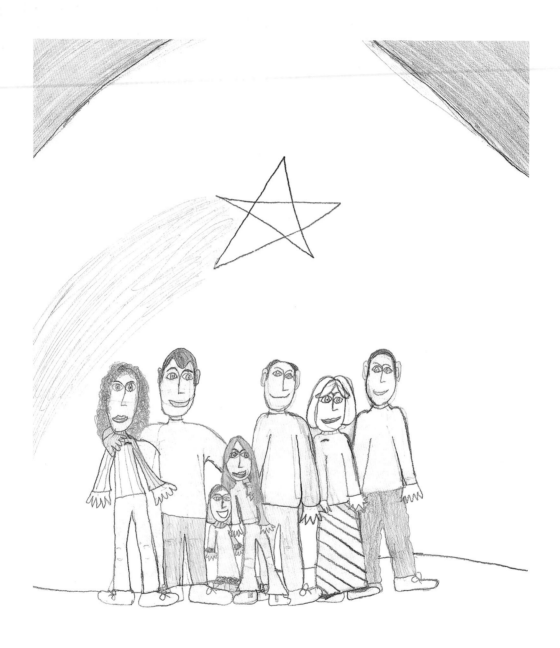

"My Family." By Robin Auerswald, age 8.

The human figure emerges by the time the child is 3½ to 4 years of age. These drawings seem to be cross-cultural in their progression toward meaningful, symbolic representation of the human figure.

Early drawings are also precursors to writing and recognizing letters. Across early and middle childhood, visual-motor integration is developing. **Visual-motor integration** refers to the brain's ability to perceive a shape or object, communicate that perception accurately to the motor planning and coordination areas of the brain, and carry out an attempt at copying the shape. In other words, it is a child's ability to copy a figure presented to them, starting as simple shapes in early childhood and evolving to complex figures in adolescence and adulthood. Deficits in visual-motor integration usually manifest as difficulty learning to write letters and can be associated with other challenges in motor planning or executive functioning.

Pediatric providers can begin to assess drawing abilities at the 2-year well-child visit by handing the child a pen or crayon and seeing what they do with it (anything from putting it in their mouth to scribbling on paper is expected). At 3 years, children may be able to copy a circle, and at 4 years, a square. Handedness is usually firmly established by these ages. Triangles are trickier and may be drawn as late as 5 years of age. Well-established norms have been documented for the sequence of copying simple geometric forms (Fig. 4.1). Engaging with children like this during visits is not for the purpose of "testing them" but for assessing their pencil grasp (Fig. 4.2), celebrating their abilities with them, and asking caregivers what opportunities for drawing the child has regularly. Some caregivers may be proud to discuss their child's ability to tap and navigate a touchscreen device to scribble, so this is a good opportunity to mention that grasping a pencil or crayon involves many more muscles and brain areas, and therefore is more supportive of early brain development.

Beginning at 4 or 5 years of age, children can be asked routinely to "draw a picture of your family" at all well-child encounters. This gives the child a chance to calm down and

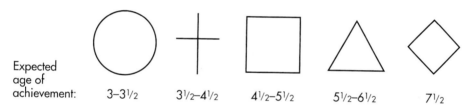

Expected age of achievement: 3–3½   3½–4½   4½–5½   5½–6½   7½

Fig. 4.1 Screening test for visual-motor integration and fine motor coordination and the expected developmental sequence for copying geometric forms.

Stages of Early Mark Making

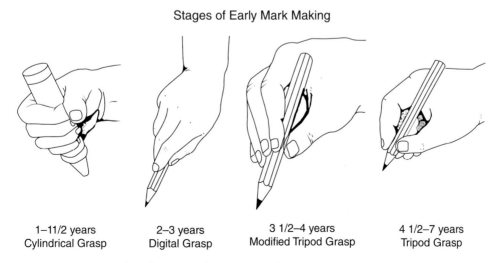

| 1–1½ years | 2–3 years | 3 1/2–4 years | 4 1/2–7 years |
| Cylindrical Grasp | Digital Grasp | Modified Tripod Grasp | Tripod Grasp |

Fig. 4.2 Development of pencil grasp between ages 1 and 7 years.

not be the center of the clinician's attention, while history is obtained from the caregiver. Some children will sit right down and start drawing, while others might throw the pen, explore the room, refuse to draw and ask for the caregivers' phone, or not appear to know how to start—all of these responses are important data for the clinician about how the child responds to a new challenge. The clinician should not coerce the child to draw, of course, but can offer a few options ("Would you like to draw with a red pen or a blue pen?") or hints ("How many people live in your home?"). If the parent seems self-conscious about the child's refusal, normalize the child's reaction by explaining that some children may not want to draw because it does not feel good to them (e.g., due to fine motor weakness) or they are anxious about the doctor's visit.

As children are invited to draw across sequential clinic encounters, they may become more comfortable with the task and even look forward to showing how their skills have improved. Drawings can be scanned into electronic medical records to document the child's abilities over time. Children are interested in their previous drawings; adolescents, in particular, are impressed with what they have done in the past, and this thread of continuity helps them to understand their personal identity. Ideally, a sense of control and ownership in the primary care visit builds a foundation for involvement in and responsibility for health and health care.

From ages 6 to 8 years, fine motor abilities and handwriting start to become more important for academic progress, and this can be monitored through drawing. Ask children to write their name on the drawing, and notice their pencil grasp, that is, how tightly they are holding the pen or pressing on the paper (both indicate fine motor coordination difficulties or weakness, as children squeeze harder to control the writing utensil). This allows discussion with the caregiver about whether teachers have expressed concerns about handwriting and whether occupational therapy support is provided in school. Intervening before a child turns 8 years is associated with better handwriting legibility and lower child frustration.

From elementary school through high school, children start to develop more focused interests in drawing—often copying comics, anime cartoons, or creating fantasy landscapes. Representations of people, objects, and events evolve from concrete to more abstract as children mature. Caregivers can be asked whether the child draws or colors "for fun" in their downtime, and this can be supported as a calming activity to replace screen media use if needed. Children who struggle with visual-motor or visual-spatial deficits might have disorganized, disproportionate representations of objects; if this cooccurs with difficulties in math, organization, or reading social cues, a related learning disability might be considered (see Chapter 19 for in-depth discussion of learning disabilities).

The Content of Children's Drawings

Since the 1950s the content of children's drawings have been analyzed as part of psychological evaluations. Sometimes termed *projective testing*, this method involves seeing how children respond to a free-form prompt (e.g., "draw your family") and assumes that implicit psychological processes—things the child may not know how to say out loud, including conflicts and personality traits—will be manifested in the drawing. The use of drawings in psychological evaluations has its roots in psychoanalytic theory, in which the goal is to identify unconscious drives and defenses to aid in diagnosis and treatment planning. However, the validity of projective tests such as the Draw-a-Person (DAP) Test (see Online Appendix) has been questioned for several reasons. First, there are significant interindividual variations in cognitive and perceptual abilities that influence how a child draws. Second, interpretation of drawings depends on the training experience and implicit biases of the interpreting clinician. Finally, empiric studies on the DAP test show that it does not predict mental health traits such as aggression (Klein, 1986). Therefore this chapter will discuss the general use of drawing in clinical encounters—for the purpose of prompting curiosity and discussion—rather than for diagnostic purposes.

For many children, drawing provides a window into their interests and experiences. From the time of early childhood, children are immersed in visual media such as books and cartoons—many of which they try to emulate through their drawings. Even if a child seems to be influenced by their favorite TV show or *anime* cartoon, something personal is infused into the drawing—these might include objects, concerns, or events that do not surface during the clinical interview (Fig. 4.3). These provide insight into the child's unique perspective and are a launching point for supportive conversation with the family.

Children at different developmental levels also have fascinating mental models of how the world works—often with magical or unexpected mental "rules" that they may not express to their caregivers. For example, they may have illogical fears about the way their body works or what happens during common experiences that they may find frightening or stressful (e.g., fear of using the toilet due to a perception that they will be flushed down, fear of going to bed at night because they worry they will not wake up). Therefore drawings provide children a way to reveal their magical explanatory models of the world—and caregivers/clinicians an opportunity for **mentalization** about how the child thinks about the world. As discussed in Chapter 2, mentalization involves understanding a child's motivations, perceptions, desires, and emotions and is crucial for

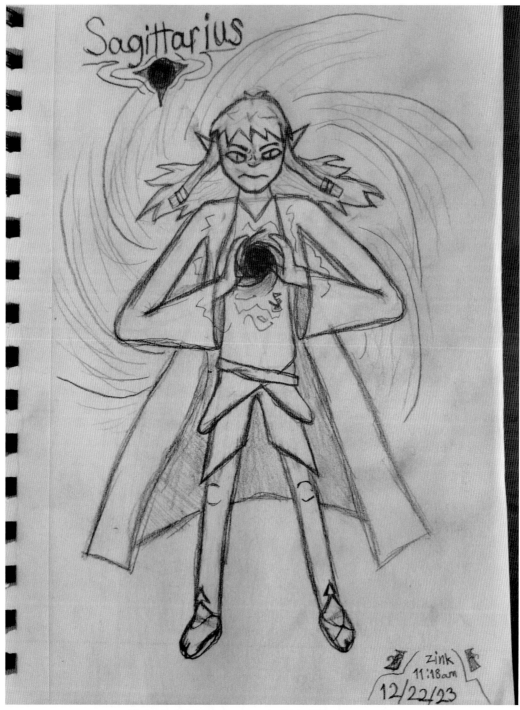

Fig. 4.3 Original character by Zeke Watson, age 14.

helping the child overcome struggles by "meeting them where they are," rather than imposing adult expectations or agendas. In this case, drawings may shed light on the child's perceptions and emotions, thus providing useful information that helps the clinician and caregiver correct any misunderstandings that contribute to illogical fears.

However, it is important not to "read" too deeply into the content of drawing, as their construction will evolve over time with the child's cognitive abilities. In early childhood, depictions in drawings are *intuitive* or *egocentric* and contain more magical components. More accurate, realistic drawings come from grade-schoolers who are in a more logical, *concrete* thinking stage (see Chapter 2). Abstractions, or conscious distortions used to convey concepts, coincide with the emergence of abstract thought in adolescence.

The development of a third dimension, depth perception, and visual occlusion (not seeing the parts of a figure through another object, so-called x-ray visibility) is a mark of an intellectual maturity that gradually develops between the ages of 7 and 8 years through 10 to 12 years, with some individual variation between children.

One common approach is to ask the child to draw a picture "with everyone in your family, all doing something." Parents are often interested in interpretation of these drawings, but it is important not to overextend their meanings—just use them as an opportunity for the parent to wonder about the child's experience and celebrate their abilities. Analysis of these drawings has historically looked at details such as where individual family members are placed, relative size and position of family members, any distortion or omission of individuals, or barriers between members. This is thought to signify the child's internal perceptions of their family and emotions that are hard for children to put into words (Figs. 4.4–4.6). When the child is able to describe

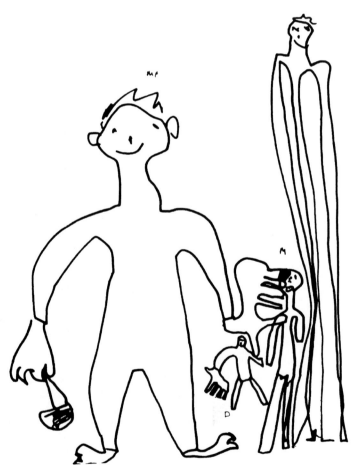

Fig. 4.4 Family drawing by a 6-year-old boy with interesting differences in the size of different family members. This offers a chance to ask the child who the different members are, what they are like, and why they are different sizes.

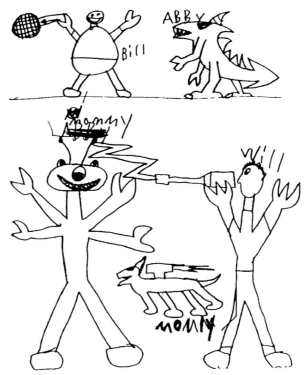

Fig. 4.5 This drawing was done by a 9-year-old boy who had been admitted to the hospital on three occasions for severe abdominal pain and vomiting in the setting of significant family stress.

their drawings, verbal explanations can assist in the interpretation and should be encouraged. The clinician can ask open-ended questions like "What's this? Who is this? Can you tell me about them? Why is he doing that?"

To caregivers, clinicians can ask questions that support mentalization, such as "I wonder what that represents in his mind?" or "What's your hunch for why she chose to draw it that way?" Finally, directing questions at a drawing on a piece of paper—rather than directly to the caregiver or child—may feel less intimidating and may open up new topics for discussion.

Children's Drawings of Their Own Body or Symptoms

Children with somatic and pain complaints can be asked to draw the location of their symptoms and what they feel like. These drawings can help children develop insight into their own symptoms and the stresses or emotions that contribute to them. (Fig. 4.7). Reviewing these drawings with the child or family often serves to open up discussion of the background and dynamics of symptoms.

The drawings of children with a serious chronic condition can illuminate the child's understanding of the illness, perceptions of being sick or injured, and feelings of isolation. Specific indicators in the drawings can help the clinician evaluate the child's degree of psychosocial adjustment. For example, unusual treatment of certain parts of the body in drawings may suggest feelings of anxiety or worry (Fig. 4.8). Threatening or scary themes (e.g., stormy weather) may suggest feelings of distress about the illness that the child may be unable or unwilling to verbalize (Fig. 4.9). Drawings of seriously ill children may demonstrate a sense of social isolation (Fig. 4.10) or feelings of being overwhelmed by the illness (Fig. 4.11). Recovery, in a psychological sense, can be seen in subsequent drawings (Fig. 4.12).

In an interesting study, children's drawings were able to help differentiate migraine from nonmigraine (tension) headaches in an outpatient pediatric clinic. Children of 4 to 19 years old were asked, "Where is your pain? What does your pain feel like? Are there any other symptoms (before or after the headache) that you can show in a

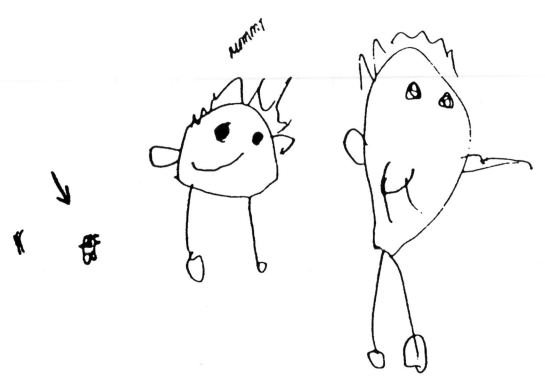

Fig. 4.6 A 7-year-old boy, depicted by the *arrow*, drew this picture during an office visit for behavioral and school challenges. The drawings of people are less developed than expected for age and might prompt a recommendation for a psychoeducational evaluation.

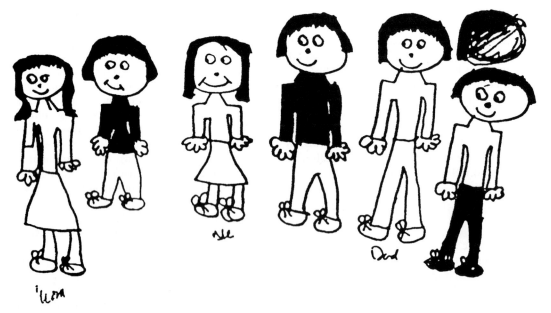

Fig. 4.7 A 9-year-old girl with several months of recurrent abdominal pain drew herself, her parents, and three siblings. The drawing is notable for the strong similarity between family members.

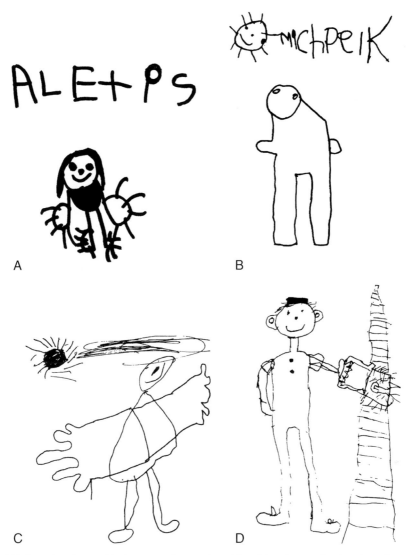

Fig. 4.8 (A) Drawing by a girl, 3 years 10 months old, with advanced school readiness skills in language, social, and motor domains. This drawing shows advanced features for a 3- to 4-year-old, with hair, nose, fingers, toes, and ability to write her name. (B) Drawing by a 6-year-old boy who was small for gestational age, had behavioral dysregulation in early childhood, and experienced delays in school readiness. His drawing is simpler than would be expected for age, with limited body parts, especially a paucity of facial features. (C) Drawing by a 6-year-old boy with attention-deficit/hyperactivity disorder associated with aggressive behavior and a history of viral encephalitis. Although the drawing shows fingers and facial features, it has disproportionate body parts and appears rapidly drawn. (D) Drawing by a boy, 6 years 4 months old, which he described as "an engineer that signals to the train." Advanced features of this drawing include ears, hair, details of clothing such as sleeves and shoelaces, and perspective on the train tracks, which get smaller as they go farther back on the page. He had advanced school readiness skills in the areas of fine motor, spatial, and conceptual skills.

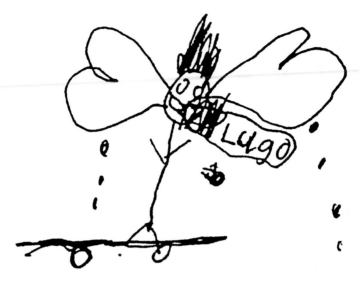

Fig. 4.9 This picture by a 9-year-old boy with hemophilia and asymptomatic human immunodeficiency virus (HIV) infection was drawn during a routine visit to the HIV clinic. The figure on a skateboard is spitting and has exaggerated ears that appear to be crying, thus suggesting feelings of distress and a need for reassurance about his diagnosis.

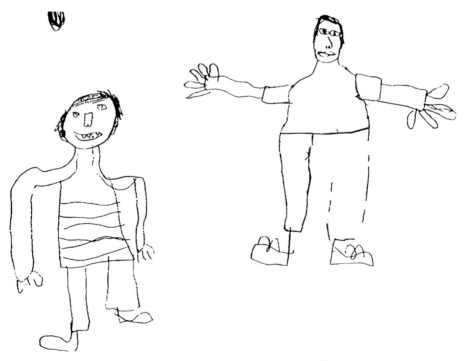

Fig. 4.10 An 8-year-old boy drew the self-portrait on the *left* that illustrates his perception of his spastic left hemiparetic cerebral palsy. After treatment and some improvement in function, he drew a picture of himself that reflects a different perception of his neurological impairment.

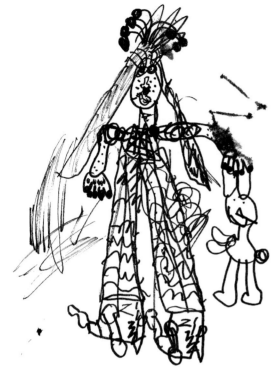

Fig. 4.11 A 10-year-old girl with high-functioning autism draws herself with incredible detail. There is a lot in this drawing that could be used to understand her unique interests and view of herself to start a conversation with her and her caregivers.

drawing?" Children were then asked to explain the drawing. Features in the drawings consistent with migraine included pounding pain, nausea/vomiting, desire to lie down, periorbital pain, photophobia, and visual scotoma. Sadness or crying did not differentiate migraine from nonmigraine headaches. Although drawings would never be the only factor used in making a diagnosis, they can help a child explain their symptoms or understand them better. In addition, the use of drawings to explain conditions the child cannot otherwise "see," such as constipation/encopresis, may help reinforce why it is important to take daily medications.

Interacting Around Books in the Office

Families often bring books as a distraction object for children at pediatric visits, but it also helps to have a supply of books that span infancy through middle childhood. *Reach Out and Read* is an evidence-based program that provides an age-appropriate book to children at each well-child encounter between birth and 5 years. The provision of books to families both endorses the fact that reading and literacy are not only important but also offers an opportunity to (1) observe the child's literacy skills together with the caregiver and (2) discuss how to get the most out of shared reading experiences.

- In infancy, before an infant can hold a chunky board book, it is worthwhile to show caregivers how reading to their child provides new ways of talking to their child and supporting serve-and-return interactions. Once the infant can hold, mouth, or bang a book, it is an opportunity to comment on the child's developing motor control and how hearing words from caregivers supports language development.
- For toddlers, hand the child a board book and see how they manipulate it, turn pages, point at pictures, or use labels. Comment on their fine motor skills, cognitive development (such as recognizing pictures and objects), and the back-and-forth interactions and snuggling with caregivers and siblings that occur around a book.
- For verbal children ages 3 to 4 years and older, show them a few different books and ask them to pick one. This allows you to see what they are attracted to and ask why. Then you can ask questions that assess verbal and early literacy skills, such as pointing to letters or colors, or open-ended questions like:
  - What do you think this book is about?
  - Can you find all the letters in your name?
  - Tell me a story about this picture. What's he doing? Do you ever do that?
- At all ages when children are verbal, ask about reading routines at home, such as:
  - Do you read books at home? What types do you like?
  - Have you read any good books or graphic novels lately? Can you tell me about them so I can recommend them to other patients?

Digital Media

Over the past few decades, it has become increasingly common to observe caregivers and children bringing mobile phones, touchscreen devices, laptop computers, handheld video game devices, and other internet-connected objects into clinical encounters. For most families, mobile devices are like an appendage: their portal into communication, information, work/school, entertainment, social support, or distraction from boredom. Although devices can feel like a barrier to clinician-caregiver or clinician-patient communication at times (just like the clinician's computer screen can), their presence is also an opportunity to talk about the ubiquitous technology that now weaves itself into families' lives.

Parent Technology Use

Most parents will put away their devices when you enter the room, but if they do not, you can make a nonjudgmental statement that normalizes the ubiquity of screens. For example, you can make a comment such as "You know, screens can make it hard to focus on what another person is saying, so I'll close my laptop and we can turn over the other screens and just chat for 10 minutes." However, also recognize that caregiver phone use can be a sign that the parent is stressed, so another option is to try engaging with the child first and then start asking the parent questions based on whatever the child is doing—in other words, refocus their attention on the child, rather than you (who may be seen as intimidating) or the phone.

Adolescents and Smartphones

For adolescents, too, using a phone during a clinical encounter can be a way to avoid interacting with other people or having uncomfortable conversations. Phone use can also simply be a habit to pass the time. Regardless, you can use the presence of a teen's phone in the room with you as a conversation starter. You can ask positive open-ended questions like *Who is the funniest/most inspirational/most creative person you follow on social media? How do you decide who to follow? What's the most amazing thing you've seen online lately?* Once you have shown your patient that you are not immediately going to judge their media use and you genuinely care that they have positive experiences online, you may be able to talk about media use in a way that gently helps the preadolescent or adolescent critically think about it. For example, you can phrase questions in a way that recognize the tensions young people feel between daily routines and all of the notifications or content that draw them into their phones. For example, *Which one usually wins, your phone or your sleep? How do you create boundaries around the things you love doing, so that technology does not get in the way? How can you tell when apps or media are trying to trick you into spending more time online or more money?* As media becomes more personalized and interactive, it is important to teach young users about the ways that technology's "persuasive design" often wants to maintain our attention as long as possible—since platforms and influencers make more money this way— sometimes at the expense of other healthy activities. Caregivers may appreciate the modeling of conversation starters that do not contain snap judgments about media and instead help the child to become a savvier consumer, such as: *How do YOU wish social media was designed better? Who do you talk to when you have online drama?*

Younger Children

For verbal children who are using a device in the examination room, try sitting next to them and watching along as they play. Ask simple questions (it is hard for children to respond when they are busy with a screen) such as *What are you playing? What is your favorite? Why? How did you find this game? What do you do when an ad pops up?* Sometimes this can reveal that the child is playing a game their caregiver thought was uninstalled or is watching an age-inappropriate video and can be an opportunity to review putting blocks and age filters on app store downloads (see Recommended Readings). It can also be a chance to reinforce positive media content decisions that families have made or suggest resources such as Common Sense Media. When it is time to transition away from the device as part of the clinical examination, this is also an opportunity to talk about how it feels to stop using media. For younger children, ask their parents: *How do you help them transition away from the screen? Do you have strategies for setting limits?* You can ask verbal children: *How do you handle it when your parent makes you stop watching videos/playing games? Do you argue? Does it help if they set a timer or give you a warning?* This type of conversation might help a patient and caregiver problem-solve about better ways of helping the child follow media limits at home rather than arguments or grabbing a device away. In the long run, our goal is to help children self-regulate their media use (and not use it compulsively), so praise younger children when they are able to put a device away without complaint.

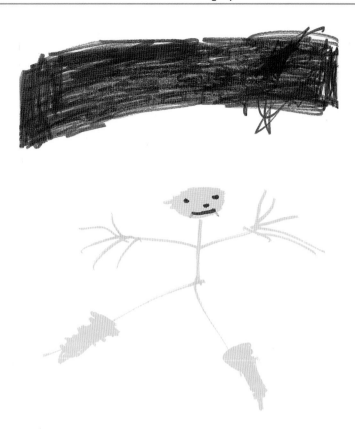

Fig. 4.12 A 9-year-old boy with attention-deficit/hyperactivity disorder hurried through this drawing of himself, which has limited detail in terms of hair, toes, clothing, or other distinguishing features. By Joshua Yudiski.

SUMMARY

Children's drawings and interactions with books are a delightful, cost-effective, low-tech way of highlighting a child's developmental progress, emotional and social concerns, and need for further evaluation. This low-cost diagnostic aid adds vitality, veracity, reflection, and insight into every pediatric encounter.

⚠ HEADS UP—USE OF DRAWINGS

- Children's drawings provide potential insight into a child's behavior and development and may launch interesting discussions with caregivers. The drawing will enhance observations of the parent-child interactions and the child's own behavior during the clinical encounter.

- Ask the child and parents what they think about the drawing. The response may surprise you and lead to areas of concern that have not been discussed.
- A child's drawing may, at times, reveal an interest, visual-motor capacity, or artistic ability that is not apparent in the typical medical encounter.
- Make the drawings a part of the medical record. Scan them into the "media" tab so that children and families can look back at them visit after visit. As the child or adolescent matures, there may be an opportunity to review the drawings with the child (or caregiver). Some college students have returned to the office requesting a look at their past drawings.

RECOMMENDED READINGS

Klass P, Dreyer BP, Mendelsohn AL. Reach out and read: literacy promotion in pediatric primary care. *Adv Pediatr*. 2009;56(1):11–27.

Uthirasamy N, Reddy M, Hemler JR, et al. Reach Out and Read implementation: a scoping review. *Acad Pediatr*. 2023;23(3):520–549.

Zuckerman B, Needlman R. 30 years of Reach Out and Read: need for a developmental perspective. *Pediatrics*. 2020;145(6): e20191958.

Erkoboni D, Radesky J. The elephant in the examination room: addressing parent and child mobile device use as a teachable moment. *J Pediatr*. 2018;198:5–6.

Milteer KR, Ginsburg DA, Mulligan N, Ameenuddin A, Brown WS, Swanson WS. Council on Communications and Media; Committee on Psychosocial Aspects of Child and Family Health The importance of play in promoting healthy child development and maintaining strong parent-child bond: focus on children in poverty. *Pediatrics*. 2012;129(1):e204–e213.

Klein RG. Questioning the clinical usefulness of projective psychological tests for children. *J Dev Behav Pediatr*. 1986;7(6):378–382.

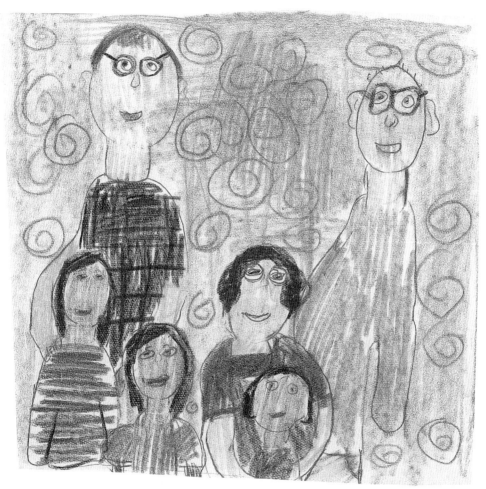

A drawing by an 11-year-old reveals that grandma was ill with cancer as she was shown without her hair. By M.D.

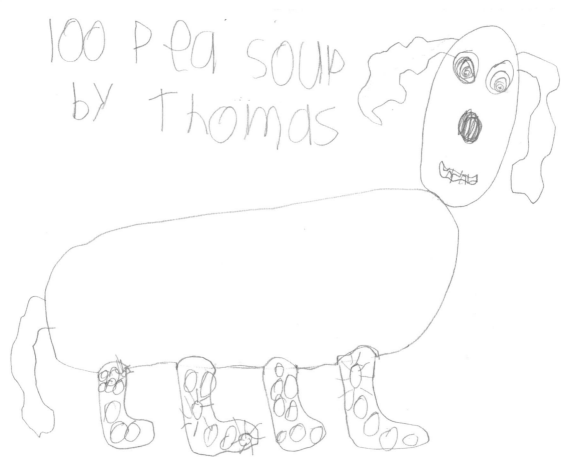

Drawing can help children express their fears. "100 Pea Soup (a dog that appeared in my night-mare, had popping corn kernels all over his body that spewed goop, who I had to sleep next to.) I was afraid of dogs and drew this right after the nightmare." By Thomas Radesky, age 8.

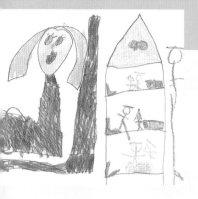

5

The Prenatal Period: Understanding Parent Stress, Mental Health, and Attachment

Yuan He

This chapter prepares the clinician to conduct an effective prenatal interview through an enhanced understanding of the developmental changes involved in becoming a parent. It also presents ways to ask about biomedical, social, and psychological information that may guide care for the family.

KEYWORDS

- Psychological changes in pregnancy
- Birth of a sibling
- Risk factors for attachment
- Fetal behavior
- Breastfeeding
- Specific health risks

The period before an infant's birth is a time of adjustment, concern, anxiety, and some adaptive stress in a family's development. The American Academy of Pediatrics recommends a prenatal visit in the third trimester of pregnancy for all expectant parents and encourages pediatricians to become more involved in prenatal anticipatory guidance. *Bright Futures* also sets the agenda for pediatric work to begin at this time. This type of prenatal encounter offers the unique opportunity to begin to build a strong working relationship with a family as well as support the family through psychological stress and changes associated with the birth of a child. While prenatal visits are offered by a majority of pediatricians, the percentage of first-time parents that report attending a visit ranges from 5% to 39%, depending on the population. For families who do not have a prenatal visit but attend a visit with an older sibling, this is also an opportunity to check in about some of the concepts covered in this chapter.

Original chapter by Suzanne D. Dixon.

PERINATAL RISK: BIOMEDICAL FACTORS

The prenatal visit often includes an assessment of medical risk in the unborn child, as well as any familial history of inherited disease, history of previous pregnancy outcomes, and the medical history of the parents. These factors are shown in Box 5.1. Most of these data can be gathered by questionnaires, with follow-up of any specific issues. A pediatric clinician's concern for these issues emphasizes to the family the continuities in prenatal and postnatal life and allows for a focused medical assessment of the infant and preparation for any known or likely special care needs.

The pediatric perspective on family medical history may vary somewhat from the obstetric perspective, with enhanced emphasis on issues affecting the fetus/infant. For example, hepatitis B carrier status in a mother requires immediate action by the child's clinician after birth and in the months following. The pediatric clinician may highlight the importance of good nutrition for optimal intrauterine development of the infant and success of lactation. Previous infertility or pregnancy loss, premature delivery, or delivery complications should alert the pediatric clinician to possible problems ahead, both physiological and psychological. A lingering sense of failure, loss, worry, and anxiety may be present for this pregnancy in the parents' minds. Getting a clear history will help deal with both. Medical records may provide important information so request a release of information to review records if there is anything complicated. However, only direct, sensitive interviewing will identify how parents perceived and experienced past events. Furthermore, it may be these perceptions that will

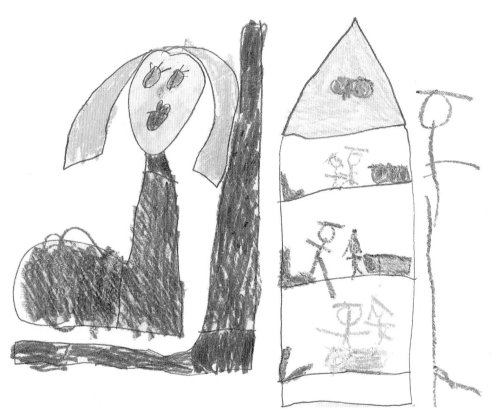

A pregnant mom with healthy baby waiting to be born. Everyone and everything is ready at home. By Briana Perkins, age 6 (her siblings were premature).

BOX 5.1 **Perinatal Risk Factors**	
• History of previous pregnancy loss or infertility, previous preterm delivery, or threatened preterm delivery • Pregnancy complications such as infections, bleeding, trauma, and/or high blood pressure • Occupational exposures, risks • Substance use, including tobacco and alcohol • Unusual or highly restricted diet, malabsorption syndrome • Thyroid disease, diabetes mellitus • Hepatitis B or human immunodeficiency virus, disease or carrier status; unknown status • Poor or excessive weight gain • Inherited diseases such as hemoglobinopathies, neurological disorders	• Prenatal lab abnormalities, such as low alpha-fetoprotein • Prenatal ultrasound abnormalities, including abnormal growth • Family history of perinatal or early neonatal illness or death • Previous birth interval of less than 18 months, multiple fetuses (e.g., twins, triplets) • Maternal age younger than 15 or older than 35 years • Maternal chronic illness (e.g., renal disease, cardiac disease, colitis) • Breast abnormalities, past surgeries, or past difficulties with breastfeeding

most influence the parents' perspective on the pregnancy, the delivery, and the child.

PSYCHOLOGICAL ADAPTATION TO PREGNANCY

The prenatal visit is an opportune time to develop a rapport and partnership with families, which clinicians can foster by actively listening and addressing questions and concerns, connecting families with community resources and supports, and introducing families to the range of pediatric care provided, including psychosocial aspects of development, family issues, and physical concerns.

It is vital for clinicians to understand the structure of each family, how it functions, and its social and cultural dimensions to address the child's issues. Now is the time to begin that understanding of the family as a whole. You will get this information through an interview that encompasses the adult development issues involved in parenting.

The adaptive psychological changes in parents during pregnancy have important implications. Some worry and anxiety are expected; after all, becoming a new parent or adding another child to the family is a big change. Pregnancy can be a time of psychological turmoil for many families, as energy is mobilized, reordered, and directed around the unborn child in a process of attachment. Anxiety, conflict, tension, and fears can be normal and necessary emotional components of even the most uncomplicated gestations for parents and other family members. Shifts in attention, time allocation, and monetary resources follow from the process of changing priorities within the whole family unit.

Excessive stress, however, may alter the family's ability to make these important developmental shifts. Severe psychological stress may directly affect fetal growth and development. Clinicians should be mindful of both interpersonal and extrapersonal sources of stress. Stress between parents or between parents and other family members may be seen to some degree in every family while individuals reorder relationships. However, extremes in conflicts may significantly impact parental health. Pregnancy is known to be a high-risk period for intimate partner violence as well as for anxiety and depression, and pediatricians should be prepared to assess parental safety and well-being and refer to supportive services as indicated. Outside of the home, families may experience other sources of stress and trauma, including community violence, racism, and other forms of discrimination and oppression that may translate into increased psychological stress.

The whole family and the pregnancy context must be taken into account if one is preparing to understand and address a child's and family's needs. Parents often reflect on and work through their relationships with their own parents with each new pregnancy. It may be important to explore who the extended family members are, how they relate, and the manner in which they will fit into the life of the expected child, especially if the extended family is either a primary source of support or of stress to the expectant parents. It may also be important to identify who else will be participating as a caregiver to the infant, including friends and family, to clarify different roles in the child's life and how they relate. If other key caregivers are identified, it is also an opportunity to invite them into the child's care, either through telephone or by including them at future child health visits.

THE DEVELOPMENTAL COURSE OF PREGNANCY

A predictable developmental course of parental adjustment during the course of pregnancy has been described through interviews with pregnant persons. Table 5.1 describes psychological stages of pregnancy.

First Trimester

In the first trimester, the experience described by pregnant persons is primarily focused on new physical sensations and changes. Some report feeling tense, edgy, nervous, irritable, and occasionally depressed. For people with a history of spontaneous abortion, previous infertility, and other perinatal problems, these feelings can be deepened and complicated by fears of loss and failure.

Second Trimester

With the onset of fetal movement in the second trimester, a marked shift in psychological processes often takes place. Dreams and awake fantasies about the child commonly begin at this time and can be positive and/or anxiety producing. No definitive data exist regarding whether prenatal identification of the sex of the child changes these fantasies, speeds attachments, or narrows the range of fantasies.

Many expectant parents increase their efforts to solidify ties with friends, community, and extended family at this time. Renewed interest in traditions, religious affiliations, or hobbies is a sign of these processes. Even in the absence of external preparations for the infant, parents are engaged in important internal preparations for the infant's arrival. Older children in the family, even toddlers, may begin to show behavioral changes during this time that indicate an awareness that their relationship with their parents is changing. This is a natural time to begin sibling preparation if this has not already happened, through age- and developmentally appropriate language and reassurance regarding the changes happening within the parent's body and within the home.

Third Trimester

The mental work of the third trimester is that of seeking a safe passage through labor and delivery. The pregnancy may become physically taxing, and many people may experience a sense of vulnerability along with an exacerbation of underlying fears and anxiety. Sleep may be erratic and

TABLE 5.1	Psychological Stages of Pregnancy
First trimester	Self-focus
	Becoming attached to the idea of pregnancy
	Pregnancy as a change—"I am pregnant"
	Ambivalence about the ability to handle the demands of (another) child
	Realignment of parenting issues, relationships of the past
	Anxiety about loss, fetal harm, or mishap
	Emotional lability
Second trimester	The fetus experienced as a separate entity; increased awareness of the fetus
	Dreams and fantasies about the unborn child
	Making changes, readjustments, plans
	Sense of well-being
	Nest building
	Increased dependence
	Interest in traditions, belief systems
	Sense of pride in the pregnancy; seeking acceptance by others
	Information seeking
Third trimester	Preparing to deliver the fetus; detachment from the idea of being pregnant
	Seeking safe passage through labor and delivery; making plans
	Attachment to the idea of being a parent
	Fears of injury to self, the partner (if applicable), and the infant
	Looking for help and support
	Vulnerability to alcohol and other drug use
	Sleep changes
	Vivid dreams
Later	Focus on details
	Fatigue, anxiety
	Putting things in order, cleaning, sorting

include shifts to a shorter sleep cycle and less deep sleep. Psychological nest building may continue through a process of inward direction of thoughts and ideations—positive and, at times, negative. The third trimester may bring specific new concerns about the child and the delivery. In addition, the actual cost of caring for a child may push some caregivers to seek extra work and to develop new strategies for financial future planning. If financial stress is identified, the clinician should ensure that parents and caregivers are aware of supports that increase access to affordable, high-quality food, housing, early childhood education, and other social determinants of health that may ease their stress during this preparation period.

In summary, pregnancy demands an important transition in adult development for caregivers, a process that is not complete at the time of the infant's birth. The parents who come in for the prenatal interview will not be the same as those the clinician will meet after the delivery. They are in the midst of a huge developmental shift. The pediatric clinician can anticipate the strength of the infant to mold some of the uncertainties, anxieties, and mild, often adaptive disorganization seen in most families at this time. Consistent, reassuring support from the clinician will be the foundation of a trusting relationship with the parents.

STRESS AND SUPPORT

Fetal well-being is affected by support from and integration into the community, and social stressors during pregnancy and the health of the infant are strongly related. Since pregnancy is a stressful time of change for all families, pediatric clinicians should ask family members about sources of stress and support, to provide resources and referrals that can help the family make a successful transition. The most common sources of stress include financial stressors, which can be exacerbated if the family anticipates a loss in the parent's income or employment following birth. The prenatal visit can be a great opportunity to ask families about the social determinants of health and explore whether they experience any barriers to food, housing, transportation, health care, childcare, or other needs that may impact their ability to adequately care for their child. The pregnancy itself can be a source of stress, especially if there are any pregnancy complications, and the family should be supported in seeking both physical and mental health care to ensure both parental and infant health. Close collaboration with obstetrics clinicians can facilitate continuity of care for families in the perinatal period, particularly for birthing parents with complex conditions, including substance use disorders, that benefit from specialized care and multidisciplinary support during and after pregnancy. Information about public programs and community resources, such as home-visiting services, doulas, parent support groups, and any other programs that may address family needs, should be shared with the family. Asking and sharing information about high-quality childcare can also be helpful anticipatory guidance. Family well-being is really a pediatric concern and should be part of the factors addressed in the prenatal interview. Such an approach in turn sets the stage for ongoing appraisal of the family as part of the child health evaluation throughout childhood, the essential microenvironment for growth and development.

ATTACHMENT—ASSESSMENT OF RISK AND RESILIENCE

Attachment is defined as a strong, affectionate connection with another person that endures over time to form that bond. As described in Chapter 2, it is the psychological process that prompts attentive care, responsive nurture, and healthy mental growth for a child. Although most families will make a strong, attached relationship with the infant, the few that will need additional help should be identified early, if possible. Helping families to develop safe, stable, and nurturing relationships with each other and with their communities can support early relational health. As discussed in Chapter 3, a trauma-informed, strengths-based approach should be used to compassionately and comprehensively address manifestations of family or adverse childhood experiences without causing additional harm. Additional resources and behavioral health referrals should be provided for families that would benefit, while working together with the family to identify and reinforce areas of strength and resilience. This approach should start in the prenatal period and carry forward at encounters after delivery. Intervention, including a recommendation to reach out to other family members and close friends, along with the support given by the primary healthcare provider and professional referrals, can promote the health of both the infant and the caregivers. Extra vigilance is needed when issues place family or individual parents at likely need for support. Some of factors that should prompt pediatricians to consider providing families with additional resources to promote healthy attachment are shown in Box 5.2.

OTHER CHILDREN

Adaptation to the impending arrival of a sibling is a hurdle for any young child. It is never easy. The birth of a sibling requires readjustment to a new place in the family. The nature of that stress depends on the child's own developmental level and temperament. The parents' pregnancy adjustment processes make a child aware of a change in the family. Young children benefit from frequent reassurance

BOX 5.2   **Prenatal Risk Factors for Attachment Disorders**

Prior or Current Sources of Trauma:
- Recent loss, death, or separation from a loved one
- Previous loss of or serious illness in another child
- Previous removal of a child
- History of depression, serious mental illness
- History of infertility, pregnancy loss
- Absence, separation from, or insecure relationship with the other parent
- Insecure or limited attachment to one's own parents

Prior or Current Stressors:
- Troubled relationships with family members or other members of the social network
- Financial stress, including unemployment, job loss, absence of paid parental leave, or difficulty paying bills
- Recent move, no community ties
- Absence of social supports
- Unintended and/or undesired pregnancy

of their parents' unwavering love and the security of their families. For a child younger than 3 years, whose capacity to understand future events is limited and whose world is largely confined to family and home, the birth of a sibling will be difficult. If changes are needed (e.g., change in beds), they should be done early to allow for accommodation. Pressure to toilet train at this time may lead to prolongation of the process. Those children younger than 3 years rarely need to be told about the pregnancy until the second trimester.

Young children may enjoy feeling the baby move in utero, looking at books, or playing with dolls, although no data suggest that these activities ease the adjustment. Rehearsal of the specific plans for a child at the time of delivery is helpful to a young child so that everyone knows what to expect. Mild regression and an increase in demands by the older child are positive signs of a child's sensitivity to the pregnancy and offer testimony to the child's attachment to their parents. Parents should be congratulated for this evidence of a positive emotional bond, even if the behavior is troublesome. Pushing the child to "grow up" will probably make the older child become more clingy, irritable, and demanding. There is no reason to expect that having to share one's parents with another child will be greeted with enthusiasm, at least not during some period of adjustment. It is a developmental crisis for the child that can be handled with support.

The central issue in the child's adjustment is the parents' continuing psychological availability. Parents may have significant feelings of loss in their relationship with the older child with the anticipated arrival of another and wonder whether they have enough time, energy, and love to share with another child. They may need to grieve this loss to move to another level of parenting. Feelings of urgency about their relationship with their older child and pressure to do all they can before the birth of their next child may be a source of additional tension in a family. The pediatric clinician should consider this family process as the basis for renewed behavioral problems, mild developmental regression, and even an increase in telephone calls to the office. Addressing the adjustment issue directly may get to the heart of the matter.

In the third trimester, parents can introduce books that deal with the birth of a sibling. Children's questions about the event should be answered clearly and honestly while bearing in mind what might be the *basis* for the specific question from the child's perspective (e.g., separation, loss of possessions, changes in special shared activities), as well as the child's developmental level. Medical details are usually of less interest to the child, so follow the child's lead through listening to questions.

Hospital visitation after the infant's birth may ameliorate some of the child's worries about separation. Acceptance of the new baby should not be the goal of this visit; reassurance of caregiver availability and intactness should be. No evidence shows that a hospital visit decreases any of the expected negative behavior at home. A tool is available to assist families with sibling adjustment (Box 5.3).

WHAT IS THE FETUS UP TO?

Helping a family learn about the developing fetus is a way to draw members into the idea of the infant as an important interactive participant in their lives. At least part of the visit should be a "did you know …" recounting of fetal behavior capabilities. This adds fuel to the attachment process, reinforces healthy lifestyle practices, and adds to understanding the individuality of the child. Importantly, it sets the stage for the newborn's arrival when these interactional capabilities are observed directly.

These capacities are summarized by Hepper, and examples are presented in Box 5.4.

PLANNING FOR BREASTFEEDING

If the parent is interested in breastfeeding, there is evidence to show that planning for breastfeeding by discussing potential barriers and approaches prenatally can lead to improved rates and duration of breastfeeding after delivery.

BOX 5.3   Helping Siblings With the Arrival of A New Baby

- Tell a young child that the baby is coming as soon as others are told.
- Provide ongoing reassurance of the parents' continuing love and care. Say it again and again.
- Use books and videos made for children on sibling births.
- Include a child older than 2 years in the prenatal visits.
- Participate in the sibling preparation classes at the delivering hospital, if applicable, or do a tour of the birthing center/hospital if not.
- Give children detailed plans for where they will be and who will take care of them during delivery.
- Include them in the plans for the new baby, such as new rooms, what the baby should wear, etc.
- Make all changes well in advance of the delivery, such as moving out of a crib, changing rooms, and arranging new preschool or daycare placements.
- Help them pick out a new gift to give the baby-to-be.
- Give them a doll or stuffed animal to take care of in parallel with the new baby. Talk about their "new baby" as the parents prepare for theirs.
- Spend some alone time each day with the older child before the baby is born and afterward as well. Keep that time sacred, even if it has to be short.
- Talk about the long-term advantages of a sibling, such as having a playmate and being seen as a "big sibling."
- Be patient with behavioral regressions in toileting, sleeping, and eating. Keep routines as much the same as possible.
- Do not scold a child for having negative feelings for a child but do prohibit acting out against the baby.
- Praise any positive attention or any help with the infant.

BOX 5.4   Fetal Behavior

Hearing
- Startles to loud sounds by 8 weeks.
- Responsiveness to sound by the fourth month.
- Turns to positive sounds by 28 weeks.
- Learns familiar sounds presented after 3 weeks.
- Becomes familiar with the rhythms and sounds of the parent's language by 32 weeks.
- By birth babies will demonstrate a preference for familiar voices, music heard in utero, and stories read before birth.

Light
- Responds to light by the 26th week.
- Will turn to light on the abdomen unless very bright—then turning away is seen.

Smell/Taste
- As evidenced by heart rate changes after birth, the fetus reacts differentially to tastes in amniotic fluid, such as the spices cumin and garlic.

Movement
- Movements begin at 8 weeks.
- Makes postural adjustments to birth parent's movements and even anticipates movement patterns by about 5 months.

- May be quite still while the pregnant female is active, only to "dance" when the pregnant female wants to rest.
- Hand to face, 10 weeks; yawn, 11 weeks; suck and swallow, 12 weeks.
- The infant sucks his thumb, fingers, and toes; rubs head; and grabs the umbilical cord. He is very active in exploring his world.

Response to Stress
- A pregnant female's stress produces changes in heart rate and activity and, if chronic, changes physiological reactivity, including cortisol secretion.
- May also result in preterm labor and low birthweight.

Novelty and Boredom
- When a light or sound stimulus is presented to the fetus over and over, the response diminishes. When the stimulus is changed to something new and "different," the fetal response comes back.

BOX 5.5   Breastfeeding Issues

Motivating Factors in the Choice to Breastfeed

Infant Health

- Most parents know that breastfeeding adds protection from disease for infants, but most are not as aware of the reduction of illness in the long term or the developmental advantage.

A Special Time

- The breastfeeding parent may enjoy the quiet time, the relaxed feelings, and the warmth and pleasure that come with breastfeeding.
- Parents may have a sense of pride in breastfeeding; they see it as a sign of responsibility and bonding.

Parental Health

- Long-term benefits in terms of reduced rates of breast cancer, osteoporosis, and arthritis.

Psychological Barriers to Breastfeeding

Lack of Confidence

- Fear of an inability to produce enough milk of high enough quality. Overemphasis on the need for a good diet that can be difficult to afford or prepare. Belief that it is hard to learn.

Embarrassment

- Fear of breast exposure in public.

Loss of Freedom

- Belief that breastfeeding will cut down on an active social or work life. Often disguises a fear of bonding or fear of that bond becoming too close because of the need to work outside the home.

Dietary and Health Practices

- Misperceptions that breastfeeding requires strict adherence to a special diet, giving up spicy foods and fast foods, that birth control pills cannot be used while breastfeeding, or that one is not healthy enough to breastfeed.
- Inability or unwillingness to forego substance use.

Influence of Family and Friends

- Family members may overtly or covertly discourage breastfeeding or give faulty advice.

Fear of Pain

- Perception that breastfeeding will be painful or disfiguring.

From Best Start: *Best Start Training Manual.* Tampa, 1997, Best Start.

The prenatal visit is also a time where any disinformation, fears, and questions about breastfeeding can be discussed. Common categories of motivators and psychological barriers to breastfeeding (Box 5.5) can be specifically and briefly addressed. Notation of these issues prenatally allows the pediatric provider to address these early insights and use them as the basis for problem solving with the family after the baby is born. The clinician can offer targeted information and help address barriers without being prescriptive or dogmatic. Encouragement to attend breastfeeding classes and identification of community resources should follow for families who are interested.

DURING THE VISIT

Setting the Stage

Each clinician will have a unique style of conducting prenatal interviews, and this style will vary according to parental factors as well. However, this encounter can be maximized by at least beginning with a set format. Many pediatric clinicians may be slightly uncomfortable at first without the presence of a child; a set agenda will help ameliorate this discomfort. The following are guidelines for a prenatal visit:

- Allow about 30 minutes for the interview, if possible.
- Invite all caregivers to participate at a time that is convenient for them and for you, typically around 4 to 8 weeks before the estimated birth date.
- Provide comfortable adult chairs in the office setting and place them in a position where eye-to-eye contact is possible.
- Ask the caregivers to fill out a medical history and identify top concerns and unmet needs—including financial strain, food insecurity, or unstable housing—before the interview, and review the information before you interact with them.

Group pediatric prenatal visits are a new option for some practices and are often attached to childbirth, breastfeeding, or sibling preparation classes. These sessions offer the opportunity to answer questions and to efficiently review your own philosophy and practice style. Information can be given to the group and productive discussion can take place. Many families enjoy the group setting, which can lay the foundation for group health supervision visits in some situations. All such group formats should include some private time with each family to address particular concerns and to begin to establish an individual relationship. The following are guidelines for a prenatal visit.

Observational Data

- Note which caregiver(s) attends the visit.
- If there are multiple caregivers, assess the interaction between them as they enter the room for the interview process.
- Be aware of the general affect; some degree of anxiety and apprehension is expected.
- Determine the degree of comfort with the pregnancy through behavioral and verbal clues from the caregiver(s).
- Note the use of pronouns or names for the unborn child and general attitudes toward the child when speaking.

What to Ask

The format of questions outlined in Table 5.2 allows control of the interaction to flow from the clinician to the parents.

A discussion of the specifics of your interactions with the family should include the following: your availability

TABLE 5.2   Questions to Be Asked at the Prenatal Visit

Question	Objective
How are you feeling?	Lay the territory to include the parent's well-being; assess the response to the situation overall
Ask how the pregnancy has gone; expand to cover medical events, life stresses, etc., as noted on the medical history form and your own individual outline (i.e., a pregnancy history from a pediatric standpoint).	Gather data for objective risk factors and the parents' perception of them, as well as assess their general response to the pregnancy and the perception of the pregnancy as high risk (whether it is by medical criteria or not)
Ask the nonpregnant parent (if available) how the pregnancy has gone.	Assess perceptions and concerns of the partner and the adjustment to the pregnancy
Was this a planned pregnancy?	Assess the place of the child in the relationship, the parent(s)' adjustment to pregnancy, and the degree and nature of adjustment for the child's health
Do you have other children at home? What are their ages and sexes? Have you cared for an infant before? What was that experience like?	Assess the family structure; note the child's place in it; assess their experience and expectations for infant care; assess the parent(s)' preparedness and give general information on the subject; create an opportunity to give information or your own preferences about the delivery event, which may tap into particular anxieties or fears in the third trimester; assess unrealistic or rigid expectations
How do you plan to feed the baby? (expand to include a diet history during pregnancy, preparation for nursing)	Assess realistic planning for the baby and advise; reaffirm the parent(s)' control of this option; emphasize the importance of nurture in general; offer the opportunity for parents to say how they feel about the situation; assess the pregnant person's nutrition vis-à-vis the infant; assess specific breastfeeding preparations; do not push a decision if the family is not ready
If the infant is male, will you have him circumcised?	Assess individuation of the baby; open this topic for a two-way discussion by providing objective information on circumcision (i.e., the lack of clear medical indications) and the procedure itself
Have you purchased a car seat?	Show interest in safety and caretaking; assess the parents' anticipation of the needs of the infant
How long have you lived in this area? Where do most of your family live? Who will be available to help you after the baby comes?	Assess family support systems; assess the realignment of old relationships; tap into parents' relationship to their own feelings
Do you have other responsibilities outside the family?	Assess other areas of responsibility and stress; what realignment of these areas is anticipated; some areas of ambivalence and concern may be discussed

Continued

TABLE 5.2   Questions to Be Asked at the Prenatal Visit—cont'd

Question	Objective
Do you work outside your home? What are your job plans? Do you have any ideas about the time you will return to work? Are you attending school? Have you made plans for the infant's care?	Assess the psychosocial situation of the family; assess perceptions of the parents' career or education and how that compares to perceptions as parents; assess realistic planning for infant care
Do you have any worries about your infant? Most parents do have some concerns about the child. Would you like to share any of those with me? Is there anything in your past history that makes you think you have some special worries about your child?	Open a discussion of concerns directly, but also use this setting to discuss normalcy of feelings and perhaps deeper concerns; provide information about common fears, fantasies, and dreams during a normal pregnancy
For families with other children: How are your other children reacting to your pregnancy? What have you done to prepare them for the birth? Most parents have some worries about how they will manage to have enough time and love for more than one child. Do you share any of these concerns? What are the specific arrangements you have made for the older child at the time of the baby's birth?	Assess the realignment of family relationships; assess the plans for readjustment around care of the infant; assess feelings toward the children who have already been born
Do you have any questions? Are you worried about or seeking help/resources for anything in particular?	Be open to questions and wait for the parents to take the lead, identifying their specific concerns while setting a model for future pediatric visits

and likelihood of seeing other providers in the office, the well-visit schedule for seeing the infant in the neonatal period and beyond, and some general statements about your own philosophy of pediatric care. This may also be a good opportunity to explore the parents' understanding and/or experiences of positive parenting techniques, recognizing that there may be cultural differences that impact each family's experience.

HEADS UP—THE PRENATAL VISIT

Infant Factors

- Are there any concerns regarding intrauterine growth? If so, investigate the cause, and plan close follow-up
- Are there any prenatally identified medical conditions that might require intervention at the time of birth, or afterwards? Identify needed evaluations, and note potential risks to growth, attachment, and healthy development

Pregnancy Factors

- Has there been a history of infertility, pregnancy loss, or pregnancy complications prior to this pregnancy?
- Are there any factors that increase the risk of pregnancy complications with this pregnancy, including age or caregiver health condition(s)?
- What are the plans or expectations for this pregnancy and delivery?

Family Factors

- Are there specific questions or concerns you have about your ability to care for yourself and your child?
- Are you worried about not having enough money to pay for food, housing, healthcare, and/or anything else that you need to care for yourself and your child?
- Who in your life do you see as a support in caring for yourself and your child? This may include family members, friends, or community members who are part of your "village."
- If you are working, do you have parental leave? Will you have any sources of income or financial assistance during this time?

HEADS UP—THE PRENATAL VISIT

- Is there anything specific on your mind that is making you feel anxious, scared, or sad? Have you ever felt scared for your safety, or worried about your child's safety?

- How would you describe your mental health? What do you do to help feel better?

- Have you experienced depression before?

- Do you have a history of drinking alcohol, smoking, or using other substances, and do you currently use any substances? If so, have you received counseling and/or treatment before?

- Are there other sources of stress you would like to share, so that I can try to find resources that may be helpful?

- Are there other supportive people you would like me to know, so that I can include them in my counseling, education, and invite them to future visits?

Special Referrals

- Call or write a note to the obstetrician regarding special concerns from a pediatric perspective. Get the records of previous pregnancies if they were complicated.

- Clarify your own availability at the time of the birth (e.g., another clinician may provide care for the baby in the hospital in some circumstances).

- Recommend prepared childbirth, breastfeeding, or other parenting classes if these issues have not already been attended to.

- Refer the patient to relevant community resources and/or social service agencies, if the family is desiring and open to receiving supports.

- Make a nutrition referral if indicated by the nutritional history or economic needs.

- Identify mental health professionals who work well with expectant or new parents. Refer as needed.

ANTICIPATORY GUIDANCE

- Encourage open discussion among all available caregivers on the subjects addressed in the interview.
- Advise the parent(s) that the immediate postnatal period can be stressful, and it may be important to seek help (e.g., from friends, a relative, or a health professional) when needed.
- Reassure parents that fears, fantasies, and feelings of loss of control are normal, adaptive, and good indicators of care.
- Emphasize good nutrition and safety planning for the infant, and congratulate the parents on advance planning and responsibility in initiating the interview process.
- Emphasize that it is important to approach the birth with flexibility to allow for unforeseen events (e.g., anesthesia, a cesarean section, or birth complications) that may need to be accommodated.
- Encourage planning for sibling response(s).
- Encourage seeking resources as needed to support child and family health and well-being.

WRAPPING UP

A summary statement about your understanding of the interview's content and process will allow a resolution of differences or highlight areas of omission. For example, "I heard you express concern about breastfeeding. We reviewed a few strategies to support lactation and will make sure to follow up at our next visit to see how things are going. Please think about the circumcision question and let me know what you decide."

Your Record

Make your own assessment of this family's strengths and vulnerabilities.
- Write down the temperamental or style characteristics of the parent(s).
- Take note of any preparations the family has made in anticipation of this child. What additional adjustments and/or supports may be important and helpful?
- Make note of the social support. Who are the members of the family? Who lives in the house?

RECOMMENDED READINGS

American Academy of Pediatrics Committee on Psychosocial Aspects of Child and Family Health The prenatal visit. *Pediatrics.* 2018;1:142.

American Academy of Pediatrics: HealthyChildren.org. https://www.healthychildren.org/English/Pages/default.aspx.

American Academy of Pediatrics. Family pediatrics. *Pediatrics.* 2003;111(6 Suppl).

American Academy of Pediatrics. The prenatal visit. In: Green M, editor. *Bright futures.* 1994. Arlington: National Center for Education in Maternal and Child Health; 2004:13–17.

Cole J. *I'm a big brother.* New York: HarperCollins; 2010.

Fifer WP, Moon CM. The effects of fetal experience with sound. In: Lecaunet JP, ed. *Fetal development: a psychological perspective.* Hillsdale: Lawrence Erlbaum Associates; 1995.

Hagan JF, Shaw JS, Duncan P, eds. *Bright futures: guidelines for health supervision of infants, children and adolescents*. ed 4. Elk Grove Village: American Academy of Pediatrics; 2017.

Mayer M. *The new baby*. New York: Golden Press; 1983.

Rusch E. *Ready, set…baby!*. Boston: Houghton Mifflin Harcourt; 2017.

Stadtler A. Fostering family adjustment prenatally. In: Jellinek M, Patel BP, Froehle MC, eds. *Bright futures in practice: mental health, vol 2, Tool Kit*. Arlington: National Center for Education in Maternal and Child Health; 2002.

www.babycenter.com: Provides information on pregnancy, names, FAQs, newsletters and chats.

Zwelling E. Psychological responses to pregnancy. In: Nichols F, Zwelling E, eds. *Maternal-newborn nursing: theory and practice*. Philadelphia: WB Saunders; 1997.

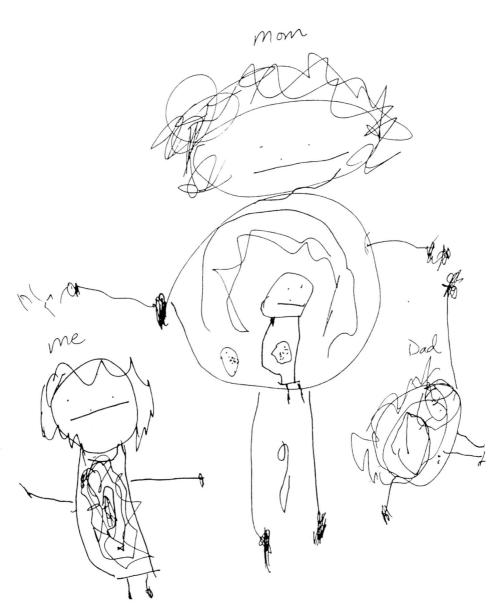

A 4-year-old girl draws her mother's pregnancy, including what she guesses the baby looks like inside her mother's belly. The drawing is notable in that no one is smiling and the Dad is very small.

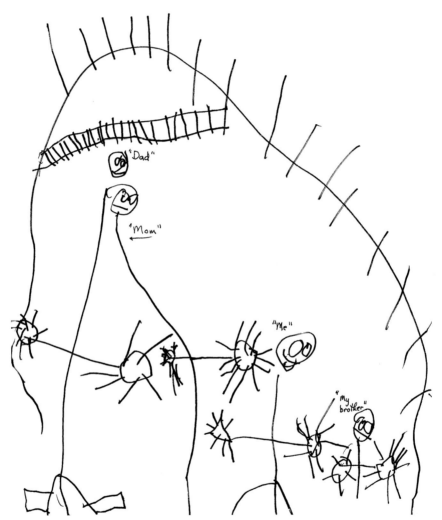

A child of 5 draws his family as he sees it when his mom, 34 weeks pregnant, is put on bed rest. Mom says she is irritable and short with the children. By Kiran Rhodes, age 5.

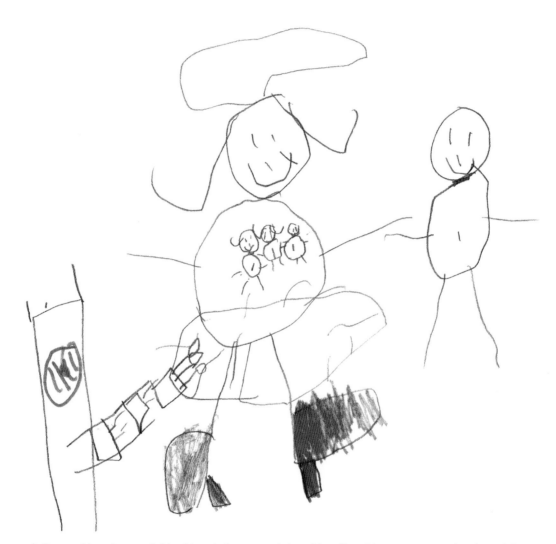

A 6-year-old portrays a bride, his relative, complete with veil and her groom nearby. A wedding cake is off to the side on a table at this reception. Note the presence of triplets still to be born. By M.H.

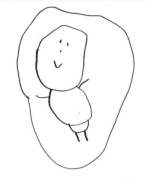

6

The Newborn: Meeting the Infant

Kelsey A. Egan

This chapter describes the neurobehavioral competencies of the newborn, the processes of adaptation to extrauterine life, and the beginnings of the family/child relationship.

KEYWORDS

- Attachment
- Sensory capacities
- Habituation
- Reflex behavior
- State organization

The full and complete examination of the newborn by a clinician usually occurs shortly after birth or within the first few days of life. The earlier the examination, the more opportunity there is to evaluate the active processes of post-birth transition and adaptation. This overlay must be taken into account when you perform your examination, for the infant will change depending on the timing after birth. For example, in the first hour or so of life, a healthy infant is likely to be quite alert and responsive. If you do the examination later in the first day, infants are likely to be a bit sleepy and slow in their responses as they rest and recover from birth. At about 18 hours to 2 to 3 days, newborns are often eager to eat and may seem a bit irritable when you bother them. When the infants are seen for the first time in the office, at about days 3 to 5, their behavior is likely to smooth out. Therefore the timing of your initial acquaintance should be factored into your evaluation and narrated to the parents as they observe you. If you perform both an initial and a follow-up or discharge examination in the hospital, the differences in behavior are important for both you and the family to notice.

Kelsey A. Egan, Original chapter by Suzanne D. Dixon.

The initial newborn examination is an important time to establish a solid relationship with families. It is also a time to reflect on and appreciate the capabilities of your new patient. Enjoy this encounter.

The goal of the newborn physical examination is to assess the neonate's general well-being and to evaluate for any evidence of systemic abnormalities or illness. The full range of infant capacities can be laid out for the family. The infant's behavior can reflect both genetic makeup and intrauterine experience. In addition, the initial visit with the newborn and their family offers the opportunity to participate in and facilitate the initial "getting acquainted" process for the infant and family. Performing the newborn examination with the parents present, with an emphasis on the behavioral component, can assure them and yourself of the infant's wellness but can also explore the unique behavior of the infant. This approach will help the family begin to form solid **attachment** and accommodate to their own child's individuality. In that sense, this visit is both an intervention and an assessment. The clinician enters into the system of the family through the shared evaluation of the infant.

The first step toward attachment and parenting requires assurance that the infant is successfully negotiating the postpartum adjustment. The second step is identifying the specialness of the infant to the family so that they can bond with the person in front of them, the real infant rather than an imagined one.

BEHAVIORAL COMPETENCIES—THE SENSES

Parents commonly have questions about their newborn's **sensory capacities**, which in general are far greater than

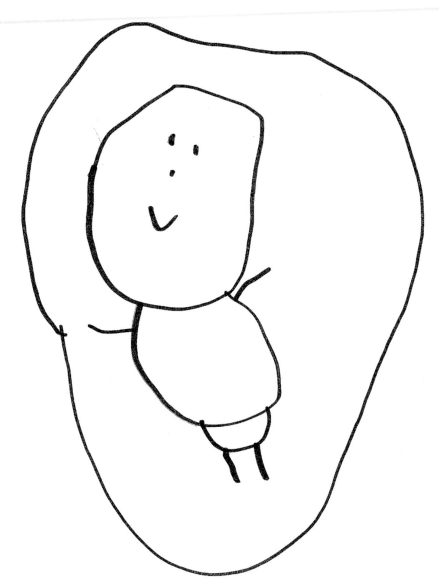

"Baby on a blanket." By Katherine Boucher, age 4 (original in a bright blue marker).

TABLE 6.1   Behavioral Competencies of the Newborn

Behavior	Expected Range of Performance	Concerning Behavior
Vision	Attends to a bright object 8–12 inches away when in an alert state	No alerting to objects
	Follows an object with eyes and perhaps with head through some arc	Very brief or no following
	Follows a face side to side	No blink with approach
	Scans the environment when alert	Dull, flat expression
	Blinks with rapid approach of a hand	
	Hands open and close with visual attention	
Hearing	Brightens to a soft sound or voice	No alerting to sound
	Turns from side to side to source of the sound or voice	No turning, even with eyes (when in a calm state)
State organization	Moves smoothly from sleep to wakefulness	Stays drowsy or irritable
	Calms self when upset	Alternates from drowsy to irritable (i.e., not alert state)
	Can be calmed by the examiner	Cries with minimal disturbance
	Comes to a bright alert state	Does not calm and quiet with calming techniques
Sucking	Roots with cheek touch	Flaccid mouth
	Brings finger into the mouth	Biting
	Coordinated suck	Disorganized suck
	Front-to-back tongue motion	

previously believed (Table 6.1). Sharing information on the infant's current and emerging vision, hearing, and other skills can help families better understand this developmental stage and what is in store as their newborn continues to grow.

Vision

The visual system has all components, peripheral and central, present at term, but substantial maturation occurs after birth, particularly in the first 6 months. Infants can see faces and objects when they are presented at their best focal distance, 8 to 12 inches, although their depth of focus may actually cover a wider range. The neonate is quite nearsighted. At birth, vision may range from about 20/200 to 20/400. Acuity is limited primarily by retinal immaturity and improves rapidly in the first 4 months. Most infants have well-developed conjugate gaze by 4 months of life, but episodic disconjugate gaze is often observed before that. Persistent, fixed limitation of eye movement is always a concern, even in the neonatal period. Full excursion of both eyes horizontally should be seen. Three-dimensional vision improves during the first 6 months through maturation of several processes, so by the time infants are crawling, they can clearly map their world visually in all dimensions. Infants demonstrate preferential attention to visual displays with high contrast, bright colors, and curved lines. Color

detection in newborns is initially very poor, though after a few weeks, infants can likely detect some amount of color, depending on saturation, size, and hue. Cone development proceeds rapidly in the first 2 months, and color detection is much more reliable after 3 to 6 months.

The human face draws much attention from infants. Neonates will preferentially look at their parents' faces, even without sound or smile. The hairline and the moving eyebrows may be the most salient features for the neonate in visually identifying familiar care providers. By about 12 weeks, this capacity is clear, and the face is the most compelling sight to the infant.

The importance of visual input for the infant is illustrated by disruptions in the visual system. An impairment in vision, such as that present with cataracts, may prevent the development of functional vision if it is not corrected early in life. Without binocular input for even short periods, long-lasting impairment may result. Children are particularly vulnerable to alterations in vision even up to 5 years of age. Early detection and remediation are imperative, so it is worth the time to observe the infant as they watch and follow you.

A newborn's visual capacities can be demonstrated at their fullest only when the infant is in a quiet, alert state and all distracting stimuli are minimized, even the child's own motor movements. Visual performance may be limited to brief periods and may be overridden, especially early on, by physiological events (e.g., bowel movements, hiccups). Visual processing is one of the most complex neonatal capacities and may be difficult to demonstrate at all times. It takes time and patience to fully bring out these capacities.

The newborn's higher visual processing and the coordination within the neurological system can be seen by observing the whole face and body when visual stimuli are presented. When attentive, the infant may initially startle slightly and then shut down body movements to focus on the visual display. Facial muscles will lift and the palpebral fissures will widen, thus giving the infant a bright, softened look. Brief periods of attention will cycle with periods of inattention, gaze aversion, and possibly even sleep. Gaze is a capacity under the infant's control from early in life. Maturation and recovery from birth or illness are characterized by increasing duration of these alert periods and the ability to respond to an increasing complexity of visual displays. This recovery of abilities is a very good attribute to demonstrate to families as you examine infants over the first weeks to months. When the same visual display is presented to infants repeatedly, they will show less and less interest in it. This process is called **habituation**. When something they perceive as new comes into their gaze, they will respond to it with renewed interest and scrutiny. This characteristic demonstrates the neonate's innate ability to seek out and preferentially attend to novelty in the world. It is also the reason why infants quiet down and attend visually to mobiles hung over their cribs, high-contrast toys, and some television programs or videos. (While caregivers may appreciate the reprieve from infant crying that TV or videos might provide, it is important to emphasize that infants cannot learn from media under age 18–24 months, and using it as a calming strategy should be avoided. See Chapters 14 and 16.)

Audition

Hearing matures earlier than vision, primarily before birth, although full development continues across the first decade of life. The infant can hear and is responsive to sounds in the second trimester, as described in Chapter 5.

An infant will respond to a pleasant auditory signal, such as a voice or soft rattle, in ways similar to the visual alerting response—an initial alerting startle, brightening of expression, and diminishing of body activity. Infants may turn their eyes and then their heads toward the sound after a short delay and will often search for the source of it. Emotionally expressive speech with higher and varied pitch, short duration, and slower rate (i.e., "baby talk" or "infant-directed speech") produces the most consistent orientation response. Hearing is not only present but is clearly discriminating from birth and even before. Soon after birth, an infant can distinguish between a parent's voice and another's. Soft, low-pitched lullabies and human heart tones produce relaxation in the newborn. Lullabies around the world have similar rhythms that appear soothing to infants. In contrast, infants often cry when another infant cries, as humans seem to be programmed to experience distress when crying is heard.

Infants may fail to respond to an auditory stimulus if it is confounded with other stimuli (e.g., loud ambient noise in the hospital). The infant can shut out these adverse auditory events very successfully and may even appear to have reduced hearing under such conditions. The clinician can be fooled by this inattention. A gentle approach (low background noise, soft sounds, and no competing visual display) may be needed to bring out these auditory capacities.

Although significant hearing differences can be identified behaviorally by the infant's failure to respond to the human voice, there is no way to completely screen behaviorally. Formal hearing screening of all neonates with the use of various technologies is recommended and nearly universal. Primary care pediatricians should be sure of the results of each child under their care before 1 month of age. Equivocal results on screenings demand prompt repeat and/or a full audiological evaluation. Never hesitate to refer a patient for diagnostic audiological evaluation if either you or the infant or child's family has any concerns for hearing, even if neonatal screening was normal. Early detection of a congenital hearing difference or progressive or acquired hearing loss allows for timely referral to interdisciplinary teams which can support a child's access to language for appropriate development, either via visual communication, such as sign languages, or hearing technologies, such as hearing aids or cochlear implants, where clinically indicated.

Some infants will be more responsive to sound than others; visual displays will produce greater behavioral attention with other infants. These individual differences may be noted even in the newborn period and will highlight the special behavioral profile of an individual child.

Taste and Smell

Newborns have a relatively well-developed sense of taste. Their taste buds are greater in number and more widely distributed than those of an adult. Preference for sweetness and aversion to bitterness are present at birth, whereas preference for salt develops at about 4 to 6 months of age, the time that solids are introduced. The infant is preprogrammed to avoid aversive tastes that in nature are largely poisonous and to seek out those that are sweet and nourishing. Complex patterns of taste preference are shaped by exposures in utero and during the first years of life. Although some infants are more sensitive to the varying tastes in breast milk based on maternal diet, it is rare for an infant to alter their nursing pattern because of the presence of a particular taste.

Smell is well developed and well used in newborns. At birth, infants will crawl up to the breast, guided by smell. Infants in the first few days of life can differentiate the smell of their parent from that of others. Parents, in turn, can recognize their own infant's smell within hours of birth, thus suggesting that each infant has a particular odor signature. Associative learning, or linking smells with events, shows the importance of olfaction in learning about the world from early infancy.

TRANSITIONAL BEHAVIOR

The ability to maintain breathing, heart rate, and temperature and to modulate peripheral perfusion improves over the first days of life with varying speed and smoothness. Infants stressed by a difficult labor or postnatal illness generally have more trouble with these physiological transitions. Late preterm infants, born at 34 to 36 weeks, and infants who are large-for-gestational-age with blood glucose irregularities also take longer to get on track. Skin color, skin perfusion, and the response to stress are important to characterize and monitor for continuing improvement. The response to, and recovery from, undressing, handling, reflex assessment, and social interaction give us an indication of the infant's stress tolerance and/or maturity. These vital observations can be made incidentally as part of every examination and provide important information. For example, if on undressing the infant, you observe that the infant turns bright red, moves their arms and legs jerkily, and quickly transitions from a sleeping to crying state, these are signs of low stress tolerance. You can narrate these observations to caregivers sensitively—so as not to lead to a perception that something is "wrong" with their child—but in a manner that helps them understand what the infant is feeling, for example, "Do you see the skin turning bright red like this and these motor movements? They show me that (infant name) is feeling stressed. It is hard to be woken up and undressed. But you can use it as a clue that their nervous system feels overloaded, so let's talk about ways to soothe them."

It is important to know that infants still grappling with organization at this basic physiological level will not be as available for auditory and visual alerting tasks because these processes are organized on a hierarchical level. When these physiological responses show greater stability, the infant will be able to more readily listen and track visually. Feeding difficulties may occur in infants who are less mature or show evidence of stress at this level of organization.

STATE BEHAVIOR

Full-term infants exist in at least six states of consciousness (Table 6.2). These states of consciousness consist of quiet sleep, active sleep, drowsiness, an alert state, an irritable

TABLE 6.2   States of Consciousness in the Newborn

State	Activity	Muscle Tone	Heart Rate	Respirations
Quiet sleep	Eyes closed, no eye movements, still with occasional startles	Steady, tonic	Regular	Regular
Active sleep	Eyes closed with globe movements Random, low-level facial movements; wiggles	Low	Variable	Irregular
Drowsy	Flat face; eyes may be open or closed Writhing movements, variable	Low, variable	Variable	Variable
Alert	Face bright Eyes open, tracking Motor movement mostly absent	Steady	First a rise, then lower than baseline	Regular
Irritable	Negative face, avoidance maneuvers, squirmy, brief whimpers, or fussy vocalizations	Slightly increased	Variable	Irregular
Crying	Crying, motor activity at high level	Increased	Slightly elevated	Irregular, with crying

Modified from Prechtl HFR: The neurological examination of the full term newborn infant. In *Clinics in developmental medicine*, vol 63, London, 1975, MacKeith Press; Brazelton TB, Nugent JK: Neonatal Behavioral Assessment Scale. In *Clinics in developmental medicine*, vol 137, London, 1995, MacKeith Press.

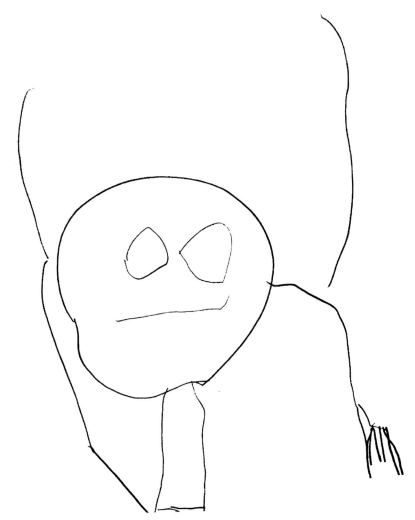

"A baby." By Heather R., age 3½.

state, and a crying state. They move through these states in cycles with some regularity. Responsiveness to some outside stimuli, motor tone, physiological processes (e.g., heart rate, breathing), and even **reflex behavior** based on motor tone vary with these variations in state. The infant's state needs to be taken into account during any examination. Clear characterization of each state and regular movement from one state to another testify to neurological competency and maturity. Noises, lights, and even painful stimuli will be ignored with successive presentation. This process is one of **habituation**, as described earlier. Infants appear to protect themselves from overwhelming or boringly repetitive noise and light stimuli through a process of selective inattention.

Many infants will show progressive gains in state stabilization in the early days after delivery. However, some infants will remain somewhat irregular and unpredictable as part of their individual temperament profile and their recovery after birth. Infants older than 3 days (and very sleepy ones before that) may benefit from a little help in establishing a regular wake-sleep cycle through the care of a regular caregiver responding to the subtle cues of early wakefulness, wiggles, and brief eye openings. Feedings geared to the infant's own shift in states are usually more successful than those attempted after a crying bout, as crying is a late sign of hunger. Regular feedings, variations in illumination and sound, and close body contact with another human being all work toward stabilization of **state organization**. In contrast, constant illumination, continuous noise, and irregular responses to restlessness, crying, and distress will make it more difficult for the infant to get organized with sleep, feeding, and alertness.

REFLEXES AND BEYOND

Newborn reflexes (Table 6.3) are indicators of general neurological integrity, and each has its own developmental course. These reflexes are based on muscle tone, which in a typical infant varies with the state of consciousness. Therefore in addition to noting the presence, absence, or asymmetry of these reflexes, the clinician should assess active and passive tone within the context of several states, including sleep and wakefulness (Table 6.4). Relative hypotonia and hypertonia are each appropriate in different states of consciousness, but the lack of variability through several states is worrisome. For example, palmar grasp should be sluggish in active sleep when tone is diminished, but brisk in a cry state when tone is increased. Abnormalities in tone may be due to transient abnormalities such as hypoglycemia or may occur as part of other conditions, such as trisomy 21. They may also

TABLE 6.3   Neonatal Reflexes

Reflex	Description
Moro	Arms and neck extend out and then arms pull back in, may look startled and cry
Trunk incurvation	In ventral suspension, trunk flexes toward the side stroked
Stepping (i.e., walking)	When held upright with feet touching a firm surface, infant appears to take steps
Tonic neck reflex (fencer's posture)	Arm extends when the head is placed to that side, contralateral arm flexes
Palmar grasp	Fingers flex when an object is placed in the palm
Rooting	Head and mouth turn to the side where the cheek is stroked
Crawling	When in the prone position with pressure on the feet, the infant pushes forward

be a sign of immaturity or an indicator of an underlying neurological condition. The observation of tone relative to the infant's other conditions, relative to their maturity, and in the context of state of consciousness, is central to the neonatal evaluation. Persistent hypertonia or hypotonia are signs that should prompt close monitoring and may require further evaluation.

All in all, the infant's perceptual and behavioral repertoire is geared toward initiating and maintaining positive interactions with the world. All of these capacities enable the infant to reach out, to become active in eliciting responsive care.

IMPACT OF THE BIRTH EXPERIENCE

The impact of perinatal events on development of the family unit is profound. Labor that is attended by supportive people tends to be shorter and less fraught with complications, and the support provided by doulas during labor has been shown to improve the experience of labor and birth outcomes. Birth is the beginning of a relationship, and as in any human relationship, it is as variable as the people involved. Sensitivity to the feelings of parents, both positive and negative, will allow the infant's clinician to support this "getting acquainted" period as it proceeds in its own individual way.

Infants belong with their parents in all circumstances except for critical illness in the infant or parent, and even

TABLE 6.4 **Motor System**		
Motor System	**Expected in Term Infants**	**Concerning**
Passive motor tone	Forced movement of arms and legs should be balanced. Return to flexion when released.	Asymmetry Flaccidity Tremulousness or jitteriness on release
Active tone	Flexion of all extremities.	Extension or flaccidity
Pull to sit	Minimal head lag behind the axis of the trunk as the examiner pulls the newborn's hands up from laying to sitting.	Significant head lag or head continues to lag after the sitting position is reached
Scarf sign	Infant's hand and arm pulled across the chest, elbow coming to the midline or less.	Elbow crosses the midline.
Suspended prone position	Infant's trunk held prone over the examiner's hand. Some straightening of the trunk, flexed limbs, and head lift.	Infant drapes over the hand with limbs dangling in extension, drooped head

then, physical contact should occur as soon and for as much time as possible. Advantages of contact include improved breastfeeding, more positive attachment, and less distress in the infant. Close physical contact enhances physiological stability.

Cesarean section, especially if it is unanticipated, may result in feelings of failure and unmet expectations on the part of parents. In addition, infants delivered by cesarean section may be drowsy and slower to feed. Birthing parents may feel more pain from the incision and have a more prolonged recovery course, and infants delivered by cesarean section often require more time and patience getting themselves behaviorally organized in the immediate newborn period.

Medications administered during labor and delivery, such as magnesium sulfate, general anesthesia, and opioids, can have an effect on the alertness and behavior of the infant and/or birthing parent. Breastfeeding may take a little more time to get started. The clinician should note the behavioral changes related to the delivery events. This sets the stage for monitoring the expected recovery process with the family in the hours and days ahead.

Newborns exposed to certain medications or substances in utero, including selective serotonin reuptake inhibitors or opioids, typically have a predictable period of withdrawal after birth that influences their behavior and reaction to stimuli. Clinicians should understand and anticipate this withdrawal and communicate with families about the expected course. The characteristics and recommended approach to neonatal opioid withdrawal syndrome are described further in Box 6.1.

THE NEWBORN EXAMINATION

What to Observe

The infant's examination in the hospital should, with rare exception, occur at the bedside with the caregivers present. This is an intervention as well as an assessment. You should narrate your observations as part of the ongoing interaction with the family. You are there to assess the infant's neurobehavioral development and individuality. Some of the details to note include the following:

- Caregiver fatigue, stress, or illness—is the birthing parent recovering from the delivery as expected? Is there untreated pain or a postpartum complication? Is a caregiver asleep or out of the room and would a different time for the examination be best for the family?
- The parents' impression and handling of the infant—this is determined by both the caretaker and the infant. Is this infant treated very tentatively or very vigorously? What do they say and do with the infant? What are their descriptions of the infant? What questions do they have for you?
- Your own responses to the infant—pay attention to your reaction to the infant throughout the examination. Do you feel concerned? Engaged? Something else? If you are feeling irritable or annoyed at a fussing infant, check in with your own state regulation. Examining your response may help you understand both the infant's state and your own role in the interactive encounter. If you are agitated from a stressful day, take some time to self-regulate when you are able to.

BOX 6.1   Neonatal Opioid Withdrawal Syndrome

The prevalence of opioid use by pregnant people has increased in the United States over the past two decades, corresponding to an increased number of newborns exposed to opioids in utero. While some pregnant people engage in illicit opioid use or misuse prescription medications, it is important to recognize that many are prescribed opioids, including methadone or buprenorphine, as the standard of care and best practice treatment for opioid use disorder in pregnancy.

Infants exposed to opioids in utero may display signs and symptoms of withdrawal after birth, now referred to as neonatal opioid withdrawal syndrome (NOWS), previously also referred to as neonatal abstinence syndrome. The timing and presentation of NOWS may vary according to opioid exposure history, metabolism (of parent and infant), and exposure to additional substances. Infants who were exposed to opioids in utero should be monitored for symptoms for at least 72 hours after delivery, longer if exposed to long-acting opioids.

NOWS signs commonly include irritability, tremors, difficulty sleeping, difficulty feeding, vomiting, diarrhea, sweating, and other signs of stress. Hospitals use different tools to monitor symptoms, including the Eat, Sleep, Console measure. Parents may feel worried, guilty, and unsure how to best support their infant during this time. Early education and continued support by clinicians and hospital staff are important for both parent and child well-being and should emphasize that NOWS is expected and treatable.

Nonpharmacologic treatment is considered the first-line approach to NOWS and includes rooming in with the birthing parent, skin-to-skin time, swaddling, and keeping the room quiet and dimly lit. Breastfeeding should be encouraged and supported, if not contraindicated for other reasons, and has been shown to decrease signs of withdrawal. Infants who continue to display signs after these approaches may require pharmacological treatment, most commonly with an oral opioid such as morphine or methadone.

Of note, many states require that all infants with prenatal substance exposure be reported to Child Protective Services (CPS), regardless of the parents' recovery status or engagement with clinical care. These policies can increase stigma and foster mistrust between families and the healthcare system. Clinicians should be familiar with state and federal requirements and should advocate for practices that center families and decrease unnecessary referrals to CPS.

- Nurse and staff observations—discuss with nurses and staff or check for documentation regarding sleep and crying, heart rate and breathing regularity, response to procedures (e.g., bath, neonatal screening tests), and any challenges faced by parents. These observations are critical for discharge planning with a family.

What to Assess

Begin assessment of the infant at the bedside, lights dim. Narrate your findings to the parents, and keep the following in mind:

- Conduct a general examination, ordering it from the least intrusive (e.g., observation of color and breathing) to the most intrusive (e.g., the Moro reflex) maneuvers. Observe the infant's color change, breathing, and awakening as you do your assessment, starting with uncovering and undressing.
- Interrupt what you are doing if the infant becomes alert. When the infant is alert, present an object such as a ball, stethoscope, or another toy at their focal distance, 8 to 12 inches. Move the object slowly along an arc in one direction, and then the other, to assess the infant's tracking and visual processing. The infant should stop moving and their face should brighten as their eyes and perhaps their head shift.
- Repeat the visual assessment using your face and then using your face and voice together. The combined stimulus is more compelling than the single one for term infants; stressed and immature infants may find the combined stimulus too complex and therefore aversive. The infant will show you that you have exceeded their limit by looking away, turning away, or becoming irritable. You and the parents will have learned the infant's limits and signaling system, and you can describe this to them.
- Hold the infant securely above eye level, swaddled as needed, and talk softly to them. Wait for the response. An alert look, turning the eyes toward you, and then turning the head toward you are the expected responses, if given time and a positive auditory cue.
- Repeat this process with parents on the other side. If the infant is in a regulated state, the infant may turn to the parents' voice instead of yours. If this occurs, point out the infant's recognition of them.
- Note the infant's irritability, changes in motor tone with state of consciousness, and the amount of tremulousness

and startles. Such assessment gives you an idea of the infant's maturity, neurological integrity, and physiological stability. This first assessment provides a basis of comparison for subsequent assessment and thus allows you to monitor the infant's recovery. Physiologically ill infants will be less available socially than those who are more organized at that level.

- A full neurological examination with careful assessments of active and passive tone and the presence, character, and vigor of the reflexes should be performed. This examination is a stressor; watch how the infant copes with it, signals distress, and recovers from the distressing maneuver.
- During periods of crying (e.g., after testing for the Moro reflex), carefully observe and assess the infant's self-quieting maneuvers and the amount of effort needed by the examiner to quiet the infant. This level of need will be replicated at home. Some infants need more help to settle down than others do. These infants can be described as "feisty or strong minded." Less perturbable infants can be described as "calm."
- The infant stepping reflex is powerful in showing the parents how much a person the infant is.
- After asking permission from the parents, put a gloved finger in the infant's mouth to assess oral-motor organization. An infant who is poorly coordinated, bites, or puts their tongue up may need extra help with feeding.
- Cuddle the infant in the crook of the arm and at the shoulder. Hypotonic infants will feel as though they are falling through; hypertonic infants will push out straight and will not curl into your arm.

HOSPITAL DISCHARGE DECISIONS AND PLANS

The timing of hospital discharge after delivery has to take into account both infant and parental well-being. Birthing parents must be sufficiently recovered to take independent care of themselves and the infant.

The infant must be stable and have negotiated the postnatal physiological and behavioral transitions. The infant must be able to signal needs, have those signals understood by care providers, and be able to feed well, which means that an experienced professional has seen the infant feed successfully and that parents also feel comfortable with the feeding. The infant should awaken to feed, and elimination should be proceeding normally. The infant should be responsive to interactions with the environment as an index of neurological intactness.

All discharge teaching should be conducted in the family's preferred language, using trained interpreters when needed. Parents should be instructed in routine care such as safe sleep, signs of illness, and car seat use. Families should have an appropriate-sized car seat and a crib or bassinet for the infant to sleep in before leaving the hospital. Families should have a rectal thermometer and be instructed to call their pediatrician for any fever. Criteria and provisions for emergency care should be explicitly laid out, including assurance of transportation.

The hospital care team should ensure families have the appropriate resources and living space to care for a newborn. Unmet social needs, including lack of access to safe and stable housing, food, and transportation, should be assessed and addressed during the newborn hospitalization. Assistance should be provided to families without safe and stable housing, which might include accessing an emergency shelter. If a family is experiencing food insecurity, information on local resources such as food pantries as well as eligibility and enrollment in government programs such as the Special Supplemental Nutrition Program for Women, Infants, and Children (WIC) and the Supplemental Nutrition Assistance Program (SNAP) should be discussed. A referral to WIC should be provided if the family qualifies, as this program provides breastfeeding support, formula, nutritious foods, and nutrition education to infants, young children, and pregnant and postpartum parents. Access to transportation for well-child appointments should be discussed and addressed.

Breastfeeding can be both rewarding and challenging for families. For breastfeeding parents, it is important to provide anticipatory guidance and resources for support after discharge, as this can be a particularly difficult time with many new responsibilities. Parents should be offered information on support groups and information on accessing lactation specialists to support their feeding goals.

Clinicians should discuss with birthing parents the risk of postpartum depression, which is higher for those with a history of depression or anxiety and/or a lack of social support. If there are any concerns for depression or anxiety during the hospitalization, the parent should be evaluated and offered the appropriate resources, including connection to a therapist and medication.

A follow-up plan should be solidly in place. A checkup within the first 3 to 5 days of life, or within 48 to 72 hours after discharge from the hospital, should be routine, perhaps coordinated with a home health visit. Problems, including breastfeeding difficulties, jaundice, and poor weight gain, may emerge and should be addressed as early as possible.

! HEADS UP—THE NEWBORN

- Infants who are preterm, late preterm, or small for gestational age are at higher risk for developmental difficulties. Close developmental tracking should be planned.
- Infants with small head circumferences need evaluation for infectious and/or toxic or structural causes. Developmental surveillance should occur at well-child visits.
- Infants with low tone and/or poor sucking are at risk for poor feeding and need more careful observation.
- Any infant with unilateral weakness of an arm or leg should be promptly evaluated for potential neurologic pathology or infection.
- Particularly irritable infants should be evaluated for the cause of their irritability, as well as extra support at home for the care provider.
- Infants who alert poorly and are marginally responsive to care need close monitoring. These infants may have a neurological, metabolic, or infectious condition.

QUICK CHECK—THE NEWBORN

- Balanced motor tone, variable across states
- Reflexes intact and symmetrical
- Turns to sound
- Follows object visually at least briefly
- Conjugate eye movements
- Mottling not excessive and shows good recovery
- Coordinated rooting and sucking
- Able to organize and sustain feedings
- Signals hunger regularly
- Weight loss of less than 10%
- Parents demonstrate the ability to feed and care for the infant

SUMMARY

The initial newborn examination is an opportunity to introduce the parents to the infant's current development and to discuss the milestones that are to come as they begin the work of caring for and connecting to the infant. It is a time to introduce the real, individual infant to the family by showing the infant's unique characteristics and abilities. Unmet expectations for the delivery or for the infant or any concerns should be discussed with families. The infant's temperament and individuality should begin to be understood in the context of the assessment, both by the clinician and parents. Finally, plans for ongoing care should be set up based on an understanding of all the individuals involved.

RECOMMENDED READINGS

Buz Harlor Allen D, Bower Charles, Committee on Practice and Ambulatory Medicine Section on Otolaryngology–Head and Neck Surgery Hearing assessment in infants and children: recommendations beyond neonatal screening. *Pediatrics.* 2009;124(4):1252–1263. https://doi.org/10.1542/peds.2009-1997.

Campbell D, American Academy of Pediatrics *Neonatology for primary care.* Itasca: American Academy of Pediatrics; 2020.

Brazelton TB. *Development of newborn behavior. Postnatal growth neurobiology.* Boston: Springer US; 1986:519–540.

HealthyChildren.Org from the American Academy of Pediatrics: *Neonatal opioid withdrawal syndrome (NOWS): what families need to know.* Available from: https://www.healthychildren.org/English/ages-stages/prenatal/Pages/Neonatal-Opioid-Withdrawal-Syndrome.aspx. Accessed July 30, 2023.

Wachman EM, Schiff DM, Silverstein M. Neonatal abstinence syndrome: advances in diagnosis and treatment. *JAMA.* 2018;319(13):1362–1374.

Patrick SW, Barfield WD, Poindexter BB. et al Neonatal opioid withdrawal syndrome. *Pediatrics.* 2020;146(5): https://doi.org/10.1542/peds.2020-029074. e2020029074.

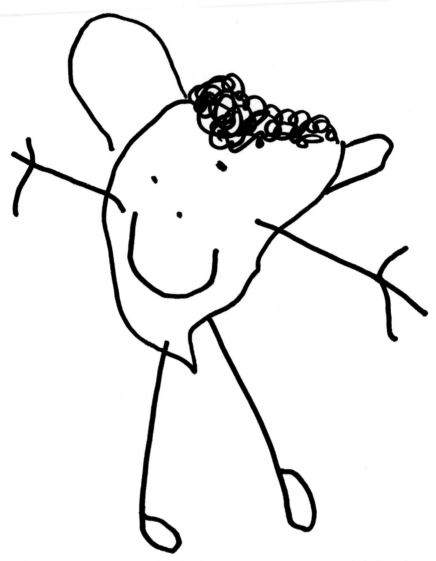

A 3-year-old draws her new little brother with prominent ears, curly hair, and out-stretched arms (original in pink marker).

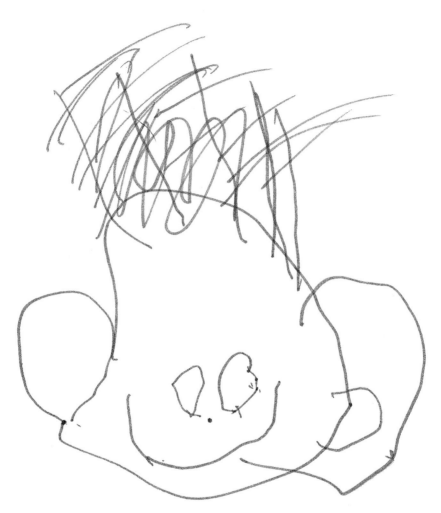

A 3-year-old draws herself. She takes in the world around her with eyes and ears attuned to her social environment. By Robin A.

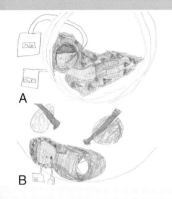

7

A

B

Neonatal Intensive Care Units: Special Issues for Medically Vulnerable Infants

Erika Gabriela Cordova Ramos

This chapter presents the special needs and concerns of the high-risk infant and family. The concept of developmental care of the premature infant is explained. The role of the pediatric clinician while the infant is in the neonatal intensive care unit (NICU) and after discharge is outlined.

KEYWORDS

- Preterm infant's behavior
- Developmental course of preemies
- Developmental care in the NICU
- Discharge planning
- Special care parenting
- Grief reactions
- NICU environment
- Multiple births
- Vulnerable child syndrome
- Kangaroo care

NEONATAL INTENSIVE CARE

The advent in the 1940s of intensive care for ill or high-risk infants began an era of dramatic change for the neonate, the family, and the healthcare provider. With increasing technological advances, we have pushed back the limits of viability, improved the chance of survival, and increased the incidence of multiple births. Families are exposed to the NICU environment for longer periods during the increasingly complex care of babies who are younger and smaller. In the course of this progress, we have learned a great deal about the neurological development of premature children,

the behavior and developmental course of preterm infants, and the impact of intensive care itself on infant physiology and family coping. We have also learned how structural racism shapes longstanding discriminatory practices that result in deprived neighborhoods, economic and educational inequalities, and differential access to healthcare, that is, the social determinants of health (SDOH). These SDOH are key drivers of disparities in premature births and health and developmental outcomes. Therefore this chapter will focus on the family as the ultimate intervention in support of high-risk infants so that nurturing the family's strengths and competencies becomes part of the care mission both before and after discharge. Lastly, for high-risk infants and families to fully benefit of the advances in neonatal care, we must all take responsibility for addressing the SDOH that influence their long-term health and well-being.

IN THE NEONATAL INTENSIVE CARE UNIT

Impact of the Neonatal Intensive Care Unit Environment on Infant Development

The NICU environment provides both sensory overload and deprivation. From the infant's perspective, the NICU is so different from the intrauterine environment that it in itself provides a source of additional stress. Data suggest associations between that environment and acute physiological fluctuations. These fluctuations, in turn, appear to alter important clinical and central nervous system parameters, including intracranial pressure changes, cerebral

---

Original chapter authors: Suzanne D. Dixon and Yvonne E. Vaucher.

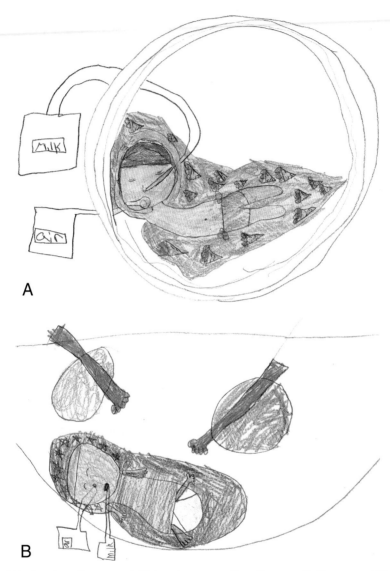

Nine-year-old twins draw the neonatal intensive care unit as they see it. They were 32-week pree-mies themselves. Mom is now a neonatal nurse practitioner. (A) "Sick baby. Milk and air keep her alive." By Ainsley Perkins. (B) "Baby with problems with her heart (like her sister)." Dad's arms are in the isolette. By Alissa Perkins.

autoregulation, brain oxygenation, hypoxemia, apnea, and bradycardia. Investigators have examined the sensory characteristics of NICUs along with infant behavioral and physiological responses to the caretaking activities in this environment. These studies found that infants experience a bombardment of stimuli from the sheer numbers of different caregivers and procedures each day. At the same time, however, very little social contact and long intervals of social isolation may also be present. From the infant's view, this may be experienced as a chaotic, nonresponsive milieu. Constant bright lights, noise, lack of diurnal variation in movement, light and sound, frequent painful procedures, and abrupt changes in position with handling are stressful factors present in the NICU that were not part of intrauterine life. Clinical practice guidelines for the individualized developmental care of infants in the NICU were established in 2007. These guidelines provide guidance on how to assess and when/how to intervene, specify the maximum intensity of sound (not to exceed 50 dB), and provide specific criteria for light levels (cycling, avoiding direct light).

Developmentally Supportive Care

Family-centered care, modifying caregiving, and reducing environmental stimuli can counter some of these aversive factors. Procedures and examinations should be scheduled so that quiet sleep times are uninterrupted, thereby improving behavioral organization and growth. Diurnal variation in lighting helps entrain a circadian rhythm, and noise reduction serves to minimize physiological stress for the immature infant. Gentle, gradual movements, soothing and holding after procedures, and providing physical boundaries to contain the infant also help improve organization. Some activities that support this process are shown in Box 7.1.

Developmentally responsive care of neonates is best carried out when the bedside nurse becomes familiar with each baby's behavioral and physiological cues and is able to arrange the baby's day for optimal well-being and interaction. As parents become increasingly active in the infant's care, nurses can help them learn to read the infant's cues and build confidence in responding to different arousal states (such as sleepy, irritable, or calm and alert). Before discharge, developmentally supportive care improves feeding and growth, decreases medical support, shortens hospital stay, facilitates maturation of motor function and state regulation, improves caregiver perception of both their own and their infant's competence, and reduces caregiver stress. In the longer term, developmental care improves neurodevelopmental outcomes up to 24 months' corrected age and decreases the likelihood of behavior problems at 5 years of age. Whether

> ### BOX 7.1 Components of an Individualized Care Plan for Infants in the Neonatal Intensive Care Unit or Special Care Nursery
>
> - Baby-specific care plans posted on each bedside, including scheduling issues, behavioral cues, likes and dislikes, stressors, and facilitators.
> - The baby's specific nonverbal vocabulary—how does the baby signal positive or negative responses?
> - Isolette covers to allow quiet, undisturbed rest.
> - Protected times for rest—posted and enforced.
> - Nesting within an isolette and the use of cloth rolls or slings to provide tactile input or containment.
> - Tapes of soft music or parental voices played *periodically* in the isolette.
> - Personalized isolette with pictures or small toys.
> - Family visiting plans stated and posted. Nurses may want to "save" feeding, bathing, and treatments for these times if possible.
> - The name of the two or three nurses who serve as primary nurses and know the family and the baby best.
> - The baby's given name clearly posted and used in the record and in conversations.
> - The baby's own clothes and blanket if the infant is stable.

developmentally supportive care improves longer term cognitive outcome is uncertain at this time, but it seems that the weight of evidence supports this type of care for the individual child.

Baby Body Language

The infant uses body language to signal both positive and negative responses to various life experiences. Even a short period of observation during rounds, treatment sessions or examinations will demonstrate many of these signs, which are listed in Boxes 7.2 and 7.3.

The behavior of a premature infant can be confusing to even an experienced caregiver. Facial expressions have a limited range, body movements may be few, and cries might be nonexistent or irritating. The latency of responses may be so long that it is difficult to connect one activity with the response. Social interactions that are perceived as exciting by a full-term infant may cause a premature infant to turn away, become mottled or red, hiccup, or even stop breathing—signs that the autonomic nervous system is temporarily dysregulated.

BOX 7.2   Behavior That Says "YES"

The following behavior signals that the baby can handle, enjoy, and gain from the current interaction with the environment:

- A relaxed posture, neither hypertonic nor limp.
- Easily flexed hands and feet.
- Grasping movements with the hands and feet opening and closing rhythmically.
- Mouthing and sucking movements when looking or listening.
- Eyes widening, face lifting, lips making an oval.
- Short, quiet vowel sounds—cooing.
- Attending to visual or auditory stimuli—looking or listening carefully.
- Decreasing body movements, wiggles, and quiet attend.
- Turning toward the phenomenon, even with long latency.
- Improved color—no mottling, duskiness, or pallor over baseline.

The caretaker should continue monitoring for signs of distress or overload.

BOX 7.3   Behavior That Says "Stop, Please"

The following behavior often signals that the interaction with the environment is overwhelming, adversive, or overly costly for the infant's coping abilities:

- Extension postures—arms out, legs straightened, neck stretched
- Arching back
- Gaze avoidance
- Turning away
- Splayed hands and feet
- Grimace, lip retraction
- Furrowed brow, a worried look
- Spitting up, gagging, onset of hiccups
- Sudden limpness
- Increasing pallor, mottling, cyanosis
- Irregular breathing, apnea

The caretaker should respond by backing off, by cutting down some aspects or intensity of the interaction and by supporting and waiting for recovery.

The baby may actively avoid eye contact, thus sending a negative message to those who would like to interact. At other times, an unremittingly irritable infant seems to resist all the usual consoling and comforting measures.

Without additional knowledge and techniques to make sense of a premature infant's behavior, caregivers may feel ineffective, frustrated, angry, perplexed, and rejected. Conversely, if the healthcare team can interpret some of the confusing messages and help a family develop effective caregiving patterns, parenting competency and confidence will be enhanced.

What is experienced as aversive stimuli will vary from infant to infant and will change as the infant matures. Aversive stimuli tend to be those that are physiologically overwhelming or involve high levels of sensory input, such as bright lights, noise, pain, rapid movements, and multiple, simultaneous inputs (e.g., movement of the infant while speech is directed at them). In addition, aversive responses emerge with rapid changes in input, even if the level of input is low. *Transitions* between one routine activity (e.g., feeding) and another (e.g., checking vital signs) may produce considerable disruptions. Even the transitions to sleep or to wakefulness may be prolonged and accompanied by much physiological instability. Times of change in activity are vulnerable periods; aversive behavior is likely to emerge at these times. To avoid instability in behavior, support for the infant *through* and immediately after the activity is needed.

Skin-to-Skin (Kangaroo) Care and the Impact of Touch

The positive role of human touch on a preterm infant is illustrated by the demonstrated benefits of skin-to-skin (kangaroo care) for an immature infant. The infant is placed in an upright, prone position on the bare chest of the caregiver and covered on the dorsal surface by a blanket. This kind of care has no minimum weight requirement and can have a very positive impact on care and outcomes. It can also be used for infants on ventilators. Many physiological and psychosocial benefits have been linked to skin-to-skin care and are shown in Box 7.4. Caregivers who can participate in this intimate care of their infant get a real sense of their own value and importance to the child. The neonatal healthcare provider can assist in this process by reinforcing the benefits of skin-to-skin care for the family and by encouraging the NICU staff to provide it when appropriate.

Breastfeeding and giving expressed breast milk reinforce the benefits of skin-to-skin care as described in Box 7.5.

Skin-to-skin care may be the single most effective developmental intervention in the NICU. Preterm-born infants exhibit lower basal stress levels (i.e., autonomic responses) during skin-to-skin care, as well as lower stress reactivity when exposed to physical stress (i.e., autonomic

BOX 7.4   Benefits of Kangaroo Care

- Decreased apnea
- Decreased bradycardia
- Less irritability
- Improved oxygenation
- Improved weight gain
- Improved temperature stability
- Improved breastfeeding
- Improved sleep cycles
- Faster autonomic maturation
- Lower basal stress levels (i.e., autonomic responses)
- Lower stress reactivity when exposed to physical stress (i.e., better state regulation)
- Improved white matter microstructural development
- More positive caregiver interaction
- Improved caregiver's mood, reduced caregiver stress, increased caregiver attachment behavior

BOX 7.5   Supporting Breastfeeding in the Neonatal Intensive Care Unit

Breastfeeding and giving expressed breast milk increase caregivers' self-esteem and confidence, the frequency of nurturing touch, and awareness of infant behavioral cues. Additionally, it provides contingent stimuli by integrating caregiver touch, en face contact, sucking, and satiation. Breastfeeding or provision of expressed breast milk is associated with a better long-term cognitive outcome in both preterm and term infants. In turn, skin-to-skin care increases the duration and exclusivity of breastfeeding. Evidence-based practices to promote breastfeeding/breast milk provision in the neonatal intensive care unit setting include:

1. Education of staff and families on the benefits of breast milk as well as training in assisting mothers with hand expression, pumping, and assessment of latch.
2. Early initiation of hand expression and/or breast pumping (<6 hours after and ideally <1 hour after delivery).
3. Frequent pumping (at least six times/day).
4. Provision of hospital-grade double electric breast pumps to mothers.
5. Skin-to-skin contact as well as pumping after skin-to-skin contact.
6. Maternal galactologue use.
   Additional practices that have been shown to reduce racial/ethnic breastfeeding disparities include peer counseling programs, assistance with breast pump acquisition, transportation, and support groups.

regulation). In addition, skin-to-skin care has a positive effect on parenting behaviors and interactions, including improved attachment behavior, affect, touch, and adaptation to infant cues, as well as lower parental stress and depression. Other sources of human touch include gentle massage by caregivers and cobedding multiples and avoiding prolonged isolation in an incubator while "feeding and growing." On the other hand, human touch in the NICU can also result in infant pain, which has been shown to result in structural changes in the brain and has a deleterious effect on long-term responses to stress and behavior. Sick preterm infants are exposed to an average of 14 painful procedures every day while acutely ill. Therefore it is important to minimize painful stimuli as much as possible and to provide physical and sensory support to reduce the physiological reactions to pain. Breastfeeding, being given expressed breast milk and skin-to-skin care, as well as sucking on a pacifier or oral sucrose, are all effective ways to reduce the distress associated with painful procedures. Specific pain medications should be used, and infants should be held and comforted whenever possible during and after all painful events.

Supporting Parents in the Neonatal Intensive Care Unit

The NICU or special care nursery may add to parents' stress by overtly or inadvertently giving the message that the parents are not capable of caring for their baby or that something they did caused the baby's difficulties. It is important not to inadvertently convey that "experts" such as nurses, therapists, and physicians must take over because the parents "have failed." After premature delivery, mothers have expressed feeling this sense of failure especially acutely, believing that their own bodies have failed to protect their fetuses from premature delivery or other adversity. This may reduce caregiver confidence and activation to engage in infant care, learn new skills, or make decisions. Even in the best of circumstances, the NICU environment itself exacerbates these feelings. This does not imply that nurses or physicians are insensitive to parents' needs; rather, the high-tech and overwhelming care requirements for sick and premature infants give these unspoken messages to families. It takes a lot of work to move away from these feelings. In addition, nurses must attach to the infants they care for if they are to give the best of care, and such attachment may lead to unconscious competitiveness with parents. As a result, parents, especially mothers, may feel both emotionally and physically inadequate, even if nothing specific is said or done to prompt such feelings.

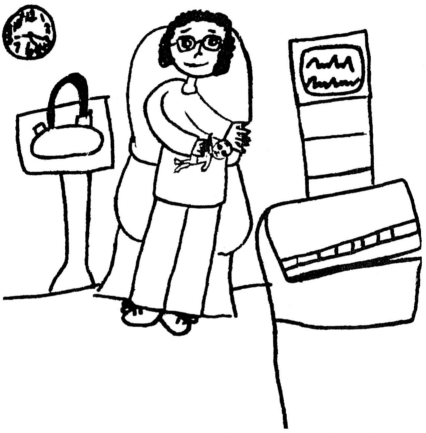

A nurse takes care of a small premature infant amid the machines, sink, and other equipment in the neonatal intensive care unit. By Carly Riehl, age 10.

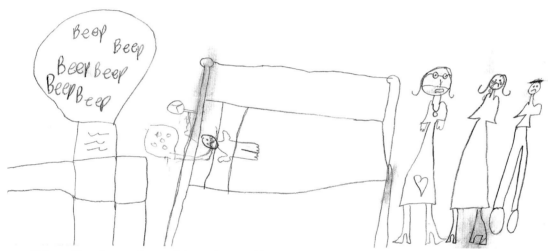

"Mom (the doctor dressed in a dress with a heart) talking to sad parents of a sick baby."
By Katie R., age 7.

The lack of opportunity to be alone with their child or to engage in any sort of caretaking without the surveillance of the nursing staff adds stress for parents. How frequently parents are able to visit, hold infants in arms, and provide skin-to-skin care in the NICU is impacted by family social factors. Most families, and particularly low-income families, experience direct and indirect financial and time costs associated with the care of their infants. Spending days to weeks to perhaps months in the NICU requires extraordinary adaptive skills at a time when parents are least able to muster these resources. Sparse visits, lack of telephone calls, lack of initiative, and angry accusations are more often maladaptive responses to these circumstances and competing demands at home rather than a measure of detachment from the infant or a lack of appreciation of the expert care. The clinician and NICU staff can help interpret such behavior correctly to one another and must demonstrate considerable empathy with families by granting the family latitude and time to recover. The NICU staff must also acknowledge the array of structural barriers that impede parental presence in the unit (e.g., costly accommodations, unreliable transportation, lack of childcare, need to return to work) and provide supports (e.g., overnight accommodations, transportation assistance) to the extent possible.

Understanding Caregiver Psychological Adjustment

The parents of a preterm infant have not completed the developmental work of pregnancy and are processing complex feelings of guilt, anger, anxiety, depression, and shame that emerge as a consequence of their infant's birth. The predictable course of response to the loss of a loved one (even an imagined person in this case) has been described in classic works. The initial responses of *denial and anger* give way to depression, guilt, and, finally, resolution. These same stages of grief reaction are apparent in the parental response to an infant born prematurely or with neonatal illness. Parents truly have lost a valued person in the form of their hoped-for or imagined child. They must resolve that grief to attach themselves to the real child who is now before them. They may require extra time to even see the infant as a separate person if the baby has been born very early. Furthermore, they may not be expected to attach to the infant until they sense a good chance for survival. Resolution of grief may be more prolonged when infants are experiencing complications that increase risk of developmental delays or long-term morbidities.

Clinicians should monitor the process of grief resolution and attachment and not be surprised at the turbulence and seemingly inappropriate responses, anger, and frustration that may be leveled at them or others. These are healthy, expected reactions that testify to the ongoing recovery process. Over the long run, these feelings help mobilize the emotional energy that will enable the family to reorganize around the child' needs. Short-term counseling may be necessary to achieve resolution of this process in some cases. Many anxious calls, repeated questions, fixation on specific laboratory values, and reluctance to be discharged from the hospital or leave the office are manifestations of this turmoil. Expect these bumps in the road. Parental "withdrawal" from the NICU as discharge nears reflects anxiety that seems overwhelming. Other signs of stress or avoidance include parents seeming to direct more attention to their phones than to their infants during NICU visits. Clinicians should avoid judging parents' behavior; rather, these behaviors can be seen as opportunities to support a parent's coping and recovery of competence and empowerment.

Nonbirthing parents may be especially uncomfortable in the NICU environment but should be encouraged to take part in care so that they can support their partner and build confidence with their infant. Grandparents and other family or community support can also add balance and energy and are particularly important for single-parent households. The clinician should look broadly for sources of support that can be mobilized.

A common defense mechanism for parents is intellectualization or overfixation on certain aspects of care so that parents perceive more control. Although social media provides parents with social support while they cope with a hospitalized child, the Internet can also be a misleading source of poorly moderated information. Although parents may challenge clinicians in care decisions, it is important to interpret these challenges as a sign of stress and avoid being drawn into prolonged technical discussions, intellectual nit-picking, or arguments. Chasing specific concerns can lead to frustration until one pulls back to identify the underlying and unvoiced worries that are the basis for most of these discussions. It is important for the nursing and medical care providers to listen and validate parent questions while using empathic and open-ended inquiry to uncover the "unvoiced" worries.

Research has shown that parents in the NICU experience high levels of psychological distress, including acute anxiety disorder, posttraumatic stress disorder, and depression, which often continue after the infant is discharged from the hospital. Consequently, interventions to provide psychosocial support to the family and enable parent coping with problems during the infant's hospitalization are undoubtedly needed. These interventions include trauma-informed care, family-centered developmental care, peer-to-peer support, mental health professionals in the NICU, palliative and bereavement care, logistical support (e.g., transportation, translation for families with limited English proficiency), and staff education and support.

Multiple Births

The number of **multiple births** is increasing as a result of fertility treatments. More than a quarter of NICU admissions now are premature multiple births. Multiple gestation increases the chance for a high-risk delivery, extremely low-birthweight babies, a prolonged stay in the NICU, and the likelihood of the family facing at least one serious neonatal complication, including neonatal death.

Even in the case of term or near-term twins, the situation has a higher risk and places greater demands on the parents. The process of attachment to two babies at the same time is more complicated than to one. For some period ranging from hours to weeks, families respond to these infants as one unit. The process of *individuation* in response and care comes on gradually in healthy circumstances and waxes and wanes. Increasing levels of recognition of individual differences, beginning with appearance and moving to behavioral characteristics, are the added dimension that should be monitored by the healthcare provider caring for multiples. Sharing observations of differences between the babies by the healthcare provider may help this process along.

Attachment difficulties get more complex if there is a discrepancy in size and vigor between the babies. Data suggest a general tendency to spend more time with the more fragile, usually lower weight baby. This child is likely to be both more irritable and more demanding. The healthcare provider can assist the family in the difficult task of balancing efforts by being sure that the one who "needs the least" does not get left out and that the parents can respond appropriately to each infant's bids for attention.

Multiple gestations increase the chance of neonatal death, either prenatally (e.g., twin-to-twin transfusion, intrauterine growth retardation), in the course of early care, or postnatally because of complications of illness or sudden infant death syndrome. The bereavement may cause parents to pull back from the process of attachment to the surviving child or children. Fear of loss of the surviving child is a natural impediment to attachment because we do not become attached to what we think we will lose; therefore parents may be appropriately guarded in their full psychological commitment to the survivor or survivors. Supportive care, including acknowledgment of the loss (no, the survivor does not "make up for" the loss of the other), patience, and a longer time frame, is needed here. A mental health referral is necessary to assist in this complex psychological adjustment.

PREPARING FOR NEONATAL INTENSIVE CARE UNIT DISCHARGE

Getting Ready to Go Home: Discharge Planning

As discharge approaches, parental anxiety increases sharply. The demands of unrelenting care, the lingering sense of inadequacy, and the fear of further damaging the infant while at home all contribute to this increased anxiety. It may be manifested as decreased visiting, anger, accusations, or the proposal of impediments to discharge. The clinician should recognize the need for the family to withdraw and consolidate before this new step, support the process, but still hold firm on the discharge plan with as specific a course as possible.

The family needs to know what the baby must be able to do to demonstrate readiness for discharge, such as the following:
- Tolerate all feedings by mouth.
- Gaining weight and maintaining body temperature in an open crib.
- Have no significant apnea and bradycardia.
- Have discharge assessments (e.g., eye examination, hearing screen, car seat test) and parent teaching completed.

The family then knows that discharge does not occur at a specific date, gestational age, or weight. Rather, it depends on the child's own maturation and recovery. To avoid disappointment, parents should be informed that the planned discharge date often changes.

Preparing a discharge repository for all instructions, appointments, important telephone numbers, and critical observations helps channel parents' anxious energy into more adaptive behaviors. This is usually compiled as printed material from an electronic repository, but parents are encouraged to keep a log wherever it suits them best. Reflection on these feelings of anxiety and inadequacy as normal and as a testimony of caring will help parents feel understood and validated.

The *explicit* agreement of *frequent, scheduled* check-ups and visits after discharge appears to generate earlier independence in a family than does an ad hoc arrangement. These postdischarge check-ups may include a call from a nurse or a home visiting nurse. So set this up ahead of time. It is very helpful if nursing care and parent education in the week before discharge are provided by nurses who know the infant and family well and with whom the family has developed a good relationship.

The family conference at discharge should be concrete. It should summarize the remaining problems briefly and focus on short-term goals, expectations, and specific care plans. Discharge skills demonstration and discharge education should be carried out in the family's preferred learning style and language. At discharge, the family should be given a copy of their baby's discharge summary to keep with them for future reference and share with the baby's PCP. At discharge, parents suddenly leave behind all the technology and experts who have safeguarded their baby. At home, they must assume their baby's care alone, which is often a very frightening prospect. Parents should be given explicit instructions on when to call their primary care doctor or nurse for advice. Social service evaluation for all families should be routine in the NICU and should focus on making sure that material needs and mental health support are lined up before discharge. It is essential for social service providers to establish a shared power dynamic with families, whereby families are well informed about their scope of work. Trust should be fostered by explicitly appreciating families' strengths and offering available support services in a timely manner. Parent-to-parent connections with families who have similar challenges can be very positive. Parenting groups, particularly for children with specific conditions (e.g., Down syndrome), may be helpful to families during this adjustment phase.

Practice Sessions

To learn the infant's signal system, parents must spend time in the NICU watching and participating in care. The parents can be asked to monitor their own infant's response to the environment, caregiving, and support (Box 7.6).

Nurses should share their own observations and care techniques and note how they change over time. The goal here is not just to provide excellent care but also to support the parents in the process of discovering their own infant. The goal is that parents see their infant as an individual with communicative intent—a person who can be known and understood. **Mentalization**, an umbrella term that encompasses mind-mindedness, parental reflective functioning, and parental insightfulness, refers to parents' tendency to regard their child as an independent psychological entity and to reflect on their child's internal states. The degree to which the parent masters showing frequent, coherent, and

appropriate appreciation of their infants' internal states is associated with infant-parent attachment security. Parents can reach this level of attachment only after they are sure that the infant will survive and are confident that they can cope with the child's practical care needs. Skills in cardiopulmonary resuscitation (CPR), feeding, and administration of medication should be seen as building tools for the parent-child relationship, as well as skills required for infant survival. Competency in skills enables parents to see their infant as manageable, understandable, and lovable. It is only with these feelings that true attachment can occur.

The following components are necessary for a successful discharge from the NICU:

- Families must have the knowledge and skills to provide physical care for infants. If this is beyond their capabilities, specialized care and/or additional resources must be mobilized. The goal of this care should be to assist families in assuming more responsibility over time. A family resource assessment, including physical assets (e.g., a car, a phone), community support (e.g., family, friends), and psychological readiness, is the first step in planning for care after discharge.
- All assessments and discharge teaching should be performed in the family's preferred language, either through an interpreter or a medical staff person who is fluent in that language. Parents with low English proficiency need additional supports to be adequately prepared for NICU discharge.
- Determining discharge readiness involves infant readiness (e.g., attainment of physiologic maturity milestones) as well as parental readiness. This process requires a reciprocal exchange of information between the medical team and the family that aligns with the infant's needs and the family's preferences, goals, and values (Table 7.1).
- Caregivers with mental health conditions, teen parents, immigrant parents, and those with substance use disorders, extreme poverty and unmet basic needs, or domestic violence may need special attention and mobilization of resources and support as part of the discharge planning process. To provide ethical care, staff should be aware of their own explicit and implicit biases to minimize their influence on the family and home assessment process.
- Families must have access to care that is acceptable to them and adequate to the needs of the infant. This means access to a working phone, Internet, heat, electricity, health insurance, and culturally sensitive, linguistically compatible ongoing healthcare. Discharge without these elements in place is likely to lead to less than optimal, if not dangerous, circumstances. Do not send the caregiver home without them; advocate for systems change when you see recurrent issues.

BOX 7.6   Bedside Observations for Clinicians and Parents

- Observe the infant's state.
- Can you see the cycles of sleep?
- Can you tell when the infant is waking?
- What soothes the child's upset?
- What are the child's responses to sight? To sound?
- What things are aversive, and what are positive?
- What kinds of movement and posture are positive, and which are stressful?

TABLE 7.1   Questions to Include in Assessment of Discharge Preparedness

Question	Observation
How is the baby doing?	Level of attachment—are the parents answering with a shrug of bewilderment, with a list of laboratory values or with personalized observations of their infant's response to them?
Is the baby ready for discharge?	Assess the parents' understanding of readiness issues; gather data from their perspective about the infant.
Are *you* ready to take (name) home?	Assess readiness and response—expand to include the specifics of readiness, special needs; assess parental adjustment.
Who will be at home to help?	Assess support systems, intrafamilial concerns, and the level of the partner's involvement; assess sibling and family needs.
Do you feel comfortable with (name)?	Evaluate feelings of inadequacy; reassure parents of the normality of anxiety; evaluate specific areas in which parents' skills are inadequate.
Do you have any questions about the infant's hospital course?	Open the discussion for any questions about the perinatal events; be honest about your level of concern vis-à-vis these events.
What things would you like to see happen before you take (name) home?	Establish the locus of control with the parents; develop a plan to meet these wishes if possible, explain if not.

- Families should have transportation plans laid out for both emergency and planned visits. Adjustment of the car seat, taxi vouchers, and other issues should be addressed.
- A brief review of the medical course, anticipated problems, and the need for specialized (e.g., ophthalmology, audiology) follow-up helps parents know what to expect and to ask questions or get clarification. Parents should be told that certain problems specifically related to the infant's condition at birth as a sick neonate *will not* recur (especially intraventricular hemorrhage, pneumothorax, etc.). Many parents continue to worry that these neonatal problems could recur or be chronic, but they never ask!
- A notebook with all the infant's needs, resources to meet those needs, warning signals, appointments, medications, and telephone numbers of specialists and staff can be most helpful. Highlight one or two resources, including the primary care provider, to work with the parents in coordinating multiple services.
- Appropriate community agency referrals should be initiated or noted even if the services may not be needed immediately.
- The NICU staff may designate one nurse to follow up with a call in 1 or 2 days to ease the family's transition to home.
- Parental expectations before discharge should be reviewed. The parents must demonstrate competency in all aspects of their infant's care. They should rehearse

what will be needed in emergencies. Instruction in infant CPR and appropriate emergency action will relieve fears rather than generate them. Videos, dolls, and pamphlets should supplement, not replace, *direct* teaching in this and other areas.
- Review nutritional needs, including vitamins and minerals. Very-low-birthweight infants may need additional protein, electrolytes, and calories in the form of special preterm discharge formulas or supplementation of breast milk with powdered preterm formula for a period. An iron-deficient infant is an irritable infant. Premature infants require additional iron supplementation up to 1 year of age. Anemia is a *late* sign of iron deficiency, which has been shown to have adverse effects on development even before the anemia surfaces. Appropriate iron supplementation should be initiated even in the absence of frank anemia. Check the hematocrit at discharge and periodically throughout the first year. Adequate vitamin D supplementation is needed to ensure optimal bone mineralization.
- **Breastfeeding**. A *realistic* postdischarge feeding plan, developed in conjunction with the family and a lactation specialist experienced with preterm infants, should be clearly laid out. If supplemental nutrition is needed after discharge to ensure adequate growth, it may be added directly to expressed breast milk or given as one or two feedings of an adapted preterm formula. A preterm infant should be able to nurse at

the breast before discharge for part of a feeding or for all of some feedings. For exclusively breastfed infants, the recommended approach for each feeding may be (1) breastfeeding at the breast, (2) supplementing with pumped breast milk, and then (3) pumping for the next feeding to keep the milk supply up and store it appropriately. Some infants, especially those born late preterm, may be able to breastfeed exclusively at the breast without the need for supplementation or pumped breast milk.

- Describe the infant's growth, behavior, and development at the *adjusted age* so that neurodevelopmental expectations are realistic. Continue to make this correction at the beginning of future encounters. Be sure that an accurate head circumference is recorded at the time of discharge. A growth chart that includes head circumference should be started and values added at the adjusted age at each visit.
- The need for ongoing longitudinal neurodevelopmental follow-up should be discussed. Every family should be assessed for Part C of Individuals with Disabilities Education Act eligibility and make a referral to qualifying families prior to discharge. Referrals and education on the value of high-risk infant follow-up clinics should also be completed prior to discharge.
- Parents often need to be reassured that their "sleepy" premature infant will become more alert and interactive with maturity. Until they understand this, their infant's apparent response to them (to sleep) is very discouraging. The irritability that may follow it can also be predicted. Parents need to understand these aspects of typical behavior for their infant.
- Routine discharge counseling includes the use of car seats and recognition of the "back-to-sleep" message. Parents should be encouraged to place their baby prone for "tummy time" when awake to strengthen the trunk and shoulder muscles, which tend to be weaker in preterm infants and thus interfere with developmental progress.
- Discuss the need for routine immunizations in the usual amounts and at the usual times. The need and schedule for respiratory syncytial virus prophylaxis should also be addressed for eligible infants.
- An explicit invitation to call or visit the NICU after discharge is also helpful as parents attempt to separate from the nursery, the staff, and the support that has been so vital.
- Parents should be encouraged to stay overnight, if possible, before discharge, or they may be accommodated for a period in nearby lodging if they are going to a rural or remote area.
- Referrals and follow-up care at discharge (Box 7.7).

BOX 7.7   Assessments

Hearing
- Discharge hearing screen (BAER or OAE) with follow-up BAER if abnormal: VRA when sitting at 6–9 months' adjusted age.
- Further follow-up if the infant has abnormal speech-language development or frequent otitis media.

Ophthalmology
- If the premature baby weighs less than 1500 g or a gestational age of 30 weeks or less, examine before discharge. The entire retina should be visualized with frequent follow-up by an experienced pediatric ophthalmologist until the retina is completely mature.
- Ophthalmology follow-up for astigmatism, amblyopia, strabismus, and refractive errors should occur within 4–6 months from discharge.

BAER, Brainstem auditory evoked response; *OAE*, otoacoustic emission; *VRA*, visual reinforced audiometry.

THE TRANSITION FROM NEONATAL INTENSIVE CARE UNIT TO HOME

How Primary Care Providers Can Help Families Adjust

The primary care clinician has important therapeutic opportunities in interactions with caregivers raising a premature infant. As important as monitoring the infant's changing capacities as they grow is the chance to observe and support the parents' growth into the role of caretakers who understand their unique infant. Supporting the caregiver-infant relationship is the most important thing a PCP can do to promote resilience and long-term developmental outcomes. On the other hand, caregivers who are overwhelmed by their child's complexity, find it difficult to read the child's signals, or are overly anxious/preoccupied or lax in their responses to infant needs, there have a higher chance that caregiver-infant attachment will be insecure. Promotion of caregiver-infant secure attachment can occur through the interview, physical examination, and follow-up care that help the parent understand the infant's unique trajectory while addressing developmental needs through therapies and resources.

Family Interview

The primary care provider will become the lead of the medical home for the high-risk infant after discharge. The primary care provider should acknowledge the

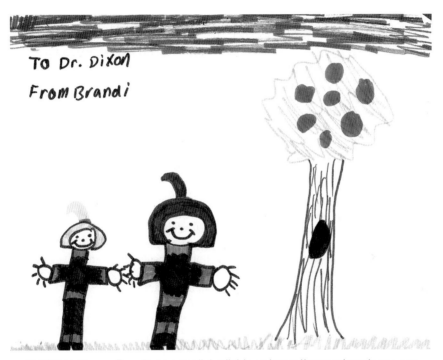

"NICU to Home: Free Resources." Available at https://www.nicutohome.org

frequent medical appointments the infant has in the first few months after discharge and assist the family with organization of subspecialty care and other community referrals (e.g., early intervention). The family interview should include an assessment on how the infant and the family are adapting to the new environment and what changes the family has noted since getting home in the infant's behavior, feeding, and sleeping patterns. It is also important to screen for postpartum depression and to assess families' coping with stress and anxiety that typically follow a NICU experience or traumatic birth. Families need to understand that posttraumatic stress disorder is not solely a military combat disorder; rather, it is a normative reaction to extraordinary circumstances. Referrals for psychosocial support and other resources (e.g., hotlines, support groups) may be needed at this time.

Many families will be unprepared to manage the financial burden associated with NICU hospitalization and follow-up care on their own. The primary care provider, social worker, or case manager should review any referrals to resources placed during hospitalization (e.g., supplemental security income). Families may benefit from help applying for assistance, financial counseling, and resources.

Physical Examination

Primary care providers should make adjustments in neurodevelopmental expectations commensurate with a child's adjusted age rather than chronological age, beginning with a correction in the physical growth chart and how we label an office visit (e.g., indicating both chronological and adjusted age). Families should be reminded of this correction to adjust their expectations accordingly. For an infant who weighed less than 1500 g, this adjustment should last for 2 years and possibly 3 years for those who were born at less than 28 weeks' gestation and weighed less than 1000 g. For higher birthweight preterm babies, the adjustment should continue for at least a year.

The clinician can observe the baby first in sleep and then through gentle talking, moving, undressing, examining, and narrating of the infant's behavior, both positive and negative. Parents should be asked to provide their observations and experiences as well so that everyone is seeing the *same* infant. For example, if the infant becomes mottled and fusses during undressing, the clinician can say something like, "I see that their skin gets mottled and face bright red when I took off their onesie. This is one sign that infants are a little stressed—do you see this during diaper changes at home? How do you help them calm?" The level of stimulation that the infant tolerates should be noted. Signals of overstimulation, physiological instability, and fatigue should be met with a rest period, a pulling back of stimulation, and a period for recovery, which can be accompanied by narration about why the clinician is doing this.

If the infant becomes alert, the clinician should demonstrate the baby's alerting and orienting to voice, then to face, and then to both together. If overload occurs, this should be pointed out to the parents as evidence of the child's limits, which should be normalized as common among premature infants. Considerable support for the extremities, head and trunk, and temperature control may be needed to demonstrate the brief periods of alertness. The *cost* to the infant or the difficulty that the infant experiences in these periods should be noted so that this may be observed at home. For example, the clinician can say "I know outings and experiences like this take a lot out of him" or "She really had to work hard to stay calm while being examined" to acknowledge that premature infants have a different threshold for becoming dysregulated. Clinicians can coach parents on noticing whether these types of experiences gradually become easier for their infant, which reflects neurological maturation.

The general pediatric examination, including a detailed neurological evaluation, should follow. Any areas of abnormality, as well as encouraging signs, should be clearly stated in an ongoing narrative of what the clinician is evaluating and what is observed, normal and abnormal. The clinician should carefully describe types of behavior that will represent things caregivers can look for in the next step in improvement—for example, increasing periods of alertness, decreased color change with undressing, and more ability to quiet self.

A summary statement by the clinician should open a discussion with the parents about the evaluation, from the infant's perspective if possible. For example, "Joey is able to really take in more of the world around him these days, and his sleep pattern is getting more regular. This is on track for his adjusted age. His legs still seem a bit tight, however, and getting a full feeding in without a break is still hard for him, so keep working on these things with his Early Intervention team." An unrushed pause and encouragement may be needed for parents to convey their own observations and concerns. It is not to be expected that all issues or concerns will be laid out and discussed at this time; rather, this discussion sets a pattern for ongoing developmental surveillance, an honest partnership in observation and care, and an individual perspective. This helps build trust between families who have been through a stressful and sometimes alienating clinical course, as well as a sense of competence in understanding their infant.

Developmental and Physical Examination Differences in Preterm Infants

A preterm infant's behavior and developmental course will not be the same as that of an infant born at term, no matter how smooth the postnatal course. Although behavioral expectations should be adjusted for the degree of prematurity (i.e., the adjusted age) as the best approximation, differences can be anticipated, including the following:

- Motor tone and posture will be altered. Many will have a pattern of passive hypotonia (i.e., floppiness or offering little resistance to passive movement). This may be accompanied by active hypertonia and brisk reflexes, especially the lower extremities. The predominance of extension postures is present in many infants throughout the first year. Although most infants will resolve these differences by the second year, some will maintain an imbalance in tone that will be seen as subtle movement or postural differences.
- Much of the development that depends on posture and tone may take a different, often delayed path if external support is not provided to these children. *Shoulder girdle weakness* and *shoulder retraction* (i.e., shoulders rolled back) may mean that the infant has difficulty with self-quieting behavior, such as hand to mouth, and will need special help to settle in a tucked, flexed position. Without support to bring the hands forward, the natural hand regard and midline play opportunities will be diminished, which is important for fostering cognitive development and visual-motor skills in which infants efficiently start to connect their visual, perceptual, and motor coordination brain pathways. Therefore helping infants bring their hands to the midline through caregiver support (e.g., supporting the trunk during play and feeding) and early intervention therapy will help prevent further cognitive delays.
- *Truncal instability* results in the infant actively resisting the prone activities that are vital to learning. They may have difficulty lifting their head during "tummy time," to be able to look up and interact with objects and people around them. These babies need physical support (e.g., rolled towel under the chest) and inducements (e.g., a toy or face in front) to enable them to tolerate prone positions. Assistance will also be needed to maintain a sitting position.
- An undifferentiated, drowsy state at about 28 weeks gradually evolves into wake and sleep at about 32 weeks' adjusted age; the pattern becomes clearer over time with the emergence of active and quiet sleep at about 36 weeks. Increasing periods of alertness can be seen by 36 weeks. Full-cry states become available to the infant after 35 to 36 weeks. However, even at term, a prematurely born infant is likely to continue to have irregular sleep and variability in the quality of alertness and spend more time in a drowsy or irritable state. These difficulties are lessened if the special care environment has quiet and dark times, if the infant is not disturbed for blocks of time and if intrusive levels of light and sound are avoided. Parents may perceive the lack of wakeful interaction as rejection and regard sleep difficulties as evidence of subtle damage or poor parenting. These misconceptions need to be directly countered with realistic explanations of the evolution of social availability and state organization in this group. Alterations in wakefulness and sleep may continue even beyond the first year.
- *Sensitivity to pain, touch of the feet, and scars from procedures* may be a source of discomfort and, later, a source of unusual aversive responses. Some infants, for example, dislike feeling certain textures or having their feet touched, perhaps an association with repeated heel sticks. This can be normalized with parents, and they can be encouraged to speak with their infant's early intervention team about helping their infant process sensory input.
- The infant's *self-protective behavior* of avoiding or ignoring intrusive stimuli may mean that the infant sends signals to care providers that are seen as confusing or counterintuitive. For example, gaze avoidance sends the message, "Leave me alone." Confusing behavioral signals, interactional availability only in short segments, and unpredictability of behavior may remain even after the baby is well. This leaves parents confused, disappointed, and often frustrated. The clinician can act as an interpreter to demystify these signals and what they mean, to avoid parents developing negative mental models of their infant.

Medical Concerns Needing Follow-Up in Premature Infants

- *Visual difficulties* are common in this group, including astigmatism, refractive errors, and strabismus. Retinopathy of prematurity may result in diminished peripheral vision after spontaneous resolution, as well as after photocoagulation. Careful visual follow-up and periodic reassessment should continue throughout early childhood, even without obvious abnormalities or visual complaints. Additionally, significant visual impairment precludes the valid use of the usual developmental tests.
- *Alterations in motor tone*, as well as anatomical changes caused by prolonged orotracheal tube placement, may result in difficulties with feeding and swallowing early on and articulation problems later because of structural

and functional changes in the mouth and palate. In addition, orthodontic care later in childhood may be needed because dental position may be altered by the architecture of the palate.

- *Recurrent otitis media* may also result from these differences in structure and function in the mouth, pharynx, and airway. Eustachian tube dysfunction may likewise contribute to this problem. Vigilance and aggressive follow-up are called for. Hearing must be monitored in these circumstances.
- *Limited energy and oxygen reserves* result in slow growth, particularly in children with bronchopulmonary dysplasia and congenital heart disease, and often lead to additional delays in motor activities because of decreased stamina and strength. The biomechanics of movement may also be altered by these delays in linear growth.
- *Feeding challenges* are common. All families should have access to lactation support to reach their breastfeeding goals. As the infant matures, lactation consultants and the medical team should support the gentle transition to feeding at the breast. Some babies may never adapt to feeding directly at the breast but can continue to receive the benefits of pumped breast milk. The emphasis on feeding and growth that is appropriate in the first year or two in this group may result in *long-term feeding issues* due to oral aversions and oral-motor dysfunction from prolonged intubation, as well as negative parent-child dynamics around feeding. Pressure to get the baby to eat is usually felt acutely by families, particularly if they mentalize the child as being vulnerable or difficult. A combination of relational and sensorimotor interventions is often needed.

Vulnerable Child Syndrome

The family's perception of the child is not always directly related to the severity of the perinatal illness. Even conditions that the clinician may regard as relatively minor or transient, such as a rule out sepsis or treatment for hyperbilirubinemia, may set the groundwork for a permanently altered perception of the child by the family. Green and Solnit in their now classic description have highlighted the important dimensions of the "**vulnerable child syndrome**." In this circumstance, a child with a perceived or serious illness in early life is the target of altered attachment by parents. The parents develop a long-term sense of the child being particularly susceptible to illness, injury, or loss. The child is viewed as fragile and incapable of age-appropriate behavioral expectations, particularly in areas of independence. This perception of vulnerability leads to ongoing intrafamilial stress, altered interaction between the child and parents, and decreased tendency to either allow age-appropriate autonomy or set limits. The clinician should be sensitive to this perception in the newborn period as the basis of many later problems (e.g., problems with sleep, eating, discipline, and school phobias).

Pediatric providers can support early relational health to promote safe, stable, and nurturing relationships among all families through developmentally appropriate anticipatory guidance and counseling on effective parenting practices. Providers should universally assess development and protective factors, including child, family, and communication factors, as well as parents' knowledge about access to support to address families' needs. Targeted relational health interventions include *Reach Out and Read, Healthy Steps, Promoting First Relationships in Pediatric Primary Care*, and *Video Interaction Project*.

Developmental Follow-up

Formal appraisal of development should be done at regular intervals through specialized programs (e.g., early intervention, NICU follow-up clinics) that offer the extended time needed to perform a comprehensive assessment of development. This follow-up should be continued through the early school years because many problems related to prematurity are not evident until school age. Across this period, the likelihood of the emergence of particular problems changes. The early motor difficulties are rarely missed; the cognitive, organizational, and linguistic concerns may be more difficult to identify in a general office setting. They require specialized evaluation tools and a family interview as the child grows and develops (Box 7.8).

Use of developmental surveillance tools at ages recommended by the American Academy of Pediatrics is important for detecting delays in different developmental delays. Major developmental delays and hearing abnormalities should elicit referral for early *intervention* before 1 year, if not earlier. Speech and language delay at 18 months to 2½ years in children born prematurely warrants early referral for formal evaluation because these children are more likely to have persistent language impairments or autism spectrum disorder. Hearing loss secondary to recurrent otitis media may also contribute to language delay.

In the preschool period, oral-motor dysfunction may result in speech articulation difficulties that may influence early letter-sound identification. Extremely preterm infants are also at risk of visual-motor cognitive delays that may appear as handwriting challenges (e.g., figure copying). Executive functioning difficulties and attention-deficit/hyperactivity disorder are often present in early childhood as impulsive and dysregulated behavior; in preschool and kindergarten as difficulty mastering or retaining early academic concepts; and in middle childhood as social challenges, disorganization, or difficulty focusing/refusing to complete academic tasks. Approaches to discussing these

BOX 7.8   Timing of the Presentation of Developmental Abnormalities for the Premature Infant

First Year[a]
- Cerebral palsy
- Severe sensory abnormalities
- Significant visual compromise
- Severe hearing loss

Second Year
- Speech and language difficulties
- Early cognitive delays
- Subtle visual and hearing difficulties
  - Autism spectrum disorder/social communication difficulties

3–5 Years
- Fine motor difficulties
- Difficulties in regulation of behavior
- Hyporesponsive or hyperresponsive behavior (i.e., attention-deficit/hyperactivity disorder)
- Motor and behavioral "immaturity"

6–8 Years
- Learning disabilities
- Sensory processing problems
- Visual-motor difficulties
- Minor degrees of compromised motor coordination

[a]Probable time frames of appearance.

challenges with families and referring for school evaluations are discussed in Chapters 18 and 19.

Sleep Difficulties

Children cared for in the bright light and continuous sound environment of the NICU will maintain immature state regulation patterns for the first several months after discharge. It may be more difficult for these infants to settle down for sleeping, they may have long periods of irritability when awakening and falling asleep, and they may find it difficult to come to a quiet/alert state for sustained periods. Cycled lighting and activity in the NICU help somewhat but do not eliminate these problems. Once removed from the stressful NICU environment, the baby will demonstrate increasing competency at state regulation in a quieter, more predictable environment, although full normalization of sleep patterns is rarely achieved in the first year. A noise machine and a dim light may help the baby make the transition from the NICU to the home environment. Sleep

disorders are more common in toddlers who had perinatal difficulties, and these disorders may persist. Difficulty in making transitions from one activity to another may also be impaired well beyond discharge from the nursery. Irritability and sleep difficulties should *start* to decrease at 3 to 4 months of adjusted age in most children. The individual child should be monitored for increasing regularity and predictability in sleep, with the infant's own behavior used as a baseline for future comparisons.

Hearing and Vision Issues

Premature or ill infants have a high incidence (2%–4%) of hearing disorders. These difficulties can rarely be detected in office settings; they require formal assessment. A brainstem auditory evoked response screen should be done just before discharge, followed by visual reinforced audiometry or other behavioral audiometry when the child is sitting stably, at about 9 months. Otoacoustic emission techniques may be used for this population. Even normal results of these early tests do not rule out a high-frequency or progressive hearing loss, which will affect language development and school performance. Recurrent or resistant otitis media may also contribute to later hearing loss. Another preschool test of hearing is advised if any speech or language difficulties persist. An audiologist who has experience with infants and young children provides the best chance for accurate results.

Infants born at less than 30 weeks' gestation and those born with less than 1500 g are at risk of developing a disorder of the developing retinal blood vessels called retinopathy of prematurity (ROP), which is the leading cause of childhood blindness. Infants born at greater than 30 weeks' gestation or between 1500 and 2000 g who were severely ill (e.g., inotropic support, prolonged oxygen supplementation) should also be screened for ROP at the discretion of the attending neonatologist. While in the NICU, a pediatric ophthalmologist performs scheduled retinal screening examinations after pupillary dilation using binocular direct ophthalmoscopy to detect ROP. The initial examination is scheduled based on postmenstrual age and chronologic age (4 weeks postnatal age or 31 weeks postmenstrual age, whichever is later). Follow-up examinations are recommended by the examining ophthalmologist based on retinal findings. If hospital discharge or transfer to another hospital is contemplated before retinal development into anterior zone III has taken place, or if the infant has been treated for ROP and there is either incomplete regression or incomplete retinal healing or maturation, follow-up must be arranged before the infant's departure from the NICU. Regardless of whether infants are at risk of developing treatment-requiring ROP, pediatric providers who care for infants who have had ROP should be aware that these infants are at increased risk for other seemingly unrelated visual disorders, such as strabismus, amblyopia, high refractive errors, cataracts, and glaucoma. Ophthalmologic follow-up for these potential problems after discharge from the NICU is indicated within 4 to 6 months after discharge.

RECOMMENDED READINGS

Bradford N, Lousada S. *Your premature baby: the first five years.* Buffalo: Firefly Books Ltd; 2003.

Davis DL, Stein MT. *Parenting Your premature baby and child: the emotional journey.* Golden: Fulcrum Publishing; 2004.

Feldman R, Eidelman AI, Sirota L, Weller A. Comparison of skin-to-skin (kangaroo) and traditional care: parenting outcomes and preterm infant development. *Pediatrics.* 2002;110(1 Pt 1):16–26. https://doi.org/10.1542/peds.110.1.16. PMID: 12093942.

Garcia-Prats JA, Hornfischer SS. *What to do when your baby is premature: a parent's handbook for coping with high-risk pregnancy and caring for the preterm infant.* New York: Three Rivers Press; 2000.

Hynan MT, Hall SL. Psychosocial program standards for NICU parents. *J Perinatol.* 2015;35(Suppl 1):S1–S4. https://doi.org/10.1038/jp.2015.141.

Hynan MT, Mounts KO, Vanderbilt DL. Screening parents of high-risk infants for emotional distress: rationale and recommendations. *J Perinatol.* 2013;33(10):748–753.

Klein AH, Ganon JA. *Caring for your premature baby: a complete resource for parents.* New York: Harper Collins; 1998.

La Leche League. *Breastfeeding your premature baby.* Schaumburg: La Leche League; 1999.

Linden DW, Paroli ET, Doron MW. *PREEMIES: the essential guide for parents of premature babies.* New York: Pocket Books; 2000.

Ludington-Hoe S. *Kangaroo care: the best you can do to help your preterm infant.* New York: Bantum Books; 1993.

MedlinePlus: *Premature babies.* Available from www.nlm.nih.gov/medlineplus/prematurebabies.html

Melnyk BM, Alpert-Gillis L, Feinstein NF, et al. Creating opportunities for parent empowerment: program effects on the mental health/coping outcomes of critically ill young children and their mothers. *Pediatrics.* 2004;113(6):e597–e607. https://doi.org/10.1542/peds.113.6.e597.

Melnyk BM, Feinstein NF, Alpert-Gillis L, et al. Reducing premature infants' length of stay and improving parents' mental health outcomes with the Creating Opportunities for Parent Empowerment (COPE) neonatal intensive care unit program: a randomized, controlled trial. *Pediatrics.* 2006;118(5):e1414–e1427. https://doi.org/10.1542/peds.2005-2580.

O'Brien K, Robson K, Bracht M, et al. Effectiveness of Family Integrated Care in neonatal intensive care units on infant and parent outcomes: a multicentre, multinational, cluster-randomised controlled trial [published correction appears in Lancet Child Adolesc Health. 2018 Aug;2(8):e20]. *Lancet Child Adolesc Health.* 2018;2(4):245–254. https://doi.org/10.1016/S2352-4642(18)30039-7.

Sears J, Sears M, Sears R, Sears W. *The premature baby book: everything you need to know about your premature baby from birth to age one.* New York: Little, Brown; 2004.

Smith VC, Love K, Goyer E. NICU discharge preparation and transition planning: guidelines and recommendations [published correction appears in J Perinatol. 2022 Mar 30]. *J Perinatol.* 2022;42(Suppl 1):7–21. https://doi.org/10.1038/s41372-022-01313-9.

Tracy AE, Maroney DI. *Your premature baby and child: helpful answers and advice for parents.* New York: Berkley Books; 1999.

Vandenberg KA. Individualized developmental care for high risk newborns in the NICU: a practice guideline. *Early Hum Dev.* 2007;83(7):433–442.

Zaichkin J. *Neonatal intensive care (Cuidado Intensivo Neonatal).* Santa Rosa: NICU Ink; 2000. (in English and Spanish).

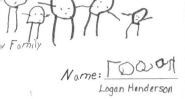

8

Name: Logan
Logan Henderson

First Days at Home: Making a Place in the Family

Anna Klunk and Shaquita Bell

This chapter describes the relational aspects of bringing a new infant home, including understanding infant behaviors, caregiver stress, postpartum support, parental leave, adjustments of siblings and other caregivers, and caregiver-infant interaction touchpoints such as feeding and soothing.

KEYWORDS

- Postpartum adjustment
- Breastfeeding
- Postpartum depression
- Sibling rivalry
- Postpartum support
- parental leave
- Infant-caregiver interaction
- Serve and return

The early neonatal period after hospital discharge is usually filled with turmoil and adjustments for all members of the family. In this chapter, in meeting families for the first time, it is important to consider inclusive definitions of "family" that include same-sex partners with a new child, individuals who may have given birth but identify as trans or nonbinary, grandparents, single fathers, and foster parents. At the same time, when these caregivers are adapting to the new member of the family, it is also important to remember that the infant is working too, using capacities for communication and coregulation to develop relationships with each caregiver. Each infant's particular temperament, physiological regulation, stamina, and behavioral characteristics determine how they communicate through their cries, body movements,

Original chapter by Suzanne D. Dixon and Martin T. Stein.

and elicit caregiver responses. The caregivers' perception of the child, as it is formed during this time, is a powerful predictor of their own interaction with the child over the long term, which, in turn, shapes the infant's social and emotional development. Caregivers' self-efficacy and competence are built on the experiences of these early days. This period has huge implications for the child and family, and thus it is a great opportunity for the healthcare provider to make a difference.

The clinician's role during the first month consists of monitoring and supporting the development of synchrony in the family unit while evaluating the infant's growth and physical well-being. Turbulence is expected as evidence of healthy developmental work as family members adjust and negotiate their new roles, and it can be normalized for families as a sign that they care deeply. In families whose members have competing stressors, particularly when no extended family members are available, the clinician has a special role of support and guidance.

This realignment within a family that occurs to adapt to the new family unit is done through experiences of success in each member's care of the infant. Through sensitive observations and some thoughtful suggestions on seemingly small matters of management, the clinician can ensure that everyone, including the infant, grows during the adjustment period. However, these interpersonal processes of family realignment may not be easy topics of conversations for caregivers during routine health supervision, so it helps if clinicians sensitively bring these issues to consciousness and a problem-solving conversation.

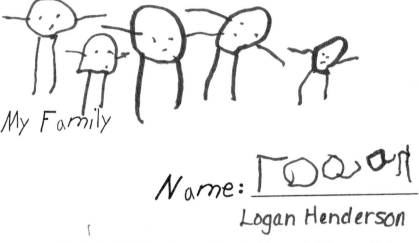

A 5-year-old draws his family, his baby sister positioned at the end of the line. He is next to his mom. By Logan Henderson.

SUPPORTING CAREGIVER-INFANT RELATIONSHIPS

Helping Caregivers Read Infant Behaviors

Infants begin life equipped to interact with the environment. Evidence of the baby actively participating in social interactions includes movement in rhythm to the human voice and visual fixation on the human face that is different from that of any other kind of stimuli (see Chapter 7). The infant's early behavioral repertoire includes socially directed behavior used both to elicit and to terminate interactions.

Generally, the baby's eyes widen and brighten as they fixate and track caregivers' movements and scan their faces. Gaze aversion, conversely, is often actively used by the infant to either avoid or take a break from an interaction. Directed gaze is thought to be important to the bonding between infant and family; however, it is important to note that related research has been primarily conducted in White, Western cultures. In other cultures, less emphasis is placed on directed gaze, and there are many other ways that infants demonstrate readiness for interaction with body language (e.g., smooth, cyclic movements of the extremities or slowing down of body movements, open hands, and mouthing). Types of behavior that signal withdrawal from caregivers, either to modulate the level of input or to avoid insensitive or overwhelming interaction, include back arching, pulling away, hand to head, increased body tension, and diffuse jittery movements of the extremities.

The first newborn visit presents a good opportunity for observing these infant cues along with caregivers. The provider can help caregivers recognize bids for attention, while also recognizing avoidance cues (and therefore not talk, shake, bounce, or nuzzle an infant who is clearly overwhelmed and is signaling that they need a break). Such lack of synchrony between the baby's body language and caregiver's behavior occurs in all dyads but is more common when infants are more dysregulated, or caregivers have their own stressors; therefore it can be a sign that increased support is needed. A list of nonverbal communication behavior is presented in Box 8.1.

Infant crying, too, can powerfully elicit both positive and negative caregiver responses. Research suggests that parents with depression are more likely to show anger, disgust, or withdrawal in response to infant crying. Therefore providing supports such as home visitation or infant mental health therapy can help support infant-caregiver synchrony and attachment. Research shows similar patterns exist across cultures in terms of longer-term relational health and attachment, but the specific caregiving behaviors vary between and within parents from different cultures.

> ### BOX 8.1   Baby Language
>
> **Come-On Behavior**
> The following types of behavior signal a positive response from the infant, saying in effect, "Keep doing this; this is great."
> - Softening of facial expression
> - Lifting of eyebrows
> - Relaxed body posture
> - Hands opening and closing
> - Feet relaxed, "grasping" with plantar flexion
> - Leaning forward with head and shoulders
> - Making an "Oohh" facial expression with the mouth in an oval
> - Mouthing, tongue going back and forth
> - Cooing sounds
>
> **Go-Away Behavior**
> The following types of behavior signal a negative response from the infant, saying, in effect, "Go away. Stop that."
> - Arching away
> - Turning the face away
> - Gaze aversion
> - Hands, feet splayed
> - Extension of the legs, pushing away
> - Downturned face
> - Lateral stretching of the mouth into a "grin"
> - Spitting up, burping, passing a bowel movement
> - Whiney sounds

From Als H: *Manual for the naturalistic observation of the newborn (preterm and fullterm)*, Boston, 1984, Children's Hospital Medical Center (revised 1997).

Smiling is a powerful social "tool" that progresses from a reflexive activity to a responsive activity prompted by external events (e.g., a human face, gaze, or voice) to spontaneous behavior produced to elicit response from others at the age of 6 to 8 weeks. A smiling infant changes a caregiver dramatically because it finally feels as though the infant is a person who is responsive to care. The first smile is a very big event in the emergence of the caregiver-child relationship.

Supporting Serve-and-Return Interaction and Communication

Newborns prefer high-pitched vocal tones with lots of modulation. Parents from different cultures with different languages instinctively use high-pitched voices when communicating with a young infant. Babies begin to "answer" in the first month with cooing sounds. These soft vocalizations come out of a positive social interaction—sometime in the first month. By the second month, most infants will engage in verbal "dialogs" with their caregivers, going back and forth in a "conversation" that is mutually regulated.

The infant's interactional pattern begins with each caregiver over the first days and weeks of life. During this acquaintance period, the family members develop reciprocal relationships that are shaped by both the infant's temperament and regulatory abilities and the caregiver's style and cultural norms of responses. The back-and-forth verbal and nonverbal interactions between infants and caregivers have been termed *serve-and-return* interactions because, like a tennis match, the partners respond to one another contingently (but also miss their serves and returns at times!). An infant's babble, cry, or movement (a "serve") is followed by a caregiver's "return" that could involve a variety of different behaviors responsive to the infant's state, from picking up the infant, talking to them, or helping reduce stimulation. Serve-and-return interactions have been shown to shape brain architecture in infants, particularly the areas of the frontal lobe that play a role in executive functioning and emotion regulation. Serve-and-return dynamics have been studied across a range of cultures, and while the specific behaviors may differ based on child-rearing norms and expectations, the main point of this concept is *reciprocity* between infant and caregiver. Caretaking activities such as feeding, diapering, playing, and sleep routines are the matrix on which this synchrony is built. Feeling successful in the infant's care and being able to see pattern and meaning in the infant's behavior enable the caregivers to grow in their role and to meet the child's physical and psychological needs. Close physical contact early helps this synchrony develop, which is essential to attachment.

Caregiver-Infant Feeding Interactions

Infants and caregivers both bring something to the table to shape feeding interactions (Table 8.1). The infant is born with reflexes, but they must be quickly adapted to the feeding interaction. The infant's temperament, state regulation, physiological vitality, and behavioral organization all contribute to that process; infants who struggle with motor coordination may have difficulty latching and coordinating sucking, while those with weaker state regulation may be easily distracted or frustrated during feeding. Likewise, the breastfeeding parent's nutrition, hydration, psychological state, and rate of recovery enter into the equation. In a variable time of adjustment for both partners, rhythms and behavioral patterns of individuals are melded into a successful interaction. Personal, cultural, and group differences are evident here, as they are in other situations of interaction. The clinician should be *very* familiar with the practical advice and support required for successful

TABLE 8.1 Interactional Nature of Breastfeeding	
Infant Characteristics	**Maternal Characteristics**
Reflexes	Nutrition
Temperament	Hydration
State regulation	Psychological state
Physiological variables	Recovery stage
Behavioral organization	Concepts of parenting
Residual of recovery from delivery influences	Extent and use of support
Neurological maturation	Psychosocial history
	Residual of pregnancy and delivery circumstances
	Role models

breastfeeding because it is important for much more than the child's physiological needs (Box 8.2).

The American Academy of Pediatrics (AAP) recognizes that support of breastfeeding has not only nutritional, immunological, and infectious disease benefits but psychosocial ones as well. The AAP recommends exclusive breastfeeding for the first 6 months of life and recognizes continued benefits of breastfeeding throughout the first 2 years of life. There are many barriers to breastfeeding including medication-assisted therapy, previous reconstructive surgery, work schedules, decreased social support, and other factors beyond parents' control. It is important to note that children of sex-diverse parents may have less access to human milk, due to a variety of constraints, and may feel more comfortable using more inclusive terminology, such as "chest feeding." If the caregiver is interested in providing breast milk for the infant but is facing barriers, national and local resources should be provided for the family. If it is not possible or too challenging for the family to breastfeed, it is important that the clinician provide reassurance that the family should not feel guilty as the infant will still receive the necessary nutrition to grow from formula feeds.

If the family chooses to breastfeed, the first 2 weeks of life are the toughest as breastfeeding patterns are established. Breastfeeding parents may feel that they have been reduced to a milk machine at this point. The clinician can help them see the broader perspective as well as provide practical management advice. The setting of family priorities (feeding for the infant, rest, and good nutrition for the breastfeeding parent) may have to be explicitly laid out.

Observation of feeding in the office offers the best opportunity to assess the synchrony that is developing between parent and infant. In addition, direct observation offers

BOX 8.2   Knowledge About Successful Breastfeeding for Pediatric Clinicians

The following specific criteria will help clinicians accurately assess the success of early breastfeeding and provide timely intervention to prevent excessive infant weight loss or diminished maternal milk supply.

Schedule of Feedings

An infrequent feeding schedule is a common, preventable cause of insufficient milk. The birth parent must be prepared to nurse the baby whenever the infant signals readiness to feed, such as increased alertness, sucking motions, or rooting. Crying is a late sign of hunger.

Breastfed newborns should nurse approximately 8 to 12 times in 24 hours, usually taking both breasts at each feeding. A breastfeeding parent should nurse their baby every 1½ to 3 hours during the early postpartum weeks. A single longer night interval of 4 or 5 hours between feedings is reasonable. Nonnutritive sucking on a pacifier should be discouraged until a consistent pattern of acceptable weight gain has been established. Nondemanding babies should be aroused to feed. The intrafeeding interval in days 2 to 4 of life and at any time of a growth spurt may be *very* short, an hour or so. The duration of feeding should be approximately 15 minutes per breast, during which the infant suckles actively with short pauses. Infants are unlikely to obtain sufficient milk by sucking less than 10 minutes per breast in the early weeks of life. Conversely, marathon feedings that last more than 50 minutes are usually indicative of ineffective nursing. Older breastfed babies often nurse very efficiently and take the bulk of their feeding in only 5 to 7 minutes per breast, although they may nurse longer for comfort. Very short feedings may mean that the infant only gets thin foremilk. The high-calorie, fat-rich hindmilk follows the sense of letdown. It is this milk that results in real weight gain.

Infant Behavior and Appearance

Reports of the infant's behavior during and after nursing can provide important clues about the quality of feedings. Well-fed infants should act satisfied after feedings and sleep contentedly. Hyperbilirubinemia in breastfed infants is a common marker for inadequate breastfeeding, a condition known as "breastfeeding jaundice."

Once milk has come in, a mother should hear her baby swallow regularly during feedings and see evidence of milk in the baby's mouth. These observations are somewhat subjective, however, and do not always correlate with objective measures of milk intake. Generally, a breastfed baby should appear satisfied after nursing and sleep contentedly until the next feeding. Persistent crying or excessive need for a pacifier often signifies infant hunger and suggests that little milk was obtained during feeding.

Exaggerated physiological jaundice in a breastfed infant is a common marker for inadequate breastfeeding. Whenever unexplained unconjugated hyperbilirubinemia is present in a breastfed infant, evaluation of the infant's nutritional status is warranted. The baby is probably getting insufficient milk to push the bilirubin out via the gut and kidneys. Strategies to improve the effectiveness of breastfeeding should be implemented whenever "breastfeeding jaundice" is diagnosed. Formula supplements may be necessary to provide adequate nutrition, but breastfeeding need not be interrupted.

Infant Elimination

A newborn's pattern of voiding and stooling provides one of the most sensitive historical indicators of the adequacy of milk intake. Always inquire about infant elimination patterns.

Shortly after the milk comes in, a thriving breastfed newborn should void colorless urine at least six to eight times daily. With inadequate infant intake, mothers often report a "brick dust" appearance in the diaper, which is caused by precipitated urate crystals. Dark yellow, scant urine or visible urate crystals beyond 3 to 4 days of life strongly suggest that a breastfed infant is not obtaining sufficient milk. *Beginning about the fourth or fifth day of life, well-nourished breastfed infants typically pass sizable (not a small stain), loose yellow "milk stools" after most feedings.* Between about 4 days and 4 weeks of age, a thriving breastfed baby should pass at least four such "milk stools" daily, often resembling a mixture of cottage cheese and mustard. Dark transition stools, infrequent bowel movements, or scant volume of stools in a young, breastfed infant are common indicators of insufficient milk intake. However, beginning around 1 month of age, stooling frequency may gradually diminish in breastfed infants, although stools remain soft and easily passed.

---

opportunities for support, specific suggestions, and direct reflection on the baby's behavior. It should be a set part of the examination at least once in the first 2 weeks of life and more often if the adjustment process seems to be progressing slowly or with difficulty. An effective way to observe nursing or feeding without altering standard office routines is for the office nurse or medical assistant to suggest that a feed occurs after measurements are taken, while waiting for the clinician or as the history is being taken. The clinician is then able to observe nursing or feeding. A planned office visit within the first week enables the clinician to intervene if difficulties are identified. Optimally, the visit should be planned within 1 week after hospital discharge for new parents and those with a rocky start and no longer than 2 weeks for mothers with previous experience. In communities where home visitation programs are available, office visits in the first few weeks may be adjusted to coordinate with the home visit.

POSTPARTUM STRESS, ANXIETY, AND DEPRESSION

Parental adjustments to a new baby do not come automatically nor do they emerge in a neutral emotional atmosphere. Some turbulence occurs in most families. Having postpartum "blues" is a normal, transient phase in the adaptation process for the birth parent that occurs within the first week after birth. Crying, confusion, mood lability, anxiety, and depressed mood are symptoms. They last a few hours to a few days and generally have few negative sequelae. Most birth parents experience this phase as a mild form of depression. It may be related to exhaustion, physical depletion, and hormonal shifts. Contributing factors are pain, sleep deprivation caused by demanding caregiving responsibilities, as well as major shifts in roles. Household and other childcare duties may be overwhelming. While letting go of the former household dynamic, the family begins to incorporate this "new person," who generally upsets most established home routines and patterns, such as mealtimes, talk times, social activities, and sexual patterns. Being home all day and pausing career or academic pursuits often add to the ambivalence and role conflict many new parents experience. Economic uncertainty may also compound the stress. A single parent's difficulty during this time may be heightened by their sense of aloneness if supporting individuals or groups are not available. Existing family stresses usually get worse rather than better at this time.

As a result of these factors, new parents must cope with many unanticipated feelings. They are often overwhelmed by the chaos that this new baby seems to have created. The clinician is an important resource during this period of heightened dependency and uncertainty. Studies have shown that birth parents who experience physical problems during pregnancy, pregnancy-related anxiety, or stressful life events in the perinatal period are more likely to struggle with postpartum adjustment and have an increased risk for antepartum and postpartum depression (PPD). However, protective factors such as social support and resilience weaken the association between these risk factors and the development of postpartum depression.

The clinical features of severe depression are quite different from these "baby blues." Postpartum depression affects up to 13% of females; however, it may be under identified, since recent research shows that one in eight mothers were not asked about symptoms of depression during a postpartum visit. Additionally, due to exclusion from research, the rates of PPD among transgender males are unknown, although in one study 35% of participants self-reported symptoms of PPD. Its symptoms may include sad mood, heightened anxiety, immobilizing indecision, attention deficits, irritability, and changes in sleep and appetite. Excessive guilt and dysphoria may also be present and last at least a week and often longer; individuals experiencing PPD may also interpret their infant's behavior in a more negative light as well. The usual onset is within the 30-day period after birth, but it may be later. Most new birth parents resolve these feelings by 6 to 8 weeks after delivery, although some studies suggest continuing symptoms at 6 months. Birth parents may experience a prolonged depressive state accompanied by sleep disturbances, anorexia, constipation, agitation, and a sluggish effect. They may develop an altered way of thinking that is a radical departure from the prenatal personality, such as talking about past, present, and future events in a negative or unrealistic way. Suicidal ideations, delusions, and hallucinations, as seen in the most severe forms of postpartum depression, may occur and can be identified through routine PPD screening (see resources).

Some caregivers will adjust over time as they build greater sense of competence, which providers can reinforce at each visit. However, many caregivers need additional supports, which can include referral to an integrated behavioral health or mental health provider; group health supervision visits; and short-term professional counseling and/or medication, even hospitalization. Psychosis is rare, but it occurs more frequently at this time than at any other point in a parent's life, and it will be the child health provider who is the most likely professional to have the opportunity to identify this serious condition. Most studies report high rates of recovery from the acute phase of this illness.

Birth parents with the following characteristics may be more vulnerable to severe depression in the postpartum period (although there is still significant disagreement within the literature on this matter):

- A history of psychiatric illness in oneself or in close relatives
- A history of substance use
- Poor marital relationship
- A recent loss (e.g., death of parent)
- A history of past or present thyroid illness
- Isolation, with other major life stressors

- Family history of severe depression
- Parents of infants born preterm or with other illnesses/conditions

Assessing Postpartum Depression

Every child healthcare provider should have available some systematic screening process to evaluate postpartum depression or the presence of caregiver depression in general. There are formal screening tools such as the Edinburgh Postnatal Depression Scale (see Appendix), as recommended by the American Academy of Pediatrics Bright Futures project.

Making it even simpler, a report by Olson and colleagues (2005) that has since been endorsed by the US Preventive Services Task Force suggests that if just two questions, requiring less than a minute, posed to a parent by the primary care physician are positive, there is a high likelihood of significant depression. These questions are: (1) During the past month, have you often been bothered by feeling down, depressed, or hopeless? (2) During the past month, have you often been bothered by having little interest or pleasure in doing things?

Caregiver depression and mental illness are pediatric issues. Although the caregiver's well-being is clearly at risk in this circumstance, the baby's is too. Mothers with depression touch their infants less, speak to them less, and are less responsive to their vocalizations. Even brief periods of depressive behavior have profound effects on the infant's behavior, including a decrease in infant's activity, less vocalization and play interaction participation, and less smiling of the infant. Poorer developmental outcomes and more behavioral problems are more likely in children of caregivers with depression. This may be indirectly caused by the lack of reciprocal, serve-and-return interactions with the infant. The infant depends on the parent to learn about their effectiveness in acting on the world to begin to establish a sense of self; when they struggle to elicit a sensitive response from their caregiver, infants may become more withdrawn or irritable. Many adverse child-rearing conditions, such as poverty, isolation, and substance use disorders, may affect the infant through the medium of caregiver depression. Therefore the pediatric clinician has enormous potential to improve the outcomes of both parent and child through addressing depression and other serious mental illnesses. Parents often ask the pediatric clinician whether it is OK to be taking antidepressants or other medications when breastfeeding. The research is very clear that preventing and treating severe depression and suicide is the most important. It is important to reassure the caregiver that they are improving the child's developmental and emotional outcomes by adequately managing their own mental health.

REACTIONS OF OLDER SIBLINGS

Sibling rivalry is a predictable, normal, and healthy response to the birth of a new brother or sister. In most families, it demonstrates that the older child is appropriately attached to their caregiver and is responsive to a perceived threat to their relationship. It is a normal response to having your place as the baby of the family usurped. In this context, the emergence of behavior that reflects sibling rivalry should be viewed positively. It is normal that older siblings will show ambivalence toward the baby, as evidenced by an ongoing shift between positive and negative behaviors.

Behavioral manifestations of sibling rivalry can take several forms, such as the following:

- *Aggressive* behavior is directed most commonly toward the mother, but it may also be directed toward the baby, other caregivers, playmates, self, or toys. Aggressive behavior most often occurs when the older sibling is a toddler. Increases in this behavior will probably occur when the new baby becomes more engaging socially at 4 to 5 months of age and again when becoming mobile during the last half of the first year. Open hostility may be reduced to more subtle behavior directed at the infant, such as pulling the pacifier out of the baby's mouth or taking a toy away.
- *Naughtiness*, or doing things contrary to family rules, occurs frequently at times when the caregivers are busy with the baby. This strategy serves to both increase tension in the household and verify the continuing power of the toddler to alter the behavior of those around them. A careful history of when such behavior occurs may highlight to the family for the first time that it is not "random," but dependent on a particular situation.
- Some children are *overly compliant* to or overly solicitous of the infant. Perhaps the child fears being totally replaced if they misbehave, so the child becomes "extra good" to ensure their place in the family.
- *Regressive and dependent behavior* is usually seen in the form of clinging and demanding. Other possible types of regressive behavior include sleep disturbances, stuttering, thumb sucking, bedwetting, eating refusals or demands, and baby talk. These responses serve to see whether one can get the same attention and care as the infant. They are also the expected response to any stress and demand for adjustment.

Behavioral manifestations of sibling rivalry generally decrease but may not entirely disappear during the year after the new sibling's birth. Eventually, the older child becomes confident of a new place in the family, with its status and privileges. Additionally, the older sibling usually develops a separate relationship with the younger child as the latter becomes more fun, more responsive, and interactive. Young babies are not much fun and are usually quite a disappointment to a child initially.

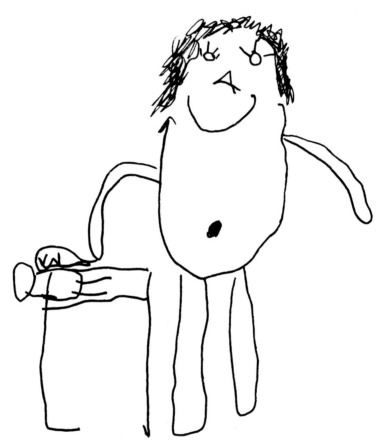

"Mom changing baby's diaper." By Eric Ries, age 6½.

The arrival of a younger sibling can evoke positive behavioral changes, as well as negative ones, even in the early get-acquainted period. Dunn and Kendrick report gains in the older child's independence and mastery, particularly with regard to self-help skills (e.g., dressing and feeding). The child may gain new skills and a growing sense of competency through participation in the baby's care. Siblings may be able to reflect on their own growth and development as they see the baby's emerging capabilities. The older sibling may try out new ways of dealing with the little stranger, such as initiating and maintaining interactions in which they bear the burden of greater understanding, or they may make the infant laugh, play games, and imitate. This is an opportunity for the reinforcement of such behavior by the caregivers. Ways to support the older child are laid out in Box 8.3.

Factors That Influence Rivalry

Certain factors have been shown to intensify an older child's *negative* responses at the time of the sibling's birth:

- A very intense, tight relationship between the first child and the parents before the baby's arrival is correlated with the child's increased hostile and aggressive behavior.
- Extremely withdrawn behavior is more likely in children whose birth parents experience severe postpartum exhaustion or depression.
- Evidence is conflicting regarding the effects of child spacing on the sibling's response, that is, whether a narrow age gap intensifies rivalrous behavior. There is, however, some general agreement that the birth of a sibling in the second year is more stressful than in the third year and beyond.

The child's own issues and coping strategies differ at varying ages, but an adjustment period appears at all ages. Temperamental characteristics (see Chapter 2) are also a major contributor to the nature and intensity of a sibling's response to the birth of a baby. Children who are adaptable to new situations, with positive or mild behavior changes when separated from a parent, usually have a similar behavioral response to the birth of a newborn. They come through with mild and/or short-lived reactions. Temperamentally challenged siblings who are less tolerant of change in routines or novel situations are more likely to have sleep problems and clinging behavior and to lack positive interest in the baby.

Several personal factors negatively affect the caregivers' own response to the child's behavior. Such factors include the caregivers' ambivalence toward the new baby, guilt in feeling less attached to the new baby, and mourning over loss of the previous family structure. Caregivers under stress and those with a strained relationship with the older

---

BOX 8.3 Ways To Help Siblings After The Arrival of A New Baby

- Make time each day for the older child all by themselves without infant demands. Have the sibling decide what to do during that time.
- Be very generous with hugs, cuddles, and kisses.
- Discuss the longer-term advantages of having a sibling, such as having a playmate and being the leader or teacher of a little one.
- Don't force the sibling to share all the toys they had as a baby. Have them decide which ones they are ready to share.
- Praise any positive attention they give the infant.
- Provide the sibling with a stuffed animal or a doll to hold, nurture, and "baby" as their own.
- Be tolerant of behavioral regressions, but keep the rules pretty much the same. Consistency will help the sibling feel safe.
- Invite the sibling to participate in age-appropriate baby care; then invite them again if they initially refuse.
- Allow the sibling to express negative feelings with words, but do not allow any physical action directed against the infant.
- Brag about the older one's accomplishments when visitors come so that the infant doesn't get all the attention.
- Bring out the older one's baby book or pictures of them as a baby so that they get the care and attention that the new child is receiving.
- Avoid pushing him into being a "big boy" or "big girl." Respect their need to try to be a baby again without abandoning the general house rules.

---

child are likely to see more rivalry. Parents may be surprised, embarrassed, or disappointed to see the older child's rivalry after their concerted prenatal efforts to prevent it. Caregiver's shame and guilt for "abandoning" the older child are confounded when the older child acts out in very negative ways. Trying to coercively control the interaction with the infant has been shown to foster a more antagonistic response between siblings. Certainly, the caregivers' physical exhaustion in caring for the new baby diminishes their ability to meet the other child's needs physically and psychologically.

Extreme responses in siblings may be markers of long-standing family adjustment problems, not just that associated with the infant's birth. The child's clinician may be the only professional to see the family at this time of crisis when the issues are very close to the surface. They are then able to suggest more extensive support for the family as a whole, such as through home visiting or family-based therapy. This may be a window in time in which parents are open to getting outside help for long-standing issues.

Social Support and Parental Leave

Specific families and cultures show wide variation in the type, extent, and duration of support given to a new family. Supportive care may include emotional support, baby care, or advice or homemaking tasks. The baby's other caregivers, extended family (especially grandparents), friends and neighbors (with or without children of their own), and various members of the healthcare team may be part of the support structure. Many studies show that the stronger the social network parents have, the better their mental health.

Despite knowledge that the early postnatal period is an important time for caregiver's recovery and parent-infant bonding, the reality for many families in the United States is that parents may be required to return to work shortly after the baby is born, often due to financial needs or a risk of losing a job. Legislation designed to protect job security during leave, such as the federal Family Medical Leave Act, does not apply to all employers or jobs. As of 2022 only 11 US states have paid parental leave policies in place. Clinicians should ask caregivers early on what their plans and needs are for return to work outside the home and should work closely with families to ensure support is in place. This may include connection to programs that can offset some financial strains (such as enrollment in Special Supplemental Nutrition Program for Women, Infants, and Children [WIC] and the Supplemental Nutrition Assistance Program [SNAP]), discussion of feeding plans that can be used when primary caregivers are not present, and an offer to follow up with additional caregivers—such as grandparents or childcare providers—who will be assuming more infant care when the parent returns to work.

Pediatric clinicians should help the parent returning to work advocate for accommodations—such as the ability to sit while doing their job while recovering from delivery or the need for several regular breaks throughout the day for pumping breast milk. Often a signed letter from the clinician can help a parent access support at work that may otherwise be denied. From a pediatric office organization perspective, flexible clinic scheduling helps caregivers who have returned to work or have inflexible work schedule. There are many routine infant visits in the first year of life, so providing additional options such as weekend or evening appointments can help.

Outside of the clinical encounter, pediatric providers should advocate for policies that support families during this key developmental stage, including paid family leave, economic supports (such as SNAP eligibility expansion), and subsidized childcare.

AT THE VISIT

History

To take the history, begin with open-ended questions about the infant—"What new things is the baby doing?" or "In what ways can you tell that the baby knows you?"—and proceed to closed-ended questions, such as the following:

- Ask more focused questions regarding hearing (Does the baby turn to sounds?), seeing (Does the baby enjoy seeing things?), and feeding behavior (How does the baby act while being fed?).
- Ask about irritability episodes and soothing preferences. What seems to work best to settle the baby down? What upsets the baby? How can you tell if they don't like something or enjoying something?
- Activity patterns. How predictable is the baby? How regular are their sleep patterns? Are they easily awakened? How long are their alert periods? Does the baby like their bath?
- Open-ended questions regarding the caregivers' adjustment are also important: How are *you* feeling? How are *you* dealing with this? Are *you* eating and sleeping well?

If any concern appears in what is said and how it is said, have the caregiver describe what happened yesterday in detail. If this elicits a minimal response, explore further by stating possible feelings they may be experiencing ("Many people describe this time as so exhausting and discouraging that they feel overwhelmed and frightened by the responsibility. Some have feelings of regret or even negative feelings about having the baby. Have you experienced any of these feelings?"). Proceed to a more structured assessment if there is any question of depression (see the earlier section "Postpartum Stress, Anxiety, and Depression").

Ask about other caregivers' reactions and involvement. If they have a partner in the home, does the partner hold the baby, change diapers, and help with the housework?

The clinician should also evaluate the siblings' responses, normalizing negative reactions. Although some siblings' adaptive behavior may not manifest until months after the birth of a baby, most have some type of behavioral change or regression. Give permission for the parent to discuss possibly negative behavior with you now or in the future ("Most children show some negative reactions to the new baby at some point. This is a normal response to feeling somewhat replaced."). If negative behavior is described, pursue how it is perceived and handled by the parent.

The availability and use of support systems should be specifically explored, including the emotions that surround those reports. Ask, "How does your family feel about the baby? How is having grandparents around, positive or negative, on a scale of 1 to 10? Are there any friends or neighbors with kids you can depend on? Who is cooking, cleaning, and shopping?" An alone and isolated parent or couple is at high risk for difficulties in the adjustment to parenthood.

The safety of the environment for the caregiver and infant should also be evaluated. It is necessary to screen for intimate partner violence (IPV) in the perinatal period. Ask indirect questions, "How does your partner treat you? Do you feel safe at home?" Once you have established a relationship, more direct questions can be asked, "Has your partner ever hit you, hurt you, or threatened you?" It is also important to ask about and document any past history of IPV the caregiver may have experienced.

Observation

Social development is sensitive to the rhythms of interaction between caregivers and the infant. Point out the infant's body language during the history-taking and examination. This is a wonderful opportunity to inform caregivers about their infant's ability to communicate with them. Note the baby's responsiveness to the caregiver. How easily is the infant consoled? The clarity of the baby's body language is important. Are needs and moods easy or difficult to read? Note the caregivers' sensitivity to the baby's cues. Do they pick up on the baby's subtle behavior that requires parent readjustment? How do they console the infant? Note their effect, level of exhaustion, and relative comfort in handling the baby. Keep in mind individual and cultural differences in the caregivers' sensory mode with the baby (e.g., talking, touching, eye contact, and grooming behavior). The feeding situation offers an excellent opportunity to observe social development and interaction between baby and parent.

If the older child is in the room, observe how this may impact the interaction between the caregiver and infant. Note mood changes in the child and the caregivers' responses. If grandparents or elders are present and they are not the primary caregiver, note their interactions with the baby, the primary caregiver, and other children; are they supportive or dismissive? How do they respond to the baby's distress (e.g., bowel movement, crying)? Are they helpful and consoling? Provide a positive comment about the value of an extended family's presence during the office visit. It is important to keep in mind that in many cultures, if there is an elder present, they speak for the family. This should not be considered a bad thing, but a supportive aspect for that family.

Examination

Direct the parent to sit with the baby on their lap to maximize your opportunity to observe their interactions. The infant should typically turn to a voice at this age, which can be nice to point out to new parents. Interact (play, smile) with the baby to evaluate responses, which you can describe out loud. Observe visual and auditory responses in this context. Encourage the parent to hold and talk with the baby often at home. Explain that narrating activities with the baby encourages and promotes language development.

Give reassurance that the baby cannot be "spoiled" at this age. Holding will, in fact, decrease crying overall. Quick responses to cries, effective soothing, and close human contact lead to less crying in the first and second years and improved emotional health and self-regulation. At this age, infants need close physical contact.

Ask caregivers specifically about their mood, feelings, and behavior and create an open and trusting space for them to express their emotions. Attempt to restore confidence (e.g., "You're doing a good job; it takes a while to adjust to this baby and to get to know one another"). Enhanced self-esteem energizes new parents. Even minor concerns (e.g., diaper rash, mild jaundice) may impinge on the caregivers' feeling of competence. Clinicians should be careful to put problems in a clear perspective and to be unequivocal in their praise and support of positive things about the infant, both physical and behavioral. Be explicit about your availability to discuss feelings further. Make it known that the topics do not necessarily have to center around that infant, but that conversations surrounding family adjustment, coping skills, and relational health are common after a new addition to the family.

Note Reactions of Older Siblings

If an older sibling is present, acknowledge and focus on them first before you go to the infant. Ask specific, separate questions of the older child rather than only asking, "Do you help with the baby?" Give praise for any recent developmental achievements the caregiver may have mentioned or any helpfulness shown toward the parent and baby. Ask about the child's interpretation of the baby (e.g., "Do they cry a lot? Are they not as much fun as you thought they'd be?").

Explain to the caregivers the positive aspects of their older child's behavioral changes. For example, you might say, "Although I'm sure it's frustrating to see your older child behaving this way, it's actually very healthy behavior. They are clearly demonstrating that they are attached to you and highly value their relationship with you." Reassure them that no matter what preparation was made before the baby's arrival, children will have hurt and resentful feelings; this is real and natural. The goal is not to minimize the negative behavior, but to help the older child get through and gain from this experience. Some of the ways to help that happen are the following:

- Acknowledge the adjustment process that everyone experiences when learning to juggle their availability with the needs of two or more children. It takes time for families to settle into new patterns and rhythms. For some families, books for caregivers and children regarding these issues can be helpful.
- Encourage caregivers to continue "special time" with the older child alone on a daily basis; a realistic time frame may be 10 to 15 minutes. Emphasize the importance of physical affection or "snuggle time."
- Encourage caregivers to discuss the new baby's needs and behavior with the older child and to allow participation in the baby's care. Children often benefit from duplicating these activities with their own dolls; these play experiences should be encouraged.
- Plan structured activities for the older child during the baby's bath and feedings so that an attractive distraction is available for the older child.
- The child should not be expected to share all toys, even if they have outgrown them. Reserving some items that are theirs alone and providing a special place in which to keep them are important. Sharing parents with the baby on a permanent basis is hard enough.
- Urge parents to minimize changes in the older child's life for a while. This is especially important for an older sibling who is temperamentally slow to adapt to change. Such changes as moving to a new bed or new room or starting nursery school should ideally occur a few months before the baby's arrival or after some weeks of adjustment.
- Displaced aggression can be released through play (e.g., with modeling clay or a foam ball and bat). Caregivers can also redirect rough affection to the new sibling (e.g., *you can't hug the baby around the neck, but you can kiss their toes*) and help the older sibling understand how the baby is feeling. This is an important opportunity to teach older siblings empathy and mentalization about other people's feelings.
- The need to be tolerant of regressive behavior should be stressed. Most caregivers will be reassured to learn that most lapses in developmental achievements are temporary.
- Review the suggestions laid out in Box 8.3.

 QUICK CHECK—FIRST DAYS AT HOME

- The infant should be alert enough to sustain feedings of at least 10 to 15 minutes.
- Alertness should be brief, at least.
- Fixes and follows a face.
- Responds to a soft voice.
- The dominant posture is flexion.
- Moves all extremities equally.
- The tonic neck response peaks at 6 weeks.
- Hands should gradually show a more open position.
- Head held up briefly when the infant is placed in a prone position.
- Evaluate jaundice and hydration status.
- The newborn hearing test should have been performed and the results should be available.

! HEADS UP—FIRST DAYS AT HOME

Infant Factors
- Does not turn to sound? Check hearing screening
- Excessive weight loss—more than 10%
- Jaundice
- Poor alerting
- Disorganized suck
- Awake/crying or sleeping excessively
- Extremely irritable and/or hypertonic child
- Lethargic and/or hypotonic child
- Any motor asymmetries on examination

Parent Factors
- Depressed (see questions and questionnaires)
- Visible change in self-care status
- Illness or extreme fatigue. Excessive pain
- Misses appointments
- Isolated family, no support
- Partner abandonment
- Suggestion of substance or alcohol use

Interaction
- Caregiver does not hold the infant or appears disengaged
- Caregiver asks few questions and offers few comments
- Caregiver is struggling to interpret the cues of the infant (e.g., has overly negative interpretation of typical infant behavior)
- No joyful play or talk while caring for the infant
- Grandmother or other support person dominating the visit (except in cultures in which that is the norm)

RECOMMENDED READINGS

Support Systems for New Families

Fussell Jill J. Committee on Early Childhood, Adoption, and Dependent Care The pediatrician's role in family support and family support programs. *Pediatrics*. 2011;128(6):e1680–e1684. https://doi.org/10.1542/peds.2011-2664.

Duffee James H, Mendelsohn Alan L, Kuo Alice A, Legano Lori A, Earls Marian F. Council on Community Pediatrics, Council on Early Childhood, Committee on Child Abuse and Neglect Early childhood home visiting. *Pediatrics*. 2017;140(3): https://doi.org/10.1542/peds.2017-2150. e2023062509.

Gedzyk-Nieman Stephanie A, McMillian-Bohler. Jacquelyn. Inclusive care for birthing transgender men: a review of the literature. *J Midwifery Womens Health*. 2022;67(5): 561–568.

Crying and Colic

American Academy of Pediatrics. *Crying and your baby: how to calm a fussy or colicky baby*. 2021. Pediatric Patient Education. 10.1542/peo_document223

Postpartum Mental Health

Biaggi Alessandra, et al. Identifying the women at risk of antenatal anxiety and depression: a systematic review. *J Affect Disord*. 2016;191:62–77.

Urizar GG, Muñoz RF. Role of maternal depression on child development: a prospective analysis from pregnancy to early childhood. *Child Psychiatry Hum Dev*. 2022;53:502–514. https://doi.org/10.1007/s10578-021-01138-1.

Markova G, Nguyen T, Hoehl S. Neurobehavioral interpersonal synchrony in early development: the role of interactional rhythms. *Front Psychol*. 2019;10:2078.

<https://www.aap.org/en/patient-care/perinatal-mental-health-and-social-support/integrating-postpartum-depression-screening-in-your-practice-in-4-steps/>

<https://www.behavioralconsultationandprimarycare.com/wp-content/uploads/2015/07/As-Indicated-Screening-Tools-Chap-8-9.pdf>

Intimate Partner Violence

Taillieu TL, Brownridge DA, Brownell M. Screening for partner violence in the early postpartum period: are we missing families most at risk of experiencing violence? *Can J Public Health*. 2020;111(2):286–296. https://doi.org/10.17269/s41997-019-00266-5.

Jonathan Thackeray, Nina Livingston, Ragavan Maya I, Schaechter Judy, Sigel Eric. Council on Child Abuse and Neglect, Council on Injury, Violence, and Poison Prevention Intimate partner violence: role of the pediatrician. *Pediatrics*. 2023;152(1): https://doi.org/10.1542/peds.2023-062509. e2023062509.

Helping Siblings Prepare

<https://childmind.org/article/preparing-child-new-sibling/#:~:text=Bringing%20a%20new%20baby%20into,few%20extra%20minutes%20of%20playtime>.

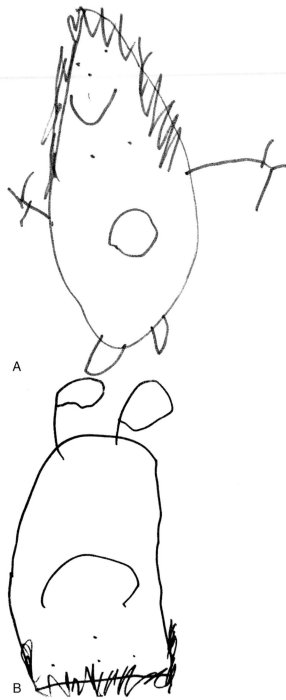

A

B

A 4-year old draws his parents topsy-turvy. Many families feel that way with the arrival of a new child.

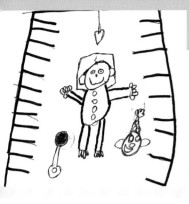

9

One to Two Months: Adjusting to the World

Caroline J. Kistin

This chapter reviews early infant feeding and growth, including physical development milestones and the determinants of inadequate growth across childhood. Infant sleep and crying behaviors are often on caregivers' minds at this age and are discussed here as well. Caregivers may experience postpartum depression or feel overwhelmed at this stage, and many may also have returned to work or be planning to return to work in the near future. The role of the clinician in supporting the infant and family is discussed in the context of parent-child interactions, family relationships, and connection to community resources.

KEYWORDS

- Feeding and growth
- Sleep behavior
- Crying/infant colic
- Caregiver well-being

IMPORTANT DEVELOPMENTAL CONCEPTS AT THIS AGE

The period of an infant's early life bounded at one end by the first month and at the other by the third month represents a transitional time. Having adjusted in the neonatal period (including postpartum physiological changes and the new environment of the family), the second month of life is often a settling-in time for the infant and parents. The baby's rapid changes in weight and length focus the caregivers' attention on feeding and physical growth, and concerns about the adequacy of the infant's intake often occupy much of their thoughts. In addition, infants at this age often start to sleep for longer stretches at night, although there is great variability at this stage. Fussiness and crying commonly peak in intensity around 6 weeks of age, between the 1-month and 2-month visits.

Original chapter by Martin T. Stein.

Increased infant alertness during the day provides many opportunities for social and verbal interactions at this age. More frequent periods of visual attention and the onset of reproducible cooing sounds join the development of a reciprocal social smile in pulling parents into an infant's world. These early developmental strides are associated with postnatal structural maturation of the brain and the rapid growth in brain volume at this time; head circumference increases by 5 cm during the first 3 months of life, the most rapid period of postnatal brain growth. The formation of new synapses occurs especially in the motor and visual cortex, and cortical maturation leads to inhibition of the more primitive brainstem functions. A spontaneous smile emerges, and maturation of the visual cortex precedes a reciprocal social smile that develops at 6 to 8 weeks of age. As the infant becomes less dependent on reflex-driven brainstem mechanisms, crying gradually becomes responsive to cortical control and environmental input.

Postnatal experience markedly alters brain development. The synaptic connections that are forming after birth are shaped and controlled by the infant's early experience. Adequate caloric intake and a steady flow of visual, auditory, tactile, and proprioceptive stimuli act together to enhance the early development of the brain. Nurturance on all levels is the theme here. During this early postnatal period, clinicians should be aware of the sensitive interplay between parent-child interactions and infant growth and development. A focus on early relational health—including

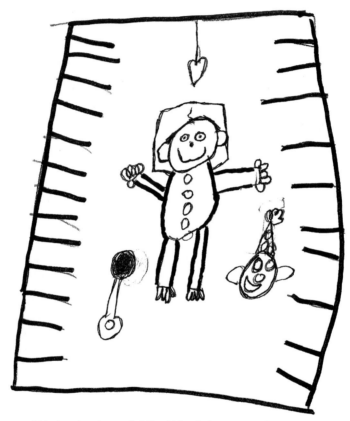

"My brother in a crib." By Abby Roberts, age 6.

supporting positive parent-child emotional interactions and centering the parent and family experience—is key to promoting both infant and caregiver well-being (see Chapters 1–3 and 10 for more detail).

GROWTH ASSESSMENT

From birth until the age of 6 months, infants experience the most rapid rate of growth of their postnatal lives (Fig. 9.1). Infants may lose around 7% to 10% of their birthweight in the days following delivery but should regain that weight by the second week of life. Children then typically gain an average of 30 g per day up to 3 months of age, followed by an average of 20 g per day from ages 3 to 6 months. Length typically increases by 3.5 cm per month for the first 3 months of life, then by 2.3 cm per month from age 3 to 6 months. Head circumference also increases considerably, by an average of 2 cm per month from birth to 3 months of age and then 1 centimeter per month from age 3 to 6 months.

Child growth is influenced by a number of factors. Population studies conducted by the World Health Organization (WHO) have demonstrated that in the first 5 years of life, children grow similarly when they have access to good nutrition and their other needs are met. Early feeding is a complex relational interplay between caregiver and child, and clinicians should work with families to understand the dynamics at play. Parents may find it challenging during this developmental stage to read their infant's hunger and satiety cues for a number of reasons, which can result in both underfeeding and overfeeding. Infants described as "fussy" or who cry a lot, for example, may temporarily soothe when feeding, prompting overfeeding by their caregiver even if hunger is not primarily driving the infant behavior.

At every routine visit, children should have their weight, height, and head circumference measured and plotted on the appropriate growth curve, with the WHO growth charts used from birth until age 2 and the Centers for Disease Control and Prevention growth charts used from age 2 onward. Children with specific diagnoses, such as trisomy 21 or DiGeorge syndrome, should have their growth plotted on condition-specific growth charts. Weights should be measured on a calibrated infant scale with the infant undressed and without a diaper. Length is best measured using a stadiometer. Infants born at a gestational age less than 37 weeks should have their weight, height, and head circumference plotted for their corrected age (current chronological age in weeks minus the number of weeks born before 40 weeks) until they reach the chronological age of 2 years. Cumulative measurements over several office visits are usually more helpful than the measurements at a single point in time in understanding a child's growth and nutrition status.

Children with weight loss after the first 2 weeks of life, a low weight-for-age or weight-for-height percentile, or less-than-expected interval weight gain should be evaluated for factors contributing to poor growth. A complete history and physical examination is the most effective way to uncover the etiologies at play, including inadequate nutritional intake, which is common, or more rare conditions such as malabsorption or increased energy demand. Laboratory studies may be helpful in confirming or ruling out a diagnosis but should be guided by the history and physical examination findings.

Infants may also present with rapid early weight gain, above the average expected in this period. Most of these children will naturally decrease their growth rate between 6 and 12 months of life and go on to exhibit normal growth patterns without any intervention. Clinicians should conduct a thorough history and physical examination. If there are no concerns and feeding appears to be going well, it is reasonable to reassess growth after 6 months without making changes to the diet.

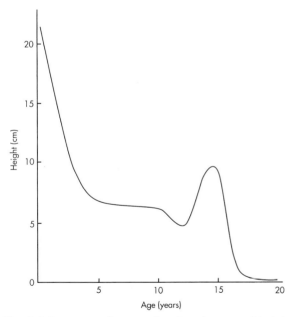

Fig. 9.1 Incremental curve showing the rate of height gain. During the first years of life, the growth rate is more rapid than in other periods. (From Valadian I, Porter D: *Physical growth and development: from conception to maturity.* Boston, 1977, Little, Brown.)

SLEEP PATTERNS

Sleep-awake cycles after the first month are highly variable and dependent on the infant's temperament and satisfaction with feedings and the parents' response to periodic awakenings. This period represents a transitional time between the neonatal sleeping pattern, characterized by shorter, multiple sleep periods, and the postnatal longer sleep periods each day. Changing sleep patterns reflect central nervous system maturation after the third month (see Chapter 10). The 2 standard deviation range of maximum longest sleep time at 6 weeks of age varies from 3 to 11 hours. No wonder parents of infants with shorter sleep times seem bewildered when sharing their infants' nighttime experience with other parents!

Since 1992 after reviewing several epidemiological studies, the American Academy of Pediatrics recommends that infants be placed on their backs to sleep in their own crib or bassinette. The data that supported this position pointed to a dramatic decrease in the incidence of sudden infant death syndrome (SIDS) when caregivers use the "back to sleep" position. After the new recommendation, the prevalence of prone sleeping dropped from 70% in 1992 to about 20% in 2000. The SIDS rate in the United States decreased by over 50%. Firm bedding, breastfeeding, and the avoidance of smoking are also important in SIDS reduction. Babies sleeping on their backs need to spend awake time in the prone position to strengthen arms and shoulder musculature and will also have less occipital flattening.

Positional plagiocephaly (unilateral flattening of the occiput) is a side effect of supine sleeping in some infants but is not associated with any adverse effect on brain development; most cases resolve by the second birthday. Recommendations for the prevention of occipital flattening in infants include prone positioning ("tummy time") when awake, alternating the supine head position (i.e., left and right occiput) during sleep, and minimal time in a car seat when not a passenger in a vehicle.

INFANT COLIC

Parents are confronted with intermittent periods of fussiness in their babies at various times during the initial few months of life. Most parents describe a period of manageable irritability beginning at about 2 weeks of age, peaking between the first and second month, and disappearing by 3 to 4 months. Typically, the fussy behavior begins in the late afternoon and resolves in the evening. Parents often find that if they hold, position, gently rock, or feed the infant, the fussy periods resolve into comfortable sleep. The predictability and inevitability of these events in all cultures and in varying caretaking patterns suggest that such diurnal behavior is part of normal development, probably mediated by the central nervous system. The infant becomes increasingly unable to modulate responses to environmental stimuli over the course of the day and expresses that overwhelm and tension through crying.

When these behavioral outbursts are either more intense or longer in duration, the term *infant colic* is used. Colic is a more severe form of the diurnal behavior seen in the majority of infants. Why certain infants at this particular age (2–3 weeks through 3–4 months) express this behavior with more intensity is unclear. Individual temperamental factors seem to be important. Before a diagnosis of infant colic is made, the clinician should have an appreciation for normal crying at this age. In a study of 80 infants, crying lasted about 2 hours daily at 2 weeks and progressed to nearly 3 hours daily by 6 weeks in healthy infants. It then gradually tapered to about 1 hour daily for 3 months. During this interval, most crying occurred in the evening. With this pattern in mind, Wessel's definition of infant colic is helpful. It says that "colic occurs when an infant, otherwise healthy and well fed, has paroxysms of irritability, fussiness or crying lasting for a total of more than 3 hours a day occurring on more than 3 days in any 1 week, for 3 or more weeks." Many families, however, will present to clinic before 3 weeks have passed, due to the distress of trying to soothe their crying infant.

The etiology of infant colic is unknown and likely represents several underlying contributing factors. Our understanding of infant temperament may provide some insight into the behavior of colicky infants. Temperament refers to an individual's behavioral style of reactivity to external events or stimuli (see Chapter 2). The normal spectrum of infant temperaments is broad. The behavior of babies with a low sensory threshold, high intensity of reaction, and difficulty with self-soothing is similar to those with colic. Babies rated by a parent at 2 weeks of age as having a "difficult" temperament were more likely to have longer and more frequent episodes of crying at 6 weeks of age.

Because colicky babies have been observed to press their flexed hips against the abdomen during the crying episode and then pass gas at the termination of the episode, it has been suggested that these babies have a form of intestinal dysmotility that produces segmental air trapping secondary to autonomic dysfunction. Research on the psychobiology of stress is beginning to describe links between different levels of reactivity and physiological responses in the cardiovascular, immunological, and neuroendocrine systems. Some circulating hormones (motilin) and neurotransmitters (serotonin) that cause enterospasm have been found to be increased in colicky babies. This conceptual framework suggests that colicky infants may tend to have hyperresponsive gastrointestinal tracts that mirror their behavioral response to external stimuli. When colic is accompanied by flecks of blood in infant stool, protein intolerance, and elimination diets for breastfeeding parents should be considered.

Whatever the cause, infant colic almost always resolves by the end of the third month. More severe or prolonged cases of colic require special attention from the child's clinician. Infants with intense crying lasting beyond 4 to 6 months have a higher likelihood of developing sleep behavioral disorders in early childhood. This may be due to inherent child temperament differences but also may be because difficult periods of crying are taxing on caregivers and can potentially disrupt caregiver-infant attachment behavior. Caregivers may develop maladaptive coping responses, such as overfeeding or the use of TV or videos to keep infants calm and quiet (Box 9.1). In extreme cases, inconsolable episodes of crying may lead to "shaken baby syndrome."

An infant mental health clinician can provide important emotional support and coping strategies for caregivers raising a fussy infant. These mental health professionals specialize in the treatment of the caregiver-infant dyad, focusing on issues such as how the caregiver perceives and responds to infant fussing, understanding of what the infant is feeling/experiencing at different developmental stages, and caregiver self-care and self-regulation. In the United States, availability varies by geography—some infant mental health providers are provided through county-level mental health services, others through private practice, and others through the Early Intervention system. It is important to know how to refer for caregiver-infant services in your area, as well as national resources from organizations such as ZERO TO THREE.

CAREGIVER WELL-BEING

Caregiver stress, anxiety, and depression (see Chapter 8) commonly persist beyond the immediate perinatal period. The American Academy of Pediatrics recommends screening for postpartum depression at the 1-, 2-, 4-, and 6-month child visits using validated tools such as the Edinburgh Postnatal Depression Scale (see Appendix). Caregivers with positive screens should be referred for treatment, which may include psychotherapy, medications, or a combination of the two.

As described in Chapter 8, many caregivers in the United States have no paid parental leave, and at the 1- and 2-month visits, parents may already have returned to work. Clinicians should offer support around this transition time and help with feeding, bonding, and sleep recommendations that can be incorporated into the family's new schedule. If the infant spends significant time with another family member or childcare provider while the parent is at work, it may

be helpful—with the parent's permission—to contact these caregivers as well to learn more about how the infant is doing.

In the United States, millions of families with young children live in poverty, which adversely impacts child growth and development. Clinicians should know about the federal antipoverty programs that have been shown to be effective, including the Earned Income Tax Credit, Temporary Assistance to Needy Families, the Supplemental Nutrition Assistance Program, and the Special Supplemental Assistance Program for Women, Infants, and Children, and should understand how to refer eligible families to these programs.

DURING THE VISIT

Observations

As you enter the examining room, observe the interaction between the infant and parents. If the infant is being held, observe the comfort of the parent in handling the baby.

- Does the infant seem at ease? The parent?
- Do the infant's posture and position appear tense with an increase in extension behavior?
- Is there evidence of visual engagement between the parent and infant?
- How does the parent talk to the baby—rhythmically and quietly or erratically and with a harsh voice?
- Is the infant responsive to the parent?

The accumulation of these observations will assist the clinician in assessing the individual style, quality, and intensity of the bond between the parents and infant.

History and Physical Examination

Table 9.1 presents questions that should be asked when taking the history and observations that should be noted during the physical examination.

MANAGEMENT AND GUIDANCE

Growth Concerns

If the measured weight, height, or head circumference are lower or higher than expected, the medical team should first repeat the measurements and ensure the data are plotted correctly on the appropriate growth chart. At this age, the WHO growth chart should be used for most infants, unless there is a condition-specific growth chart, like the Trisomy 21 chart, that should be used instead. Corrected gestational age should be used to plot growth for infants born prematurely.

For infants with weight loss after the first 2 weeks of life or less-than-expected interval weight gain, the most common underlying cause is insufficient nutritional intake. Explore the infant's feeding behavior and schedule with the parent in detail, including what the infant is fed and how it is prepared (if drinking bottles of formula or expressed

BOX 9.1   Infant Fussing/Crying and Screen Media

Screen media—such as televisions, smartphones, or iPads/tablets—provide lights and sounds that infants can entrain their attention on but do not yet learn from. Similar to the effect of visual stimulation from a mobile over a crib, infants looking at a screen may reduce their motor movement and vocalizations—thus appearing "calm." For this reason, TV or videos have become a strategy used by many parents to calm down infant fussing or keep them occupied. Population-based studies estimate that about half of infants watch 1 or more hours of TV/videos per day. In low-income populations, some studies suggest that over half of infants regularly start watching TV by 3 months of age. While some of this screen media use is driven by caregiver factors, including the presence of postpartum depression or having a "media-centric" household (meaning, caregivers and other family members enjoy using lots of media)—some is driven by infant factors. Multiple studies have shown that infants with more difficult temperament, fussing, or intense crying watch more TV/videos in early infancy and into the toddler years. Caregivers may choose to sit their infant in front of TV shows or YouTube videos in an effort to take a break, with the hope that the shows are educational (as many are marketed as such), or because they otherwise feel overwhelmed with managing their household and need a safe way to keep the infant occupied.

However, early introduction of screen media use in infancy has been associated with delays in language, social-emotional skills, and executive functioning. The use of educational programs—such as PBS KIDS or Sesame Street—is protective against these delays, as is shorter usage (<1 hour/day) and when caregivers talk or sing to infants during media use.

What You Can Do

- Start talking about screen media use in infancy; don't assume caregivers will wait until the toddler or preschooler years to start a regular media habit or to get their infant a tablet.
- Rather than asking about "screen time," which can make caregivers feel guilty or defensive, ask about: (1) how they usually get the infant to calm down, (2) how they are adjusting to the new baby with their other life demands, or (3) what their usual morning or afternoon routine is like. These may reveal the ways TV/videos are woven into a family's day, the motivators for screen use, as well as potential points of intervention.
- If caregivers endorse media use in their infant, ask what types of shows they watch. Encourage switching from lower quality videos (e.g., YouTube videos with nursery rhymes, toys, or kid influencers) to high-quality shows from PBS KIDS. Free internet videos or apps are usually created by people with no developmental backgrounds, who aim to make money off of caregiver exhaustion! In contrast, PBS KIDS and Sesame Street have teams of developmental experts who make sure their programs are educational.
- Similarly, encourage verbal interaction such as talking or singing if an infant is watching TV/videos; this helps protect against language delays. Remind caregivers that infants learn *much* better from in-person interactions with their favorite adults compared to images or characters on a flat screen.
- Overall, provide practical and strengths-based ideas for how the caregiver can help the infant calm down, play with the infant, and build their bond without media. Also help caregivers understand that media use in infancy is not educational (because infant brains cannot yet understand it all) and is linked to later developmental delays.
- Use open-minded inquiry to explore with the caregiver how they themselves use media, including when it feels positive and supportive versus when it feels like a waste of time or an avoidant coping strategy for them. Assess their motivation for making feasible media habit changes in the home.
- Offer other ideas for keeping infants occupied while a caregiver gets things done, such as setting them in a high chair with a few toys in the kitchen while the caregiver cooks.
- Involve all family members/caregivers in the conversation, since screen media practices may differ between them.
- If you are concerned about the caregiver-infant relationship and stress in the home, encouraging healthier media use is only a small piece of the solution. Refer for infant mental health therapy or other community-based supports.

TABLE 9.1   History Taking and Examination

History Taking

Clinician's Question or Action	Objective
How are you (parent) doing?	Follow the parent's lead based on how they respond—some may answer with a simple "good" or "fine," while others may take this opportunity to describe their own health or questions they have about their child.
Can you describe your baby's personality? What is the baby like most of the time?	Understand the parent's view of the infant's temperament and style. This question may prompt the parent to describe the parent-child relationship and any stressors as well—some parents may describe their child as "easy" or "difficult," which can open an opportunity for further exploration.
How is feeding going?	Listen carefully to the response to this open-ended question; follow up as needed with specific questions about what the infant is eating, how much, how often, who typically feeds the infant, and how the infant shows they are hungry. If the parent is breastfeeding, ask as well about how they are doing and whether they are having any difficulties. If formula fed, ask how the bottles are prepared.
Does the baby have a fussy time on most days? Can you describe it to me?	Assess colic-like behavior.
Do you think that your baby cries longer than most infants? What do you do when the baby cries?	Help the parent adapt to periods of difficult infant behavior; explain the expected amount of crying.

Physical Examination

Clinician's Question or Action	Objective
Obtain accurate measurements of weight, length, and head circumference plotted on standard growth curves	Assess the adequacy of growth and demonstrate rates of growth on chart to parent.

Clinician's Question or Action	Objective
Complete physical examination.	Although always important at a health supervision visit, performing a careful physical examination while demonstrating normal findings is particularly important to parents with concerns about feeding or a colicky baby at this age.
If colic appears likely from the history, rule out during routine physical examination the following: inguinal hernia, corneal abrasion, otitis media, or a thread wrapped tightly around a finger or toe.	Note: These are uncommon causes of paroxysmal crying at this age.

breast milk), how often they feed, how much they take in or how long they feed at each time, and whether the parent has any additional thoughts or observations about feeding. Of note, when detailing a child's recent intake, a 24-hour recall period is typically more accurate than a longer recall. Parents should be asked about other factors that can impact intake, such as recent illness, or any increased losses, such as vomiting and diarrhea.

Poor growth in infancy is rarely due to a serious underlying illness or condition that has not previously been diagnosed. A thorough history and physical examination should be done at each visit, however. Concerning symptoms such as decreased activity levels or signs such as decreased or increased muscle tone, certain heart murmurs, congenital anomalies, and other findings should be worked up further. Gastroesophageal reflux is common in infancy and does not typically result in weight loss or failure to gain weight. If the infant is vomiting or spitting up after every feed and also has poor weight gain, this should be investigated further.

In breastfed infants, problems with latching on or continuously ineffective sucking are common. Observing a feeding may be helpful. Improving the mechanics of nursing often resolves the problem, such as suggesting pillow support for the baby, helping the infant to latch on effectively, or providing a reassuring comment that it is normal for the baby to suck vigorously, followed by a brief rest period before sucking is resumed. Formula-fed infants may not be receiving enough milk at each feeding, they may be fed too infrequently or the milk may be inappropriately mixed and overdiluted, sometimes in a family's attempt to make formula powder last longer.

Infants with rapid weight gain should similarly have their measurements repeated for accuracy, followed by a detailed feeding history. Signs of overfeeding can include frequent reflux after feeding and feeding primarily to soothe, especially if there are significantly more feedings or volume of intake in 24 hours compared to the expected intake.

Colic ("Paroxysmal Fussing")

The following steps can assist the clinician in treating an infant with colic:

1. Begin with *reassurance*, when appropriate, that the findings of the baby's physical examination are normal. Narrating your normal findings for the parents as you examine each body part may be particularly reassuring.
2. Discuss *"fussiness" and crying at this age in terms of normal patterns of behavior*. A parent with a colicky baby may find it helpful to see the infant as a variation of what is expected rather than as someone who is abnormal. Clinicians can share that colic occurs as part of brain development at this age, as their infant starts taking in more of the surrounding world. This framing can support the caregiver's **mentalization** about the infant's experience and perspective.
3. Recognize how stressful persistent infant crying can be for parents and spend time identifying how parents can take time away when needed. *A frequent antecedent to the shaken baby syndrome is prolonged crying in a healthy infant.* The National Center on Shaken Baby Syndrome developed the pneumonic "PURPLE" as a useful educational tool to inform parents (see Box 9.2).
4. Consider the following recommendations, which may give parents some additional ways to respond:
   - Review soothing behavior, such as swaddling, gentle rocking, or the use of a pacifier. Some infants may be soothed by holding the baby parallel to the

floor and gently and slowly moving them back and forth; this can be demonstrated in the examination room.
   - White noise (a hair dryer or vacuum cleaner) placed near the crib is found helpful by some parents.
   - A mechanical swing may soothe some infants, but with the caveat that infants need monitoring while in swings—due to hunched posture that can compromise their airway—and these swings should not be used for overnight sleep.
   - Formula change is almost never helpful; these babies are not allergic or intolerant of various formulas for the most part. A double-blind crossover study demonstrated that any initial decrease in colic after elimination of cow's milk diminished rapidly and that only infrequently was the effect reproducible. Lactose intolerance is rare at this age.
5. *A positive and optimistic approach is beneficial.* Parents should be reassured that colic is common and time limited. Some measures can be tried, and improvement and resolution may occur. It often means that the parents have discovered new ways to relate to and settle their baby. Frequent follow-up telephone calls are usually helpful and serve to enhance the therapeutic relationship.

BOX 9.2   The Color Purple (Mnemonic: An Educational Tool for Parents to Prevent the Shaken Baby Syndrome)

P—Peak pattern: crying peaks around 2 months **U—Unpredictable:** crying can come and go unexpectedly with no apparent reason **R—Resistant to soothing:** crying continues despite soothing efforts of caregivers **P—Pain-like face:** healthy infants can look like they are in pain when crying even though they are not **L—Long bouts:** crying can go on for 30 to 40 minutes and longer **E—Evening crying:** crying occurs more often in the afternoon and evening

Parent Action Steps to Prevent Shaken Baby Syndrome

1. Discover ways to comfort baby: carry-walk-talk responses to crying.
2. If crying persists and you get frustrated, it is okay to put the baby down in the crib and walk away for a brief time.
3. Never shake or hurt your baby.
4. More information for parents: www.dontshake.com.

QUICK CHECK—1 TO 2 MONTHS

- Hands becoming open, unfisted most of the time.
- A tonic neck peaks at 6 weeks and then decreases.
- By 2 months, briefly holding head up in the prone position.
- Symmetrical motor movements of arms and legs when the head is in the midline.
- Visual tracking to 180 degrees horizontally, briefly vertically.
- Alerts to pleasant sounds.
- Cooing sounds.
- Spontaneous smile.
- More awake time during the day; moving the longest sleep time to night.
- Alert periods increase in length and predictability.
- At 6 weeks, the range of the longest sleep time is 3 to 11 hours.

HEADS UP—1 TO 2 MONTHS

- Postpartum weight loss: up to 7% to 10% of birthweight. Infants typically regain birthweight by 2 weeks.
- After the reacquisition of birthweight, most babies will grow at approximately 30 g per day for the first 3 months of life.
- Occasionally, a baby with a head circumference in the usual or upper range at birth crosses percentile lines in the first few months and is at or above the 95th percentile. When this curve is maintained in the absence of any evidence of increased intracranial pressure, it usually represents familial macrocephaly, a benign, dominantly inherited condition. The measurement of parental head circumference can help with the diagnosis. Rapidly increasing head circumference should prompt additional evaluation, however, including imaging to assess for signs of hydrocephalus and consultation with neurology.
- Any emerging motor asymmetry is abnormal and suggests an upper motor neuron problem (possible perinatal stroke) or a previously undetected peripheral nerve injury.
- Any dysconjugate eye movements should be transitional; fixed strabismus needs evaluation.

RECOMMENDED READINGS

For Clinicians

American Academy of Pediatrics Changing concepts of sudden infant death syndrome: implications for infant sleep environment and sleep position. *Pediatrics*. 2000;105:650.

Barr RG, Hopkins B, Green JA. *Crying as a sign, a symptom, & a signal: clinical, emotional and developmental aspects of infant and toddler crying*. London: Cambridge Press; 2000.

Carey WB, McDevitt SC. *Coping with children's temperament: a guide for professionals*. New York: Basic Books; 1995.

Cohen GM, Albertini LW. Colic. *Pediatr Rev*. 2012;33(7):332–333. https://doi.org/10.1542/pir.33-7-332.

James-Roberts IS. Helping parents to manage infant crying and sleeping: a review of the evidence and its implications for services. *Child Abuse Rev*. 2007;16(1):47–69.

Moon RY, Carlin RF, Hand I. The Task Force on Sudden Infant Death Syndrome and the Committee on Fetus and Newborn; Sleep-Related Infant Deaths: Updated 2022 recommendations for reducing infant deaths in the sleep environment. *Pediatrics*. 2022;150(1): https://doi.org/10.1542/peds.2022-057990. e2022057990.

Pak-Gorstein S, Haq A, Graham EA. Cultural influences on infant feeding practices. *Pediatr. Review*. 2009;30(3):e11.

Shonkoff J, Phillips D. *From neurons to neighborhood: the science of early child development*. National Research Council, National Academic Press; 2000.

For Parents

Karp Harvey. *The happiest baby on the block. The new way to calm crying and help your newborn baby sleep longer*. fully revised and updated ed 2. Bantam; 2015.

Karp Harvey. *The happiest baby guide to great sleep: simple solutions for kids from birth to 5 years*. Harper Collins; 2012.

Murkoff H. *What to Expect the First Year*, ed 2. New York: Workman Publishing; 2003.

National Center on Shaken Baby Syndrome. http://www.dontshake.com/.

Satter Ellyn. *Child of mine: feeding with love and good sense*. Bull Publishing Company; 2012.

Weissbluth M. *Healthy sleep habits, happy child*. New York: Ballantine Books; 1999.

American Academy of Pediatrics: *Depression during and after pregnancy: you are not alone. Healthy children*. https://healthychildren.org/English/ages-stages/prenatal/delivery-beyond/Pages/understanding-motherhood-and-mood-baby-blues-and-beyond.aspx

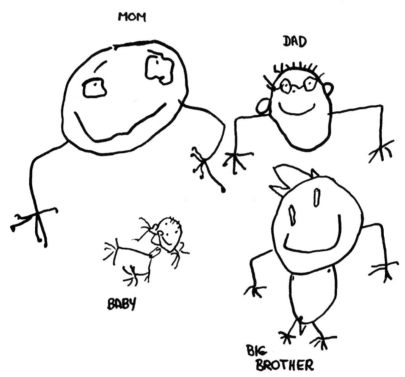

"Our family with our baby." By "Big Brother," age 4¾.

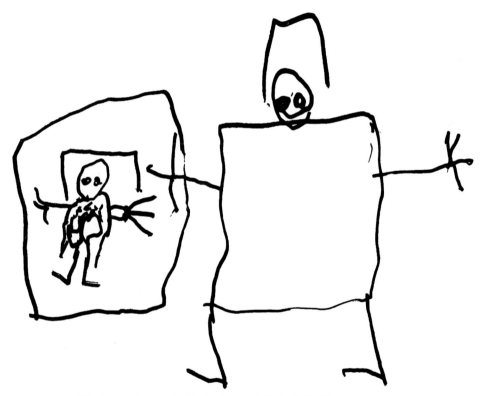

"Dad goes to comfort baby in cradle." By Colin Hennessy, age 4.

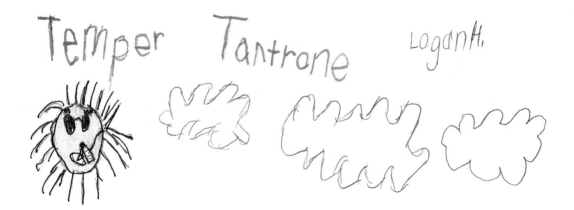

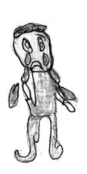
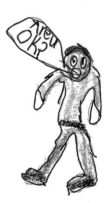

An older boy captures the spectacle of a temper tantrum in a younger family member. By L. H.

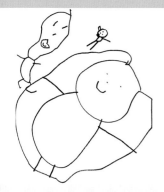

10

Three to Four Months: Smiles and Laughs

Caroline J. Kistin

This chapter examines the role of social interactions in early child development. The importance of learning how to play interactive games as a core prompt to cognitive and emotional development is explored. The impact of caregiver depression on the development of a child is discussed. The emergence of night awakenings at this age and across early childhood is explained.

KEYWORDS

- Social interaction
- Social play
- Temperamental differences
- Sleep organization in infancy
- Night awakenings
- Caregiver depression

A child 3 to 4 months of age is a delightful, engaging creature. A big shift in responsiveness, an expanded behavioral repertoire, social needs, and a unique personality draw caregivers into playful interactions. A decrease in reflex-determined behavior and more predictability in routine often frees up everyone for the next level of parenting, which includes real social interaction. If a caregiver is not going along with this shift or is not having fun with a baby this age, there may be additional factors at play or stressors in the home. Caregivers typically enjoy the baby very much at this stage, and this is often a delightful visit for the clinician. An emphasis on the importance of play and social interaction should be the main focus of this visit.

IMPORTANT DEVELOPMENTAL CONCEPTS

Neurological Maturation

The central nervous system changes occurring at this time prompt both shifts in sleep and new social skills. Increases

Original chapter by Suzanne D. Dixon

in myelination, synaptogenesis (the establishment of connections between neurons with the formation of new synapses), and maturation of the electroencephalogram attest to these processes. Increases in the mobility of the lens in the eye and better optic muscle control mean that the baby can see and track a person close up and across the room. Children can watch their own hands and their actions in the environment while experimenting with distance, size, and depth perception. Refinements in vocalization and facial movements allow a wider range of emotional expressiveness. As psychologist Hanuš Papoušek has stated, there is "a marked qualitative change in higher nervous function at the third month." This organizational level enables the child to interact with the family in new and elaborate ways.

Cognitive Growth

New cognitive skills are evident in the infant's ability to momentarily delay gratification and to make linkages in life events. For example, a child of 3 months will stop crying when placed in the nursing or feeding position and may hold back on vigorous sucking at the breast for a few minutes until milk letdown begins, content in the anticipation of the reward. The infant may smile while being eased into a front pack, linking that event to an expected adventure, and may flex the hips readily when placed on a changing table. All such behavior indicate that children this age have been mentally active in assimilating events that occur consistently. They are observing patterns of association and can anticipate and wait. This behavior can be observed easily during dressing, feeding, or a play session.

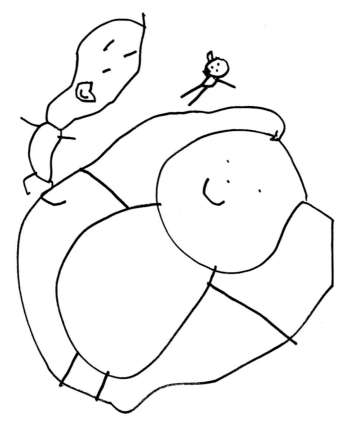

"Happy baby on a blanket with family all around." By Katherine Boucher, age 4½. The baby's presence is large and everyone is gathered around.

Social Skills

The human drive for **social interaction** is never more obvious than in the behavior of a 3-month-old infant. The presence of people is more compelling than any other phenomenon. A 2-month-old infant participates in social exchanges; a 3-month-old can actively *initiate* the interaction with wiggles, smiles, and soft cooing—a whole range of social behavior. The infant draws people into play because that is the fuel for development.

Although studies of parent-infant interactions confirm that infants know their specific parents from the earliest weeks of life, a 3-month-old infant offers very dramatic testimony even to the most skeptical parent. At this age, children will visually search a room until they find familiar care providers, will move all extremities in excitement, and will arch forward with outstretched arms to urge their caregivers to notice, talk, and touch them. Even a temperamentally quiet infant will stop all activity and increase visual regard in their parents' presence. Vocalizing in different ways, such as squeals, laughs, and phony coughs, serves to initiate and sustain an interaction. A 3-month-old has a whole new series of facial expressions to indicate an expanded range of emotional responses and individual personality: pouting, coyness, disgruntlement, teasing, wariness, appearing to be insulted, fearful, bored, and so forth. The infant explores the caregivers' faces through looking at their facial components and then swipes, pokes, and pulls toward them. Parents' clothes, hair, glasses, and skin offer new, safe opportunities to explore the most important part of the environment, the family.

Social Play

In an interactive setting an infant has incredible abilities to respond to subtle behavior (e.g., glances away for fractions of a second) or underlying emotional tones (e.g., frustration, tension). A baby is like a sponge for the emotional tones of the environment. This awareness and sensitivity set the stage for more complex patterns of interaction. The development of "the game" as a concept is strong at this age and is a foundation for later cognitive and emotional growth. A child learns how to prompt and respond to reliable exchanges with the caregiver. Finding the world predictably responsive is the key at this age. Verbal, tactile, vestibular, and motor games are the elements through which the child learns about affecting the behavior of others and that their own behavior has meaning and effectiveness. The infant is developing a sense of self through seeing the results of actions on people and objects. Social game interactions, delivered in the context of caretaking, are the main event of the infant's day. Responsive caretaking is essential for cognitive and emotional growth. The infant needs ready partners for all these games, day in and day out. There is no idle chitchat here; it is all essential for development.

Rhythms, styles, content of games, and the intensity of interactions vary across individuals, socioeconomic groups, and cultures and subcultures, but the basic pattern of game playing with its reciprocal nature, mutually regulated, seems to be a universal pattern of human development.

Infants work hard at **social play**. They are motivated to attend to the social behavior around them and modify their own behavior in response. Familiar people call forth the most attention; unfamiliar adults elicit wariness, an initial unbroken gaze, a tentative bright smile, and then avoidance behavior such as gaze aversion and head turning. A baby will make new relationships with regular interaction, so this is a good time to introduce alternative care providers. A baby will hook new adults into a relationship at this age without the stranger anxiety that will come later. Any caretaker should be attentive to the baby in this need for social interaction, as well as for care.

A caregiver's ability to engage with their child's bids for social play may be disrupted due to a number of factors, including the caregiver's own physical and mental health. Caregivers who are in pain, depressed, experiencing posttraumatic stress disorder after trauma, or coping with additional stressors may have altered sensitivity and responsivity to their infant's activities, which can in turn change the child's behavior and development. Caregiver engagement may also be disrupted by mobile device use, which has been shown to draw adult attention away from the playful infant in front of them.

"SPOILING" BABY

For social interactions and game playing to be successful and meet the infant's needs for responsive caretaking at this stage, some elements are required. The adult must be convinced that these affectionate interchanges are worthwhile. Playing with the infant and holding, massaging, moving, talking to, and nuzzling the baby are not **"spoiling"** the child (i.e., making the infant more dependent or demanding). Babies at this age do not act with premeditation to manipulate and cannot disobey. In fact, the more that caregivers play with the baby, the more the infant will learn ways to amuse themselves. Play is a way of learning, building basic trust, and improving self-esteem. Prompt and appropriate responses build self-sufficiency, not dependency. The world is experienced as a safe, responsive, predictable, and exciting place to be.

Mealtime Adjustments

The extent of the infant's drive for social interaction is very evident in feeding behavior at this age. The baby simply cannot resist looking around, **smiling**, cooing, and poking at their parent's face during a feeding. Distracted by every sound or sight, the child may even stop feeding just to look around. This can be frustrating for parents, as feeding will inevitably take longer. Caregivers may not be entirely ready to change their parenting from the "symbiosis" or tight biological bond of the early newborn period, but they must make this shift and appreciate their children's need for social time during feedings, not just physical nurturance.

The child's new social interest should be highlighted, as well as the tendency to overdose on excitement if given the opportunity. At least two feedings per day should take place in a quiet room without distractions. Television and other media may particularly draw infant attention away from food, and devices should be kept away from the table. Other types of vigorous social interactions should be enjoyed at other times. The social agenda has to be added to the feeding one. Families should adjust to these new demands and see the interactions and the games with the baby as being vital as food. This is a basic change period or "touchpoint" in development, when changes in abilities require changes in parenting.

When Fun Becomes Overwhelming

The seductive behavior of a 3-month-old infant is hard to resist. The baby's smiles, laughs, and total body wiggles are a terrific reward for a few tickles or a play face expression. Some parents, probably most parents some of the time, can push the infant beyond the limits of what the child can tolerate in the way of excitement. Overstimulation can occur if the infant's body language is not heard. Clinicians can coach caregivers in being sensitive to the infant's behavioral cues and recognize signs of "overload" when play must slow down. This pause allows organization of the experience, recovery of attentional energy, and some physiological rest. The required pause may be seconds or hours. Each child manifests stress and overstimulation in different ways. Some children will be more clear in signaling their overload than others.

Some parents may easily pick up on their infant's behavioral signals and pull back; others may need help in understanding the baby's needs and recognizing their child's specific "back off" signals. When a baby disengages, or even cries, parents may feel as though they are a failure. During the course of a clinical examination the clinician can demonstrate a play interaction that is responsive to the individual baby and support parents in recognizing child cues.

Some child behavioral changes at this age are situational and predictable. Young children who are brought for long periods to large gatherings, on prolonged trips to large shopping centers, to siblings' schools, or on long car rides may have a decreased capacity to handle further stress. Sleep and feeding difficulties can be anticipated in these contexts, and quiet containment by a calm adult will help the infant get back under control. This kind of responsiveness restores energy to the child; it does not "spoil" them. Parents who are upset themselves by a child's crying episode should put the baby down or hand him over to another person if they feel out of control.

Temperamental Differences

Temperamental differences in infants' personalities make some babies' bids for social interaction difficult to interpret. For example, one infant may signal interactional readiness by serious regard and be overloaded by all but the most gentle play. This child may be perceived as unhappy or unappreciative of the parents' efforts at interaction. The parents may even feel that the child does not like them. This situation may evolve into a "difficult" or "slow to warm up" style that will continue to challenge parents and clinicians in the days ahead. Sensitivity and low-key responsiveness ought to be pointed out and a subtler style modeled. Reassurances about the child's normalcy and competency must be given.

For most infants, classic "colic" has disappeared by this age, but what may not have disappeared is the highly responsive, intense, and overly reactive characteristics in a previously colicky infant. This temperamental profile may now be evident in an infant who is easily overwhelmed by exciting days, who reacts strongly to changes in routines, and who may have difficulty in falling asleep or restless, disturbed sleep. Vomiting may follow feedings that are frantic and fast, or feedings may be full of wiggles and distractions. The need to anticipate and bypass these buildups, give support at the time of change in routine, and provide quiet times for winding down is evident now. Such actions will establish the healthy interactional patterns that will be needed later and which will support the development of self-regulation in these more dysregulated infants. Individual differences get clearer every day as a child's temperament unfolds. The earlier these profiles are understood, the smoother things will go (see Chapter 2).

SLEEP PATTERNS

By the third or fourth month the state organization and the wake-sleep cycles of the child have shown increased stability and reliability. Most infants have shifted their longest sleep time to nighttime hours and have developed reasonably set nap times. This may be called "sleeping through the night," although a 5- to 6-hour stretch is more usual. Most children do not require a night feeding at this age and can learn ways to settle themselves. Routines for settling to sleep have usually developed between the child and parents, and this predictability gives parents a sense of competence, as well as less fatigue. The child, if left alone, can usually settle back to sleep after the periodic awakenings that occur every 1½ to 3 hours during sleep times. Individual, biologically determined differences are now manifested in these sleep patterns: some children are short sleepers and some are long sleepers. They are likely to maintain these characteristics through the lifespan. An infant at this age usually has two to four naps per day, gradually moving toward two naps throughout the first year and consolidating to one regular nap per day from 18 to 36 months, or longer if a strong environmental push to a nap at midday exists. This pattern varies considerably. Total sleep time, including nighttime and naptime, decreases gradually across toddlerhood, but the actual amount varies from child to child. As children give up naps, their nighttime sleep commonly increases. Sleep at this stage of infancy is less automatic than it was earlier, and its patterns are now altered by care practices. This neurological change means that the family is at a critical juncture at which parents have choices about where and when their child sleeps.

Regularity in the environment helps with sleep organization; a regular bedtime, a regular ritual, and clear expectations are helpful throughout childhood, beginning now, in facilitating good sleep organization (Box 10.1).

Premature infants, even those without serious perinatal complications, may have less regular sleep and have more difficulty falling asleep throughout the first year. Some active children are predictably wiggly at night, and others have a pattern of difficulty settling to sleep. These children need more support from the environment, but *not* qualitatively different interventions. Good sleep hygiene applies to all.

Up at Night

Sleep can be disturbed by periodic awakening at all ages. Some children are able to quietly settle themselves back to sleep without awakening their parents. These children are said to sleep through the night. Individual differences exist in children, in parents, in families, in household layouts and schedules, and even in cultural expectations. In cultures where infants are expected to demonstrate substantial independence in the matter of sleeping, including in much of the United States, being awakened by an infant at night is a violation of these expectations, of the infant and the parent, who it is felt should be able to get bedtime organized. Therefore infants who do not "sleep through the night" may be viewed as developmentally delayed or as a source of stress. In other cultures, where schedules are more fluid and sleep independence is not a goal, "sleep problems" do not exist in the same way. **Night awakenings** are the usual occurrence in all groups because awakenings are biologically based. The introduction of solid food *does not* result in longer sleep times. Most infants by 3 to 4 months of age do not *need* to be fed during the night to maintain nutrition, although many of them and their parents may choose to provide nighttime feedings. Parents can prolong the awakening and sustain this pattern of waking others by responding with an elaborate interaction with the infant at that time. Talk, activities, and game playing will all communicate to the infant that this is a time for play. Quiet comforting, perhaps a quiet feeding, dim lights, and silent rhythmic soothing (e.g., patting, rocking) will signal the infant that this is the time to sleep.

BOX 10.1   Assisting Sleep Organization for Young Infants

- Back to sleep (prone position) in the baby's own crib is the safest sleep position.
- Put the infant to bed when drowsy, not fully asleep, so that the baby gets used to fully settling on their own.
- Put the infant to sleep where you want them to sleep all night long. Falling asleep in one place and trying to get back to sleep in another is confusing.
- Be consistent as possible with sleep times and places. Start a routine.
- Do not respond to the baby's every whimper at night. Give them a chance to settle back down on their own.
- Make your evenings calm and relaxing.

- Examine your own nighttime behavior. Does your vigorous handling and talk give the infant the idea that it is play time? Calm, quiet responses are best. Avoid lifting the infant out of the bed if they sleep on their own.
- Be generous with a bedtime feeding, but limit middle-of-the-night feedings (unless you are consciously strengthening breastfeeding with nighttime nursing). This is a type of trained night wakening.
- If the infant is an early riser but sleeps 6 hours or more, consider a later bedtime. Shift gradually, 30 minutes earlier every 5 days or so.

Sleep at 3 to 4 months of age becomes more vulnerable to outside disturbances, such as loud sounds or bright lights in the room. The excitement of the day's activities may infiltrate sleep time, so settling in for the night or staying asleep may be a new problem when there is a change in routine or household excitement. Some parents who do not get enough time alone with their infants during the day may choose, consciously or unconsciously, to use the night as a private time to get and stay close. For working parents, those without partners, or parents who have experienced a lot of loss, nighttime separation may be challenging. Identifying consistent routines that work for caregivers will help the child organize their sleep behavior at this stage and in the months to come.

Each family must decide a sleep management plan with each child. The clinician should offer information on infancy sleep issues and options and should support families in the development of their own solutions, while providing information and guidance on safe sleep practices including "back to sleep" supine positioning. Questions about what has been going on sleep-wise up to now and the sleep traditions and expectations of the family and their culture are important. The clinician should find out the sleep goals for each so that assistance can be given to reach these goals. This leads to the important choices parents have at this juncture. The age of 4 months is the time to highlight this decision point because a change in pattern will be much more difficult later. A prescriptive approach is to be avoided, but a choice will be made, either actively or by default (see Box 10.1). Consistency in the expectations and the environment is the key from the child's perspective.

THE FAMILY AT 3 MONTHS

Parents should generally be having fun with their infants at this time and are often on or moving toward a new level of parenting—that of attention to the individuality of the infant through playful responsiveness and care. Parents typically both enjoy and appreciate the infant as an individual at this time. Parents of ill or preterm infants, as well as parents who are isolated, stressed, or depressed, may instead experience a lack of joy or engagement in their interactions with their babies, which should prompt additional support, as well as referral to appropriate clinical and community services.

Siblings may reach a new level of organization at this time as well. The baby is now able to enjoy the older child's antics and bids for interaction, provided that they are not too vigorous or overwhelming. The infant will prefer to watch the other child if not overloaded or stressed. The infant's sleep stability and the parents' more rested state allow a little more time for the older child's separate time with the parents. The infant should be adding energy to the family at this time in the form of love, delight, and active appreciation of the life around them.

Caregiver Depression and Altered Interaction

Maternal depression, and the association with child development, has been studied more than paternal or other caregiver depression. Maternal depression may be influenced by poverty, family stress, and other difficulties, which are also known to have an adverse effect on a child's development. Depressed caregivers may be less likely to respond to infant bids for attention, which can lead to altered interaction patterns.

It is also clear that depression (maternal or otherwise) is a treatable condition, with positive outcomes for both parents and children. It is vital to identify and intervene with a parent and infant who are not having fun with each other. Joy in the interaction is an important observation; its absence is a signal for prompt intervention. This is probably the core evaluation to be done at this stage of infancy. The American Academy of Pediatrics recommends screening for postpartum depression at the 1-, 2-, 4-, and 6-month infant visits, using the validated Edinburgh Postpartum Depression Scale or the Patient Health Questionnaire. Caregivers with concern for depression on screening, by history, or during the clinical encounter should be referred to behavioral health services for further assessment and treatment. In addition, clinicians should screen for food security and other basic needs and connect families with supportive community resources which may help with necessities and decrease overall stress.

SUMMARY

The visit at 3 to 4 months is about joy, delight, and fun. This is not a frivolous agenda. When we look at the essential tasks of infancy—the development of trust, a sense of self-effectiveness, and a positive emotional state for learning and growth—this visit gives us a chance to look at the emergence of these core developmental tasks. With these insights, we have a chance for long-lasting positive intervention. It is through parent-infant exchanges that these vital forces for growth are activated. As stated by Stanley Greenspan in a reflection on the importance of these early interactions in infancy:

The self now exists in relation to others. It is aware of shared pleasures and joys and even of loss and despair, as when the caregiver doesn't return the infant's overtures. the consciousness that (now) embraces the human world—the sense of shared personhood as critical to the development of an individual's feeling part of the human community—flowers out of these early and enduring interchanges.

The clinician has the chance to observe, support, and even participate in these most vital processes.

DURING THE VISIT

What to Observe

- Are the caregiver-infant interactions in the examination room, including undressing, holding, and waiting, sprinkled with game playing, dialogues, and toy object play?
- Does the infant visually scan and auditorially monitor the room with an active search?
- Does the infant monitor your approach and initiate an interaction on a smile cue alone?
- Are the infant's hands open, active, and meeting in the midline?
- Is the infant beginning to make verbal exchanges with the parent?
- Does the baby invite interaction? How? What's the baby's style?

What to Ask

The following are questions the clinician should ask the parents during the visit:
- Are you enjoying the baby?
- What games do you play together?
- Describe the baby's personality. Are they like you? Like others in the family?
- Has the baby's schedule changed? In what way?
- Has your schedule changed (e.g., returning to work)?
- Can you predict the infant's behavior from day to day?
- What things does the baby do to settle into sleep? What are your bedtime routines?
- Can the baby amuse themself for a time?
- Can the baby wait for feedings if you call or pick them up? Does the baby stop crying just with anticipation?
- Does the baby awaken during the night?
- What does the baby do to settle back down to sleep?
- Has the baby discovered hands and feet?
- Does the baby play with both hands together?
- Does the baby respond to sound and visual objects easily?

- Does the baby bat at things?
- Can the baby hold onto simple toys?

Examination

During the examination the clinician should ask herself the following questions:
- Does the baby coo (ahs, ows, i.e., open vowel sounds with the beginning of labial consonants), smile, or laugh? Does the baby do this without a prompt?
- Are the baby's hands active? When visually regarding things, does the baby swipe, reach, or grasp at things?
- Are the baby's reach attempts symmetrical?
- Have the primitive reflexes disappeared (e.g., tonic neck reflex, grasp reflex, Moro reflex, and walk-in-place reflexes)?
- Can the child lift head and hands up when prone?
- Does the baby look at and follow you across the room?

Modeling of play interactions during the examination—or noting how nicely the caregiver is playing with the infant—may be particularly important to parents. Point out the baby's smiles as social elicitations. Develop a verbal or tactile game with the infant to see the response. Point out the infant's signs of overload or avoidance during the course of the physical examination or even with undressing. Does the child look away, arch the back, change color to pale or mottled, or get fussy or frantic in movement? Consciously stop, pull back, and point out the infant's behavioral recovery. When is the baby ready to deal with you again?

> ### QUICK CHECK—3 TO 4 MONTHS
> - Waves hands and arms at the sight of a toy
> - Bats at object (such as a stethoscope) and may grab it
> - Holds onto a toy placed in hand. Shakes a rattle
> - Holds head steady when held in a sitting position
> - Head up to 90 degrees when in a prone position, up on hands
> - Rolls back to abdomen
> - Laughs and squeals
> - Initiates smiling
> - Symmetrical postures and movements
> - Follow a person across the room with eyes and head
> - Brings toy to mouth
> - Alerts or turns to sounds at the sides
> - Holds and examines own hands, scratches, clutches at clothes or examination table paper
> - Has a variety of facial expressions

⚠ HEADS UP—3 TO 4 MONTHS

- Infant Issues (Based on Corrected Gestational Age)
- Be alert to any asymmetry in movement. Hemiparesis shows up at this time with asymmetrical arm or leg movement.
- A hypervigilant infant may have compromised hearing. Check the neonatal screen, test sound localization with your voice but without vision, and order a hearing test if there is any doubt in any of these.
- If babbling shows a decline instead of an increase, also consider hearing loss.
- Hands should be open and all extremities in an easy, flexed position. If not, consider abnormalities in the neuromotor system.
- The infant should have enough head control to come up with a pull to sit and should maintain head control in a supported sit position.
- The infant should notice and follow a person across the room. Consider visual or generalized neurological concerns if not.
- The infant should be having their longest sleep at night with a pretty predictable schedule overall. If not, discuss care practices and expectations.

Parent Issues

- The parents should be enjoying the infant. If not, ask open-ended questions like "How is it being [name's] parent?" to explore the parent's mental model of their infant, any perceived difficulty, or difficulty reflecting on their experience as a parent. These may be signs of depression or trauma.
- Parents with concerns about sleep problems need to have this situation assessed and some intervention performed. Sleep difficulties may stem from difficulty with sleep routines and environmental factors including crowded housing or noise and light in the home. Spend time exploring potential contributors.
- Does the parent respond specifically to the infant's style and behavioral cues? Observations during weighing and measuring and after immunizations may reveal the parent's response to various stresses.

- Parents should be cautioned about overstimulation in toys, lots of background television (i.e., keeping the TV on when no one is watching), social interactions, and stressful events. Excess fatigue because of loss of the ability to handle environmental disturbances is a pitfall to be avoided. In considering any changes, think of ways to make the least number of alterations.
- The surge in activity often produces an increase in appetite and growth. It also means feedings may be more disrupted by wiggles and giggles.
- Emphasize the importance of holding and playing. Infants cannot be spoiled at this age. The baby should be near someone whenever awake.
- Siblings should receive cautious permission to interact with the baby under supervision. Help them learn what is too much.
- Babies at this age do not typically need to be fed at night, although their parents may wish to do so to maintain milk production if breastfeeding.
- Good sleep rituals begin at this age. The baby should be put to bed in a drowsy state without a bottle and with a quiet, calming song, poem, or pat.

RECOMMENDED READINGS

Erickson N, Julian M, Muzik M. Perinatal depression, PTSD, and trauma: impact on mother–infant attachment and interventions to mitigate the transmission of risk. *Int Rev Psychiatry.* 2019;31(3):245–263.

Field T. Infant sleep problems and interventions: a review. *Infant Behav Dev.* 2017;47:40–53.

Muzik M, Borovska S. Perinatal depression: implications for child mental health. *Ment Health Fam Med.* 2010;7(4):239.

Moon RY, Darnall RA, Feldman-Winter L, Goodstein MH, Hauck FR, Task Force on Sudden Infant Death Syndrome SIDS and other sleep-related infant deaths: evidence base for 2016 updated recommendations for a safe infant sleeping environment. *Pediatrics.* 2016;138(5): e20162940.

Rafferty J, Mattson G, Earls MF, Committee on Psychosocial Aspects of Child and Family Health, et al. Incorporating recognition and management of perinatal depression into pediatric practice. *Pediatrics.* 2019;143(1): e20183260.

ANTICIPATORY GUIDANCE

The clinician can offer parents advice and assurance about a variety of issues that arise at this age:

- The importance of the child's own active exploration of the world should be emphasized.

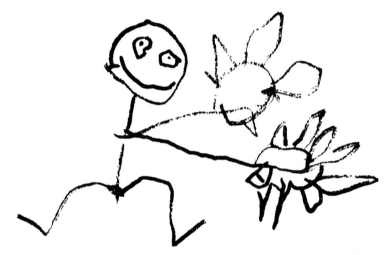

"Smiling kid." By girl, age 5½.

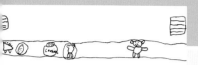

11

Six Months: Reaching Out

Caroline J. Kistin

The chapter describes the general principles of motor development and tracks the emergence of reaching, grasping, and hand movements from infancy to the preschool period. Sitting, self-feeding, and the importance of tummy time are discussed.

With discovery of their hands and the power of a simple grasp, the 5- to 6-month-old infant goes on to learn what to do with these new skills. Anything the infant sees can now be explored in an active way. The texture, temperature, shape, and malleability of objects become new dimensions of the world that add interest and excitement to the child's life, as well as enhanced learning opportunities. The eyes, hands, and mouth work together in this exploration. Reaching and grasping have a direct link to cognitive growth because such skills allow for the active learning that is fuel for mental growth in infancy. The specific way that the skills of reach and grasp are refined during infancy and how these changes make interaction with the external world possible are the focus of this visit. Observing child's hand movements and skills at this age and beyond will not only tell us about motor development but also allow us a window on cognitive development and social engagement with the environment. This chapter is designed to build clinical skills in the monitoring of manipulative behavior in early childhood.

Original chapter by Suzanne D. Dixon and Michael J. Hennessy.

BASIC PRINCIPLES OF MOTOR DEVELOPMENT

The pattern of acquisition of skills in this area illustrates several observations about **motor development** in general:

- *Primitive* reflexes disappear before *voluntary* behavior appears. For example, the grasp reflexes must be gone before voluntary grasp begins. It is not clear whether these reflexes are subsumed into voluntary patterns or disappear to set the stage for non–reflex-driven behavior.
- Development follows a *proximal-to-distal* progression. This is evident in control proceeding from the shoulder to the fingers. **Reach** with shoulder muscles precedes **grasp** with forearm and hand muscles. Control moves from the shoulder down to the fingers and from the hip to the ankle (see Chapter 13).
- The emergence of motor skills follows a relatively predictable sequence, but the timing and style show variation from child to child. Some environmental supports or constraints influence this process, although the sequence remains constant.
- Variation in motor development occurs in the *rate* of maturation of skills, with the timing at each stage being poorly predictive of the time at which the next stage will emerge.
- *Pronation precedes supination*. Palm-down maneuvers, such as picking up objects, occur before palm-up maneuvers, such as putting objects in the mouth or transferring objects.
- *Action and movement precede inhibition*. A child holds onto objects before being able to release them. Inhibition of a movement already started is harder than

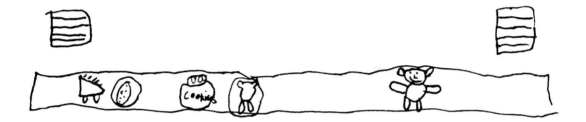

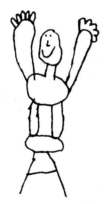

"Reaching out." By boy, age 7.

never moving in the first place. Once a reach is initiated, it is difficult for the child to stop. Once an early walker takes off, it is hard for the young child to readily stop. Starting and moving come under the child's control before stopping or changing course.

- The *exact* way a skill (e.g., grasping, forward progression) is completed each time varies; every attempt is a new behavior in that sense. In fact, *lack* of variability in such behavior, with rigid or stereotyped patterns of reach, may indicate an underlying developmental delay or disability. The ability to modify motor actions in an ongoing process of learning and adaptation is a characteristic seen in infancy and throughout life in the course of skill development.

CHANGED PERSPECTIVES ON MOTOR DEVELOPMENT

The process of motor development is no longer conceived of as the inevitable rolling out of skills based solely on neuromotor competencies but rather an interactive process influenced by the child and their environment. Physical growth coupled with neural maturation, the child's internal motivation, and their drive to mastery create new movement possibilities and patterns. New skills then emerge within the context of the child's physical environment and social-emotional interactions with caregivers and others. Old skills evolve into new skills as these forces work together to prompt growth in an ever-changing way. This view of a *dynamic systems approach* to motor development, nested within the *relational system* of the caregiving interactions, allows us to see the vital interplay between child, caregiver, and environment in the emergence of motor skills (see Chapter 2).

Opportunities to exercise and use new skills in ever-changing ways and circumstances are created by a supportive environment, in which caregivers support the active practice of skills and **scaffold** adaptation to mildly challenging conditions through play. This can be accomplished by ensuring infants have ample safe space to move on the floor and by encouraging them to build on motor skills they have already mastered. Once a child is able to grasp and lift a rattle, for example, their caregiver can then provide them with an object that is slightly heavier, differently shaped, or further away. Children develop and hone motor skills by using internal drive, maturing motor competencies, changing physical characteristics, and environmental prompts. Adaptation is specific to the mix of these factors within each child and the active interplay with their surroundings.

THE REFLEXES

The grasp reflexes are presented in Table 11.1 and Fig. 11.1. These reflexes have a predictable course related to central nervous system (CNS) maturation. From the child's vantage point, these reflexes allow tactile interaction with the

TABLE 11.1 Types of Grasp Reflexes

Reflex	Elicitation	Response	Emerges	Disappears
Mental	Touch chin	Hands close	Birth	At 6 weeks
Palmar	Touch palm between thumb and index finger	Hands close	28 weeks of gestation	2 months
Traction	Stretch shoulder adductors and flexors	All joints of the arm flex	2–3 weeks, weakens at 6 weeks	Up to 5 months
Instinctive grasp reaction, orientation A	Light touch to radial side of the hand	Open and supinate hand	3–4½ months	4–5 months
Instinctive grasp reaction, orientation B	Light touch to ulnar side of the hand	Open and pronate hand	5½–6 months	6 (?) months
Groping	Light touch to hand on the side	Hand will move toward stimulus	6–7 months	7 months (onset of reliable volitional grasp)
Grasping	Light touch to side of the hand	Hand will grasp object	6–7 months	7 months (onset of reliable volitional grasp)

surrounding world (Fig. 11.2). The asymmetrical tonic neck response, which peaks at about 6 weeks of age, facilitates the infant's exploration of the hands. The infant is able to see what interesting things the hands are by turning the head to the outstretched hand even before having the strength and coordination to bring the hands up in front of the face in the midline. The influence of the tonic neck reflex either before its full peak or after it wanes is such that muscle tone increases on the side of the body to which the head is turned. This means that all neurological maneuvers during a physical examination should be done with the head secured in the midline so that extremity motor tone is symmetrical. Consistent asymmetry in reflexes or their persistence beyond the expected departure date should cause the clinician to evaluate the child's overall neuromuscular development.

DEVELOPMENT OF REACH AND GRASP

Early Infancy

The precursors of reach and grasp are in the form of coordination of visual processing with hand activity, the presence of grasp reflexes, and some early reaching behavior. A newborn in the quiet/alert state who visually fixates on a pleasant sight will begin to have mouthing movements, the hands will open and close, and after considerable latency, the infant will swipe toward the midline with the hand and arm working as a unit. The feet and toes may also be activated in this process, closing and opening. A neonate will reach up to touch the breast or bottle while feeding, a skill that goes away in a month or two. Infants as young as 4 weeks respond differently to objects that are in their range of reach than to those that are beyond that range;

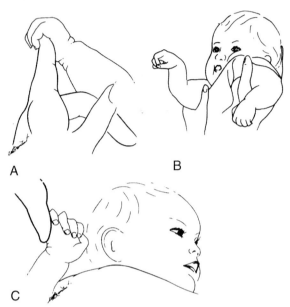

Fig. 11.1 Grasp reflexes. (A) Reflex palmar grasp. (B) Traction orientation grasp, type B, ulnar. (C) Instinctive orientation grasp.

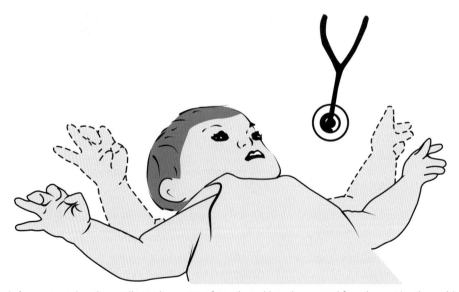

Fig. 11.2 Early infancy contains the earliest elements of reach and hand-arm and foot-leg activation with the presentation of interesting sights.

BOX 11.1 Reach

- Arm and hand activation: 6 weeks–2½ months
- Closed hand reaching: 2–3 months
- Hands open with reach: 4 months
- Accurate reaching: 6 months
- Anticipatory hand shape and movement: 9 months
- Coordinated timing of hand closure with reach: 13 months

they will swipe at reachable and touchable objects but not at those that are out of range. Such behavior shows a primitive visual-motor linkage. Infants may even show the ability to differentiate their manual approach to two-dimensional versus three-dimensional objects with a curved swipe to the latter and a flat swipe to the former. Coordination of systems is present from the start, even though accurate completion of the task and efficient control of hand movements may be months down the road (Box 11.1).

In this earliest form of infant reach, vision may initiate the reach but does not control it accurately: the infant cannot make ongoing corrections of efforts toward an object after starting a swipe toward it. This lack of fully mature coordination ability makes success very unlikely at this stage. Additionally, a young infant will reach out in the dark for a pleasant sound, although success is unlikely here as well. In later infancy, reach becomes more finely tuned with vision and more adjustable based on visual input. Reach in the dark without vision will rarely occur after 6 months of age.

An infant initially swipes with the whole hand and arm as a unit, with initiation of movement at the shoulder. Hand grasp will occur only if the hand touches something. This early type of volitional reach disappears at about 7 weeks of age. In a typical clinical setting, we rarely see it because we do not wait out the long latency period needed for this behavior to emerge, unbind the infant's arms, or provide the truncal support that is needed to see these skills. Caregivers may note that the baby reaches up to touch the breast or bottle when feeding or swipes at a mobile or toy while lying in a crib. The **development of reach and grasp** is detailed in the following milestones:

- *Mutual hand grasp* is observed around 2 to 3 months of age after a decrease in the tonic neck response. The infant really starts to explore their hands when this happens.
- By 5 months the automatic grasp responses to objects touching the hand have largely disappeared, although remnants may linger for years. *Volitional grasp* is prominent now and acts independently from reach (i.e., the

hand moves separately from the shoulder). Increasing bulk and control of the shoulder musculature, as well as truncal strength and stability (i.e., sitting with slight or no support), enable reach to be more reliable at this age as well.

- Fixed-extension postures at the shoulders or weakness of the shoulder girdle musculature, often present in a premature infant, may prevent the child from reaching out. Applying external support with an increase in flexion at the shoulder (e.g., a rolled towel or small blanket behind the shoulders) often helps this group of children develop these reaching abilities. For children with persistent truncal hypotonia, external supports may be needed to free up the hands for exploratory work.
- By 3 to 6 months the hands should be loosely fisted at rest and both hands activated when the infant attempts to reach. Repeated failure to see one arm or hand move when the other extends should prompt further evaluation, as should persistently tightly fisted hands, with thumbs tucked inside.
- By 6 months the child should *reach across the midline* when the contralateral hand is restrained, although both hands are usually activated when a reach is started.
- By 6 months the *thumb fully participates* in grasp, although full thumb opposition may not be present until 2 to 3 months later.
- A few simple items in the office allow the clinician to be a good hand watcher with minimal effort. For a child in an alert state and comfortably supported, these observations are easy to set up (see Box 11.3).

Grasp Development

Volitional grasp matures with increasing control at the wrist and with increasing use of the fingers as separate units. A grasp with the whole hand is typically used for medium objects, and a raking grasp is used for small objects at first. Control of grasp then moves to the fingers as a unit, including the thumb, which is kept to the side of the hand; the result is an "inferior pincer" for small objects and a flat rather than cupped-hand grasp for larger items. When the tips of the fingers are used to deftly pick up a small object with the thumb across from the index finger ("opposed"), this is termed a pincer grasp. The pincer grasp is used naturally only with visual coordination; we all revert to raking for small objects in the dark (Fig. 11.3).

Even before the complete pincer grasp is evident, the *index finger* takes the lead in grasping and exploring objects. Poking at things, particularly into holes at 8 to 9 months old, testifies to this maturation of specific finger skills and is usually coincident with the pincer grasp. It also means that electrical outlets, buttons, cracks, and other dangers become very attractive for this exploring first finger.

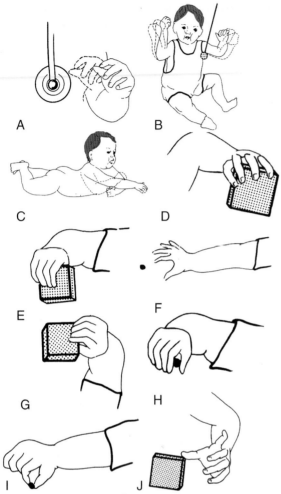

Fig. 11.3 Progression of reach and grasp. (A) Nondirected swiping, 1 month. (B) Swiping, about 4 months. (C) Corralling, about 4 months. (D) Ulnar-palmar grasp of a cube, 4–5 months. (E) Radial-palmar grasp of a cube, 6–7 months. (F) Raking of a pellet, 6–7 months. (G) Radial-digital grasp of a cube, 7–8 months. (H) Scissors grasp of a pellet, 7–9 months. (I) Pincer grasp of a pellet, 9–10 months. (J) Voluntary release, 9–10 months.

Grasp of medium-sized objects, such as small blocks, shows a similar progression from use of the whole hand and palm at 7 months to increasing use of the fingertips and finally to use of the index finger and thumb to stack the blocks "deftly and directly" (see Fig. 11.3). The hand goes from a flat approach to a cupped position as the thumb moves down and around an object and the fingers splay out around the object.

The child shows increasing ability to anticipate the shape and weight of an object (Table 11.2; see Fig. 11.3). That is, as the child begins consistent grasp or reach, near the age of 6 to 8 months, the hand position and the arc of movement of the arm and hand reflect the shape and distance away from the object sought, as shown in Fig. 11.4. As the baby begins to go after an object, the hand position, angle of arm movement, and postural adjustment show that the properties of the desired object are understood and that these concepts are transferred from the visual system to the motor system. This system coordination, vision and reach, and the higher level of integration that it implies can be seen even in children who cannot successfully execute a reach or a grasp, such as a child with athetoid movements, weakness, hypertonicity, or an arm in a cast or splint (see Fig. 11.4). The clinician should look at the *quality* of the grasp attempt and the basis for it even when task accomplishment remains incomplete. Although difficulties with visual-motor tasks will be more obvious as the child becomes capable of drawing tasks (see Chapter 4), they may be evident at this age if the clinician watches these aspects of reach and grasp.

After 6 months of age, reach and grasp are separate. That is, the child can grasp a nearby object without a reach and can first reach for an object and grasp it only when it is near. This uncoupling is an example of the increasing efficiency of the motor system with maturation.

Between *5 and 7 months*, visually directed corrective movements can be seen in patterns of grasp. That is, the child watches the hand and alters its moves to more closely accommodate the object's shape, distance, and texture, even if these change while reaching. These ongoing corrections affect both the direction and the velocity of movement. Grasp is more specific, efficient, and smooth.

Volitional reach at this time is two handed and symmetrical, at least at its start. The child "misses" and "overshoots," occasionally getting the object batted into the opposite, available hand.

Between *7 and 11 months*, diminishing dependency on bimanual reach can be demonstrated and consistent single-hand reach becomes evident. The transfer of objects is an outgrowth of these midline activities (Fig. 11.5). Wrist movement comes in *after 1 year* and wrist rotation *at about age 2*. Doorknobs and other latches become vulnerable after that time.

The interest and vigor in the infant's investment in the manipulation of objects at this age make it both easy and exciting for parents and clinicians to begin to be "hand watchers." Point out these signs of visual-motor development during your examination, to help caregivers understand how the brain is developing. A dangling stethoscope, a red ball of yarn, or even a pencil can be used to watch the emergence of these hand and hand-eye skills throughout the first year (Box 11.2).

TABLE 11.2   Progression of Grasp

Age (months)	Term	Pattern Components
1	Nondirected swiping	Arms and legs activated, often beginning with a startle; long latency; hands and mouth may open
3–4	Swiping	Moving arm up and down in an attempt to contact objects
4	Corralling	Reaching out with an entire arm and hand and sweeping the arm toward the body
4–5	Ulnar-palmar grasp of a cube; rotates the wrist	Fingers on the top surface of an object press it into the center of the palm, thumb adducted, wrist flexed
6–7	Radial-palmar grasp of a cube	Fingers on the far side of an object press against the opposed thumb and radial side of the palm, wrist straight
6–7	Raking grasp of a pellet	Raking an object into the palm with an adducted, totally flexed thumb and fingers
7–8	Radial-digital grasp of a cube	Object held with opposed thumb and fingertips; space visible between
7–9	Scissors grasp of a pellet	Object held between the ventral surfaces of the thumb and index finger
9–10	Pincer grasp of a pellet	Object held between the distal pad of the thumb and index finger
9–10	Voluntary release	Drops objects when desired

Modified from Bayley N: *Bayley Scales of Infant Development*, New York, 1969, Psychological Corp; Erhardt RP: *Developmental hand dysfunction: theory, assessment, treatment*, Laurel, 1982, RAMSCO; Knobloch H, Stevens F, Malone A: *Manual of developmental diagnosis: the administration and interpretation of the revised Gesell and Amatruda developmental and neurologic examination*, New York, 1980, Harper & Row.

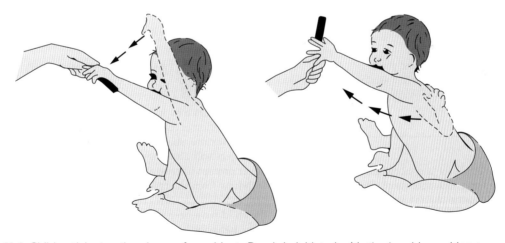

Fig. 11.4 Child anticipates the shape of an object. Reach is initiated with the hand in position to grasp the object, dependent upon the object's shape and position.

USE OF TOOLS

The use of tools to extend, amplify, and specialize our hand movement distinguishes humans from most lower animals. After a child learns how to use the hands well—reaching, grasping, transferring, manipulating—they learn to extend the functions of the hand through the use of objects. These instruments or tools allow them to reach farther, to act on things in new ways, and to do things that would be impossible through the use of hands alone. Although this seems

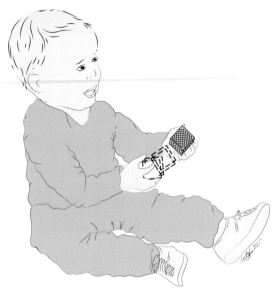

Fig. 11.5 Transfer of objects from one hand to the other.

BOX 11.2   Grasp

- Regards toy: newborn
- Activates with reachable toy: 1–4 weeks
- Holds onto toy: 1–2 months
- Hands open: 2½–3½ months
- Grasps toy near hand, palm: 4–5 months
- Two-hand grasp: 4–5 months
- Rotates wrist: 5–7 months
- Unilateral reaching: 6–7 months
- Grasps two things in each hand: 7–8 months
- Scoops (rakes) a pellet: 6–8 months
- Inferior pincer: 6–10 months
- Pincer: 7–12 months

---

like a simple progression, it is conceptually an enormous developmental step that allows for more elaborate exploration of objects. It is, at the child's level, the dawning of the age of technology. Progression of the *use of instruments* at this new age is shown in the following stages:

- First comes the discovery that banging one thing against another makes an interesting sight and sound. Putting objects together in the midline and banging one object on the table demonstrate this first step.
- The second stage is the realization that an object extends reach, such as seeing that a stick can get a toy that otherwise would be out of range. The instrument becomes a *hand extender*, doing the same thing as the hand, only farther afield.

- The next stage is the finding that a tool can do something *different than the hand*. This progression goes on through childhood with increasing agility with specialized tools that do more and more complex things, farther removed from the simple actions capable of the hand alone. For example, the child discovers that a spoon can scoop material that would otherwise squish between the fingers on the way to the mouth. Children start to use spoons at around 1 year, but they are rarely adept at doing so until closer to 2. Forks do things very differently than hands do and are generally used by 3 to 4 years of age. Skill with a knife, which requires both hands doing different but coordinated actions, will take years, into school age at 5 to 6 years. Scissors are commonly used at 3 years.
- Over time, the child's hands become more adept at using these specialized tools, with more coordination between the hands, increasingly separate use of the fingers, and each hand separately and differently threading objects; the use of simple musical instruments is an example of these "tool tasks." The developmental course of figure copying and other paper and pencil tasks is presented in Chapter 4.

At each stage, caregivers may observe that frustration, fatigue, and stress cause children to go backward in the demonstration of skills. For example, they may use their hands to eat or may tear something rather than cut it, even when they have previously successfully used utensils and scissors. This is an expected, temporary occurrence that usually resolves after a brief period.

ENVIRONMENTAL FACILITATORS AND DETRACTORS

Several factors may influence both the emergence and the demonstration of reach and grasp behavior. Characteristics such as texture, shape, thickness, distance, and density of the object will also play a part because these factors will either prompt interest and adaptation or cause the child to withdraw from the task. Objects with varying shapes, colors, and characteristics that can be perceived as novel by the child have been shown to provoke the most manipulative behavior by infants (Fig. 11.6). As in other areas of mental development, *moderate novelty* elicits more activity on the child's part. An environment filled with a variety of safe, reachable, graspable objects provides fuel for development in this area. For some children who are more sensitive to all or some textures, this means a gradual, gentle approach to the consistent presentation of a variety of types of these objects.

Some infants may show specific delays in visual-motor activities even when other areas of development have

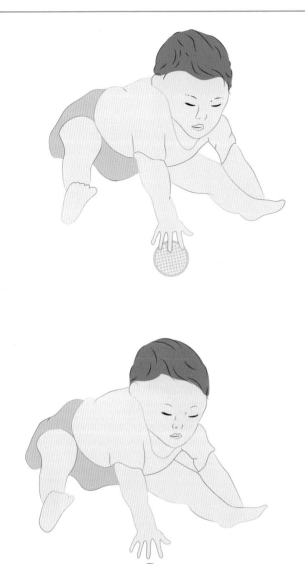

Fig. 11.6 Sitting steadily with the hips abducted enables a child to stretch to the limits of his play space and use vision effectively in going after objects of varying size and texture. Adjustment to the size of the object will only occur when the child actually touches the object.

appeared to follow expected patterns. Infants with even mild shoulder girdle weakness, which may not have previously been appreciated, may present with a lack of hand monitoring, for example. The clinician should pay particular attention to visual-motor coordination during routine visits from infancy into school age. Practice with hand/eye tasks should be included in any intervention program for children with delayed skills.

Tummy time, where the child spends time on their stomach in the prone position, is essential to develop good visual-motor skills and can progress as the child grows. This position is illustrated in Fig. 11.7. In early infancy, tummy time is often best done with the infant on the caregiver's chest. As the child develops the ability to lift and control the head, they may be placed in the prone position on a mat on the floor, initially with a rolled blanket or other support under the upper chest and then on their own. Tummy time should start off in short intervals and gradually increase as the child develops strength and skills. Caregivers can support their infants by getting down on the floor face to face and talking or by holding up a mirror or other interesting toy for the child to watch.

MOUTHING BEHAVIOR

Mouthing of and at objects should be expected in the majority of young children because it is an integral part of the infant's early exploration of objects, as part of the reach and grasp sequence. A child at 3 to 5 months and beyond goes after things with hands and mouth together, sucking at things that look interesting and bringing everything to the mouth when able. As reaching and grasping skills mature, children learn to explore their world with increasing hand-to-mouth activity. Within limits of cleanliness and safety, it should be praised and encouraged. With cognitive growth the child learns more specific and complex ways to explore particular objects, and mouthing behavior disappears in typically developing children (Fig. 11.8).

Feeding provides the optimal exercise for these emerging fine motor skills (Fig. 11.9), but hunger or lack of food is not the usual reason for mouthing. Foods with varying texture and size are a great way to get a child interested in **self-feeding**, as well as in learning more about the world. As soon as a child can sit with stability and is eating solids, self-feeding should become another laboratory for cognitive growth. If this period of maximal interest in hand activities and hand-to-mouth behavior passes without such an opportunity, a long-term diminution in hand-to-mouth behavior may result. Self-feeding will then become a struggle rather than an opportunity.

ASYMMETRIES

Motor asymmetry of reach or grasp in the first 3 to 4 months of life is unusual and may be due to a peripheral nerve deficit or some bone or joint impairment or injury. The signs of CNS injuries, such as those seen after perinatal stroke, may become more pronounced between 3 and 6 months with increasing asymmetry of spontaneous arm and hand movement, an asymmetrical residual Moro reflex, exclusive

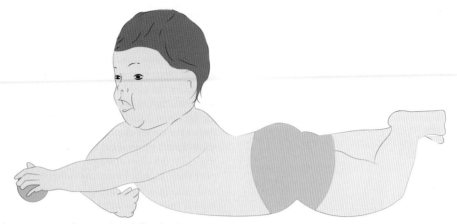

Fig. 11.7 The importance of truncal stability in the prone posture is seen in situations in which the child is unwilling or unable to assume this posture. Reach and grasp are facilitated in the prone position.

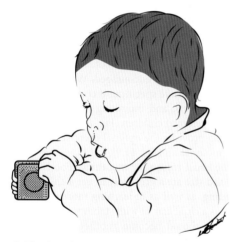

Fig. 11.8 The hands and mouth work together to explore the world, independent of hunger and adequacy of the feeding situation; this is to be encouraged.

use of one hand, or asymmetries in movement when the child is upset. Differences in the maturation of reach and grasp between one side of the body and the other, from reflexes to volitional movement, may also signal a central lesion. Such differences may be observed in free play and exaggerated when the child is crying. Failure to use both hands to pull a cloth off the face also adds to evidence of central dysfunction in this age range. Asymmetries of this type should always be evaluated further. By 6 months both hands should be used in this maneuver, perhaps with one

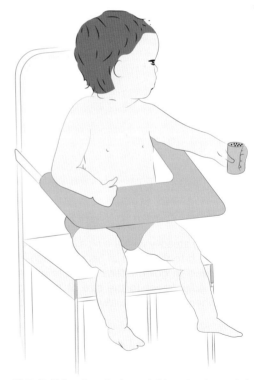

Fig. 11.9 Self-feeding is best initiated when sitting is steady, reach is unilateral, and grasp is at least scissors in type. The multiple sensory inputs in this situation and opportunities for exploration make it an exciting (though messy) part of the day.

predominating or leading as part of the early emergence of **handedness**. The lead hand can usually be identified by careful observation, but clear hand dominance before 18 months is not typical and calls for additional evaluation.

HANDEDNESS

A child gradually comes to use one hand more frequently than the other; this hand is termed *dominant*. There are many ways to define dominance. A practical definition for the pediatric clinician, though somewhat arbitrary, is that the dominant hand is the hand used consistently to hold a spoon, preferred to stack blocks, hold a crayon, or throw a ball. It may or may not be the strongest hand.

Handedness is the most commonly observed manifestation of lateralization in the brain. In a child between 1 and 3 years the dominant hand becomes more and more apparent. Dominance appearing earlier than that most often indicates impaired peripheral or central control of the other hand. Normally, clear and consistent handedness is not fully established until 4 to 6 years of age, with most children being right handed. Mixed or indeterminate dominance is seen in a higher proportion of children than adults, thus suggesting a continuum of increasing lateralization with age. This process is related to differential functional maturation of the cerebral hemispheres. About 15% to 18% of children will still not have established clear dominance of one hand by school entry.

A strong genetic predisposition to dominance exists. Only 2% of children of right-handed parents are left handed, whereas 42% of children with left-handed parents are left handed. The whole body participates in this laterality of function (e.g., eye, leg, arm, ear), but we focus on hand function because of its central importance in fine motor functioning.

SITTING

With increasing truncal strength and stability a child is able to sit upright with decreasing amounts of support for increasing amounts of time. As **sitting** evolves, the spine increasingly straightens and the hands are used less and less for balance and support. When the hands are needed forward for balance and support, the position is called a *tripod sit* (5–7 months); this gradually emerges to an independent, stable sitting position, first on a regular surface (6–8 months) and then on an irregular or soft one (6–9 months).

As soon as independent sitting is established, the hands are freed to manipulate objects, with gravity as a help rather than the hindrance it was when the baby was confined to their back. Object manipulation takes off when sitting is established, and the two motor milestones are intertwined.

For children with truncal weakness or with hypotonic or hypertonic postures, a delay in the ability to sit means that the learning opportunities provided by object manipulation are curtailed. Devices and activities that give the child support while sitting are worth pursuing so that these play opportunities are available.

The visual world changes greatly when sitting is established. The child now has at least a 90-degree horizontal horizon, which may extend to as far as 270 degrees once the infant can pivot. Truncal strength and flexibility allow increasing control over what is in visual range and what can be reached by hand. When sitting is well established, the child begins to map three-dimensional space. The child turns to follow and then gets a toy going behind them (8–9 months), provided that pivoting is stable. Turning to get an object behind with only a sound cue takes place at 8 to 9 months, as does throwing toys from a high chair to see where they go and, of course, who will retrieve them (Fig. 11.10). Increasing gross motor competency, including stable sitting and hand control, sets the stage for new learning opportunities and novel ways to interact with the environment.

SUMMARY

The emergence of voluntary reach and grasp is the time to look at motor competency, visual-motor coordination, and the relational environment that scaffolds the infant in exploring the object world.

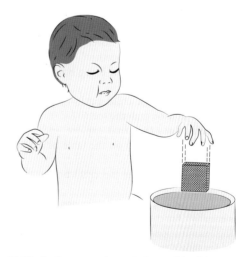

Fig. 11.10 Active experimentation with objects serves the important cognitive work of play. Simple objects allow basic principles to be clear to a young child.

TABLE 11.3   Reach Progression

Action	Age
Visual object pursuit	Birth
Arm/body activation (long latency)	2 weeks–2 months
Sustained hand regard	2–4 months
Arm swipes, bilateral	2–3 months
Alternating glances	2½–4 months
Unilateral arm activity	3 months
Reliable reach to midline	4 months
Reach for object disappearing beyond the visual field	4–5 months
Unilateral reach	4–7 months
Hand-to-hand transfer	5½–6 months
Finger poke	8–10 months
Plays midline games	8–12 months
Visual anticipation of object shape	9–10 months
Throwing objects	9–18 months

BOX 11.3   Reach and Grasp Behavior Sequence: Use of Simple Objects in Assessment

Raisin Behavior

5 months: regards, mouthing, activation
6 months: rakes
7 months: inferior pincer
9 months: pincer

Pencil Behavior

2 months: follows with eyes horizontally
3 months: activates hands, follows vertically
4 months: bimanual reach, opens hands if touching
7 months: anticipates shape with hand opening at the start of reach
8 months: unilateral grasp
9 months: reaches across midline
12 months: makes marks on paper
18–24 months: imitates stroke on paper
30 months: imitates circle
3–5 years: mature hold on pencil

Stethoscope Behavior

2 months: regards across midline, follows vertically
3 months: bimanually swipes; brings to mouth if caught
5–6 months: reliable reach, hands open on contact
6–7 months: reaches across midline if restrained
9–10 months: unilateral reach, with mirroring movements
13 months: unilateral reach with contralateral opening/closing

Block (1×1×1 Inch) Behavior While Sitting

3–4 months: waves at block on the table, holds onto one if placed in the hand
4–5 months: brings both hands to the block
5–6 months: brings block to mouth
6–7 months: picks up with one hand; holds onto one in each hand
7–8 months: bangs block on table
9–10 months: bangs 2 blocks together
10–13 months: stacks 2 blocks
15 months: stacks 3 blocks
18 months: stacks 4 blocks
24 months: stacks 7 blocks
36 months: stacks 10 blocks

DURING THE VISIT

Observations

The clinician should pay attention to how the child uses their hands and mouth in exploration, which will change with age. Age-appropriate motor milestones as delineated in Table 11.3 can provide an assessment scale, along with the following:

- At 1 to 2 months, does the child move the hands and mouth to go after an object?
- At 2 to 3 months, does the infant increase motor activity (wiggle) when looking at a novel object nearby? Does the baby hold both hands together?
- At 4 months, does the child bring both hands to the midline?
- At 6 months, does the child rattle the paper on the examination table or grab the feet?
- At 7 months, does the child explore and manipulate toys, such as hitting them on the table or banging two blocks together?
- At 10 to 11 months, does the child hold a toy out to show you?
- At each time period, does the child use both hands and arms equally? Are the movements smooth?

During examinations from birth through the third year the examiner should present objects toward which the child can reach. Four clean objects are suggested (Box 11.3): (1) a dangling stethoscope; (2) 1-inch cubed blocks with up to six available, beginning at 2 months; (3) a raisin or round cereal bit, beginning at 5 months; and (4) an unsharpened pencil, beginning at 4 months.

The **raisin** offers the child the opportunity to demonstrate fine motor activity with increasing use of the fingers. The pincer grasp should be seen by 8 months. The use of both hands equally during the course of this play should be seen.

An unsharpened pencil or stick can be presented in the midline horizontally and then vertically to induce reach. A 4-month-old should have a bimanual reach and close the grasp if contact is made. A 6-month-old should anticipate the shape at the beginning of shoulder movement by shaping their hand to an accommodating posture. After 1 year the child will readily transfer the pencil and will begin to direct it downward to write. Going from a fisted grasp to an increasingly mature finger hold should be mapped across this time. By 5 years of age, if not earlier, a mature "writing" grasp of the pencil may be the single best predictor of adequate **fine motor skills** for school achievement. Motor tone, the child's posture, and strength and control in the trunk, shoulders, and extremities should be noted throughout the course of the examination. Disappearance of the reflex grasp should be noted to follow the course outlined in Table 11.1.

A dangling **stethoscope** should elicit increasingly smooth tracking with activation of the mouth, hands, arms, and lower extremities in the newborn period. Swiping should begin at 3 to 4 months of age. Reach should be reliable by 5 to 6 months of age, with both arms participating and the hands opening on contact. With one arm restrained the child should reach across the midline. By 9 to 10 months of age the reach should be quite unilateral, although mirroring will be common. Reaching across the midline may not be seen reliably until the second year of life. Movements should be increasingly smooth with increasing use of the elbow and wrist.

A small block should be placed before the child on a surface while the child is sitting on the caretaker's lap. The grasp efforts should proceed as shown in Table 11.2 and Box 11.2. This activity can be done during the history taking. In the second year and beyond, this activity can move along the continuum of stacking blocks and building imagined structures, bridges, trains, and then stairs.

Observe delays or abnormal patterns of the infant's fine motor behavior. Persistence of primitive reflexes will interfere with the emergence of purposeful fine motor skills.

In addition to observing laterality, observe what the other hand is doing. For example, at 7 months, are the hands equal in skill? At 10 to 11 months, is the other hand mirroring the active hand? At 12 to 13 months, is the other hand passive but fisted during a manipulation? At 4 to 6 years, is the other hand passive during a manipulation?

What to Ask

The pediatric clinician should inquire about the infant achieving developmental milestones for reach and grasp as indicated in Tables 11.1 and 11.2 and Box 11.3. These are minimal competencies, and failure to achieve these milestones calls for further evaluation. The following are specific questions to ask parents during office visits (after starting with open-ended questions about how the child is moving and interacting, what new skills the parents have observed since the last visit, and whether the parents have any concerns):

- At 1 to 3 months: Does the baby look at their hands?
- At 4 months: Does the baby swipe at objects within their visual space?
- At 5 months: Can the baby reach for and hold onto toys?
- At 6 months: Can the baby transfer an object from one hand to the other?
- At 7 to 9 months: Does the baby feed themself crackers or other foods?
- At 9 to 11 months: Can the baby pick up a pea, raisin, or a cereal bit between the thumb and forefinger?
- Are there any imbalances, weaknesses, or asymmetries that caregivers notice?

ANTICIPATORY GUIDANCE

Activities at Home

Motor development in infancy and early childhood is promoted and supported through play with caregivers. The child should spend time in a comfortable, safe space on the floor, where there is room to move. Parents can place a variety of simple items nearby to see, touch, and mouth, and the office can model this activity with safe, washable toys.

The parental role as primary teachers for their child is one of facilitating the child's own efforts through careful observation and developing a safe environment for the child's own free exploration. Many "developmentally appropriate" toys are available for purchase, but they do not possess magical qualities in themselves. Good toys are simple, safe, and brightly colored (e.g., blocks and balls) and provide a variety of textures and actions. They also leave room for the child's imagination. Other recommendations at this age include:

- When "table" foods, or foods with more texture than purees are introduced, the child should be free to explore them with their hands. When the pincer grasp appears, the child will participate in self-feeding and effectively reach for and consume small, soft pieces of cooked vegetables, dry cereal, cooked rice, and pasta and cheese. Failure to start allowing participation in and relinquish some control in this area spells the beginning of feeding difficulties.

- Asymmetry of reach or grasp should be taken seriously because it may signal underlying neurological difficulty. Although subtle differences may be apparent, very evident persistent or worsening differences must be investigated. Parents should provide ample opportunities for the child to use the "less mature" hand. However, if these differences persist for 1 to 2 months, further evaluation is indicated; a short reevaluation time is needed in these matters.
- A premature infant or any child with altered tone or strength should be placed with forward shoulder support to allow for good visual monitoring of hand activity. Prone positioning is particularly important in these groups, even though it may take the child a while to accept this position. Chest support will help. When the child is seated, a towel under the thighs flexes the hips, thereby relaxing the trunk and facilitating hand movement.

QUICK CHECK—6 MONTHS

- Sits with minimal support
- Bears weight on feet when held upright
- Rotates wrist
- Picks up a cube from the table
- Rakes a pellet
- Reaches and grasps an object
- Transfers objects from hand to hand
- Grasps and brings feet to his mouth, lying supine
- Makes the phonemes "ba," "ga," "da"
- Up on arms when in the prone position
- Makes sounds with objects (shake, rattle, or bang)

! HEADS UP—6 MONTHS

Motor Delays at This Age

- Children with poor truncal tone or head control, who cannot sit without significant support, are behind in a motor sense. Central and peripheral etiologies should be considered, as well as general physical well-being and strength.
- Both hands should be active, and there should be accurate reaching in the midline.
- Objects should be manipulated in the midline.
- Asymmetrical reaching is unusual and should be investigated further.

Other

- Babbling, or sound units with a consonant and a vowel, should be heard at this age, perhaps even strung together in "phrases." Watch a child who has not said any "ba's" or "ma's."
- Any child with a decrease in vocalizations at this time (or any other) needs a hearing test.
- Children at this age should have a wary look when strangers first approach. Failure to "glare" raises a question of delay in social development.
- Six-month-olds should be very interested in and going after interesting people and objects in the environment.
- Dysconjugate gaze should be resolved at this time. If not, an ophthalmological referral is indicated.
- Solid foods should be started between 4 and 6 months of age. If tongue thrust persists at this age after 2 to 3 weeks of solid feeding, a closer look at pharyngeal function and development is generally necessary.

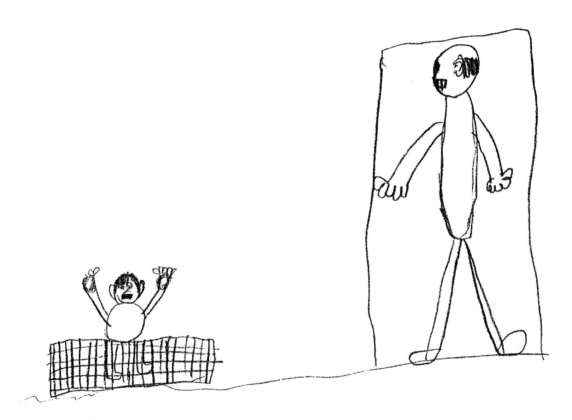

"Dad goes to the playpen to get the baby, who is reaching to be picked up."

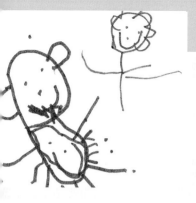

12

Eight to Nine Months: Exploring and Clinging

Caroline J. Kistin and Jenny S. Radesky

This chapter discusses the social and emotional changes occurring in early childhood as attachment with primary caregivers continues to develop and deepen. New cognitive abilities and motor skills at this age provide opportunities for different parent-child interactions and are also associated with stranger anxiety, new safety considerations, and night wakening. Simple play activities are presented as ways to probe a child's development in clinical settings, at this age and beyond.

KEYWORDS

- Stranger anxiety and separation
- Attachment
- The strange situation
- Motor development and exploration
- Child safety
- Feeding and eating
- Sleep and night wakening
- Help with separations
- Assessment through play

The landmark of social development described by Rene Spitz as "stranger anxiety" is reached after the midpoint of the first year. This change from the happy-to-be-with-anyone baby to the screaming child may not appear to be a developmental advancement when first encountered, but it really is a sign of cognitive maturation. This behavior calls for some explanation, requires awareness by all who care for and make decisions about children, and testifies to the huge leaps in development that occur at this age. Play at this age offers a window to look at these new cognitive gains and better understand or mentalize the thoughts, feelings, and desires underlying new child behaviors. Parents can

be reassured that separations, strangers, and mild stressors are opportunities for growth that will support their child's development of coping strategies.

IMPORTANT DEVELOPMENTAL CONCEPTS

Stranger Anxiety

Until now, the infant has been sensitive to the differences between parents and strangers since the earliest weeks of life and has shown real preference for the company of parents and other predictable adults. This continuum of development accelerates in the second half of the first year. Fear of being touched or picked up when approached by a stranger typically occurs at about 6 months, with an even more overtly negative reaction known as **stranger anxiety** appearing around 8 months and lasting until 18 to 24 months. This encompasses the period during which the child misses their regular care providers (a cognitive skill we call "**object permanence** for people") but does not have the linguistic and social skills to easily negotiate a relationship with new people, the strangers. In addition, other cognitive capabilities such as the ability to categorize and remember allow the child to notice very quickly and become acutely distressed by the appearance, sound, and touch of unfamiliar people. Well-established routines of interaction and care are now in place, and the child becomes exquisitely sensitive to any differences from these expectations. Although children much older than 2 are still appropriately wary around people they do not know, the

---

Original chapter by Maria Trozzi and Suzanne D. Dixon.

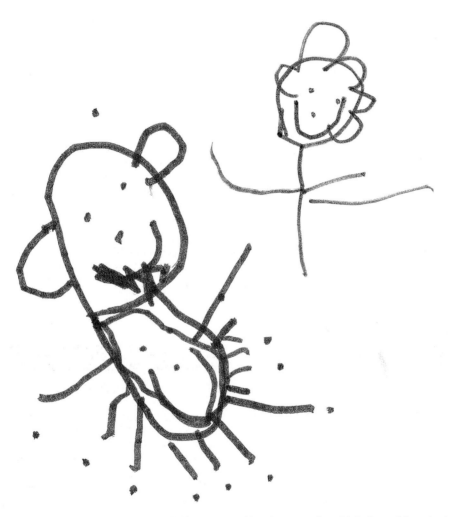

"The active movement of a young child is conveyed by the use of multiple legs. Mom looks on, dancing herself." By Katherine Baucher, age 4.

degree and intensity of stress are much less than during this stage around the first birthday.

If separated from a parent at the age of 8 to 9 months, particularly if left in the presence of strangers, the child becomes very upset. This reliance is evidence of secure attachment to loved ones, as well as the child's new cognitive skills in visualizing them and wishing they were present when they are not. Cross-cultural work provides evidence of this process being universal in healthy human development. The intensity and form of the behavior may vary around the world, but this pattern between child and care provider has been observed everywhere it has been studied.

At this stage, the opportunity to interact with adults outside the immediate family offers the infant new perspectives and the chance to learn about other people and themselves through these social interactions. The child also learns over time that other people can be trusted and enjoyed. Alternative caregivers or important people in the family's community can be introduced in a way that supports the child's efforts at social expansion without unduly stressing the child. A time of familiarization with the new caretaker, maintaining regular routines, and the initiation of leave-taking routines all make brief separations easier.

It is worth noting that another peak of stranger anxiety often occurs at 18 to 20 months of age, usually just before the development of real language competency. The toddler relies heavily on the nonverbal communication patterns established with their close caregivers, but strangers will have social cues that are less familiar. This second peak of stranger anxiety diminishes as the child's mastery of language skills allows communication with unknown people. By 2 to 3 years of age, the child begins to show decreased distress and increased friendliness with strangers, which makes it easier to enter longer days at preschool and other environments where increasing socialization and independence are expected. These examples illustrate how a child's changing developmental skills will shape their attachment and separation patterns with their caregivers and exploration of the larger world. By understanding these attachment concepts (see below and Chapter 2), pediatric clinicians can help caregivers navigate their child's shifts in emotional reaction and distress to new situations.

WHAT IS ATTACHMENT?

Attachment is the enduring emotional bond that humans feel toward special people in their lives. It encompasses trust that the other will be attentive and responsive to one's needs and emotional state. It leads to types of behavior that keep us close to the attachment figure. Absence from that person creates distress to some degree, and reunion

> ### BOX 12.1   Safety First for Baby on the Move
>
> - Cupboard doors should have safety stoppers.
> - Household cleaning products should be put up out of baby's reach.
> - All stairways should be blocked by attached gates.
> - Outside doors should be closed tightly, perhaps with plastic sealers, or for older children, high hooks.
> - The crib mattress should be at the lowest level.
> - The diaper-changing area should be safe in the event of falls, which may mean a pad on the floor or on a low bed.
> - Baby walkers should not be used at all.
> - The car seat should be adjusted for size and never ignored. Watch for the child wriggling out of it.
> - The garage and bathroom should be off-limits unless an adult, focused on the child, is present at all times.
> - Sharp corners of tables and cabinets should have protectors on them.
> - Poisonous plants should be removed from the house and yard.
> - Attached gates at staircases and to block off rooms.
> - Bathrooms should be off-limits.
> - Any body of water should be removed or blocked. Buckets and toilets are bodies of water.

brings relief from that distress. Much of the key developmental work of the first year is to develop and deepen the attachment to one's care providers. This forms a model for other attachments throughout life and is the foundation for healthy emotional development. Multiple factors influence attachment across the socioecological continuum, as shown in Box 12.1.

WHAT DOES SECURE ATTACHMENT LOOK LIKE?

Child development researchers have used several different approaches to classify whether young children and their primary caregivers have a secure or insecure attachment. This has included self-report surveys, videotapes of caregiver-child interaction at home, and laboratory experiments in which children are briefly separated from their caregivers and then reunited. This latter approach, called the "**The Strange Situation**," is sometimes used by early childhood clinicians to understand the nature of a child's relationship to caregivers. It involves having a child and caregiver play in a room with toys, a stranger enters the room and talks to the caregiver, the caregiver leaves, the stranger attempts to comfort or play with the child, the caregiver returns and comforts the child, and the stranger leaves.

Developmental psychologists have identified varying profiles in the Strange Situation that represent the child's general strategy for having their emotional needs met when they are stressed. These include:

- A *securely attached* child of 8 to 24 months plays eagerly with new toys when a caregiver is present but looks wary at the approach of a stranger and will turn or move away with approach or touch. The child will protest, may or may not cry, and will try to follow the departing caregiver. On the caregiver's return, the child will go to them for comfort, and crying is reduced, illustrating that seeking out care is their strategy for emotion regulation. This is the most common type of attachment, occurring in an estimated 65% of caregiver-child dyads in research studies. Caregivers with secure attachment generally show consistent and sensitive responses to a child's cues, and in turn, the child comes to internalize the belief that their physical and emotional needs will generally be met.

- An *avoidant* child seems unresponsive to the caregiver and demonstrates little distress when they leave. The child reacts to the stranger in the same way as to the caregiver and at reunion avoids the caregiver or is very slow to approach. The child may resist being picked up and does not cling. Avoidant styles of attachment, which studies estimate occur in about 20% of dyads, often occur when caregivers are more distant and disengaged, or the child's distress has been met with emotional distancing in the past, so infants may internalize the idea that their needs may not be consistently met.

- An *ambivalently attached* child appears insecure and clings to the caregiver and does not explore the room at all. The child becomes dysregulated and may cry intensely on separation and shows inconsistent responses on reunification with hitting, pushing, and failure to be comforted easily when picked up. This type of attachment is estimated to occur in 10% to 15% of dyads and is linked with inconsistent responsiveness from caregivers—sometimes sensitive, sometimes intrusive, and sometimes distant—so infants are thought to use intense crying to elicit caregiving responses.

- *Disorganized* attachment is evident in a child who shows a flat or passive affect throughout the procedure and shows little response to the caregiver leaving or returning, often failing to cry or crying at odd times. Gaze avoidance with the caregiver may be seen. Little or no toy exploration takes place. Children with disorganized attachment (10%–15% prevalence) are thought to have no consistent strategy for getting their needs met; this is often due to erratic, extreme, frightening, abusive, or passive caregiving responses.

Although pediatric clinicians will not carry out the Strange Situation, the clinical encounter can sometimes provide opportunities to observe an infant or young child's responses to strangers, a brief separation from the caregiver, or ease of soothing during a clinical encounter.

VARIATIONS IN ATTACHMENT BEHAVIOR AND RESPONSE TO STRESS

When assessing child development at this age, especially when observing parent-child interactions and talking to families about how a child responds to separation and reunion, some additional factors should be taken into consideration.

First, some children sail through this developmental period with only a mild behavior change over a short period of time. Other children exhibit significant recurrent fear responses that continue until the end of the second year. Strong negative responses are not typically the result of bad experiences in the past or lack of parental support in the regular environment, but rather most often due to normal variations in temperament and sensitivity to change. It can be helpful for parents to understand that for sensitive children, transitions with people and events may require additional time and support, in the first year and beyond.

Second, cross-cultural investigations suggest that infants of all groups studied have the onset and first peak of stranger anxiety at about 8 months of age. However, in cultures in which infants are regularly exposed to many caregivers and members of their community, the response was less intense, was more easily overcome with a brief familiarization time, and lasted for a shorter period into the second year. In all cultures studied, the strongest infant response came with separation from the primary caregiver. Infants have been found to securely attach to their parents, even those working outside the home full time, if the parents' care is responsive and if time spent with the parents early in the infant's life has helped a relationship to start.

The healthcare encounter allows the clinician to make observations of attachment styles. Every visit can invite the child to explore, includes the approach of a stranger (the clinician), and may include some separation. The quality of the reaction to strangers is influenced by the infant's developmental age, temperament, presence of illness, hunger, or fatigue, the stranger's demeanor, and the presence or absence of familiar figures. Clinic-based conditions that heighten the fear response are unfamiliar surroundings (e.g., an examining room), active approach by the stranger (e.g., moving in quickly to examine the child), and close proximity to the stranger, especially with eye-to-eye contact. In addition, the response to the stranger is more dramatic when the parent is present but not in physical contact with the infant (e.g., parent in chair and child on examining table). Factors that lessen fearful behavior in the clinic setting include a position close to or in contact with the parent, familiarization time in a new setting, and a stranger who approaches with toys and responds to the infant's cues.

During the visit, the clinician can point out these natural responses to stranger anxiety, describe the developmental reasons they occur, and comment on how the infant's unique temperamental style influences their reaction to this minor stress. For example, with a child who fusses with the clinician's approach but calms with being placed in the lap of the caregiver, you can say something like, "At 9 months, infants start to have stranger anxiety because their brain now realizes that they are separated from the parent they love, and they can now recognize me as a different adult from you. It feels a little stressful to him, but he coped well by looking to you and calming down once you hugged him a bit. It's a great sign that he's cognitively on track and very attached to you."

For infants who are dysregulated or avoidant during the visit, it can help to ask a few questions, including whether the responses observed in clinic are common for the child or have been noticed by the parent in other settings, and whether the family has had any concerns or observations they would like to discuss.

HELP WITH SEPARATION

Transitional Objects

Bowlby and Winnicott have pointed out that a young child's attachment to a cuddly object, which they called the **transitional object**, is part of the developmental process of becoming independent, of separating from parents psychologically. These first treasured possessions are frequently capable of filling the role of an important, though subsidiary attachment when the primary attachment person is not there. The object can provide particular comfort when the child is hungry, tired, or distressed.

Transitional objects, or "loveys," are effectively used by children to calm themselves when upset. Selection of a special object may occur as early as 7 to 8 months but usually takes place between 1 and 2 years of age. This object may take many forms—a blanket, doll, toy, or piece of the child's or parent's clothing. Although most children discard the transitional object as they approach 3 or 4 years of age, when the separation process is farther along and peer pressure mounts, some children retain these attachments into their school years.

Some parents may perceive the ever-present cuddly object as a weakness, a crutch rather than a strength. Embarrassment may develop if they view it as a negative reflection on their parenting or on the child's ability to cope. The parents and the child may also receive pressure from extended family or childcare providers to "give up that thing." The child's clinician can help parents appreciate their child's resourcefulness and emerging independence. Having a duplicate for washing or replacement is wise because these treasured items get heavy use.

Comfort Habits

Most children rock on occasion (usually when falling asleep), do some head banging or later twirl hair, pull at their ears, or rub their faces. These comfort habits, along with the use of transitional objects, are common ways to settle down, cope with stress, or fill in quiet time. These are positive steps in learning ways to solve life's little problems. Use of these comfort habits is healthy most of the time but may be a concern if the child will not usually stop to acknowledge or respond to a parent when using the lovey or comfort routine or if the child hurts herself with the lovey or other comfort habit. If such behavior is noted, further evaluation of development and the environment should take place.

MOTOR DEVELOPMENT AND EXPLORATION

Moving in space is the motor milestone that comes in at this age and exploration of the world becomes the goal. Some children roll, others scoot along while sitting, others creep by pulling with their arms and still others eventually get up on hands and knees and crawl. The exploration of space at this age is vital to cognitive growth. Interesting sights at a distance, objects that disappear, and the joy of moving prompt this forward progression. Getting a chance to move and explore opens up opportunities to refine motor skills and to learn from these explorations.

As new motor competencies are discovered and practiced, the child can also now start to move farther away from a parent. This can be both exciting and alarming for a child. The internal drive for mastery and discovery is tempered by the realization that approaching new things or people in the environment increases one's distance from familiar providers. *Internal security is needed to go forward on these adventures.* A child who is anxious will not explore as widely, as often, or as confidently. Being free to explore requires the relationship with the caregiver to be secure. The caregiver's presence must be seen as a reliable place to which the child can return physically and psychologically if they need safety and assurance.

In addition to increased mobility, children learn to use the index finger as a separate "pointer finger" and to use the index and thumb together in a "pincer grasp" around 9 months of age (see Chapter 11 for a discussion of the emergence of hand skills). Opposition of the thumb sets the stage for the sophisticated use of the hand and allows the child to pick up very small objects and explore them in complex ways. Moreover, the ability to put one thing into another that emerges at this time sets the stage for more elaborate ways to play and explore.

A very young infant acts as though objects cease to exist when they are not visible; now, a child will pursue a disappearing object—uncovering a block or moving to get a car behind a chair. Such behavior is called object permanence, a key cognitive building block. Children love peek-a-boo at this age because this game plays into this new mental ability to remember and anticipate. They will nearly shake with anticipation when a parent disappears behind a screen, just waiting for them to reappear. In fact, children's own play at this age will include experiments with hiding and finding, putting one thing into another, and then retrieving it. Play, at this age and at all ages, reflects the child's newly emerging cognitive and physical abilities.

CHILD SAFETY

At 8 to 9 months, the emergence of mobility and the more adept use of fingers and hands mean more fun, learning, and potential trouble. Parents can try exploring their home space on their hands and knees to see the world—and potential safety hazards—from the child's point of view. If the parents can see the world from their child's perspective, they can anticipate how to make the environment safe while offering the child the chance to explore and learn to use their new skills. This is a broader perspective than merely a list of safety issues or a checklist given at each visit. Box 12.2 shows some of the safety precautions appropriate for a newly mobile child who can now change location, and Box 12.2 shows some of the safety precautions to keep in mind for a child who now has enhanced grasp, reach, and manipulative skills.

FEEDING AND EATING

With each new developmental gain, the child can explore **food** in new ways. Table 12.1 presents the developmental stages related to feeding at different ages. At 8 months, with development of the pincer grasp and improved eye-hand coordination, the child can be given finger foods and encouraged to explore the feel and texture of food. Most children at this age can now grasp a spoon but have a hard time manipulating it effectively. Children

> ### BOX 12.2   Safety First for Active Hands
>
> - All electrical outlets should be plugged or covered.
> - Electrical cords should not hang down.
> - All breakables should be put away.
> - Residents' and visitors' purses should be placed out of the child's reach.
> - All medicines must have safety caps that are kept on.
> - All siblings' toys with small pieces should be put away.
> - All houseplants should be checked for poisonous components and removed if present. If safe ones are kept, be ready for pruning that you did not count on and roughage (i.e., dirt) for the baby that you did not plan.
> - Cat and dog food should be kept out of the child's reach.
> - Anything tiny should be kept off the floor.
> - Sandboxes, beaches, and playgrounds should be inspected for tiny undesirables such as cigarette butts, coins, and buttons.

this age should participate in self-feeding activities but will still require caregiver feeding as well to take in adequate nutrients. Different flavors and types of food should be introduced, and textures should advance from the smooth purees given at months 4 to 6 to more textured soft foods and foods with lumps. Difficult-to-chew items, like chicken or beef, should be cut into very small pieces, as should other foods, like grapes, that pose a choking risk.

SLEEP AND NIGHT WAKENING

Night wakening often returns at this age. To parents, this may feel like a step backward or like something is wrong. Before the clinician advises families about possible next steps, it is important to understand what current bedtime routines look like, where the infant is sleeping, how family members feel about the awakenings, and what the caregivers would like to be different.

It can help to start with reassurance that night wakening is common and predictable at this developmental stage. Some believe that the basis for this is the child's increased ability to miss the parents when they are not present. In addition, the emerging ability to pull to stand means that the child can really wake up completely by trying out new motor skills at night and may cry out for attention and reassurance. In addition, sleep regression is often observed during times of rapid cognitive and physical development throughout early childhood and then improves again.

TABLE 12.1	Behavioral and Developmental Abilities Related to Feeding in Young Children
Newborn–2 months	Primitive reflexes (rooting, sucking, swallowing) facilitate feeding and quickly become organized into a wide pattern of behavior; a hunger cry initiates feeding interaction; minimal vocal, visual, or motor activity during feeding
2–4 months	More alert and interactive during feeding; explosive cough to protect self from aspiration; beginning ability to wait for food; associates mother's smell, voice, and cradling with feeding; hand-to-mouth behavior quiets infants and increases interest in mouthing activities
4–6 months	Readiness for solids; excellent head and trunk control; reaching for objects; raking grasp; increased hand-to-mouth facility; loss of extrusion reflex of the tongue; may purposefully spit out food as part of food exploration; adaptation to introduction of solids may be affected by infant's temperament
6–8 months	Sits alone with a steady head during seated feedings; chewing mechanism developed; holds bottle; vocal eagerness during meal preparation; much more motor activity during feeding
8–10 months	Finger food readiness; thumb-forefinger grasp (i.e., inferior pincer); grasps spoon but cannot use it effectively; enjoys new textures, tastes; emerging independence
10–12 months	Increasing determination to feed self; neat pincer grasp; drops food off highchair onto floor to see where it goes; holds cup but frequently spills it; more verbal and motor behavior during feeding
12–15 months	Demands to feed self without help; decreased appetite and nutritional requirements; improved cup use (both hands); uses spoon, fills poorly, spills, turns at mouth; can use spoon as extension of the hand; messy play
15–18 months	Eats rapidly, with short feeding sessions; wants to be physically active (too busy to eat); fairly good use of spoon and cup; enhanced ability to wait for food; plays with or throws food to elicit response from parent
18–24 months	Feeds self with combination of utensils and fingers; verbalizes "eat, all gone," asks for food; negativism emerges, says no when really wanting offered food; wants control over feeding situation
2–3 years	Uses fork; ritualistic, repetitive at mealtimes; food jags, all one food at a time; dawdles; likes to help set and clear table; may begin to help self to refrigerator contents
3–4 years	Spills little; uses utensils well; washes hands with minimal help; likes food preparation; reasonable table manners while eating out
4–5 years	Serves self; choosy about food; resists some textures; makes menu suggestions; likes to assist in washing dishes; helps in food preparation

Oftentimes, children of this age are able to settle themselves back to sleep after a minute or two of crying. If this does not occur, some quiet, brief reassurance from a parent may help. Cuddly "loveys" may help children self-soothe and return to sleep as well. Overall, consistent bedtime routines that involve putting the child to bed drowsy but still awake appear to still be effective at this age.

Children in Stressful Situations

Loss of a caregiver is hard on children at any age but may be particularly stressful at times of enhanced stranger anxiety. Young children do not have the cognitive and linguistic skills to understand explanations of the situation and have no sense of time to understand if or when their caregivers may be coming back. Clinicians may have to be advocates for young children with social service agencies and the courts regarding shifts in care during this critical interval. Children who require hospitalization at this developmental stage may also experience emotional distress and disruptions in attachment, especially if there are barriers that prevent their caregivers from staying with them at the bedside. Every effort should be made to make parent involvement easier for such patients. See Chapters 25 and 27 for more detail on these topics.

PLAY AS ASSESSMENT AT THIS VISIT

Children will demonstrate the cutting edge of their developmental competency in their **play** if we give them a few props, a lot of support, and protection from stressors. The 9-month visit, because it occurs at a time of great developmental change, is the perfect time to pay attention to how the child plays. Referrals for additional evaluations and enrollment in early intervention programs can all be completed before the first birthday if concerns are found at this assessment.

Formal assessments are done by only a few primary care clinicians. Most are left to specialists, special programs, or clinics. However, certain easy-to-clean play activities inform the observer quite readily of where the child is on the developmental continuum, from newborn through adolescence:

- Blocks (1-inch cubes)
- Stethoscope
- Markers for drawing on paper

With a few simple items, including some 1-inch blocks, a stethoscope, and markers and paper for drawing, it is possible to get a fairly accurate estimate of development across childhood with minimal time. Blocks can be brought out at the beginning of the visit, while you are talking to the caregivers. Depending on what is observed with the blocks, a decision can be made about whether to spend more time on evaluation or to bring in additional tools and structure. Tables 12.2 and 12.3 lay out typical ways children interact with stethoscopes and blocks at different developmental ages.

TABLE 12.2   Stethoscope Play Continuum

Action	Age
Regards in the midline	Birth–1 month
Follows to at least 90 degrees	2–6 weeks
Swipes at it	2–4 months
Reaches for it	4–5 months
Brings it to the mouth	5–8 months
Reaches across the midline	6–8 months
Pivots to get it while seated	8–11 months
Unilateral reach	9–11 months
Examines parts of it	12–15 months
Imitates use	15–19 months
Pretends with others	2 years
Knows where the heart is and perhaps what it does	3–5 years

TABLE 12.3   Block Play

Action	Age
Regards the block at 8–10 inches	Birth–1 month
Follows the block to at least 45 degrees while supine	Birth–2 months
Mouth, hands, and feet activate, go after the block	1–3 months
Swipes at the block	2–4 months
Holds the block placed in the hand	3–5 months
Holds two blocks	5–7 months
Bangs two blocks together	7–8 months
Releases the block to put it in a cup	11 months
Builds tower of 2	15 months
Builds tower of 6	20 months
Builds tower of 8	25 months
Builds bridge of 3	30 months
Builds stairs of 6	35 months
Counts one block	36 months
Knows four different colors of the blocks	3½ years
Counts five blocks	4–4½ years
Can add two sets of blocks (i.e., 2 + 3 = 5)	5–7 years
Can calculate take away to 10	7–8 years

DURING THE VISIT

Observation

On entering the examination room at the beginning of the office visit when the infant is 8 to 9 months old, you may observe a wary expression on the child's face. Observe the child's *social distance*—the limits of proximity that the child allows before showing signs of distress. Within the visit, pay attention to the parent's response to the child's distress.

History Taking

Several issues can be addressed while taking the child's and family's history by asking questions such as the following:

Stranger Anxiety

- How does the baby respond to seeing new people?
- If the child seems upset at these encounters, how do you respond?

Transitional Objects

- Does the child have a "lovey," a special toy or object?
- Ask whether the parent notes any pattern to the child's associated behavior when she wants the object (e.g., fatigue, hunger, stress).

- How do you feel about use of the object?

Other caregivers. At this office visit or earlier, the parents' activities outside the home should be discussed in terms of their impact on the child:
- Is the child left with a regular caregiver?
- What is the leave-taking routine?
- Is the baby's response different now than before?
- What helps the baby with these transitions?
- Do you plan any changes in the future?

Observation

Sitting down on the floor or with the child on some surface will get you ready to look at how the baby explores the world. At 8 months of age, in a *free play session*, we would expect the child to do the following:
- Sit without support
- Reach around the side to get a toy
- Reach for objects with both hands
- Anticipate the shape of an object with shaping of the hand while reaching. Use a pencil or the stethoscope
- Transfer objects from hand to hand
- Stand while holding on (i.e., weight bearing)
- Move in some way—scooting, creeping, crawling
- Use a pincer grasp for small objects
- String phonemes together, such as "mamamama," "dadadada"
- May do pat-a-cake or wave bye-bye
- Hold a cube in each hand
- Bang cubes together
- Go after the stethoscope with one hand at a time, may imitate the dangling
- Be unable to let go of a cube to put it in a cup or hand
- Look wary at first approach
- Cry when the parent leaves or moves away
- Require help to sit and stand
- Try to put the ball and the cube together

QUICK CHECKS TO 9 MONTHS

✓ Sits: Gets there, sits steadily, pivots
✓ Moves forward: Scoots, creeps, crawls, rolls, cruises or walks
✓ Says: Phonemes, strung together, jabbers, gestures
✓ Understands: Name, "no," familiar objects or people, "bye, bye"
✓ Games: Peek-a-boo, pat-a-cake, waves "bye, bye"
✓ Finds a hidden object she has seen disappear
✓ Hands: Shapes hands to objects, transfers, has pincer grasp, pokes with fingers coming apart, used separately
✓ Stranger response: Wary, worried or distressed
✓ Feeding: Feeds self with hands, fingers
✓ Sleeping: 1–2 naps. Expect night wakening

! HEADS UP—8 TO 9 MONTHS

Signs of Attachment Concerns

- A child who shows no differential response to strangers by 1 year of age.
- A child who is extremely fearful and clingy in all circumstances and does not change by age 2.
- A child becomes so upset with a brief separation that she repeatedly refuses to eat or to stop crying.
- A child who does not notice or becomes upset with departure of the parent or care provider.
- A child who never checks back with the parent when exploring a new environment.
- A child older than 8 months who goes to anyone without preference.
- An extreme response to a stranger, e.g., extreme fear.

Note: The child's current caretaking environment and medical, developmental, and social history should be explored if such responses are present. Children with developmental delays have a delayed onset of stranger awareness in line with their cognitive level. Those with disorders in the autism spectrum will start to have both delayed and atypical responses to separations around 9–12 months of age.

ANTICIPATORY GUIDANCE

The cognitive basis for emerging stranger anxiety should be clearly explained. This puts it in a positive, normative framework. The clinician can offer guidance for dealing with separation issues:
- Children should never be forced to show affection for a new person if they are distressed. This protest behavior must be seen as developmentally based and protective. Give children a chance to see the stranger in a familiar context for a period.
- Leave-taking rituals and routines help children cope with separations. This includes sleep; bedtime rituals are vital.
- When moving from room to room, parents should keep voice contact with children and reappear regularly.
- Baby-sitters should be introduced while the child is in the parent's arms, should approach slowly, and should give the child a chance to look them over.
- If a child needs a medical procedure, encourage the parent to stay with the child. The child may cry *more*, but the stress of the situation will be *less*. Decreased crying is not necessarily the desired endpoint.
- Suggest sharing the infant's care with other adults if no other adults are regulars in the family. Introductions to friendly strangers are opportunities for growth.

- Discuss the night awakenings often seen at this age. Discuss management by allowing the child the opportunity to get back to sleep.
- Suggest establishing falling-asleep rituals that can be replicated by the child when he awakens in the night.
- Suggest support in choosing a transitional object for a child or family who is having trouble with separations.

ACKNOWLEDGMENT

The previous editions of this work are benefited from the contributions of Pamela Kaiser, PNP, PhD.

RECOMMENDED READINGS

Zeanah CH, Berlin LJ, Boris NW. Practitioner review: clinical applications of attachment theory and research for infants and young children. *J Child Psychol Psychiatry Allied Discip*. 2011;52(8):819.

Zeanah Charles H, Smyke Anna T. Attachment disorders in family and social context. *Infant Mental Health J*. 2008;29(3):219–233.

Rosenblum KL, Dayton CJ, Muzik M. Infant social and emotional development: The emergence of self in a relational context. CH Zeanah, *Handbook of infant mental health*. 2009:80–103. ed 3, Guilford Press: New York. Available at http://digitalcommons.wayne.edu/soc_work_pubs/43

Pak-Gorstein S, Haq A, Graham EA. Cultural influences on infant feeding practices. *Pediatr Rev*. 2009;30(3):e11.

Field T. Infant sleep problems and interventions: a review. *Infant Behav Dev*. 2017;47:40–53.

Circle of Security (Attachment Intervention) Resources for Parents: Resources for Parents - Circle of Security International. Available at https://www.circleofsecurityinternational.com/resources-for-parents/ (last accessed 6/26/24).

ZERO TO THREE Resources for Families: For Families | ZERO TO THREE. Available at https://www.zerotothree.org/resources/for-families/ last accessed 6/26/24

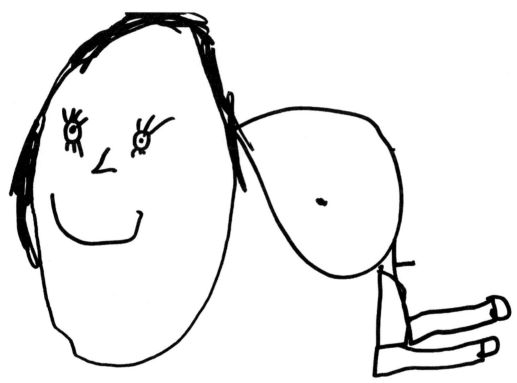

"My brother crawling." By Anne Atkinson, age 5½.

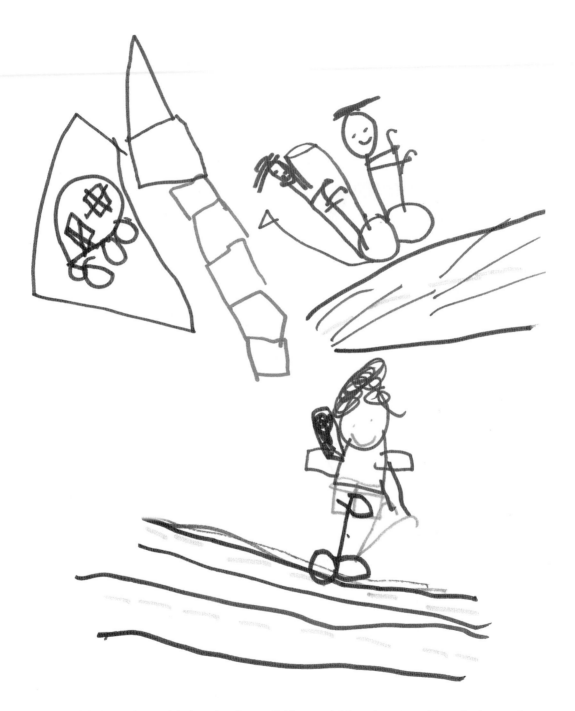

"This child shows the world of exploration available to a child as she grows. Note the house, the walk, and the garage with car as the child moves out with a parent and sibling on the back of a bike." By Hannahmarie Zambroski, age 8.

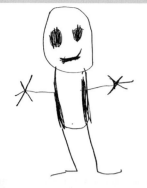

13

One Year: One Giant Step Forward

Jenny S. Radesky

This chapter explores gross motor development broadly, with a special focus on the emergence and refinement of walking as it progresses from infancy into middle childhood. Complex motor skill development is described. The cognitive and social-emotional changes in the child that are prompted by the ability to walk are explained.

KEYWORDS

- Walking
- Gross motor development
- Gait cycle
- Running
- Developmental coordination disorder
- Atypical motor development
- Sports
- Shoes

When children can start **walking** independently, their whole perspective on the world changes. With their body held upright, moving around home and community spaces, they can now explore in new ways. Walking is also one of the clearest milestones apparent to caregivers and one that they remember the best. Independent gait is greeted by parents as a source of pride and assurance that the child is developing typically, while delays may trigger worry. The visit of a 1-year-old offers the opportunity to look at the development of ambulation and **gross motor processes** in general that emerge both before and after the start of walking. The goal of this chapter is to see this area of development in the broader context of the whole child, their other developmental processes, and the context of the family.

The neuromaturational model (see Chapter 2) first described the predictable progression of motor skills

Previous edition chapter by Suzanne D. Dixon and Michael J. Hennessy.

in infants and young children. Although we now know that not every aspect of gross motor development can be accounted for by this model, the regularity and the readily observable nature of these motor achievements form a core of basic developmental assessment, as shown in Figs. 13.1 and 13.2. Physical milestones in infancy are presented in Table 13.1. These milestones are easy to observe, readily reported by parents, and easier than most to remember.

MOTOR SKILLS: GENERAL PRINCIPLES

Walking must be seen in the context of other gross motor abilities. These all share, in addition to their regular sequence, certain characteristics:

- Gross motor skills are shaped by the child's *neuromotor tone*. Hypotonic children, from whatever cause, will have delays in postural maturation and skill acquisition. Hypertonic children, with prominence of extensor postures, will have both "pseudo-accelerations" (e.g., rolling over, weight bearing on legs, and pull to stand sooner than expected) and delays (e.g., sitting).
- *Reflex behavior precedes volitional behavior.* For example, the newborn reflex patterns of reciprocal kicking and automatic stepping clearly foreshadow the movements of walking seen near the end of the first year. These early patterns usually disappear clinically at approximately 2 months of age, only to later reappear in the progressive emergence of independent gait. This sequence is thought to result from increasing suppression of the primitive reflexes by maturing cortical centers and their subsequent reorganization into volitional

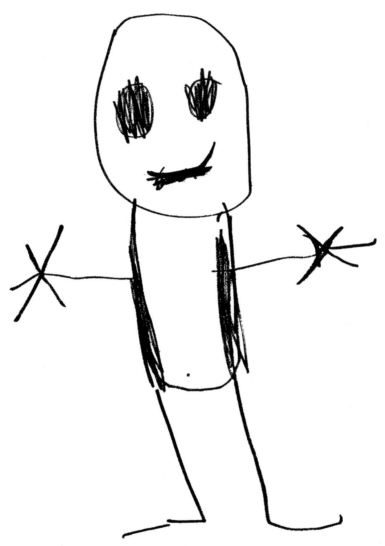

"'Getting up on your own two feet' gives a sense of independence and an urge to explore." By Colin Hennessy, age 3½.

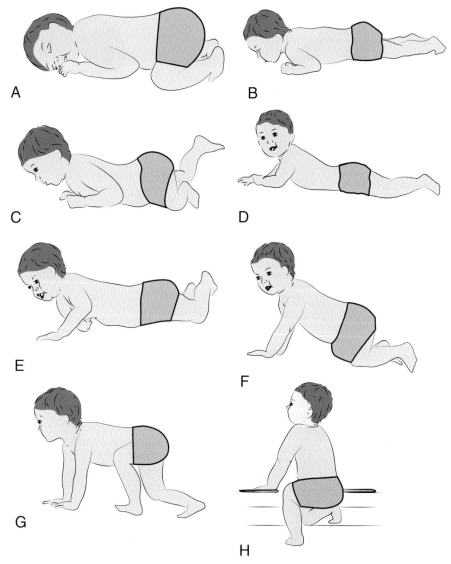

Fig. 13.1 Progression of prone posture. (A) Newborn in a flexed posture. (B) Infant at about 1 month of age, head up briefly, some extension at the hips and knees. (C) Infant about 1–2 months old, head up to about 45 degrees, active legs. (D) Infant about 3–4 months old, up easily on forearms, head steady, and able to be turned with minimal bobbing. (E) Infant about 5–9 months old, up on hands; may use arm to pull self forward; may push with thighs and knees, creeping. (F) Infant 7–11 months old, crawling; reciprocal movement of legs and legs with hands. (G) Crawling on feet. (H) Child 8–18 months of age, climbs stairs.

movement patterns. Concomitant with increased strength and improved balance, the child learns to control the reflex pattern and use it in a more complex and flexible pattern.

- *Maturation entails increasing efficiency in the energy expenditure that is required to move through space.*

The child becomes an increasingly efficient movement machine. The biomechanical parameters ensure that with maturation and practice, forward movement is achieved with less change in the center of gravity, less overall joint movement, and refinement of muscle movement. This means more efficient movement.

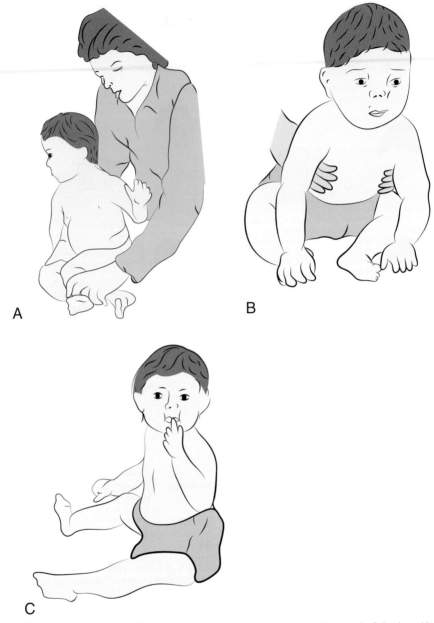

A

B

C

Fig. 13.2 Sitting progression. With each time period, steadiness, and control of the head increase, the back becomes straighter from the upper portion down, and the arms are held naturally further back, with external rotation at the shoulder. (A) Age 1–2 months, sits with truncal support, head and shoulders steady, lower part of the back still rounded. (B) Age 4–7 months, sits in a pivot position with slight truncal support; all energy is directed at maintaining posture. (C) Age 5–9 months, independent sitting, back straight, able to pivot without losing balance.

- *The progression of control is from more proximal joint movement to recruitment of more distal movement.* This usually means a refinement, a fine-tuning of movement because the more distal joint can make adjustments with less movement and more accuracy, as seen in the development of reach (see Chapter 12). Control of reach moves from the shoulder to the wrist; control of gait is transferred in part to the knee and then to the ankle

TABLE 13.1   U.S. Centers for Disease Control and Prevention Movement/Physical Development Milestones in Infancy

Age	What most babies do by this age
2 months	Holds head up when on tummy
	Moves both arms and both legs
	Opens hands briefly
4 months	Holds head steady without support when you are holding them
	Holds a toy when you put it in their hand
	Uses their arm to swing at toys
	Brings hands to mouth
	Pushes up onto elbows/forearms when on tummy
6 months	Rolls from tummy to back
	Pushes up with straight arms when on tummy
	Leans on hands to support self while sitting
9 months	Gets to a sitting position by self
	Moves things from one hand to other hand
	Uses fingers to "rake" food towards self
	Sits without support
12 months	Pulls up to a stand
	Walks, holding on to furniture
	Drinks from a cup without a lid, as you hold it
	Picks things up between thumb and pointer finger, like small bits of food
15 months	Takes a few steps on their own
	Uses fingers to feed self some food
18 months	Walks without holding on to anyone or anything
	Scribbles
	Drinks from a cup without a lid and may spill sometimes
	Feeds self with fingers
	Tries to use a spoon
	Climbs on and off a couch or chair without help
24 months	Kicks a ball
	Runs
	Walks (not climbs) up a few stairs with or without help
	Eats with a spoon
30 months	Uses hands to twist things, like turning doorknobs or unscrewing lids
	Takes some clothes off by self, like loose pants or an open jacket
	Jumps off the ground with both feet
	Turns book pages, one at a time, while you read to them
36 months	Strings items together, like large beads or macaroni
	Puts on some clothes by self, like loose pants or a jacket
	Uses a fork

with maturation. This is an example of the general principle of cephalocaudal direction of development that began in fetal life.

- *The child increases in both speed and accuracy of movement with time.* These last characteristics (gains in efficiency, accuracy, and speed) are demonstrated in the specific developmental course of gait. Overshooting or undershooting and less well-directed movements are characteristics of immature movement. Fewer mistakes and greater accuracy evolve with maturation.

- *Moving is easier than stopping; going up is easier than going down.* Acceleration, in biomechanical terms, is less complex and matures earlier, whereas deceleration requires more energy and organization. In simple language, kids develop a gas pedal before brakes.

WALKING: A CHANGE IN PERSPECTIVES

New motor competencies dramatically change a child's view of themselves and the world. Placement in space is now under the child's own control, and hands are free to explore the new sights. The child can now choose (within limits) *what* to explore, not just *how* to investigate the objects within vision or reach. These skills allow the child to perceive, learn, and experience in entirely new ways by movement through space, such as choosing to go away from or toward caregivers. That new option is both exciting and scary. Everything changes because of this new perspective. Selma Fraiberg describes the overwhelming world and self-view changes that a child experiences when they learn to walk:

> In the last quarter of the first year, the baby is no longer an observer of a passing scene. He is in it. Travel changes one's perspective. A chair, for example, is an object of one dimension when viewed by a 6-month-old baby propped up on a sofa ... It's when you start to get around under your own steam that you discover what a chair really is.

> The first time the baby stands unsupported and the first wobbly independent steps are milestones in personality development, as well as in motor development. To stand unsupported, to take that first step is a brave and lonely thing to do.

All development is fueled by the ability to change position in space and to move away from a completely dependent vantage point. Or as pointed out again by Fraiberg:

> The discovery of independent locomotion and the discovery of a new self usher in a new phase in personality development. The toddler is quite giddy with his new achievements. He behaves as if he had invented this new mode of locomotion and he is quite in love with himself for being so clever. From dawn to dusk he marches around in an ecstatic, drunken dance, which ends only when he collapses with fatigue.

A child with a motor disability is therefore at risk of additional delays because of limitations in visual, perceptual, and tactile experiences when compared with walking and moving peers. Seen in this context, therapies, surgical procedures, and external supports and braces are even more important interventions for children who are nonambulatory.

THE DEVELOPMENT OF GAIT

Fig. 13.3 illustrates the gait cycle of events that occur from heel strike to the next heel strike. The observation of gait throughout these phases allows a more accurate characterization of gait and how it matures over time, as shown in Table 13.2. All these gait parameters are geared toward maximal displacement in space with a minimum of energy expenditure. The body's center of gravity moves forward in nearly a straight line in a mature gait, the path of least

TABLE 13.2 **Walking Chart**	
Stepping movements	6–12 months
Walks holding onto furniture	7¼–12¾ months
Walks with help	7–12 months
Walks independently	9–17 months
Walks well	11–14½ months
Walks sideways and backward	10–20 months

TYPICAL NORMAL WALK CYCLE

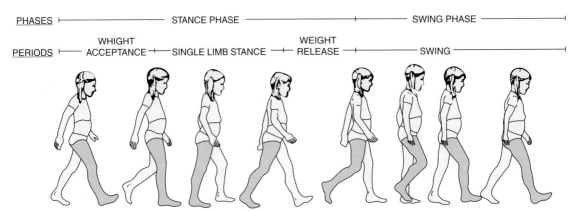

Fig. 13.3 Phases of the normal gait in childhood. (From Hennessy M, Dixon S, Simon S: The development of gait: a study in African children ages one to five. *Child Dev* 55:844–853, 1984.)

energy expenditure. Extremity movements work together toward that end. Each of these parameters has its own developmental course; the following are characteristics of walking in a young child (Figs. 13.4–13.6):

- A toddler's stance is *broad based*. As the child matures, the stance will narrow in absolute measure and in proportion to leg length. The narrower the base, the more mature the gait.
- A young child's *knees and hips are flexed*, even while standing, and remain so as the toddler waddles with one leg forward and a twist of the trunk and a swing of the hip. Hip movement involving alternating flexion and extension and a locked knee will emerge with maturation.
- A child's belly and bottom stick out because of the increased lordotic curve of the lower part of the back. This provides balance in an immature walker. As the hips straighten (i.e., extend), with time the child will tuck in the tummy and straighten the back. The "S" curve of the body viewed from the side will become less pronounced.
- Ankle movement is minimal at first with flat-footed foot placement. As a child matures, the ankle will dorsiflex and plantarflex. The child will develop a consistent heel strike to start his step after 30 months and a reliable lift-off with the forefoot and toes after that. A toddler's foot moves very little in early walking but becomes active during walking between 2½ and 3 years. *Walking with the toe striking first ("toe leads") is never part of normal gait progression.*
- When the child is first walking, the arms are abducted (out to the sides) and flexed at the elbow. The arms move little throughout the gait cycle, providing balance only. The arms first come down, the hands go from fisted or splayed to relaxed, and then reciprocal arm movements are added. The higher and more fixed the arms, the less mature the gait.
- Feet go out nearly sideways at first. With maturation, they turn more straight ahead—from a "duck walk" to a people walk.
- The center of gravity in a toddler just starting to walk shifts markedly up and down and side to side, an observation you can note if you just watch the umbilicus move throughout the gait cycle. This movement stabilizes throughout gait maturation, and truncal rotation decreases. At first, the whole body goes back and forth, up and down, side to side. With maturation, the movement is more and more isolated to the extremities. Watching the belly button helps identify this maturational point.
- Angles of displacement at all joints decrease with time. Less overshooting or excess movement occurs. Things become smoother, targeted, and graceful. Lurching,

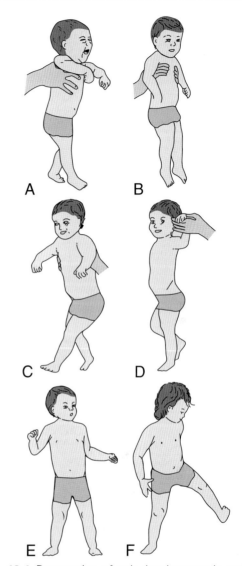

Fig. 13.4 Progression of gait development in toddlers and preschoolers. (A) Reflex walk of the newborn, which usually disappears at 3–4 weeks of age. (B) Before 3 months, an infant bears little weight on legs. (C) After 7 months, an infant will walk with much truncal support. Excessive hip flexion with a forwardly displaced center of gravity means that the child is not ready for walking. (D) Near 1 year of age, a child's center of gravity is over the hips, and the child can walk with help. (E) During the toddler years, the position of the child's arm and feet testifies to the level of maturity of gait. (F) It is not until 3–5 years of age that a child can balance steadily on one foot with all the reciprocal truncal, hip and arm adjustments that are required.

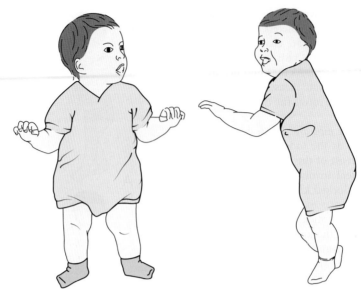

Fig. 13.5 Toddler's gait: wide based, flexion at the hip and knees, abducted feet, and arms up and fixed.

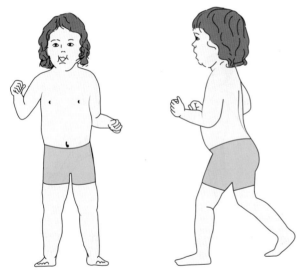

Fig. 13.6 Gait of an older toddler: arms still used as part of balance, feet turned out, and relative lordosis with the trunk over the hips.

waddling, and swaying become less as this joint movement is minimized.

- Acceleration forces are stronger than deceleration forces, so forward momentum is hard to check at first. Stopping is much harder than starting for a young child. Only later can stopping be combined with a pivot.

- For the same reason, going down an incline is much harder than going up. A child cannot check their speed.
- Step length and walking speed increase, and cadence decreases with time, gradually approaching a fixed mathematical relationship between these biomechanical aspects of gait. Older children take fewer steps to walk at a given speed, largely because of an increase in step length. This, in turn, is related to leg length; shorter children have a faster cadence, whereas those with longer legs have a slower cadence.

By 5 years of age, gait has matured to nearly adult patterns clinically and biomechanically (Fig. 13.7). Electromyography tracings show adult patterns of muscle firing by this age as well. Although increasing refinements emerge slowly and allow for more complex movements to develop, the mature biomechanical aspects of gait are established by school age.

Running emerges about 6 months after independent walking is well established. This involves a reduction in stance time (time with weight on both feet) to less than 50% of the gait cycle. Young children do not increase their stride length when they run as toddlers; they just take more steps to go at a running speed. They keep the knees at a fixed flexion and do not use their feet to initiate a lift-off. Hip movement is as inefficient with running as it is for walking in the younger ages. This means that running requires a lot of effort for a toddler, although most find the effort worth it. All of the run parameters gradually shift to more mature forms across the preschool years. Children will learn how to increase stride length, will add a "flight" phase when

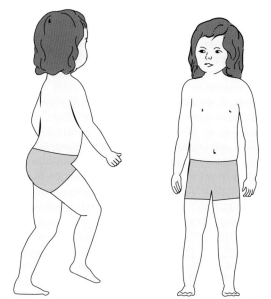

Fig. 13.7 Gait of a preschooler: biomechanically, nearly at adult patterns; heel strike present; and neck, shoulder, hips, and knees nearly vertical.

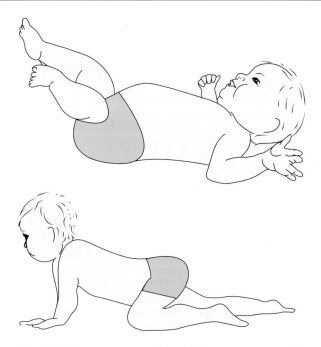

Fig. 13.8 Spontaneous reciprocal hip movements take a variety of forms. Practice opportunities are provided in the prone position.

they lift off the ground briefly, and will learn to use reciprocal arm movement to propel themselves forward. With less extraneous movement, the run is smooth and straight and has much less sideways movement in an older child. Running should be very smooth by school age.

PREWALKING

The biomechanical precursors of gait are actually the reciprocal hip and leg movements of a kicking and crawling child, not standing or pulling to stand. These early spontaneous movements have the biomechanical characteristics, interrelationships, coordination, and rhythm of gait. However, not every child will crawl, and this does not reflect either motor or cognitive development. In fact, crawling may be the most overrated motor milestone in the first year. However, all typical children will demonstrate ongoing reciprocal movement of the lower extremities that becomes smoother and more rhythmic and efficient from 9 to 12 months of age (Fig. 13.8). Spontaneous "swimming" movements are seen during bathing at about 9 months and can also be seen when a child is supine on an examining table. These back-and-forth movements are the precursors of gait. Practicing walking—for example, with a walker or bouncer toy, or through holding caregiver's hands—has not been shown to accelerate or decelerate the emergence

of walking. Freedom to move in the prone position and enticements to explore in space by whatever means form the prompts for walking.

GETTING STARTED AND REFINING SKILLS

Most children will cruise by 12 months, walking while holding onto objects at shoulder height, as shown in Fig. 13.9. Some children may resist any attempts at stepping if their hands are held up because this eliminates the usefulness of arm position and truncal rotation, which provide stability. Cruising *on one's own* provides opportunity for real practice and the development of firm prototypes of movement that can be applied to varying demands, such as walking on a carpet versus walking on grass and going up the stairs or down an incline versus walking on a flat plane. The child is experimenting with new approaches to motor activity rather than simply repeating fixed actions. It is not rote repetition of a single activity in a single circumstance many times over, but the accumulation of experiences that demands the ongoing accommodation that forms the basis of gait development. For example, an adult could not claim competency in skiing after going down only one hill, no matter how expertly that hill had been skied. Learning the skill (in the child's case, walking; for the adult, skiing)

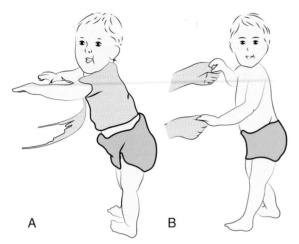

Fig. 13.9 Getting upright, cruising. (A) Cruising on one's own provides opportunities to practice and explore. Most children do this by 12 months. (B) Walking with help. Many families enjoy this activity. No evidence shows that walking with help harms the child or accelerates walking. Some children resist holding on with both hands.

includes actively assimilated experiences in many circumstances and conditions. Passive practice or repetitive exercise of motor skills in isolation (e.g., infant walkers or exercise classes) has no effect on skill acquisition; however, passive range of motion and strengthening exercises are important for children with identified motor disabilities. *Self-initiated actions, active movement, and exploration of the possibilities of movement are the necessary components of motor development.*

Most children are *not* walking on their first birthday. The mean age for walking is about 60 weeks, with a 2 standard deviation range of 9 to 17 months. The misconception that a child will walk by age 1 leads caregivers to feel worried and disappointed if the first steps have not appeared by the first birthday. The clinician should mention these averages if the child is not walking, regardless of whether the caregivers bring up the issue. If caregivers express worry, the clinician can explain that as long as tone is within a normal range, the child has unrestricted joint movement and has shown some reciprocal leg movements, it is safe to watch and wait at age 1.

The biomechanical aspects of gait in a child younger than 2 years may vary widely from child to child and will change from month to month. This is as dynamic and wobbly a process as the version of the early walker suggests. It is like each child finds his own course and reinvents himself over and over.

INDIVIDUAL DIFFERENCES

Peripheral nerve myelinization and cerebellar growth increase rapidly from 6 to 12 months, and these changes appear to coincide with the movement changes that occur during that time. These processes in the CNS set up basic readiness. Premature infants will develop gross motor milestones at approximately their corrected age, not chronological age, at the earliest. Physical growth factors such as height and leg length may influence patterns of motor development through biomechanical relationships that are necessary to get walking going. Any condition that delays growth, undermines nutrition, or produces muscle weakness will probably delay motor achievement. Balance and strength are important as well.

An internal consistency within a child allows some anticipation of gross motor skills. For example, a late sitter is likely to be a late walker. Alterations in general tone, though still within the range of normal, may set the stage for this delay.

The style with which a child approaches motor skill development is also consistent. Some children charge ahead to pull to stand, cruise, and walk with lots of energy and lots of falls. Others will take a more contemplative approach: they study the task well, wind up slowly, and feel assured of each step before trying the next. The clinician will learn more about a child by monitoring *how* they achieve gross motor skills than by focusing exclusively on the timing of such behavior.

LEARNING COMPLEX MOTOR SKILLS

Although we often place the greatest emphasis on gross motor development in the first 2 years of life, this sequence continues beyond walking. These competencies are based on an increasing ability to *balance* on one side and *ater-alize* more and on other varying motor activities (Box 13.3). Children should be able to ride a big wheel or tricycle adeptly at 4 years of age and should be able to ride a bicycle at 7. Observations of jumping, skipping, hopping, ball catching, and throwing, as well as specific questions about the handling of stairs and riding a bike, will usually help you assess a child's gross motor competencies. For children who struggle to learn these skills, particularly those that integrate movements from both sides of the body (e.g., pedaling a bike, swimming with crawl stroke), with or without abnormalities in pencil grasp (see Chapter 4), consider a referral to occupational or physical therapy. Some children with **developmental coordination disorder** come to attention in kindergarten and elementary school years when they experience challenges participating in physical education class or joining sports teams. Children with motor coordination deficits have lower core and extremity tone, more ligamentous laxity, and may avoid physical activity because it requires more effort and feels more frustrating. Treating motor coordination challenges before age 8 can help children build skills, motor tone, stamina, and strength that will allow greater physical activity participation, while decreasing obesity risk.

Motor skills do not exist in isolation. Cognitive competencies have an impact on when and how a child learns new motor skills. Similarly, motor movement and related sensory input help improve focus and emotional regulation. Many children with attention-deficit/hyperactivity disorder and autism spectrum disorder have motor coordination deficits and challenges in proprioception (i.e., sensing where their body is in space). They benefit from occupational therapy to not only improve motor coordination but also learn strategies to regulate their attention and behavior.

It is not until midlatency or even adolescence that a young person can use preknowledge of outcome to improve motor performance, such as verbal coaching or step-by-step instructions. Younger children must experience the outcome of their motor activities to alter them, and they need considerable practice before they can do that. The ability to sequence concepts parallels the ability to sequence motor behavior; only an older grade-schooler or high school student can do this reliably if the sequence is longer than two to three movements. This has implications for participation in classes and coaching of **sports**, which not only provide fun and mastery for children but also important social skills and behavioral self-control learning opportunities.

ATYPICAL GAIT AND MOTOR DEVELOPMENT

Though awkward at first, the gait of a young child should follow the sequence described previously and should show symmetry. Red flags for atypical motor development are listed in Box 13.1.

Motor delays accompanied by alterations in motor tone—hypotonia or hypertonia—are generally more worrisome than a delay in one or more landmarks alone with normal tone and reflexes. Postures or positions not seen in the normal sequence should elicit concern, such as a frog-leg position in the supine posture. Late integration of primitive reflexes with delays in several areas is of more concern regarding slowed central CNS maturation. Finally, some milestones should be weighted more than others. *Unsupported sitting* is a strong indicator of general developmental progress because it involves balanced truncal tone, good hip flexion and abduction, and excellent head control. In contrast, creeping and crawling are poor indicators because some children never perform these activities and the timing and form are highly variable. With these general considerations in mind, some clinical precision points may be considered (Box 13.2).

The differential diagnosis for abnormal motor development is broad and includes disorders of the central and peripheral nervous system, musculoskeletal system, metabolism/genetics, nutrition, endocrine, and deconditioning from other chronic diseases. Most of these conditions will require evaluation by pediatric subspecialists, but the most important motor-related issues for primary care clinicians to identify include:

- **Cerebral palsy:** Cerebral palsy is usually characterized by lower tone earlier in infancy, followed by hypertonia, spasticity, and hyperreflexia in later infancy and toddler years. Differences may be seen on one side of the body (arm and leg; hemiplegia), legs only (diplegia), or bilateral arms and legs (quadriplegia). Physical examination findings concerning for cerebral palsy are described in the section "During the Visit" and warrant referral to a neurologist or physical medicine specialist, in addition to Early Intervention and physical therapy.

BOX 13.1   Red Flags in Motor Development[a]

- No rolling prone to supine by 7 months
- No rolling supine to prone by 9 months
- No unsupported sitting by 10 months
- No independent steps by 18 months
- No running by 2 years
- No jumping by 2½ to 3 years
- No pedaling of a tricycle or big wheel by 4 years
- No bike riding by age 10

[a]These time frames should alert the clinician to problems that clearly call for more evaluation.

BOX 13.2   Observations that Trigger Concern about Walking

- A "limp" at any time
- Gait asymmetry, including asymmetry of the arms
- Persistent toe walking or the appearance of toe walking after 2 years
- A decline in performance, ability, coordination, or endurance
- A persistent waddling gait
- Refusal to walk or bear weight
- Persistent forward falling

- **Sequelae of prematurity.** Even correcting for gestational age, premature infants walk later and also seem to lack some of the coordination and efficiency that are age appropriate. These factors in themselves do not predict other areas of development, but all children born prematurely are generally at risk for developmental concerns. Although they might even show early standing, the reciprocal hip movements, the experience in the prone position, and tightness at the hips and knees may make walking more of a challenge. Truncal weakness, any degree of slow weight gain, reductions in linear growth, and the stress of chronic illness mean that strength and truncal tone will compromise walking further. Clinicians can ensure that premature infants are enrolled in Early Intervention (see Chapter 15) and have referrals to high-risk infant follow-up clinics and developmental therapies, if needed.

ALTERED PERCEPTUAL DEVELOPMENT: CHANGES IN MOTOR TIMETABLE

The impact of perceptual input on gross motor development is illustrated through the motor development of infants with congenital **blindness.** These infants demonstrate all the postural readiness (e.g., excellent truncal tone) and acquisition of static skills (e.g., stepping in place with support) at the same time as sighted children do. However, they are predictably delayed in any movement through space, such as crawling, walking, and climbing. These skills do not begin to emerge until the child can reach toward sound cues alone, a landmark met by *all* children between 10 and 15 months. Some children with blindness will not crawl at all, will not walk until they are 2 or older, and may even begin sitting or standing late, although they may have the ability to maintain these postures. Until these children are able to use perceptual input other than vision to map their environment and are able to understand the consistency of three-dimensional space, they may be uncomfortable moving about. In addition, the fueling that walking typically receives by way of visual input does not sustain the efforts of children with blindness through all the falls and uncertainties of early movement.

THE LARGER CONTEXT OF LEARNING TO WALK

Behavioral Changes

The drive to mastery that energizes all of development is never more obvious than in a child just learning to walk. The revelation that one's placement in space can be changed while visually monitoring and even holding onto an object is so overwhelming for a child that all else pales by comparison. Routine things such as feeding, diaper changes, and sleeping are terrible interferences with this new activity from the child's viewpoint. A child's new interest in motor activities may even invade sleep time with wakefulness and restlessness. The child may pull to stand and cruise around the bed with every night waking. Difficulties, as well as regressions, in other areas of functioning should be anticipated at the time of learning to walk. The child may be less interested in learning new words or engaging in sustained toy play. This will require adaptations in caregivers' approaches to the child, including a new round of safety-proofing the home.

Caregivers' Role

The sparkle of joy testifies to a walking child's own sense of internal reward for a growing sense of mastery. An internal reward system is fueled as the child learns to walk for walking's sake. An external reward system cannot have the energy or longevity of an internal one. The parents' role is to encourage, ensure safety in exploration, prevent overtiredness, and enjoy (Fig. 13.10). A parent's praise is welcome if not overwhelming, but it is not the key motivating factor.

Walking changes a child's perspective on self and those around them. It literally makes the child a new person.

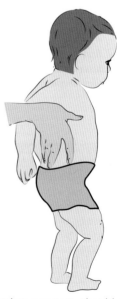

Fig. 13.10 Parenting support should be gentle, well placed, but not compelling.

A sense of independence and ability to separate from caregivers are enhanced by this accomplishment. Some caregivers are thrilled. Others are surprised and many are sad. Most have all these emotions. The child can play by roaming the environment with clear planning and direction and is no longer dependent on caregivers to deliver toys and orchestrate their whereabouts. The child can get into more trouble and have more fun. The ability to ambulate independently heralds a whole new era, including temper tantrums (see Chapter 14), the word *no*, and the thrill of running away. The infant becomes a toddler.

A Word About Shoes and Walkers

The role of **shoes** is to protect the child from sharp, rough, hot, or cold surfaces. They do not shape the foot or assist in gait development. Barefoot walking best develops the lower part of the leg, foot, and particularly the arch and, thus, avoiding shoes when it is safe to do so is best. The arch develops with foot movement, so rigid shoes do not further this process. In typically developing children, high tops, wedges, inserts, and other expensive foot devices are not needed. Shoes should be changed frequently to accommodate rapidly growing feet. Those made of soft material that allows flexing by the child and monitoring of fit by the parent are best. Orthotics for children should be reserved for those with clear neuromuscular problems and should be used only with the advice of a clinician or physical therapist trained to evaluate and monitor these conditions.

The use of **infant walkers** in particular does not improve but, in fact, delays motor and mental development. Safety may be seriously impaired in children using these devices, and injury and death may occur. They are *not* recommended. Extensor postures may be solidified in children with lower extremity hypertonia, thereby undermining rather than facilitating walking in these youngsters. If a parent insists on using a walker, it should be wider than 36 inches, too wide to go through a door. Stationary activity centers contain a child without risk of injury, so these are preferred as a safer alternative to walkers.

DURING THE VISIT

What to Observe

The following are actions the clinician should observe to track the development of motor skills:

- At every encounter during the first 5 years, the child should be allowed free movement so that the clinician can observe the child's motor competencies. Place the child both supine and prone on the examining table to observe increasing head control, truncal stability, arm support, movement at the hip, and the smoothness and rhythmicity of the movement. Symmetry in movement is a vital observation.
- A line on the floor provides guidance for the child's directed walking. An area of some reasonable length (e.g., a hallway) must be provided for free-walking assessment. A child will not be able to follow a line exactly until age 2 or older.
- Observe the amount of support the child requires to do other things, such as reach for a stethoscope. Note a decreasing need for support with sitting and increasing weight bearing on the lower extremities across the first year.
- Observation of the child walking with help and then alone should begin when the child is 9 months of age and continue until school age or beyond if there is a question. The walking base, the foot position, truncal rotation, and movement at the knee should be observed and should change along the lines presented earlier. The hand and arm position should change over time. The child's stopping and pivoting should improve. Rising to stand, stooping, and recovering will become smoother with time.
- The style, interest, and excitement of a child with motor activities should be noted at every encounter.
- At 3 years of age, knee and ankle motion should be good, and heel strike should be present.

Climbing: A simple two-step climbing device kept in the examining room against the examining table can provide observation of increasing motor competencies. This apparatus will allow the demonstration of lower extremity movement, proximal muscle strength, and coordination in climbing. Walking up and downstairs should follow age expectations (Box 13.3).

Caregiver's Handling: A caregiver's handling of a child can give clues to both the child's competencies and the child's motor abilities. A caregiver who carefully supports the infant's head at all times when the child is 3 months or older may rightfully anticipate that this infant's head control is poor. Children around the world will be ready for upright packaging with or without attachment (e.g., backpacks, wrapping on the hip or back, cradle boarding) by 3 to 4 months. If a child is being carried like a neonate, something is wrong, either in the child's development or in the caregiver's ability to alter caretaking based on the child's competencies.

Caregivers who cannot allow a 4-year-old to climb up on an examining table may anticipate that the child will be unsuccessful or awkward. Excessive "coaching" of a child during the motor assessment may also be a clue that the caregiver has a worry about functioning in this area.

BOX 13.3   Later Gross Motor Skill Progression

2–3 Years
- Both feet on each stair, up and down
- Full-arm swing
- True run begins
- Jumps down a step
- Jumps up stiffly
- Hops 1–3 times
- Throws ball with forearm extension only
- Catches ball with fixed, outstretched arms
- Pushes riding toy with feet, no steering

3–4 Years
- Alternates feet upstairs
- Walks in a straight line
- Jumps, using arms
- Broad jump, about 1 foot
- Hops 4–6 times, arms and body helping
- Catches ball against chest
- Pedals and steers tricycle

4–5 Years
- Alternates feet downstairs
- Smooth run
- Gallops and does 1-foot skip
- Hops 7–9 times on one foot smoothly
- Throws the ball with shift of body
- Catches ball with hands
- Rides tricycle very well

5–6 Years
- Gallops and skips smoothly
- Jumps up 1 foot
- Broad jumps 3 feet
- Mature throwing with shift of weight
- Adjusts body, arms, hands to catch
- Rides bicycle

Modified from Berk LE: *Infants, children and adolescents,* ed 3. Boston, 1999, Allyn & Bacon.

What to Ask

Caregivers will usually find the reporting of gross motor skills the easiest of all areas of development. In addition to asking what the child can do, ask *how* the child approaches the task (i.e., with caution at one extreme or with abandon and impulsivity at the other). The manner or style in which these skills are performed may reflect the emerging personality, family expectations, or difficulty with motor coordination.

The caregivers' response about the child's accomplishments may provide data about any underlying anxiety or specific worries. By beginning questions at a lower level of functioning than anticipated, the clinician can find the floor of the child's performance and convey the importance of individual expectations in motor development.

Children readily practice newly emerging skills in motor development, as well as in other areas of development. The relatively invariant order of motor skill acquisition allows a clinician taking the history of a child whose development is on track to simply ask what kind of new movements or activities the child is doing. The internally regulated and self-fueling nature of this area of development is highlighted in this approach.

A child whose motor development is not synchronous with other areas of development or is delayed beyond levels of normal variation (see Box 13.1) needs a more detailed history. Disorders of movement versus disorders of tone and posture can be specified through the history, coupled with a careful examination. Perinatal difficulties must alert the clinician to the need for careful evaluation of gross motor competencies, particularly if walking is delayed beyond 18 months.

Examination

Most of the gross motor examination is best moved to the end of the assessment because these activities usually energize kids, who are then difficult to calm down. The following are other things to keep in mind about the examination:

- The clinician should assess the passive motor tone of all extremities throughout the first 3 years. Move all four extremities as part of a playful game.
- Both slow and rapid motions should be applied to the limbs to elicit any lowered threshold for a stretch reflex.
- Deep tendon reflexes should be monitored.
- Asymmetries in tone, reflexes, or movement provided that the child's head is in the midline should receive very careful follow-up. Persistence of these signs may require further neurological evaluation.
- Early evidence of spastic cerebral palsy is tight heel cords with limited dorsiflexion of the foot or a "catch" in the Achilles tendon.
- Scissoring of the lower extremities when the child is held upright reflects adductor spasm.
- A limp requires a complete neurological and orthopedic assessment by an experienced specialist.
- Head and truncal tone should be assessed through the pull-to-sit and prone positions, as well as the position

of a child being held over the hand. In addition, the child's head and body control when being held upright, at the shoulder, or under the arms in front of the examiner should be assessed during the first year. Truncal tone is often reflected in how the child responds to handling and holding by the examiner. It is a perfect excuse to hold and handle the baby as part of every assessment until that is too troublesome, often at 15 to 18 months.

- Placing the baby both prone and supine offers the chance to assess increasing shoulder girdle tone and strength, as well as control of the lower part of the body.
- Alternating hip movements appear at 5 months of age, but they significantly increase in some form after 9 months.
- Weight bearing on the feet is observed in children from the age of 5 months to walking.
- Persistent standing on tiptoe is abnormal after 9 months.
- Walking with help should be attempted after 9 months but may not be present until after the first birthday.
- Climbing upstairs is seen from 8 to 18 months. After the age of 2 years, children will attempt to do this with only their feet, two feet on the step. Only after 2 to 3 years of age do children alternate feet on steps.
- Gait should be observed during the second through the sixth years and beyond if indicated. As the toddler begins to walk independently, gait is typically wide based, accompanied by waddling hips and intermittent toe walking. With each observation, the base should narrow, the arms should come down, and reciprocal movement should be added. Waddling at the hip should decrease, the knees should move a bit more, ankle movement should increase, and heel strike should be present at the age of 3 years. By the age of 5 years, the child's umbilicus should move very little except forward as the child walks. Forward movement, either walking or crawling, should be smooth and rhythmic by and large. Any asymmetry in gait is always cause for concern.
- Children can stoop about 6 months after independent walking. They bounce to music at 15 to 18 months of age. Getting up to sit or stand should be accomplished by a smooth roll to the side by 15 months.
- A soft foam ball provides an easy way to assess catching skills (see Box 13.3). This game can be done at the end of the examination or as part of the weight-measure procedure of the nurse.
- Children who are consistently 3 to 6 months behind on motor skill acquisition need a second look. Muscle tone, deep tendon reflexes, and the persistence of primitive reflexes and postures should be evaluated carefully. Cerebral palsy, hypotonia and muscular and metabolic diseases must be considered. Through a careful history and assessment over time, the primary care provider may determine whether the delays are global or confined to the motor area. Further evaluation and intervention can become more focused with this in mind.

QUICK CHECK—1 YEAR

- Pulls to stand, cruises, and takes (maybe) a few steps
- Refined pincer grasp; points with the index finger
- One word plus "mama" and "dada"
- Waves "bye, bye"
- Tries to pull off clothes
- Feeds self, with hands
- Drinks from a cup
- Imitates vocalizations
- Understands simple requests, phrases, and familiar objects
- Points at objects desired (proto-naming)
- Watches and imitates older children and adults, single actions

---

ANTICIPATORY GUIDANCE

- The clinician can support the caregivers' feelings of assurance and pride in their child's motor accomplishments and can highlight the individual **temperamental characteristics** of the child that affect all areas of development, including the style of motor achievements. Careful assessment should appropriately diffuse anxiety about individual patterns of development and confirm the child's progress.
- Caregivers support development of gross motor skills by providing opportunities for free exploration of the environment within safe limits.
- A safe play area and encouragement of daily gross motor activities in nonrestrictive clothes support development.
- Playing on the floor, wrestling sessions, and ball playing are good activities if they are done in a relaxed, social manner. Baby gymnastics, yoga, swimming classes, and therapy programs are fine if they are done with these principles in mind; the activities themselves do not magically enhance development.

! HEADS UP—1 YEAR

- A child who is not moving in space in some manner needs evaluation, including a broad assessment of development with emphasis on the neuromotor system.
- Asymmetries in movement must be taken seriously at this age. The arms and hands, legs and feet should be working in a parallel, balanced way. If not, hemiparesis must be considered. Hand preference is not yet expected at this age.
- A child who cannot pick up a raisin or pellet needs an extra look at this age. This may indicate general delays or specific neuromotor concerns.
- Children should be starting to point at objects. If not, suspect language delay or emerging autism spectrum disorder and arrange follow-up 2 to 3 months later.
- A drop-off in the amount and complexity of vocalizations may signal hearing loss or emerging autism spectrum disorder.
- Insecurely attached children (see Chapter 2) show either no or a frantic response to separations, cling to or avoid the parent or are "too friendly" to strangers.
- Children not feeding themselves at this time may be due to developmental delays or parental desire to control feeding (see Chapter 14).

- Sleep should generally extend through the night, and naps should generally consolidated to one a day.
- Lead exposure becomes a real possibility as children become mobile. Screen children based on risk level (e.g., housing, lead in drinking water) and local recommendations. Even low levels are associated with declines in cognitive abilities.
- Uneven gait or a limp always needs evaluation for hip and structural problems, intraarticular pathology, or abnormalities in neuromotor functioning. Toddling should be symmetrical.
- Early walkers generally fall backward and land on their bottoms. A consistent "forward faller" needs evaluation of motor tone and Achilles' tendon tightness.
- Bruises on early walkers are on the bottom, forehead, and, occasionally, the anterior tibial surfaces. Investigate atypical bruise patterns or injuries because nonaccidental injury must be suspected.
- A 1-year-old should be exuberant, active, avoidant, and wiggly—in other words, very difficult to examine. If your examination is too easy, look again at developmental delays and social/emotional processes.

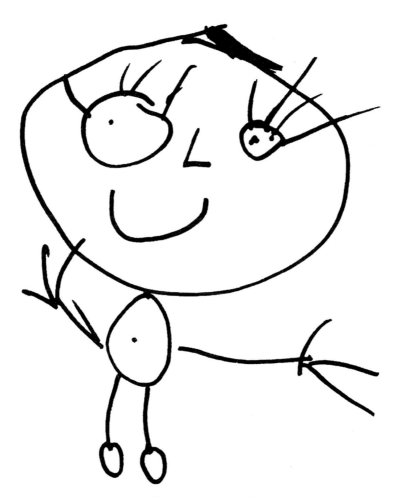

"A girl-baby walking." By Anne Atkinson, age 5.

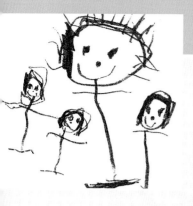

14

Fifteen to Eighteen Months: Declaring Independence and Pushing the Limits

Jenny S. Radesky and Caroline J. Kistin

Fifteen to 18 months is a period of language and cognitive development accompanied by an increasing drive for independence. Temper tantrums, temporary regressions in development, and other negative behavior should be interpreted in the context of a toddler's quest for autonomy; this age range is an important opportunity for helping caregivers mentalize about what is driving their child's changing behavior and provide responsive support. Experience with toilet training, discipline, and learning self-feeding skills are discussed in the context of changes in cognitive development and the drive to independence. Early recognition of autism spectrum disorder (ASD) at this age is reviewed and supported with specific screening tools.

KEYWORDS

- Autonomy
- Attachment
- Mentalization
- Discipline
- Regressions
- Self-feeding
- Rapprochement
- Transitional object
- Behavior modification
- Autism spectrum disorder
- Temper tantrums
- Toilet training
- Mobile devices

IMPORTANT DEVELOPMENTAL CONCEPTS

The middle of the second year often presents a shift in language, cognition, and behavior that caregivers may find both delightful and stressful. Well-child visits between

Previous chapter by Maria Trozzi and Martin T. Stein.

15 and 18 months therefore present an opportunity to wonder, along with the caregiver, about what their child understands, thinks, wants, and feels. At this age, toddlers have an expanding receptive language vocabulary (meaning, words that they understand)—primarily labels of things important to them such as "bottle" or "cookie," but also familiar commands such as "bring that to me." Their improving motor control (most should now be walking, bending down to pick things up, and getting back up again—a major way of exploring the world around you!) means that they might now be able to feed themselves by hand or get a toy that they want. Toddlers are still very much dependent on caregivers for reaching things, opening them, and doing daily activities like getting dressed, so they start to develop single words or eventually two-word combinations that help them express what they want (including "no!"). Many neurotypical toddlers also can learn hand gestures and signs for requests such as "more" or "hungry." Therefore toddlers at this age have several new skills that allow them to explore their worlds and exert their agency.

From an attachment perspective, this increased autonomy is coupled with a need to use their caregiver as a "secure base" to which they can return after brief explorations on their own. A child might appear eager and confident in running into their favorite playground or library

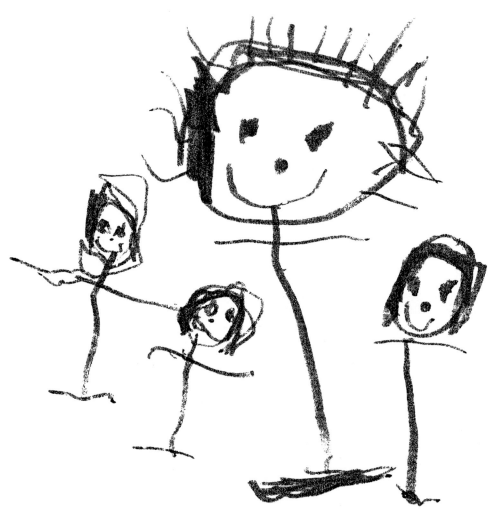

This picture shows the preschooler's perspective on the world. This girl shows herself as the largest and central figure. Mom, Dad, and sister are also pictured. By Louise Dixon, age 3½.

but then after some time turns around and seeks their caregiver, often running up for a hug or a "check in," almost to ask "Is this all ok?" This "secure base" behavior can be explained to caregivers in several ways.

First, caregivers can be praised for the fact that, through serve-and-return interactions and general responsiveness to their child's needs and cues during infancy, their child now sees them as a trusted source of security, organization, and emotional "holding." (See Chapter 2 for more description of these aspects of attachment theory.) Toddlers who have experienced trauma or neglect, or who have disorganized attachment, may not as consistently return to check in with their caregiver or may show more unclear social cues or dysregulation when they do. Relationship-based dyadic therapy is an important intervention for caregivers and toddlers with attachment insecurity, and pediatric providers should be familiar with the programs and clinicians who see infants and toddlers.

Second, caregivers may benefit from understanding that their child seeks to be more independent by using newly attained skills but needs additional nurturance to refuel the push toward **autonomy or self-regulation**. Children need caregivers for additional security but at the same time may show new assertiveness and negativism. This push-pull behavior can be confusing and frustrating, especially to caregivers who have trauma histories or mental health challenges.

The negativism toddlers exhibit at this age comes from a mismatch between their drive to explore and master new skills, with their still-developing attention span, social-emotional skills, motor dexterity, and frustration tolerance. Clinicians can help by framing negative, aggressive, or dysregulated behavior as *a sign that the child needs help but does not know how to communicate what they need*. This can help caregivers not interpret negative behavior at "face value" (e.g., reacting to a toddler's hitting by saying "he's violent") and can prevent caregivers from misattributing their child's behavior to malicious intent (e.g., interpreting their child's hitting as "he wants to upset me, just like his dad did"). The practice of **mentalizing**, or pausing to wonder about what the toddler is thinking or feeling during a difficult moment, can help caregivers more accurately interpret their child's behaviors in an developmentally appropriate way.

Cognitively, most 18-month-olds are starting to be more aware of the external world (e.g., other children, other adults, toys, furniture), and this awareness now comes into conflict with a previously secure environment modulated by their caregiver. Cognitive skills have matured enough that a child can imagine a threat and appreciate more subtle dissonance with what is familiar. This stage, called "**rapprochement**," may exhibit as clinging to a parent, crying in the presence of a stranger or refusing the approach of their pediatrician. It signifies attachment to the caregiver, the person who helps them communicate and navigate the world.

Helping a caregiver through this period is easier when the clinician's observations and expectations of behavior are informed by these developmental phenomena. The clinician can help support caregiver patterns of interaction with the child, informed by how they think about what the child is feeling, thinking, and trying to master, which have considerable longevity. Caregivers must see the struggles for mastery and independence as both inevitable and a positive sign of the child's emotional and social growth. As in adolescence (another developmental window in which children seek more independence), caregivers who respond with anxiety, overcontrol, and overprotection do not allow room for the psychological growth that is appropriate at this age.

Three aspects of behavior and development often surface at this age, either in the questions parents bring to the office visit or in what a clinician observes in the office setting: (1) discipline and temper tantrums, (2) toilet training, and (3) changes in feeding patterns. All of these issues can be interpreted with a mentalizing approach, grounded in the child's developmental stage, and seen within the context of a drive for independence.

DISCIPLINE

The newly discovered capacity to walk, run, and climb opens up new pathways of exploration for the toddler. Not only can they get to things through curiosity and self-discovery, but they can also manipulate objects into new forms that follow from imagination. Fine motor and visual-perceptual skills allow the toddler to shape, invent, and explore objects; these manipulations give definition and form to the child's world. Interestingly, hands-on play with manipulatives also helps toddlers create visual-spatial mental maps that go on to support development of math skills—another reason why only two-dimensional play with TV or touchscreens does not provide as much support for brain development. Simultaneously, receptive language function is developing rapidly; the child now *understands* many words, follows simple directions, and can even point to some parts of the body when a parent sounds its name.

These new skills emerge rapidly and must be incorporated into a psychological framework that was previously dependent solely on caretakers' manipulation of the child's environment. The awareness that through language, motor, and perceptual skills the child can shape and pattern their own world brings about inner conflict for most children. These conflicts can be seen when a tower of neatly stacked blocks falls; when a playmate, cooperative at one moment, suddenly touches a child's favorite toys; or when a parent removes a child from one enjoyable activity and moves them to another place (e.g., from playing with toys to sitting in the highchair). The toddler can now make a choice about a toy, a playmate, or a meal. Infringement on these choices produces inner disharmony that may lead to anger and aggression. A young toddler does not possess the psychological structure or frontal lobe development to delay gratification, to suppress or displace angry feelings, or to manage these difficult situations through verbal communication. The child cannot wait, see things from another's point of view, anticipate compound effects of actions, or cope effectively. An explosion is predictable.

Seeking alternative responses consistent with developmental capacities, the child pouts, cries, becomes morose, or has a temper tantrum. Behavior outbursts by an 18-month-old can be viewed as developmentally predictable (Fig. 14.1). The frequency and intensity with which an individual child manifests such behavior is dependent on many factors, including (1) the security of attachment to caregivers, (2) the toddler's individual temperament (including emotional intensity, sensory profile, and distractibility) and way of adapting to new and stressful situations, and (3) the caregivers' style of responding to various behavior in the child.

Attachment (the enduring emotional bond that people feel toward special people in their lives; see Chapter 2) directed to caregivers is a major goal of the first year of life; in the second year, children need to be encouraged to broaden the focus of that attachment and become more independent. Caregivers can be encouraged to allow self-play, mistakes, natural consequences, and learning opportunities in their child and can anticipate that this independence will, at times, be accompanied by frustration and negative affect. Piaget pointed out that children at this age learn through the experience of their own errors and successes in problem solving and exploration. "Mistakes" during play give clues about how children work to understand their experience with others and objects.

If a parent limits the development of independent skills by providing an overly protective environment, infantile attachment behavior becomes more locked into an earlier phase of development. New situations—without caregivers or when frustration is inevitable—become intolerable. When a toddler is allowed, even encouraged, to experience moderate amounts of frustration during the course of play, the child learns to manage angry feelings, feelings that may be directed toward caregivers, play objects, or a playmate. These kinds of experiences assist the child in the gradual journey to becoming more independent from caregivers and more self-regulated. These experiences also give the caregivers practice in tolerating their child's negativity,

realizing that it will eventually pass or represent a learning opportunity for the child. If the child is frustrated because they are trying to do something they are not yet developmentally capable of, then scaffolding by the caregiver can teach the child how to do it or how to ask for help.

A toddler's *temperament* is reflected in how they respond to these daily moments of friction, frustration, or adaptation (see Chapter 2). Toddlers vary significantly in the energy released when a frustrating experience arises. A child with a high level of adaptability to change and a positive approach to new stimuli will probably move quickly from a conflictual situation to one that is harmonious. At the opposite end of the spectrum is a child with intense expressions of mood and withdrawal responses to new situations. This child may be easily frustrated at seemingly minor disruptions, going from "0 to 60" before a caregiver can even observe what it was that frustrated them. A child with a more sensory-seeking profile may hit, bite, scratch, or crash their body into things when frustrated and may need other outlets for this energy. The intensity and duration of crying and screaming, as well as the level of consolability, will, in part, relate to these innate aspects of temperament. Although most children are somewhere between these temperamental extremes, a clinical appreciation for them can be helpful in assessing a particular child and the caregivers' responses to that child.

Caregiver styles of responding to a toddler's tantrums affect the resolution of the episode, as well as the nature of future tantrums. Children are sponges of adult attitudes and actions at this age. Through social learning (see Chapter 2), they slowly learn how to handle their own anger, aggression and frustration by observing parents and other caretakers. Frequently, caregivers who seem able to manage toddler tantrums are less threatened or dysregulated by their child's aggressive moments and push-pull behavior. They generally do not get drawn into the struggle themselves or yell in a manner that might escalate the child's behavior (either through reinforcement or by making the child feel more overwhelmed). Caregivers who can try to understand the drivers underlying the child's behavior can usually assist the child in handling the frustration or big feelings. Styles of parenting the child at this age often reflect a parent's own sense of self-effectiveness and own experiences from childhood. A toddler can call forth feelings and responses that many caregivers did not even know were within them; for this reason, parent-toddler dyadic psychotherapy can be helpful for caregivers to process and understand their own emotional reactions to their child.

Discipline at this age should not mean punishment, or the caregivers' response to a tantrum, but rather the approach to guiding behavior and showing the child how to cooperate. When viewed constructively, discipline can be seen as a

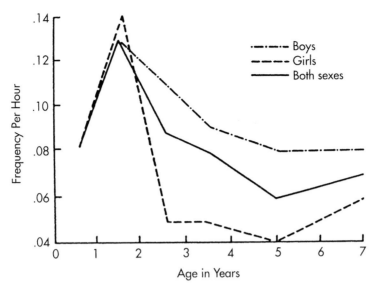

Fig. 14.1 Frequency of anger outbursts, with a peak between 18 months and 2 years. (Modified from Goodenough FL: *Anger in young children*, St. Paul, 1931, University of Minnesota Press.)

process of *teaching* the toddler to place limits or boundaries on behavior within family and cultural expectations, to learn to "use words" to express anger, to feel comfortable with feelings of anger and to learn to cope with the inevitable frustrations of normal life. It may be useful to compare tantrums with a blown fuse. The tantrum serves a purpose in itself; it releases tension by providing an exit for bound-up energy that momentarily finds no other outlet. Occasional toddler tantrums viewed in this manner can be accepted, understood and allowed to occur by an understanding caregiver. In a healthy toddler, occasional tantrums cannot usually be stopped and should even be seen as helpful.

From another perspective, teaching children what to do, rather than only admonishing them for what not to do, helps children internalize boundaries and norms, define their sense of self, and develop a sense of competence regarding who they are and what they can handle. These internalized boundaries and concepts are laid down over time from early childhood through emerging adulthood, but the 15- to 18-month window is when the first struggles are often experienced by families.

Harsh discipline, including physical punishment like spanking and verbal threats or insults, has been shown to be ineffective in changing child behavior in the long run and is associated with an increased risk of child maltreatment and child externalizing and internalizing behavioral symptoms. The majority of families in the United States report using a combination of discipline approaches, which may include both positive, nonviolent approaches as well as harsh discipline. While some parents may use physical punishment or other harsh approaches in the heat of the moment, many report using harsh discipline approaches deliberately because they believe it will benefit their children in some way in the future (e.g., getting their child to follow rules or show respect).

At the pediatric visit, the clinician can start with open-ended questions about how the parent responds when their toddler tantrums or misbehaves, what the parent observes in their child in response to their discipline, and what their hopes are in general with regards to their child's behavior. It may also be useful to ask parents what they worry will happen if they do not respond to their child with a certain discipline approach. Parents often report feeling like they need to respond in certain ways in different situations, such as feeling compelled to stop a child's tantrum quickly when at the store or out in public, when they would otherwise allow a child to finish their outburst and calm down on their own when in the home. Understanding the context in which harsh discipline is used will allow the clinician to problem solve with the family and better provide guidance around nonviolent discipline approaches.

TOILET TRAINING

Four milestones must be reached before a toddler is ready to master bowel and bladder control. They are a result of

BOX 14.1   Developmental Prerequisites for Bowel and Bladder Control

- Maturation of the central and peripheral nervous systems to the degree that voluntary control of the anal and urethral sphincters is possible; ability to sense and signal the urge to go.
- Ability to sit on a potty seat quietly for a moderate amount of time with the conscious intent to have a bowel movement or urinate.
- Desire to gain satisfaction from the successful completion of defecation and urination and recognize the pleasure in the supervising parent and within oneself through growth in competency as a form of positive reinforcement.
- Ability to understand the sequence of requirements of the task.
- Drive to imitate greater than drive to oppose parents.

neurological maturation, increased attention span, attachment to a caretaker whom they want to please, and the emerging ability to sequence events (Box 14.1).

These milestones of development reflect mastery of the motor, social, and language skills that usually come together after the second birthday. For some, it may be a few months earlier; for others, developmental readiness may not be apparent until 3 or more years of age (Table 14.1). From the child's viewpoint, toilet training that is too early or too rapid has no advantages. Indeed, from a child's perspective, there is not much to be recommended in stopping play, going to the toilet, giving up part of yourself, and then watching it summarily flushed. The process may be detrimental if it creates expectations the child cannot handle. When viewed from the standpoint of the child's needs, toilet training demands a level of complex, multistep, voluntary control that could not be obtained previously. Motor, social, and receptive language skills necessary for toilet training come together at different ages for different children, so appropriate timing of toilet training

TABLE 14.1   Guide to Toilet Training Readiness: A Developmental Approach

Child's Behavior/Competencies	Caregiver Response
Complex, multistep behavior; completing household tasks; completing tasks in sequence	Narrate the process while the child is watching a parent or siblings at the toilet
Undresses self	Allow child to undress self; loose, easily removed clothes are preferred; praise the child while mentioning that they will soon use a potty seat
Shows interest in a potty seat. Demonstrates an ability to understand the requirements of various tasks	Keep a potty seat in a regular place in the bathroom; let the child know that they can sit on it and what it is used for; some children can learn about the seat initially by sitting on it with a diaper on
Points to, looks at, or announces a BM in their diaper	Put the diaper/BM in the seat; dispose of it later; acknowledge the production
Increasing periods of daytime dryness	Use training pants during the day
Ability to sit quietly on the potty seat for a moderate period	Praise the child for knowing about the seat and discuss its use; encourage sitting on the seat
Shows satisfaction in having a BM	Praise moderately by showing pleasure in completion of the task
Asks to use the potty seat or uses it in a self-directed manner	Encourage use of the potty seat after a meal (gastrocolic reflex) or (for some children) at a time when the child usually has a BM
Desire to please by imitating parents	Praise the child by pointing out that "you're growing so big—now you're ready to use your potty seat"
Partial voluntary control of anal and urethral sphincters, as demonstrated by having a BM or urinating at a planned time on the potty seat	Show pleasure in task completion while expecting setbacks, both at times of stress and spontaneously
Interest in successful use of a potty seat	Try training pants; encourage the child to remove the training pants by self

BM, Bowel movement.

is needed to avoid struggles with the child and resulting decreases in self-esteem.

As a form of anticipatory guidance, it is helpful to discuss toilet training at the visit when the child is between 15 and 18 months old for three reasons: (1) to prevent parents from rushing into training before the child is ready, (2) to bring out the developmental significance of training as a way to assist parents in understanding and responding to the broader (and invisible, in terms of genitourinary and pelvic floor motor maturation) developmental events at this age, and (3) to help parents begin to set the stage for this process later on. It can be helpful to provide links to trusted sources of information about toilet training (e.g., the American Academy of Pediatrics [AAP] website HealthyChildren.org) so the family has access proactively.

Clues that a child is physically and emotionally ready for potty training may be observed sometime between 18 months and 2 years of age in most typically developing children. The following are examples of such clues:

- The child will demonstrate having made the connection between the feeling (muscular contractions) of urination or defecation and what is produced. This connection is communicated to the caregiver as the child points or looks at the urine or bowel movement.
- The child has increased periods of daytime dryness (i.e., increased bladder capacity and sphincter control), tells the parent after having a bowel movement or urinating, and can sit quietly for a period.
- The child shows interest in the toilet, shows imitative behavior in other areas (e.g., dressing, household tasks, washing hands), and is not otherwise showing oppositional or dysregulated behavior.

At this time, caregivers can be encouraged to introduce a potty seat, explain its function to the child, and make it available. Caregivers can take the child into the bathroom and discuss and demonstrate the process. Having the child sit on a potty chair (initially with the diaper attached) is a first step in getting acquainted with the chair and the sensory experience of sitting on it. The caregivers should be positive toward the behavior and the product (feces). The child will see the bowel movement as a part of themself; caregivers should not regard it as "yucky." Caregivers can be encouraged to show their pleasure at a successful movement, but overenthusiasm is not warranted because this makes successful stooling too "high stakes"—in other words, anxious or inconsistent children struggling to attain continence may react negatively when they "fail." Conversely, caregivers whose 2-year-old does not seem interested in a potty chair should be encouraged to wait a few months. It is often helpful to point out to caregivers that just as some neurotypical children do not walk until

after 15 months, some toddlers require more time to attain consistent voluntary sphincter control and to be willing to exercise it. It is not a measure of intelligence on the child's part or of adequacy of child rearing on the caregivers' part. Caregivers should be informed that there is immense variability in the timing and pace of this process, with boys and firstborn children generally training later. Therefore this should be seen as not something caregivers should try to exercise control over. Harsh, shaming, or overly rigid approaches to toilet training can contribute to withholding.

Initiation and continuation of toilet training are dependent on the child's personal health and environmental events. External events such as intercurrent illness, birth of a new sibling, a family vacation, or absence of a caregiver for a prolonged period can be expected to delay or cause a setback in the mastery of toilet training. When some of these events are predictable, potty training may be delayed by the caregivers. **Regressions** without any explanations should also be expected. The child's self-respect should be preserved in these circumstances. Caregivers may be very disappointed or overwhelmed with suddenly having to clean up accidents or putting a child back in expensive diapers but encourage them to try to stay supportive and calm with their child.

FEEDING AND SELF-DETERMINATION

As fine motor manipulations and visual-motor coordination advance, an 18-month-old learns to use these skills and enjoys the use of a cup and spoon. Self-feeding represents a significant form of mastery in the use of an instrument to extend and expand the abilities of the hand and in the honing of visual-motor skills (Box 14.2). It is also another psychological separation from dependency on caregivers. It is helpful to point out to caregivers that although messy and seemingly disorganized, allowing a child the freedom to feed themself assists development and mastery at several levels.

> **BOX 14.2 Developmental Skills Enhanced by Self-Feeding**
>
> - Fine motor skills
> - Hand-to-eye coordination
> - Independent actions yielding an enjoyable response
> - Learning to choose and enjoy different food textures and colors

From American Academy of Pediatrics, Committee on Psychosocial Aspects of Child and Family Health: Policy statement on guidance for effective discipline, *Pediatrics* 101:723, 1998.

As with any new skill, learning may progress at different rates in children of various temperaments, and setbacks (or regressions) may occur after intercurrent events in the family. As with most new experiences that require mastery, feeding is particularly vulnerable to individual differences and fluctuations. Particular attractions or dislikes for certain foods are frequently seen at this time, often driven by sensory differences and age-appropriate resistance to trying new things. Prolonged periods of refusing one food group are common (i.e., food jags). Excessive intake of juice, soda, or milk, on the other hand, can make a toddler feel full, even though they have not taken in the nutrients required for growth, and can lead to undernutrition. However, as long as the child's physical growth has not been compromised, parents can be reassure that fluctuations in diet are normal and self-limited. Demonstrating the child's rate of growth on a standard growth curve is often helpful for a caregiver who perceives the toddler as "too picky." Food refusal in a child who is otherwise growing normally provides an opportunity to explain to caregivers the importance of self-directed feeding in terms of a child's need for emotional independence, recognizing their own satiety cues and regulating intake, and, eventually, better eating habits. The more the clinician can do to assist the caregiver of a toddler in understanding new feeding behaviors and skills as a reflection of mastery and "separation" from infantile dependency on the parent, the better equipped they will be to support their child through continued guidance and surveillance without squelching further growth.

Transitional Object

About two-thirds of toddlers will have an inanimate **transitional object** that is used for comforting, especially when they are falling asleep and at times of stress. Their use may persist until the third or fourth birthday and occasionally later. There are several reasons why transitional objects can be helpful at this age. Cognitively, toddlers have object permanence and therefore may have separation anxiety when they are not with their caregiver, yet they know the caregiver still exists somewhere else. Toddlers and young children have weaker mental flexibility, which is why transitions from one activity to another can be challenging. The transitional object, often a blanket or doll, can have a comforting presence in these scenarios. Transitional objects can also be built into calming routines, such as going to bed, taking deep breaths when upset, or to help children be brave when trying new things. Caregivers can therefore be reassured that these objects are not a sign of immaturity.

Summary

The "push-pull" process that characterizes this stage of development can be viewed as one of daily increments of psychological growth achieved by mastery of more complicated skills. These skills require adequate maturation of the toddler's nervous system and the caregivers' ability to simultaneously stimulate and pull back, that is, to encourage self-feeding, potty seat recognition, and creative play while letting the child master these objects and events independently. To be sure, it is a delicate balance that requires caregiver skill that will vary in different families. The child's clinician can point out the developmental necessity of this balance. It can be demonstrated with a "teachable moment" during the physical examination with toys or examining instruments or when observing the child's play during the interview with the caregiver.

AUTISM SPECTRUM DISORDER: EARLY DETECTION MAKES A DIFFERENCE

ASD is a neurodevelopmental disorder that is characterized by challenges in social reciprocity, verbal and non-verbal communication, developing peer relationships, and restricted and repetitive patterns of behavior. ASD incidence has been rising steadily over the past decades to a current rate of 1 in 36 US children, according to 2023 data from the Centers for Disease Control and Prevention. This increase has been attributed to diagnostic shift (in other words, children who used to be diagnosed with intellectual disability now are more likely to also have an ASD diagnosis), recognition of milder cases of ASD that nonetheless warrant treatment, and increased screening and family/clinician recognition. It is also possible that there is a true increase in ASD incidence, which could be due to multiple factors including higher rates of premature birth and older paternal age. Environmental toxicants such as phthalates have also been implicated in raising ASD risk on a population level. In contrast, multiple high-quality studies have demonstrated that vaccines are *not* linked with autism risk.

Our understanding of ASD has evolved significantly since Kanner first described autism in 1943. Autism self-advocates describe ASD as being "a neuro-developmental disability that generally leads to differences in communication and social skills, unique patterns of thought and behavior, and divergent sensory experiences. It is a neurological difference that can present difficulties, but also advantages" (Autistic Self-Advocacy Network). Indeed, many people with ASD have excellent memory, visual-spatial skills (e.g., drawing or remembering numerical details), and sense of humor, among other unique abilities.

Toddlers with ASD usually present with a constellation of developmental differences that come to light between 12 months and preschool age range (Tables 14.2 and 14.3), although some individuals are not diagnosed with autism

TABLE 14.2   Parental Concerns That Are Red Flags for Autism Spectrum Disorder in Toddlers

Communication Concerns
Does not respond to name when called
Cannot communicate what they want
Language is delayed or repetitive (e.g., quotes favorite videos/songs)
Does not point, reach to be picked up, or wave bye-bye
Used to say a few words but now does not

Social Concerns
Does not smile at other people socially
Prefers to play alone
Gets things for themselves rather than asking for help
Is very independent
Has limited eye contact (may be stronger with caregivers than new people)
Is in their "own world" or "tunes people out"
Is not interested in other children or is overwhelmed by them

Behavioral Concerns
Tantrums with transitions or changes
Seeks movement through running, swinging, spinning, or deep pressure
Plays with toys in atypical ways, such as lining up or dumping in and out of containers
Looks closely at objects
Gets stuck on the same activity over and over
Unusual movement patterns such as toe walking, hand flapping, or twiddling fingers
Has unusual attachments to toys (e.g., is always holding a certain object)
Is oversensitive to certain textures or sounds

until the school-age years, adolescence, or even adulthood. Research has shown that ASD can be reliably diagnosed as young as 14 months of age, so it is important to identify, refer, and treat ASD early so that children can benefit most from therapies while their brain has the most neuroplasticity (i.e., under 5 years of age). A common misconception is that the toddler years are "too young" to diagnose autism. In actuality, the earlier a child starts autism-specific therapies and school supports, the better their prognosis. Therefore the 15- and 18-month health supervision visits should include specific observations and questions directed to parents that screen for autism.

The AAP recommends administering a validated ASD screening instrument at 18- and 24-month well-child visits and whenever a concern is raised by caregivers or teachers/childcare providers. ASD has a strong genetic component, so it is particularly important to perform surveillance if there is a family history of ASD. It is important for pediatric clinicians to know that commonly used screening instruments such as the MCHAT (Modified Checklist for Autism in Toddlers) do not have 100% sensitivity or specificity, and they therefore may miss some children with ASD. This is why repeated screening is recommended at two different points in the toddler years, and clinicians may choose to

refer for a developmental evaluation even with a negative MCHAT if history is concerning (i.e., see questions in Table 14.3) or parent, teacher, or clinician concern for ASD is present.

Adjusting to the possibility of an autism diagnosis is challenging for most caregivers. The development of most children with autism often appears typical to parents and clinicians in the first year of life. By the toddler years, many caregivers recognize that something is different, but they just are not sure how to make sense of it. Toddlers' challenges in social communication can be subtle, vary in different settings, or are more apparent to caregivers only in retrospect. For example, when home videotapes of first birthday parties in infants with autism were compared with those of infants who had typical development, four aspects of behavior correctly identified over 90% of infants with ASD:

- Diminished eye contact
- Lack of orienting to their name being called
- Infrequent pointing with a finger to indicate interest in something
- Not showing an object by bringing it to a person

Delays in pointing and showing are early signs of atypical development in "joint attention" behavior that are seen in toddlers with autism. Indications for immediate referral

TABLE 14.3 **Screening and Diagnosis of Autistic Spectrum Disorders**	
Ask Specific Development Probes: "Does She or He ... " or "Is There ..."	
Socialization	Look at you when you are talking or playing?
	Smile in response to a smile from others?
	Engage in reciprocal, back-and-forth play?
	Play simple imitation games, such as pat-a-cake or peek-a-boo?
	Show interest in other children?
Communication	Point with their finger?
	Gesture? Nod yes and no?
	Direct your attention by holding up objects for you to see?
	Anything odd about his/her speech?
	Show things to people?
	Lead an adult by the hand?
	Give inconsistent responses to name? To commands?
	Use rote, repetitive, or echolalic speech?
	Memorize strings of words or scripts?
Behavior	Have repetitive, stereotyped, or odd motor behavior?
	Have preoccupations or a narrow range of interests?
	Attend more to parts of objects (e.g., wheels)?
	Have limited or absent pretend play?
	Imitate other people's actions?
	Play with toys in the exact same way each time?
	Have a strong attachment to a specific unusual object?

From Filipek PA, Pasquale JA, Baranek GT, et al: The screening and diagnosis of autistic spectrum disorders, *J Autism Dev Disord* 29:6, 1999.

to Early Intervention and diagnostic evaluation during the second year of life include:

- No babbling by 12 months
- No gesturing (pointing, waving bye-bye) by 12 months
- No single words by 16 months
- No two-word spontaneous (not just echolalia) phrases by 23 months
- Any loss of any language or social skills at any age

Clinicians often worry they should "watch and wait" when autism concerns are detected, particularly if the family expresses resistance to the possibility of the diagnosis. In recent research, pediatric primary care providers have expressed feeling uncertain about mentioning the "A-word" to families, with fear of loss of trust or rapport with families who are not yet ready. Another source of resistance is the long wait times for diagnostic and treatment services; primary care clinicians express hesitation of sending families into a "labyrinth" of appointments and services if they are unsure about an ASD diagnosis. For this reason, many academic medical centers and states have been piloting tiered autism diagnostic systems that allow clear-cut cases to be diagnosed by specially trained general pediatricians, reducing wait times considerably. Until these systems are more widespread, pediatric clinicians should work on motivating parents to pursue an autism diagnostic evaluation as soon as a concern is identified; while the family waits for an evaluation, the child can enroll in Early Intervention, school services, and/or speech-language therapy. It does no harm to start developmental therapies early; in fact, even if an ASD diagnosis is not made, most caregivers report feeling that Early Intervention and therapies helped them understand their child better and have more tools for supporting their communication and behavior. Pediatric clinicians should also familiarize themselves with culturally responsive information about ASD in multiple languages, as is available through the AAP and Autism Speaks, so that the diagnosis and its treatment can be demystified and destigmatized for caregivers.

DURING THE VISIT

Observations

Watching an 18-month-old child, both during independent play and while interacting with the caregiver, provides insight into the developmental goals of this age. As the history is recorded, helpful observations include the following:

- Does the child play independently, making use of toys in the examining room?
- Fine motor dexterity and visual-motor skills can be observed through play. Does the child play spontaneously with toys in the office, make a tower out of four cubes, scribble spontaneously, or try to remove clothes by themself?
- Does the child have a transitional object? Was it brought to the office? If so, how is it used by the child?
- Does the caregiver allow the child to move around the examining room independently, to experiment with the available toys?
- How does the caregiver scaffold the child's play, verbally and nonverbally?
- When you walk into the room, what is the child doing? Does the activity change in your presence?
- What is the intensity and duration with which the child clings to the caregiver? How does the caregiver respond?
- What is the content and style of the caregiver's verbal interactions with the child?
- Assess the child's response to your examination.

History

To determine the point on the developmental pathway from dependency to autonomy for a particular toddler, the clinician may ask a caregiver to describe a typical morning at home with the child. Within this description, caregivers usually provide some examples of motor, language, and social milestones, how the child plays, what they eat, as well as how structured their routines typically are—and how much of a role TV or media play in the child's routines. If the caregiver does not provide these details in their account, focused questions can be directed to the caregivers, with the goal of assessing psychological independence:

- Does the child play alone for short periods? What kind of toys are of interest? Does the home have safe places for exploration? Is there a place for the child in every room?
- Does the child experience temper tantrums? What appears to set them off? When do they occur? How intense are they and how long do they last? What are your usual responses, and what do you do when you are in different settings (such as home vs. the store)? What happens afterward? How do they make you feel?
- What are your hopes for your child's behavior? Do you and your partner agree on expectations for and management of the child's behavior? Is your management plan different from the way you were raised?
- Does the child have a favorite thing to carry around or take to bed? How do you feel about it? Do you always make it available?
- When the child is doing something that is off limits, how do you respond? What do you say? What do you do? What do you worry will happen if you do not respond?

- Many caregivers of toddlers find it hard to say *no* so many times each day. How do you manage to change behavior without always saying *no*?
- Have you thought about toilet training? If so, what ideas do you have about when and how to accomplish it?

Examination

Approach the child gently. If when you enter the examination room, the toddler is on the floor or at a table playing with toys, you might bend down to the child's level. Sitting on the floor and engaging the child with a ball or other toy may yield a temporary alliance and permit effective interaction with the child. A simple, brief comment about the toy the child is playing with or a color (or pattern) on clothes may be helpful.

Frequently at this age a toddler may react with alarm at your entrance into the examining room, usually seeking out the caregivers and either clinging to them or sitting quietly on their lap. Reassure the caregiver that this is expected behavior at this age. In fact, it represents an emotionally close attachment between the child and caregiver. It also gives the examiner an opportunity to observe how the child communicates their distress to their caregiver, whether they show social referencing (e.g., looking to their caregiver to check their reaction to a new situation), and how the caregiver soothes them (or appears overwhelmed).

The physical examination is usually performed optimally with the child in caregiver's lap. Stranger awareness is lessened in this more secure position. Physical differences (e.g., facial features, extremities) can be assessed accurately while the parent holds the child. In the same manner, assessment of language, motor, and social skills can be successful when the child is sitting on the parent's lap. Children with ASD may show very little eye contact with the examiner, or eye contact that is not well modulated (e.g., has a staring quality; is only present when the child initiates the interaction, but not in response to the examiner); therefore do not use eye contact as the only marker of possible ASD. At 15 to 18 months, other signs to look for include lack of gestures (e.g., waving, pointing, reaching), repetitive body movements (e.g., hand flapping, finger twiddling), or atypical interests (e.g., focused interest in the wheels of a car or the leg of a table rather than playing or interacting).

Some neurotypical children, those with trauma, and those with ASD may show behavior dysregulation during parts of the examination, so their developmental skills may be difficult to assess. If they brought a transitional object, you can pretend to examine the toy first, narrating that their favorite object is OK and has no "owies." You can also give them a break and provide a book while you continue to talk to the caregiver; you can reassure the caregiver that they do not need to feel embarrassed when their toddler screams and clings to them, since doctor's visits are stressful for toddlers and it is a sign that they are seeking comfort with the person they are most attached to. A comment such as "Maggie certainly knows who is important in her life!" will go a long way to ease any tension the caregiver may experience.

If the caregiver brings out a **mobile device** such as iPad or phone for the toddler to use, there are a few ways you can handle this. First, you can ask "What do they like to watch? Can I suggest something?" Then, see if the caregiver can put on a video that includes music or nursery rhymes (e.g., Itsy Bitsy Spider; Wheels on the Bus). This may be a good opportunity to sign and gesture along with the child and caregiver, which may generate more shared enjoyment and eye contact. You can also let the child watch something to calm down and then perhaps get a better listen to their heart sounds. It is worth (nonjudgmentally) letting the caregiver know that using a screen can make it harder to interact with the child (since kids rarely want to look up from the screen!), so you'll want to transition away from it later to try to play with the child again. This is a good opportunity to ask the caregiver how they usually get their child to disengage from a screen as well as discuss strategies that might help (such as timers, countdowns, and immediately transitioning to a new activity).

ANTICIPATORY GUIDANCE

Caregiver education at this examination should focus on the following:
1. Anticipating behavioral or developmental problems based on the clinician's findings during the interview and physical examination
2. Assisting caregivers with the next developmental stage by pointing to new milestones and anticipated behavior

The child's temperament, behavioral responses to new situations, progress in self-directed feeding, and independent play will guide the discussion of anticipatory guidance. Not every visit at 18 months will require the discussion offered in these guidelines. For some caregivers, reassurance that development is on track will suffice. However, insight into broader meanings of new skills is appreciated by all caregivers.

Behavioral and developmental education for caregivers of an 18-month-old may include the following topics:

Self-feeding as an Expression of Control and Independence

The clinician can help caregivers see mealtime as important in the child's growing expression of control and independence.

- Talk about feeding time in terms of the *child's* needs, not only the need for nutrients but also the need for self-directed mastery over an important part of the environment.
- Point out that appetites are often erratic at this age, but that given the availability of nutritious foods, an 18-month-old will choose adequate nutrients over time. Recommend limited juice intake, 4 ounces a day or less. If appetite seems low, offer food before drinks and feed more often—three meals and two to three balanced snacks per day—instead of unlimited grazing on low-calorie snacks throughout the day.
- Discourage forced feeding or battles over food intake. Redirect the discussion to help the caregivers view feeding in developmental terms, as an expression of learning to be satisfied through a self-directed task. This can sometimes be difficult for caregivers who focus on observable evidence of their success as parents (e.g., my child cleaned their plate; my child's face and clothes were clean) rather than the qualitative process of seeing new developmental skills emerge and flux.
- Let caregivers know that messy feeding behavior is both expected and appropriate at this age.
- Praise caregivers for allowing the toddler to exercise new visual-motor skills that provide the hand-eye coordination for successful use of a cup and spoon. Socially accepted eating patterns are nurtured over time by a positive approach to these social situations.
- Explain that foods that the family eats should make up most of the toddler's diet.

Toilet Training Readiness

This examination (usually the last health supervision visit before the second birthday) is an ideal time to anticipate the caregivers' expectations, knowledge, and plans for the initiation of toilet training. If there are no developmental concerns identified at the visit, you can ask the caregivers, "What are your thoughts about toilet training?" Providing developmentally appropriate information at this time in terms of motor, social, and receptive language skills goes a long way in preventing either a too rigid or a too lenient program for the child. Table 14.1 provides guidelines for the early stages of the process. It is helpful to teach parents that learning to use a potty seat is an important milestone in the toddler's ability to take control of the environment while gaining a sense of mastery and feeling good about oneself. The focus should be on the *child's* control, not the parents'.

Anticipating Disciplinary Problems

Assisting caregivers in understanding the expected development of negative behavior in the form of emotional outbursts is a significant task for the child's clinician at this time. It should be explained and interpreted in terms of the toddler's striving for psychological independence while the ability to manage anger and frustrations is limited by their language and social-emotional skills. A tantrum is communication: it is the child's bid to have a say in what is going on, to have his or her perspective appreciated.

Discipline approach is shaped by many factors, including personal history, social norms, and the parent's hopes and fears about their child's behavior in the long run. The majority of parents in the US report using more than one discipline approach, most commonly combining positive, nonviolent approaches with harsher discipline at times, including yelling at or threatening their child. While spanking is less common than it used to be, it is still used by many families.

The AAP recognizes that harsh discipline carries significant risks to a child's psychological and physical development (see the "Recommended Readings"). After asking open-ended questions to better understand the family's current approach, hopes, and fears about their child's behavior, it may be helpful to provide parents with guidelines to assist them in clarifying their perception of the child's problem and a strategy for intervention. Box 14.3

BOX 14.3   Trauma-Informed Approaches for Helping Parents Reflect On their Experience as a Parent, Emotional Reaction to their Child, and Child Behavior

- What am I trying to teach my child? What values do I want to impart on them?
- Why is this important to me?
- How am I trying to teach it?
- What is my child learning from what I say and from my role modeling?
  - What is my child's behavior trying to communicate to me?
  - Is my child's behavior triggering a reaction in me because of my past experiences?
  - How am I interpreting my child's behavior, and how is that affected by my past experiences?
  - How was I parented as a child, and what parts of that approach do I want to carry forward in how I parent? What parts do I not want to repeat with my children?
  - How does my reaction to my child vary based on how tired or stressed I am?
  - What times of day do I feel most emotionally available and ready to teach? What times of day do I most need a break?
  - How can I take care of myself so that I can adapt to my child's changing development and behaviors?

---

gives critical questions for effective interactions by parents. Parents may have questions about whether or how to use "time out," which is the removal of positive parental attention for a period of time, in an effort to stop a current behavior and serve as a deterrent for future similar behaviors. While this may seem like a good alternative to spanking or yelling on the surface, it is important to share with parents that toddlers do not throw tantrums or misbehave to bother them or because they are malicious. A time out will not give them the ability to control their future behavior at this age. While it may be appropriate to leave a child alone for a few minutes while they are highly dysregulated, particularly if the parent needs a minute to calm down as well, prolonged time alone can actually exacerbate the behavior as the child continues to struggle to express their needs.

Anticipating Frustration and Tantrums

Many children at this age experience a tantrum when their immediate environment overheats (e.g., a supermarket, a large family gathering, dinner preparations at the end of a busy day). The excessive sensory stimulation may be visual, auditory, tactile, or, as is often the case, a combination of sensory inputs. There are often predictable patterns when parents know their child is highly likely to tantrum (such as in the morning when everyone is busy preparing for work or school, at the end of the day when parents and older siblings return home, or at bedtime). While some modifications to the family schedule may be possible, this pattern recognition in and of itself can help parents think about how they want to respond in moment, even if the tantrum or inciting events cannot be avoided. Ask parents whether there are times of day that seem to be the hardest—both for the toddler and the parent—and talk through what could be helpful to anticipate and prepare for those times.

Prevention of tantrums also depends on communication. It can be helpful to discuss how to deliver clear instructions to toddlers and model these approaches in a visit. Young children respond best to clear, brief explanations of what to do, accompanied by a visual signal such as a gesture (e.g., "step right here on this blue dot" while pointing at the office scale). Getting on the child's level and maintaining eye contact helps direct the child's attention. If the child brings a transitional object, such as its name, and involves it in the physical examination or playful interactions, you can even explain what is going to happen by first showing a favorite stuffed animal. For children struggling with a transition, use a "first-then" approach to help them understand your instructions (e.g., "first sit, then shoes").

When a tantrum occurs, removing the toddler from the conflictual environment and sitting with them in a quiet place is a good first step. Physical affection such as hugging is calming for some children, while others will not want to feel restrained. Making a statement that reflects the child's feelings at the moment gives the child a growing vocabulary for what they are feeling (Box 14.4). Examples of this form of communication are shown in Box 14.5. Although the intensity of the tantrum, the child's temperament, and the parent's ability to mentalize about the child's emotional state will predict the effect of this method, it is a very powerful tool, not only as a method of response to negative behavior but, more significantly, as a potential foundation for parent-child communication about feelings.

Distraction with another activity, toy, or book is another effective method for short-circuiting some tantrums, since toddlers have a relatively short attention span and are fascinated by novelty. However, caregivers should be advised to not use television or mobile devices to distract a child from a tantrum, since this has been linked with worse emotion regulation skills over time. It is possible that, because children quiet down so quickly when watching preferred media, children and caregivers do not get the practice of managing emotion dysregulation through communicating about feelings or using a calming activity (e.g., breathing, hugs, blowing bubbles). Young children may also start to expect that their negative behavior will be answered with turning on a TV show or being handed a mobile device.

Behavior Modification Principles for Caregivers to Know

Reinforcement of positive behavior and ignoring minor negative behavior form the core of **behavior modification**.

BOX 14.4   EXPRESSING EMOTIONS THROUGH IDEAS

Greenspan's model for child development emphasized the interaction between emerging emotional capacities and thought processes at different ages. He has pointed out that an 18-month-old exhibits **specific behavior to express emotions through ideas and play:**

- *Dependency and security*—Caring for and holding a doll or stuffed toy.
- *Pleasure*—Showing smiles and excitement to accompany play; indicating fondness for certain food or a special toy.
- *Curiosity*—Hide-and-seek or exploring drawers or closets; search play with dolls or stuffed toys.
- *Assertiveness*—Making needs known verbally; putting a doll or stuffed toy in charge of activities of other toys.
- *Protest and anger*—Using words such as *mad* to express anger; getting mad at an uncooperative toy.
- *Setting self-limits*—Punishing a doll or stuffed toy for being naughty; responding to parental "no."
- In this model, "a tantrum is seen as the result of a frustration—an inability to master a task, to communicate a desire, to understand why things are as they are." After a calming-down period, the parent can then reengage the child in the world of ideas and teach a valuable lesson: closeness between parent and child can occur even after a disruptive emotional experience. By teaching a child to label feelings and learn to make use of pretend play and by using words to discipline, the child's emotional and cognitive skills are blended to encourage growth. Greenspan offers the following example of managing a toddler temper tantrum: "Jimmy enjoys taking care of his stuffed dog in pretend play, but has temper tantrums when frustrated. Today, his mother cannot find his green car just when he wants it. He manages to say, 'Car. Green', and then when it does not instantly appear, he turns red in the face and starts kicking, stomping, and throwing things all over the place in a full-fledged tantrum. At moments of rage like this, your teaching about ideas obviously needs to wait until you have calmed the child down. So Jimmy's mother yells a little, threatens a little and physically stops Jimmy from kicking until he quiets down. The two then sulk in mutual annoyance for a few minutes with Jimmy going off by himself and starting to play. At this point, his mother sits next to him, becomes a partner in his play and then gives him a hug to show that everything is all right. While she is giving him a hug, she also says, Are you still angry?' This gives the child a chance to learn the word for the emotions he felt, as well as the idea that emotions can be labeled. Gradually, his mother explains about patience and how to look for things he cannot find right away. Later on, when he wants his green car again, his mother might be able to convince him to be patient and look further. She can show him, even in hide-and-seek fashion, how to look. 'Is Mr. Green Car in the closet? No, he's not here. Under the chair?' etc. This use of ideas will probably not work each time, but he may be willing to wait and look rather than throw a tantrum at least some of the time. Your ability to tolerate intense emotion and to reconnect with your child will encourage his use of ideas to express feelings."

Modified from Greenspan SI: *Psychopathology and adaptation in infancy and early childhood: principles of clinical diagnosis and preventive intervention*, New York, 1981, International Universities Press; Greenspan S, Greenspan NT: *First feelings: milestones in the emotional development of your baby and child*, New York, 1985, Penguin Books.

Some caregivers encourage negative behavior unconsciously by showing a big reaction, whether positive (e.g., laughing when a child says a rude word) or negative (e.g., yelling when a child hits or throws). Point out that a young child may see this type of big reaction as reinforcing, and that it is more effective to (1) calmly ignore minor negative behavior, (2) calmly and firmly set a limit (e.g., "no running; hold my hand in the parking lot"), and/or (3) immediately teach the child a positive replacement for the negative behavior (e.g.,

"no hitting. Tap my arm like this if you want attention"). The latter strategy allows the child to "redo" their negative behavior and use an approach that is more effective at communicating their need. At the same, specific praise for positive behavior teaches the child that parental attention and appreciation are the reward for showing positive behaviors, such as asking for help, transitioning away from a fun activity, or making something with toys.

Immediate reinforcement or teaching is important due to toddlers' stage of cognitive development. Delayed rewards are not as effective because toddlers do not operate according to rule-based thinking (a cognitive achievement that emerges several years in the future). They may respond to an adult's direction but not learn the rule behind the direction until it has been repeated and explained many times. Helping parents understand these limitations of toddler cognition and memory will reduce frustration when caregivers find they need to repeat themselves over and over. Additional concepts and recommended approaches to discipline and teaching for young children are presented in Boxes 14.6 and 14.7.

BOX 14.5 Tantrums: Statements that Reflect A Child's Feelings

- "Gee, you sure are upset right now!"
- "Sometimes we get real angry and upset inside us when things aren't going well."
- "Isn't it awful when you can't do something you really want to do?"
- "You seem really mad at me now."

BOX 14.6 Discipline in Early Childhood Management: Concepts for Clinician

- *Achieving a trusting relationship*—Caregiver perceives the child's clinician as someone available to discuss behavioral outbursts and other negative behavior—ideally a safe place to discuss their own frustrations as a caregiver.
- *Identifying problem areas*—Through a screening checklist or focused questions, developmentally predictable behavioral problems should be queried.
- *Exploring historical and social predisposing factors*—Include questions on maternal depression, prenatal events, perinatal stress, the health of siblings, the vulnerable child syndrome, substance abuse, and the parents' own childhood memories.
- *Viewing parenthood as a developmental process*—Recognize that parenting skills are established through maturation, knowledge, experience, and guidance. Development of effective parenting skills takes time.
- *Encouraging parents to take an active role in deciding how to manage the child's behavior*—Explore methods previously used by the caregivers and provide support for their methods or suggest modifications that might be more effective.
- *Respecting different parenting styles*—Cultural, societal, and past experience provide caregivers with variable responses to child behavior. Variations in child rearing in families can be instructive for the clinician. A "best" way to manage a behavioral problem does not exist.

- *Providing appropriate models*—Increase caregiver awareness that children imitate and identify with their caregivers' behavior. While modeling healthy adult behavior, the clinician can be a useful guide to the caregiver.
- *Consistency*—Rules are essential for discipline. For toddlers, the number of rules should be limited and caregivers should enforce only the important ones. This should help with consistency.
- *Talking about discipline*—Parents (and other childcare providers) should discuss with each other expectations for the child's behavior and agree on management approaches. Discuss approaches that have worked in the past for the child's specific temperament and emotion regulation needs.
- *Rewarding appropriate behavior*—Praise, encouragement, and naturalistic rewards increase a child's happiness, security, and sense of self.
- *Natural consequences to discourage some behavior*—Consistency is important. Design natural consequences to motivate socially approved behavior and to help a child learn from their experience. Carry out as soon as possible after inappropriate behavior and allow for "repair" between the child and other person whom they have hurt or offended.

Modified from Smith EE, Van Tassel E: Problems of discipline in early childhood, *Pediatr Clin North Am* 29:167, 1982.

BOX 14.7	Discipline in Early Childhood Management: Concepts for Parents

- Role modeling is important. Children are watching *what we do* as much as *what we say*.
- Set expectations for behavior in clear, simple language. Visual examples such as pictures (e.g., a visual schedule for morning or bedtime routines) or breaking down the behavior step by step can help all children comprehend instructions, particularly those with language delay.
- Teaching is most effective when children are calm, not in the midst of a tantrum or when they are hungry or tired.
- Repetition of an expected behavior, with specific praise or reinforcement after, is usually needed for a toddler to learn to do it without your help.
- Set children up for success by maintaining low-stress, predictable schedules and routines, especially around sleep, eating, and screen media. This is how children internalize and learn self-regulation.
- Give children advanced warning before transitions. Visual schedules and timers can help provide the child a sense of what is happening next. Allowing your child to take a transitional object from activity to activity can also help.
- Give your child choices around things like clothing, which cup to use, which stuffed animal to bring, or what activity they want to do first. This feeling of control can help them not try to exert control through tantrums in other situations.
- Know which daily experiences make your child frustrated, such as buckling in a car seat, waiting for a snack, or brushing teeth. For any of these tiny dramas, singing a song or counting how much time is left (e.g., counting down from 10) will help the child get through it.
- Do not take negative behavior personally. It is a sign the child does not know how else to express themselves or is wanting your attention. Use it as a teaching moment to help the child express themselves or solve a problem.
- Read books that teach about emotions, toilet training, bedtime, and other daily challenges. Children learn from storytelling.
  - If you show a big reaction such as yelling or laughing in response to a negative behavior, it is OK, but it might reinforce that behavior. Next time, use ignoring for minor annoying behaviors, teaching or "redos" for negative behaviors where you can teach them a replacement behavior, and calm/clear limit setting for unsafe behaviors.
- Understand the evidence that harsh discipline does not work well to support positive behavior in the long run and can cause harm by teaching children that yelling or hitting is the way to solve a problem. It also makes children feel ashamed or afraid of their emotions and impulses, rather than feeling that they are manageable.
- Discipline approaches are going to change over time as your child's language, cognitive, and social-emotional skills develop.
- Use consistent approaches across homes, caregivers, and childcare settings.

Anticipating Parental Distress

The rapid changes in the development of a toddler may be overwhelming for single parents, those with less social support, families experiencing economic stress, and families undergoing a significant life event (e.g., divorce, illness, or an unplanned move).

Young children are barometers of the family's emotional life. Although regressions in recently acquired milestones are common in all children at this stage, they are predictable in children of families experiencing increased stress. Developmental regressions in toddlers include refusal to use the potty seat, throwing food when in the highchair, screaming with seemingly mild frustration, and increased periods of night awakening. Although these types of behavior are transient setbacks in development, they are particularly frustrating to the caregiver in distress. The child's demands may be just too much for

the caregiver to handle, who may not be able to mentalize beyond the behavior. Some caregivers internalize the child's behavior and seem to see it as a failure in parenting ("She was so good at eating by herself and using the potty seat a few weeks ago. What have I done to cause this new behavior?"). Along with guilt, these caregivers experience anger and fatigue as the toddler's infantile responses become more difficult to manage in the presence of acute or chronic family distress. Some parents with their own traumatic childhood or adult experiences will have more difficulty tolerating child distress, negativity, or aggression. It is important to anticipate or recognize the accompanying anxiety, reactivity, or emotional distancing that may be present in the caregiver. When appropriate, offer assistance in the form of referral to a behavioral resource or dyadic therapy that involves both the caregiver and child.

QUICK CHECK—15 TO 18 MONTHS

✓ Walks and runs.
✓ Climbs.
✓ Uses both hands equally.
✓ Says more than 10 words. Understands one-step commands.
✓ Plays game: peek-a-boo.
✓ Imitates household tasks.
✓ Takes off some clothing.
✓ Uses a spoon.
✓ Drinks from a cup.
✓ The emergence of self-regulatory skills (feeding, falling and staying asleep, walking, talking) encourages autonomy.
✓ Anger outbursts peak between 18 months and 2 years.

✓ Developmental prerequisites to toilet training include voluntary control of anal and urethral sphincters, ability to sit on the potty quietly with intent to have a bowel movement, desire to please the parent and self as positive reinforcement, ability to sequence the events.
✓ Self-feeding requires and enhances fine motor skills, hand-eye coordination, autonomy, and learning to choose and enjoy different textures and colors of foods.
✓ Anticipating tantrums and short-circuiting excessive frustration by distraction and talking (expressing to the child their feelings when angry) are effective responses to tantrums.

HEADS UP—15 TO 18 MONTHS

• Social interactions should include well-modulated eye contact, gesturing with hands/fingers, social referencing (i.e., looking at the caregiver in response to an experience), and a desire to show the caregiver an object.
• An expressive vocabulary of fewer than five words is a significant delay. Regression in language can be associated with ASD.
• If a child does not point to a body part when asked, consider hearing loss or receptive language delay.
• A toddler who has difficulty learning self-feeding, sleeping alone, and limited exploratory play may not be reaching the expected goals for autonomy.
• Recognize the value of a "teachable moment" when a parent disciplines a child with physical force or harsh

language. Try mentalizing about the child's emotions, reflecting the parent's emotional experience, and modeling alternative methods. Use the visit as an opportunity to better understand the parent's understanding of the child's behavior and what their hopes and fears are that are underpinning their choice of discipline approach.
• Take notice if a parent seems embarrassed by a transitional object. Another teachable moment.
• Caregivers may be anxious about single isolated delays in development (e.g., refusal to use a cup, preference for self-play in a temperamentally shy toddler, insistence on sleeping in the parent's bed). A comprehensive developmental history and observations are required to sort out a delay in achieving autonomy.

RECOMMENDED READINGS

For Parents

Brazelton TB, Sparrow JD. *Discipline: the Brazelton way.* Cambridge: Da Capo Press; 2003.
Brazelton TB, Sparrow JD. *Feeding: the Brazelton way.* Cambridge: Da Capo Press; 2004.
Brazelton TB, Sparrow JD. *Toilet training: the Brazelton way.* Cambridge: Da Capo Press; 2004.
What's the best way to discipline my child?— HealthyChildren.org
Self-feeding—HealthyChildren.org
Potty training—HealthyChildren.org
Autism—HealthyChildren.org
Non-English Resources | Autism Speaks
An early start for your child with autism. By Sally Rogers, Geraldine Dawson, and Laurie Vismara.
Good inside: a guide to becoming the parent you want to be. By Becky Kennedy.
The whole-brain child: 12 revolutionary strategies to nurture your child's developing mind. By Daniel Siegel and Tina Payne Bryson.
No-drama discipline: the whole-brain way to calm the chaos and nuture your child's developing mind. By Daniel Siegel and Tina Payne Bryson.

For Clinicians

Emotional Life of the Toddler by Alicia Lieberman
Kiddoo DA. Toilet training children: when to start and how to train. *CMAJ.* 2012;184(5):511.
Sege RD, Siegel BS, Council on Child Abuse and Neglect, Committee on Psychosocial Aspects of Child and Family Health, et al.Flaherty EG, Gavril AR, Idzerda SM, Laskey A, et al. Effective discipline to raise healthy children. *Pediatrics.* 2018;142(6): no.

Smith AB. How do infants and toddlers learn the rules? Family discipline and young children. *Int J Early Childhood*. 2004;36:27–41.

Kohlhoff J, Cibralic S. *The impact of attachment-based parenting interventions on externalizing behaviors in toddlers and preschoolers: a systematic narrative review. Child Youth Care Forum*. Springer US; 2022:1–25.

Dozier M, Bernard K. Attachment and biobehavioral catch-up: addressing the needs of infants and toddlers exposed to inadequate or problematic caregiving. *Curr Opin Psychol*. 2017;15:111–117.

Lappé M, Lau L, Dudovitz RN, Nelson BB, Karp EA, Kuo AA. The diagnostic odyssey of autism spectrum disorder. *Pediatrics*. 2018;141(Suppl 4):S272–279.

Hamp N, DeHaan SL, Cerf CM, Radesky JS. Primary care pediatricians' perspectives on autism care. *Pediatrics*. 2023;151(1): e2022057712.

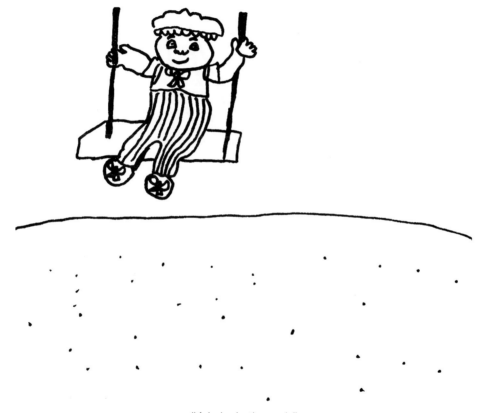

"A baby in the park."

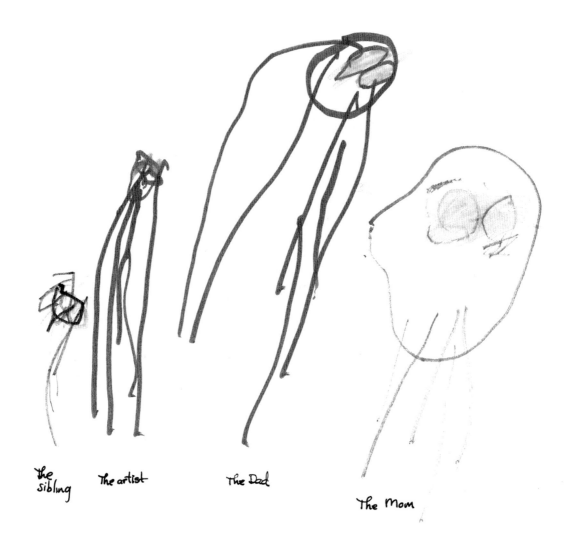

the
sibling   The artist   The Dad

The Mom

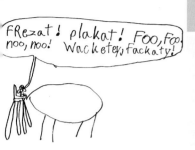

15

Two Years: Language Leaps

Jenny S. Radesky

This chapter focuses on the development of language from infancy onward. It provides the cognitive and social context of language development and looks at variations in language. Atypical language development is discussed.

KEYWORDS

- Language development
- Late talker
- Language delays
- Gestures
- Bilingualism
- Hearing
- Speech difficulties
  - Apraxia of speech
  - Autism spectrum disorder
  - Joint attention
  - Early intervention
- Symbolic function

DEVELOPMENTAL CONCEPTS IMPORTANT AT THIS AGE

The second birthday falls in a period when a whole new set of capabilities emerge, including the core concept of one thing standing for another, called **symbolic function**. Another closely aligned concept is the ability to understand rules that generalize from one situation to another. Language comes out of and further fuels these basic cognitive processes. Major reorganization of brain systems at this time coincides with this behavioral shift. **Language development** and growth in cognitive abilities

Previous chapter by Suzanne D. Dixon.

together allow the child to interact with the world in new ways, and their appearance represents a big transition in development, from infancy to childhood. A new plateau is reached—the era of the talkative, questioning, and active 2-year-old.

Cognitive Abilities

Language and cognitive abilities are strongly linked. A child's "language age" is likely to predict their cognitive abilities and functional level. A look at language is a look at the mental structures that may be critical to the skills needed now and in the school years and beyond. Language also forecasts later school concern. For example, although a child who is a **late talker** (a child who scores <10th percentile, often defined as children who are not combining words into phrases by 24 months) may not have continuing **language delays** per se by school entry, they may have other language-related challenges. These include verbally based learning disabilities, difficulties in speed and accuracy of verbal processing, and social adjustment problems (due to difficulties expressing themselves in complex ways during social interactions). Early identification and remediation through the provision of appropriate services may prevent school failure and its emotional sequelae.

Second, the chief complaint of language delay may identify young children with atypical development, such as with autism spectrum disorder (ASD; see Chapter 14). For children with ASD, early intervention through speech-language therapy, occupational therapy, applied behavioral analysis, play-based therapy, and social skills building before the age of 5 gives them a substantially improved prognosis.

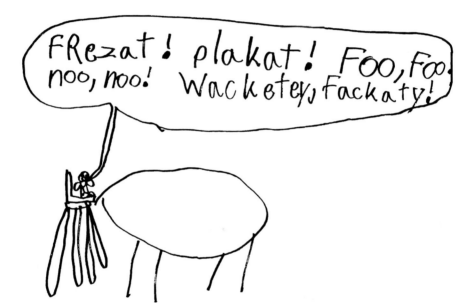

"A baby learning to talk." By Ryan Hennessy.

Finally, global developmental delay that has no major motoric component is often manifested in the second year as language delay. *Child health care providers rarely miss disabilities in the motor sphere, but those involving cognition and language are often missed or dismissed despite the fact that they are among the most common of developmental disorders.* This will not happen if the clinical setting is set up to regularly evaluate language and if the clinician has a strong sense of how language develops, including the limits of variability. To dismiss a concern about language without careful appraisal means that many types of problems, now and in the future, might be missed.

THE BRAIN BASIS OF LANGUAGE

The processes of learning words, word order and the semantic cues of language appear to reside in several areas of the brain, including the right and left parietotemporal and the frontal areas. In contrast to adults, in whom language function is nearly exclusively left sided, children have an evolving brain geography for these functions. As a word or phrase is learned and becomes part of the established language bank, the left temporal area becomes the site for this ongoing use of language. Word retrieval and the rapid recognition of words and utterances become available at this time of brain reorganization, at about 18 months to 2½ years old. The laying down of language subsumes bilateral brain systems, whereas the ongoing use of previously learned language is increasingly localized to the left temporal lobe.

LANGUAGE DEVELOPMENT COURSE

The specific patterns of early childhood language development have been summarized by many psychologists and speech-language pathologists. The following represents a synthesis of these works (Table 15.1).

Prenatal and Infancy

Language development begins before birth as the fetus perceives the sounds transmitted to the uterus, quiets or alerts to them and begins to synchronize movements to the birth parent's voice and body sounds. Increasing evidence suggests that the fetus responds to environmental sounds long before birth and begins to develop some memory of these auditory experiences. Specific pieces of music may result in the fetus turning toward the source and showing heart rate changes suggestive of alerting and awareness.

Responsiveness to specific sounds and interactional synchrony between infant movement and caregiver voices and rhythm are well developed at birth. Discrimination of even similar sounds (e.g., pa, ba) is present in the first weeks of life, although this ability may be lost later in the

first year if a specific sound is not present in that child's language. This is true, for example, with the "r" and "l" sounds, which are not differentiated in Japanese. A selective attention to one's own language, caregivers' voices, and changes in tone or prosody in the surrounding language has been seen in newborns. Infants give selective attention to speech sounds and normal phrasing and recognize violations in their native language by the second half of the first year. Children in the first year acquire a sense of what sounds are words or the units of their language. They pay more attention to real words than to nonsense sounds or sounds that do not occur in their own language. They are building a storehouse of words that will serve them in the second year when they begin to develop an expressive vocabulary of their own. (Important to note: research shows that infants do not pay as much attention to sounds or learn words that they hear through audio recordings or video, which is why they cannot learn language from TV or media.)

Expressive language also begins early; cooing, the production of vowel sounds without the formation of syllable units, begins in the first 2 months of life. The loudness of cooing starts to vary at about 1 month of age, and pitch variation develops between 2 and 4 months of age. "Conversations" with 2-month-olds should thus show some variation in tone, as well as sound. Cooing sounds are heard from children who are completely deaf, though with decreased frequency and not in a conversational or interactive setting. Babbling, the production of sounds containing both vowels and consonants, is heard starting at 4 months and continues to increase in quantity and complexity with age. Babbling is heard in a similar manner in all language groups around the world. Babbling requires a marked increase in motor control of all the oropharyngeal musculature; it exercises the coordination of these speech organs and allows the child to discover the ability to talk. The quantity and quality of babble, but not its presence, are less in children who have reduced or no hearing or who are rarely interacted with verbally. Deaf children also do not have the same tonal variation to their babble.

Imitation of adult speech, called jargon or jabber, with the phonetic and intonational features of the child's native language starts at about 7 months and occurs regularly by the ninth month. This precedes the first words by 4 to 5 months. Jabber is not nonsense, but a real step along the road to real language.

It is important to note that the above description of receptive and expressive language development applies only to infants with *normal hearing*. As described in Chapter 6, hearing loss needs to be identified through technology-based (not behaviorally based) screening before 1 month

TABLE 15.1   Clinical Evaluation of Language Skills

Age	Receptive Skills	Expressive Skills	Specific Indications for Referral
0–1 months	Recognizes sound with startle; turns to sound and looks for source; quiets motor activity to sound; "prefers" human speech with high inflection	Differentiated crying; body language showing positive and negative response	No response to pleasing sound when alert; risk factor for deafness (neonatal sepsis; meningitis; neonatal asphyxia; prematurity; congenital infection; familial deafness; renal abnormalities; aminoglycoside therapy)
2–4 months	Prolonged attention to sounds; responds to familiar voice; watches the speaking mouth; enjoys rattle; attempts to repeat pleasing sounds with objects; shifts gaze back and forth between sounds	"Eh, ih, uh" (hind mouth vowels); cooing, blows bubbles; enjoys using tongue and lips; reciprocal cooing; play dialogs; loudness varies	No response to pleasing sounds; does not attend to voices
5–7 months	Seeks out speaker; localizes sounds; understands own name, familiar words; associates word with activity (e.g., bath, car)	Initiates sounds; pitch varies; babbles with labial consonants ("ba, ma, ga"); uses sounds to get attention, express feeling; sounds directed at object	Decreased or absence of vocalizations
8–12 months	Begins word comprehension; responds to simple commands—"point to your nose," "say bye-bye"; knows names of family members; responds to a few words, those associated with specific objects	First words; "mama, dada"; inflected vocal play; repeats sounds and words made by others; "oo, ee" (foremouth vowels); intentional gestures	No babbling with consonant sounds; no response to music
13–20 months	Single-step/element commands; identifies familiar objects	Points to objects with vocalization; vocabulary of 10–50 words; rate and content vary	No comprehension of words; does not understand simple requests
18–24 months	Recognizes many nouns; understands simple questions	Telegraphic speech; vocabulary of 50–75 words; 2-word sentences, phrases; stuttering common	Vowel sounds, but no consonants; no words
24–36 months	Understands prepositions; can follow story with pictures	Identifies body parts; vocabulary of 200 words; dependent on phrases, 3-word sentences; uses words for expressive needs; pronouns; early grammar	No words; does not follow simple directions; no phrases or sentences
30–36 months	Understands some syntax (difference between car hit train and train hit car); understands opposites; understands action in pictures	Sentences of 4 or 5 words, three elements; tells stories; uses "what" and "where" questions; uses negation; uses progressive and past tense, all regular form; uses plurals, regular form	Speech largely unintelligible to stranger; dropout of initial consonants; no sentences

TABLE 15.1   Clinical Evaluation of Language Skills—cont'd

Age	Receptive Skills	Expressive Skills	Specific Indications for Referral
3–4 years	Understands three-element commands	Talks about what they are doing; uses "I" with grammar by own rules; vocabulary of 40–1500 words; speech intelligible to strangers; "why" questions; commands; uses past and present tense; passive speech in spontaneous speech; nursery rhymes; says colors, numbers 1–4, full name, sex; articulation of "m, n, p, h, and w"; four-word sentences	Speech not comprehended by strangers; still dependent on gestures; consistently holds hands over ears; speech without modulation
4–5 years	Understands four-element commands; links past and present events; decreasing ability for second language acquisition	2700-word vocabulary; defines simple words; auxiliary verbs "has" and "had"; conversation mature with "how" and "why" questions in response to others; articulation of "b, k, g, and f"; five-word sentences; "normalizes" irregular verbs and nouns; increases in accessibility of forms	Stuttering; consistently avoids loud places
5–6 years	Understands five-element commands; can follow a story without pictures; enjoys jokes and riddles; can comprehend two meanings of a single word	Correct use of all parts of speech; vocabulary of 5000 words; articulation of "y, ng, and d"; six-word sentences; corrects own errors in speech; can use logic in recounting story plots	Word endings dropped; faulty sentence structure; abnormal rate, rhythm or inflection
6–7 years	Asks for motivation and explanation of events; understands time intervals (months, seasons); right and left differences	Articulation of "l, r, t, sh, ch, dr, cl, bl, gl, and cr"; has formal adult speech patterns	Poor voice quality, articulation
7–8 years	Can use language alone to tell a story sequentially; reasons using language	Articulation of "v, th, j, s, z, tr, st, sl, sw, and sp"	
8–9 years		Articulation of "th, sc, and sh"	

of age, and any time thereafter if you or the infant's family have any concerns for hearing, even if neonatal screening was normal.

Gestures

Pointing at objects begins between 9 and 12 months and is a very important language milestone. It always precedes the naming of objects and is the gesture language equivalent of naming. Linguistics calls touching, pointing at and holding up objects "proto-declarative," thus emphasizing this linguistic importance.

It also testifies to the child's ability to engage in shared social attention, also called **joint attention**, which in turn tells us that a child has a sense of self as separate from another. Children with autism have delays in theory of mind (see Chapter 14), which means they have difficulty seeing things from another person's perspective. For this reason, they are delayed in pointing and other proto-declarative gestures because they do not realize that they need to bring another person's attention to something they see. Todders with autism may assume their caregivers see and know everything that the toddler does, or they have no concept of the other's perspective. Children with autism also show limited conventional gestures such as nodding or shaking their head ("yes" or "no") or shrugging their shoulders, as well as descriptive gestures (e.g., showing with their hands how big something is), since children learn these in part through imitation—which is also delayed in autism.

Gestures are part of emerging language abilities. Whereas pointing is the precursor to naming, some gestures may be the precursors to asking. These are called instrumental gestures or "proto-imperatives." For example, a toddler's pointing and grunting at the cookie jar is a request for the contents. Symbolic gestures used in play at 13 months are highly correlated with later language ability (e.g., recognizing a telephone by lifting it toward the ear, categorizing a shoe by touching it to the foot, or labeling a toy car by moving it back and forth on the floor). These gestures then expand to be even more elaborate pantomimes, demonstrating a connection between two events, imitating an event and developing themes in play. They are analogous to short descriptions or stories. *Children who can say or wave "bye-bye" or do "pat-a-cake" with a verbal prompt are testifying to emergent cognitive and language skills.* Children with a rich gesture communication system in toddlerhood are likely to develop typical linguistic skills even if they are late bloomers in terms of verbal language production itself. The earlier these gestures occur, the sooner the combining of words will begin. Children without such gestures are likely to have persistent language difficulties. The clinician is well advised to ask about, observe, and engage in gesture games with the infant and toddler. Always wave "bye, bye" and do "pat-a-cake" or "so big" with small patients.

First Words

By the age of 1 year, a child usually has two to eight "words," short utterances that are produced in a specific context or to identify a specific person, event, or object. The minimum competency would be **one word** other than "mama" and "dada" and following **one-step commands** and **pointing**.

A toddler both overextends (e.g., using the word "doggy" for all interesting animals) and overly restricts (e.g., using the word "doggy" only for the family dog) the meaning of these early utterances in the struggle to order and understand the world. The child is experimenting with the rules and structure of language and will gradually refine this so that "dogs" are the creatures we identify as such and Fido will get his own proper name. Feedback is absorbed from listening to others' use of language rather than specific teaching about terms or words. The child may point

and look for an affirmation of naming. From this feedback and attention to the language around him, as well as joint attention while caregivers label objects, the toddler puts the linguistic puzzle together. Being immersed in a rich verbal environment facilitates this process, but excessive background TV or parent technology use can displace it, so families should be supported in creating technology-free times and routines with their infant.

The acquisition of expressed new words during the period from about 12 to 18 months tends to be quite slow. These words are likely to be simple, salient, and overgeneralized naming that allows the child's needs to be met and permits sharing of simple observations; these are called the nominative and instrumental functions of these early utterances, and they always come before the sharing of observations or describing of people or events. This is true in both typically developing children and those with language delays. Things that a child can act on ("ba" for ball) or things that change or move ("ca" for car) are usually the first named. The size of the average spoken vocabulary of an 18-month-old is between 50 and 100 words, but this is extremely variable between children and may even fluctuate periodically within a given child, who may use a word only in a special context and not anywhere else. Words may appear and disappear in seemingly random fashion during the first part of the second year; this is important to distinguish from a true language regression that manifests as a loss of many or all words at the same.

There is much families can do to support their young child's language development. Talking to children, responding to their utterances as though they had full communicative intent, and avoiding overcorrection of word attempts will boost language skills. A caregiver can help by being overly dramatic in using gestures, providing emphasis on important words, and repeating phrases for clarity. Expansion of the child's utterances to full sentences provides a model and acknowledges the child's communication. For example, if a 2-year-old says "Soo on" while grabbing her shoe at the doctor's office, a caregiver might reflect back: "Yes, I know you'd like to put your shoes on and go home. But you have to be checked first." Most caregivers do this spontaneously because it gets a child's interest and attention; if you notice this during a pediatric visit, reinforce it by commenting on how that type of verbal exchange helps build the language centers of the brain. Box 15.1 provides ideas to suggest to caregivers on how to provide a rich, responsive language environment.

Putting Words Together

After 18 months of age, children usually experience rapid increases in vocabulary and the use of verbs, adjectives, and even some adverbs. The most significant event in

BOX 15.1   Supporting Language Development in Typically Developing Young Children

- **Talk to the child**. Beginning in infancy, talk to the baby, naming things in the environment and narrating the events of the day. A rich verbal environment supports language development all the way to college.
- **Speak slowly** and in short phrases to a young child and give emphasis to particular words. Higher pitch gets a young child's attention.
- **Talk in regular language forms**, including complex sentences, to provide good models to imitate. Children with more advanced language forms have families who speak to them in longer utterances. Use pronouns as appropriate; do not substitute proper names.
- **Talk and read to the child in your native language**. Caregivers will speak in more rich sentences, tell more meaningful stories, and provide stronger language input if they speak to children primarily in the language they know best.
- **Respond to the child's speech** as though it has meaning. Beginning at 2 months, respond to the baby's sounds with an echo or an enhancement. The baby will learn that their noises create a response.
- **Repeat what a child says** often so that the child experiences being heard.
- **Respond to the meaning** and not the form of the child's speech. Expand on what is said; do not correct the attempts. Help the child get ideas across.
- **Ask questions and wait for an answer**. Language development is enhanced by giving kids a prompt and time to respond. Children who are expected to answer will have enhanced language competency.
- **Look at books together**, name the pictures, and talk about the images and the stories. Let the child start to tell the story their way when ready.
- **Never punish or shame** a child for any language effort. Give a new model if needed but do not overcorrect or drill.
- **Increase interest in language** with exposure to music and rhymes that you do together. Just hearing the music or nursery rhymes on a video will not build the same language and social skills that singing with a caregiver does.
- **Encourage gestures** to communicate and to use in games. These will enhance not detract from the development of speech.

this period is the creation of original linkages of words into phrases that express a complete and original thought (e.g., "da da come," "dight hot," "now nigh dark"). These combinations imply, but may not explicitly have a subject, verb and perhaps an object or modifying word, but often do not have linking words in between. They are in contrast to the simple naming of objects or expression of simple demands (e.g., "doggy," "wa-wa") that are characteristic of the "prelanguage" heard earlier. Some prelanguage may have sentence forms (e.g., "I wanna," "ah done"), but because these phrases are always used all together in a single utterance, they are called *holophrases* and are not real sentences. True sentences show original linkages and associations and involve the interchange of word combinations across differing circumstances. They generally emerge when the vocabulary reaches a threshold of at least 50 words, often reported by caregivers as "too many words to count." Between 2 and 2½, the child starts to add some modifiers (e.g., "big truck"), some possessives (e.g., "my car"), and some functional words such as "on" (e.g., "shoes on"). Other prepositions blossom between 2½ and 3. Words expressing time and sequence come in between 3 and 5 (e.g., "I do bath, then do story").

A 2-year-old shows an understanding of the rules of language through the differential ordering of words to alter their meanings, such as "go car" versus "car go." Even with their *telegraphic speech* (i.e., with some parts missing from a sentence), toddlers know word order. More than 90% of utterances in a 3-year-old are grammatically correct in terms of word order and sequence. New constructions (e.g., "I like it.") for a child of this age are sometimes learned in their entirety and applied in several contexts as an experiment.

Sentences and Beyond

The years between ages 2 and 5 are characterized by a gradual expansion in sentence complexity (i.e., words or word-like utterances). The length of a child's phrases and sentences increases dramatically during this time from an average of one or two elements at younger than 2 years up to three to five elements by age 4. Linguists use this measure, mean length of utterance, to evaluate language maturity. Clinicians can write down the longest thing a child says during their appointment to get an approximation of this measure. *It should increase at every visit between the ages of 2 and 5, roughly corresponding to a child's age as a minimum competency.*

Rules are overapplied after children start to put words together, so "mistakes" are made that did not appear earlier. The first sentences are experiments in grammar and syntax. "He has two feets," "The mices are teasing the cat," and "The boy putted the cars away" are all examples of these expected errors. This represents linguistic progress, not regression. A late preschooler is now conscious of rules governing language and is overly fastidious in their application. They will self-correct these irregularities over time without teaching; no didactic instruction is needed here.

Verb tenses are added in orderly sequence; systems of negation and the form of questions also have their own specific developmental course. The "w" words ("what," "when," and the perennial favorite "why") appear in a 3-year-old's talk.

The regularity of these processes is quite striking. A 2-year-old can communicate with family members easily; a 4-year-old should be intelligible to almost anyone who speaks the child's language 100% of the time.

After 5 years of age, all the basic components of language are in place, although these forms become more accessible and usable with time. A vocabulary of 800 to 14,000 words is common by age 6. Poetry, puns, and jokes, all subtle turns on language, are enjoyed by early grade school. The study of grammar is appreciated with relish in the early school years, and foreign languages have particular interest for the child at this time. Foreign languages learned early create at least bilingual people and facilitate the later learning of other languages. Vocabulary increases should be a lifelong process, and sentence complexity increases into adult life. Table 15.1 shows the developmental progression of these language milestones.

School systems are heavily biased toward verbal skills, so it is not surprising that school performance and linguistic abilities are linked. Early language disorders are highly predictive of learning difficulties in school, and most studies show that greater than 40% of children with early language difficulties will have learning difficulties in school and should be monitored through ongoing developmental surveillance. Therefore, supporting language development in infancy and early childhood is an important investment in longer term academic achievement.

RECEPTIVE LANGUAGE: UNDERSTANDING OTHERS

Receptive language is always ahead of expressive language, so a child always understands more than they can say. This usually results in a mild-to-moderate degree of frustration, which is a source of energy for a child trying to expand linguistic skills. It can also lead to developmental stuttering, the verbal tumbling over words that will not come out fast enough to satisfy a busy preschooler's mind. This is very different from the stuttering that is a block in speech production, usually with an initial sound of a word that emerges in the late preschool and early school-age years. A little help with slowing down best guesses about what the wanted word really is and the avoidance of pressure or

embarrassment will help a young child get their mouth in line with their mind while learning to speak.

Receptive language is usually more regular in its development than expressive language because it is more closely linked with cognitive development. It is a better predictor of both long-term language competency and general cognitive abilities in most children. Expressive language is more variable because it is influenced by individual temperament, environmental prompts and constraints, and even the interpretive skills of the listener. The clinician should be much more worried about a child who has difficulty understanding age-appropriate utterances that are presented without visual prompts than about a child who has little to say but does follow verbal input at an age-appropriate level.

LINKS BETWEEN LANGUAGE AND EMOTIONS

Expressive language is an "acute phase reactant" that stagnates or even regresses in the face of any stressor, such as illness, separations from primary caregivers, and family changes. Because these are the times and circumstances during which clinicians often see children, it is even more imperative that a good assessment of language be achieved at the regular health supervision visits, when stressors are at a minimum.

Conversely, when children learn language, it supports their developing emotional awareness and regulation. Once toddlers and preschoolers can *think of emotions in terms of words*, it allows them to hold these concepts in mind—even briefly—rather than just reacting to emotional drives with behaviors. By understanding a feeling state as "sad" or "frustrated" or "silly," a child can then eventually communicate that feeling to someone else. Behavioral challenges like prolonged tantrums or aggression often improve as children with language delays receive speech-language therapy and develop a wider expressive and receptive vocabulary. This fact might motivate exhausted parents into keeping their weekly therapy visits!

LANGUAGE DELAYS

A clinician should be concerned about the child who fails to reach the minimum competencies shown in the checklist in Table 15.2. Standardized screening instruments (see Appendix) should be administered at well child visits in early childhood to identify children at risk of language delay. Language delays may also come to light through caregiver, childcare provider, or teacher concern that the child is not speaking at age-appropriate levels (including delays or atypical speech such as echolalia). When delays in language are identified, it is important to explain to caregivers that intervention as early as possible helps

TABLE 15.2 Language Milestones That Call for Referral If Not Met

Age	Milestone
Newborn	Turns to a soft voice, especially the caregivers'
By 3 months	Cooing sounds. Looks alert, interactive, smiles
By 6 months	Coos and jabbers and does more every day. Turns to a new sound and familiar voices, laughs
By 9 months	Babbles mamamama, babababa Knows name, turns when called
By 12 months	Points at objects
	Has 1 word in addition to "mama" and "dada"
	Follows one-step commands
	Gives or shows objects to the caretaker
By 18 months	Produces four or more words
	Comprehends more than 50 words
By 2 years	Produces more than 50 words
	Puts two words together
	Follows two-step commands
	Points at pictures in a book
	Names or attempts to name objects
	Uses "words" to request things
By 3 years	Talks in sentences most of the time
	Is understood by strangers at least half the time
	Says name, age, sex, and birthday month
	Names most objects in her daily life and at least three body parts
	Tells stories in three-sentence or three-phrase "paragraphs"
	Knows one color
By 4 years	Sustains a conversation
	Understood by a stranger
	Uses pronouns

children achieve the best outcomes. Prognosis is unclear at the time a language delay is identified—in other words, whether a child will "catch up" over time or continue to have significant delays—and the only way to know is to observe how the child responds to intervention.

DIFFERENTIAL DIAGNOSIS

The primary care clinician should consider other conditions for which language delay could be a symptom:
- Hearing loss
- Global developmental delay
- ASD
- Chronic illness
- Selective mutism
- Developmental language disorder

Although these categories are not mutually exclusive, they do provide direction for further assessment and intervention.

MISCONCEPTIONS ABOUT LANGUAGE DELAY

Caregivers and clinicians alike may explain a child's language delay with a narrative or understanding based on their family's experience (e.g., having siblings whose language "caught up"), defensiveness/worry about their child being "different," or feeling that 2 years old is "too young" to diagnose a language delay or autism. Additional examples of such misconceptions include the following:
- *Their older siblings get them everything they want, so they do not have to talk.* Although children lower in the birth order, when compared with firstborn children, show a slight delay in expressive language in terms of the quantity of utterances, they should have no such delay at all in receptive language or gestures. In addition, the type and complexity, if not the quantity, of things said should follow developmental expectations for age. Siblings can prompt language a bit and may provide vocabulary, both good and bad. However, birth order effects do

not account for significant delays or atypical language progress.

- *He is a boy, so what do you expect?* The gender difference in language development is small, with girls being ahead of boys in both quantitative speech measures and complexity after the first birthday. As a group, girls retain the advantage in verbal tasks throughout school. Again, this is a subtle difference of weeks to months, and it applies to groups. There is much individual difference. Significant delays cannot be explained by gender. Many detailed tests of early language have different norms for boys and girls to account for these small differences. If a screening test does show delay, further specialized evaluation should take gender into account. In a pediatric setting, gender issues should be ignored.

- *They are in a bilingual household, so we expect them to be delayed.* A common myth is that exposure to multiple languages is "confusing" for infants. As reviewed earlier in this chapter, the opposite is true: birth to age 3 represents a sensitive window for language acquisition, a time when rich exposure to multiple languages is more likely to lead to fluency in each. Exposure to a second language should therefore not be delayed. Children raised in **bilingual** households have the same rates of language disorders as monolingual children. At age 2, they may mix the syntax and vocabulary of both languages, perhaps using both languages in a single utterance. After that, children are able to switch appropriately from one language to another in context and have a *combined* vocabulary that meets the usual expectations. Bilingual exposure actually facilitates language development and executive functioning (specifically task switching) rather than hampering them over the long term. If delays are recognized through screening, referral should be made, ideally to an Early Intervention specialist or speech-language pathologist who is also bilingual. Strategies for supporting bilingual language development are described in Box 15.2.

- *They are independent or lazy.* Young children have an internal drive to mastery in this area and all others (see Chapter 2), which means that they exercise newly developing skills as they emerge. If a child is performing below age level, it is because that is the best the child can do at that time. Parents of children with autism sometimes attribute their child's lack of requests or initiation of joint attention to having an "independent" personality in which the child prefers to get things done themselves. In both of these cases, it can help to ask more questions to identify points in the day when the child's language delay is getting in the way of daily functioning (e.g., tantrums due to communication frustration; not being able to tell the caregiver what they want)—which

may help the clinician and caregiver see the problem from the same perspective.

- *They will grow out of it.* Although it is true that most children with language delays make progress over time, their trajectory of progress is much faster when they receive appropriate therapy. In addition, children with early or continuing delays are at risk in early childhood for emotional difficulties, for behavioral problems and, over the longer term, for subtle or not-so-subtle language and learning difficulties because of what the lack of language prevents them from doing. Investing in stronger language skills at an early age may help prevent school problems down the line, which may help motivate parents to pursue therapy.

SPEECH DIFFICULTIES

Clear articulation of the sounds of speech is distinct from the content and form of these utterances, which is language (Table 15.3). The ability to reproduce the sounds of one's native language has its own developmental course. A child in the first year of life can distinguish all the sounds that exist in their language (losing the ability to hear the sounds that are not in the native tongue before 9 months of age). However, the child may not be able to say all the complex blends of sounds until school age. Intelligibility by an unfamiliar adult (i.e., the clinician) should increase with the child's age, being about 50% of the time for a 2-year-old, 75% for a 3-year-old, and 100% for a 4-year-old. By 2 years of age, beginning consonants should not be omitted ("oy" for "boy"). By 3½ years, the ending consonants should always be present ("did" should not sound like "di"). The "th" sound will not be present until age 3; the "r" and "l" sounds will be mixed until age 5.

If speech in general sounds babyish or immature for the child's age although the form and complexity are at age level, an articulation problem is probable. However, language and **speech difficulties** often overlap.

Some general irregularities in speech require referral or further evaluation, such as the following:

- A decrease in the amount of speech
- Lack of change in speech for 3 to 6 months in a child younger than 5 years
- Explosive or constantly loud speech
- Hoarseness
- Awkward, unusual cadence or lack of prosody (emotionality) in speech
- A child being embarrassed by speech

Some speech irregularities should draw the clinician's attention to oral-motor function and, perhaps, motor function overall. Poor articulation of frontal consonants, which gives the speech a garbled or swallowed character, may

BOX 15.2 Supporting Language Development in Bilingual Children by Mariana Glusman, MD

Many infants and young children grow up bilingual or multilingual, but their experiences—including how languages are used and who speaks them—vary considerably based on caregivers' language abilities and preferences, family structure (e.g., exposure to extended family and older siblings), community characteristics (e.g., language(s) spoken, predominantly monolingual vs. multilingual countries), and sociopolitical factors (e.g., attitudes toward "minority" language). Caregivers may receive conflicting messages about the benefits/risks of exposing their child to the family's heritage language and wonder whether they should raise their child speaking the often higher status community language (which is taught in school and more prevalent on media) rather than their heritage language, which they may perceive as having a lower status. The pediatric provider can play an important role in dispelling misinformation and supporting a child's regular exposure to heritage languages and culture, which has a positive impact on family dynamics and the child's cultural/ethnic identity.

- Encourage regular exposure to all caregivers' languages from the prenatal and infancy periods. There is no need to only use one language around an infant, since this is a sensitive window of development in which infants can retain different speech sounds that are more difficult to acquire later in childhood.
- If parents ask what ratio of languages to expose a child to, research suggests that at least 10% to 25% of overall language exposure is necessary for a child to achieve fluency in a specific language. Therefore it does not need to be a strict 50-50 ratio. However, if the goal is to maintain the family's heritage language, the more exposure the better, as children's expressive language skills become more English-dominant with longitudinal exposure to English (in the United States).
- Encourage serve-and-return interactions in whatever language (or languages) the caregiver is most proficient, to promote the child's exposure to the most complex vocabulary and syntax possible
- Shared book reading in the caregiver's heritage language should be encouraged, to promote increased verbal interaction, relational health, and shared enjoyment of reading. In addition, research shows that oral and literacy skills in children's home language transfer to their English literacy skills, so promoting early literacy skills in the child's heritage language is also helpful for school readiness regardless of the language(s) spoken at school. If possible, provide books and other literacy materials (e.g., library resources, audiobooks) in the family's heritage language. If not possible, encourage caregivers to talk about the pictures and make up their own stories in the language most comfortable for them.

- Affirm that it is good to speak the heritage language at home and the community language outside the home. The more native speakers of a language that the child is exposed to the better the language learning.
- If grandparents or other caregivers speak another language, encourage speaking to the child in that language. This not only promotes language development but also socioemotional development and family connectedness.
- If available, encourage childcare resources that provide exposure to the caregivers' heritage language and culture.
- Provide resources about community centers, libraries, and online support for raising bilingual children.
- When bilingual children have language delays, it is ideal for therapeutic support to occur in both of their languages. If this is not possible, encourage caregivers to advocate for printed/online materials with language activities in their heritage language, for them to perform at home. Children with developmental delays, language disorders, or cognitive disabilities benefit from exposure to their family's heritage language and need not be restricted to English ("to avoid confusion").
- Code switching (the practice of alternating between two or more languages in conversation) is the norm for many multilingual families and communities and need not be discouraged. It is also common in children exposed to multiple languages. Code switching is a useful tool to fill language gaps and not a sign of confusion. In fact, increased code switching has been associated with larger expressive and receptive vocabularies.
- Each family has unique needs and goals for their children, so listening with cultural humility is important to make a shared plan toward their goals.
- It is also important to be aware of the sociopolitical context where children are being raised and help dispel myths that may discourage caregivers from using their heritage language. Promoting cultural pride through the use of heritage languages is an effective strategy (Baralt, 2020).

Modified from Fibla L, et al: Bilingual language development in infancy: what can we do to support bilingual families? *Policy Insights Behav Brain Sci* 9(1):35–43, 2022.

provide a clue to hypotonia or mild cerebral palsy, particularly if accompanied by drooling or difficulty swallowing. An overly nasal quality of speech may suggest palatine dysfunction, perhaps a submucosal cleft palate. Hearing loss must be considered with any speech concern.

Additionally, if the child regularly experiences frustration in trying to get the meaning across, a formal evaluation is needed. Children with **apraxia of speech**, in which errors in articulation are inconsistent and pervasive, often experience significant frustration when trying to be understood. This condition is caused by brain-based motor planning deficits that affect coordination of the oral musculature. Compared to children with articulation deficits, who make consistent errors (e.g., always saying "tup" instead of "cup"), apraxia is characterized by variable distortions in both vowels and consonants, pauses between syllables or words, difficulty moving smoothly from one sound to another, using the wrong emphasis in a word (e.g., "BUH-nan-uh" instead of "buh-NAN-uh"), and having a hard time imitating words. Although apraxia usually appears at first as a language delay between 12 and 18 months, its presentation becomes clearer after the second birthday when vocabulary increases. Children with apraxia of speech may start avoiding speaking due to their frustration with producing intelligible sounds, so intensive therapy several times per week with an experienced speech-language pathologist is needed.

DURING THE VISIT

What to Observe

An office visit offers an important opportunity for the evaluation of language development. Observing the following will help in such an evaluation:

- What does the child say in terms of amount, clarity, prosody, and length?
- How much of what the child says do you understand?
- How much does the parent interact with and speak to the child? In what language? What kinds of things are said? Is the child provided an opportunity to answer?
  - Does the parent try to step in and do things for the child? The parent may already know that the child cannot understand your requests and that in itself is a clue that you are asking for something beyond the child's linguistic ability.
- What does the child understand? Give one-, two-, and three-step commands to see what the child can do. Children may signal their difficulty by ignoring you, looking at you very intently, changing the task, trying to guess what you want or leaving the scene.

- What verbal output accompanies play in the waiting or examining rooms?

What to Ask

The following are examples of questions to ask the parents:
- What can the child say now? Words? Phrases? Sentences?
- What is the longest thing the child says?
- How many words does the child know? (Expect a number up to about 20, "a lot" usually indicates 20 to 50, and "too many to count" generally means more than 50.)
- Can the child follow one-, two-, and three-step commands? (Be sure you leave out gestures and visual support.)
- Does the child know their name? Siblings? Age? Pets?
- Ask the following of the child, using picture books, simple toys, and pictures on the walls:
- What is that? (pointing to a picture)
- Which one is the _____? (in a book)
- Give me the _____ (from among the objects).
- What is your name, and so on? Start a conversation.
- After age 3, ask a child to describe an experience, such as a birthday, an outing.
- Present one- to three-step commands as part of the physical examination.

Assessment

Use Table 15.2 to look at a child's language. If that raises a warning flag, look at Table 15.1 to help gauge your level of concern. Also ask about:
- General development, including motor coordination, oral-motor function (e.g., chewing, using a straw, blowing bubbles), social-emotional development, and any seizure-like behaviors.
- More details of the family history and medical risk factors for hearing loss, developmental delay, or learning problems.
- The amount of screen media the child is exposed to per day, including TV being left on in the background. Some caregivers provide more TV, videos, or YouTube when children have language delays, in an attempt to teach the child more language; however, heavy use of media at this age is associated with higher risk of language delay.

REFERRALS

If data indicate the need for further examination and possibly treatment, consider the following specialists:
- An audiology evaluation is needed for any child with language delay. If hearing loss is found, it is *never too early* for hearing augmentation.

TABLE 15.3 Speech-Sound Disorders

Type	Description
Deficits in resonance	Disorders are characterized by abnormal oronasal sound balance. Deficits most commonly appear as hypernasality (e.g., in cleft palate) or hyponasality (e.g., in adenoid hypertrophy)
Voice	Problems appear as deviation in the quality, pitch, or volume of sound production. Such impairments have either psychological or physiological bases. Thyroid disease and laryngeal polyps from overuse are some considerations
Fluency	Disorders reflect disruption in the natural flow of connected speech. The most common type of fluency disorder is stuttering
Articulation	Disorders include a large group of problems characterized by imprecise production of speech sounds. Most articulation "problems" are common at certain ages and are, in fact, normal. However, their persistence often requires intervention

From Levine M, Brooks R, Shonkoff JP: *A pediatric approach to learning disorders*, New York, 1980, John Wiley & Sons.

- A speech and language pathologist familiar with young children should be involved early for evaluation and treatment.
- For concerns about autism, refer your clinic's autism assessment program or one in the community/at a local medical center. Wait lists can often be long, so it helps to refer so the child can receive speech-language therapy and occupational therapy while the family waits for an ASD evaluation. Early intervention may also be able to provide additional ASD evaluation or treatments. Websites and books also provide interim guidance (see Recommended Readings).
- Any suggestion of hearing loss requires the consultation of an ear, nose, and throat physician, as well as an audiologist experienced with children—even if the child does not have an apparent language delay.

- Early intervention services, special education, or a language enhancement program should be consulted, depending on the specifics and the services available.
- Loss of language skills, severe language difficulties, or the presence of seizures require an electroencephalogram with consideration of Landau-Kleffner syndrome.

Helping Families Engage With Early Intervention

When a possible language or speech-sound disorder is detected, some caregivers may be eager to enroll their child in therapy, but others may be hesitant. This hesitancy can arise from the worry and stigma associated with developmental delays, caregiver beliefs that it is "too early" to diagnose a developmental condition and desire to wait and see if the child catches up, or concern about engaging with public Early Intervention agencies. Families feeling overwhelmed with childrearing may be anxious about inviting strangers into their home to observe and measure their child's abilities. Research has shown that immigrant families may engage less with Early Intervention or early childhood therapies out of concern that interventionists might report them to immigration officials or child protective services. Families from traditionally marginalized communities may feel less trust in public educational systems (see Chapter 18) or less engaged when therapists are not racially or culturally concordant with their family.

To help families engage with Early Intervention, the pediatric provider can:
- Demystify what Early Intervention (EI) is, who runs it (e.g., the county, a local nonprofit agency), and what the first visit will feel like.
- Place a referral directly to EI, with an explanation of next steps (e.g., an intake coordinator will call you and a home visit will be scheduled).
- Provide a brochure or website for the local EI agency, possibly mentioning positive experiences other patients have had.
- Reassure the caregiver that Early Intervention personnel are specially trained to work with young children, are not going to judge or report the family, and should feel like a partner. If the family does not feel this partnership with their EI personnel comfortable, let them know that they have the right to request a new provider.
- Discuss the long-term benefits of engaging with EI. These include an easier transition to preschool, more developmental progress, behavioral improvement, and better child academic progress in the long run.

ANTICIPATORY GUIDANCE

Offer parents the following guidelines regarding their children's language:

- Parents can support language development by talking *with* their children, engaging them in dialogs, asking questions and encouraging them to narrate experiences. The linkage of tactile and verbal games and the reading of body language cues in the first year begin this process.
- The playful use of language in the second year through rhymes and jingles fuels interest in words. Play and turn-taking allow the combination of language, joint attention, and serve-and-return interactions.
- Expanding the child's expressions and speaking clearly and simply with correct words and grammar are also important.
- When talking about a present object or event, beginning the description with "look" or another orienting word allows the child to focus attention. Important words should be repeated.
- Narration of parental activities and caretaking events provides a rich verbal environment.
- Encourage the use of words rather than actions to express feelings and wishes. Caregivers can narrate what they are feeling, or what they think their child is feeling, in simple terms that support emotion socialization.
- Encourage coviewing of TV or videos so that the caregiver can talk about what the child is viewing and ease the transition away from the screen to hands-on play.

READING TOGETHER

Reading of stories from infancy onward enhances language, literacy, and school performance and should be consciously encouraged by the clinician. Reading together supports language with its own developmental course. Parents who may find it awkward to know what to say to their young children may be supported in their efforts at verbal exchange through the specific use of books together. Offer parents the following types of advice on the progression of reading together:

- Beginning in the first year, parents may point to objects in books and identify them.
- Parental pointing progresses to the child's pointing and naming things in the early second year of life.
- Explanation of a picture with brief descriptions of the immediate action grows into short storytelling by 2 to 3 years of age.
- Children who are 3 and 4 years old will expand the action beyond the picture, can follow stories, and can anticipate events through the medium of books.

- Children older than 7 years regularly enjoy stories without pictures.
- Jokes and riddles for 5- and 6-year-olds are often based on words with double meanings or vagaries of language. Enjoyment of these by parents and kids reinforces this new plateau of language development.
- Poetry and other interesting uses of language can be introduced at this time, if not earlier. The clinician should have a stock of simple jokes and puns in mind to highlight this new skill in a clinical setting.

SUMMARY

The language of the second year of life is a landmark of change for the child and the family. The child can now share observations of events, recall past events to self and others, and communicate original thoughts and feelings to others. For most children, this is a liberating and exciting event. For caregivers, this often marks the undeniable end of infancy. Their child becomes more of an individual and an active participant in family life. Much of the work of exposing the child to objects and events, talking to them without obvious responses, and learning about the child through body language and nonverbal responses now pays off as the child speaks. Language acquisition marks another step in individuation for the child and growing abilities to emotionally regulate. It may also represent the single most significant developmental process in that it may be unmatched in its complexity and in the fact that it makes the child particularly human.

QUICK CHECK—2 YEARS

- Can be understood by strangers about half the time
- Uses two-word phrases
- Follows two-step command
- Has a vocabulary of 20 to 50 words or more
- Stacks at least five cubes
- Makes horizontal lines and circular shapes with paper and marker
- Can kick a ball
- Uses a spoon and fork
- Goes up and down stairs, two feet on each step
- Names seven body parts
- Runs easily and often
- Takes off clothes and helps with dressing
- Washes hands
- Points at pictures in a book
- Imaginary play, combining two or more objects

! HEADS UP—2 YEARS

- Children with autism spectrum disorder may have the following:
- Absent, atypical, and/or substantially delayed language that encompasses receptive and expressive gesture language.
- Language that is overly repetitive, formal, echolalic, or stereotyped (e.g., only speaks in quotes from TV shows).
- Difficulty with eye contact and other nonverbal ways of communicating, such as gestures or facial expressions.
- Limited back-and-forth conversation or play, imitation, or social referencing/joint attention.
- At older ages, difficulties understanding the feelings of others or understanding that others have different thoughts and perspectives.
- Restricted range of interests and/or atypical interests and activities.
- Stereotypical movements such as spinning, hand flapping, and toe walking.
- Interest in the parts of objects such as the wheels on a toy car, the knob of a door, the legs of a toy dog.
- Delay in imaginative play.

RECOMMENDED READINGS

For Parents

It Takes Two to Talk: A Practical Guide for Parents of Children With Language Delays by Elaine Weitzman and Pat Cupples.

An Early Start for Your Child with Autism: Using Everyday Activities to Help Kids Connect, Communicate, and Learn by Sally J. Rogers, Geraldine Dawson, and Laurie Vismara.
7 Steps to Raising a Bilingual Child by Naomi Steiner and Susan Hayes.
Speaking of Apraxia (Second Edition): A Parents' Guide to Childhood Apraxia of Speech by Leslie A. Lindsay.

For Clinicians

Feldman HM. How young children learn language and speech. *Pediatr Rev.* 2019;40(8):398–411.

Rose L, Herzig LD, Hussey-Gardner B. Early intervention and the role of pediatricians. *Pediatr Rev.* 2014;35(1):e1–0.

Khetani MA, Richardson Z, McManus BM. Social disparities in early intervention service use and provider-reported outcomes. *J Dev Behav Pediatr.* 2017;38(7):501.

Jimenez ME, Barg FK, Guevara JP, Gerdes M, Fiks AG. Barriers to evaluation for early intervention services: parent and early intervention employee perspectives. *Acad Pediatr.* 2012;12(6):551–557.

Council on Early Childhood High PC, Klass P, Donoghue E, Glassy D, DelConte B, Earls M, Lieser D, McFadden T, Mendelsohn A, Scholer S. Literacy promotion: an essential component of primary care pediatric practice. *Pediatrics.* 2014;134(2):404–409.

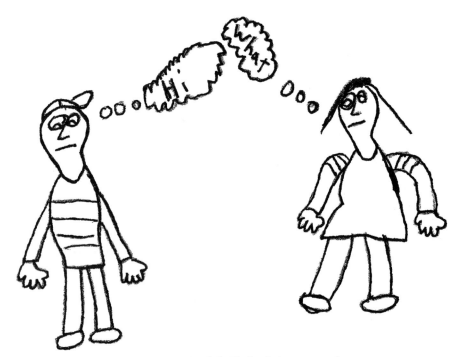

"Two kids talking." By Taylor Roberts, age 9.

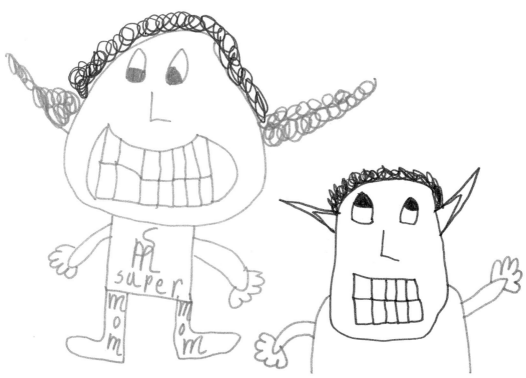

A drawing of a child and his mother, "super mom."

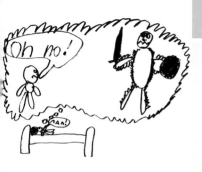

Three Years: Emergence of Magic

Lauren K. O'Connell

This chapter looks at how the world of a 3-year-old is expanding. Their inner world grows through fantasy and imagination, which affects behaviors day and night. At the same time, the 3-year-old enters a wider external world, demonstrating increasing interest in their peers and in stories while engaging in new experiences and influences through early education and media. This chapter outlines the cognitive function of representation and how it contributes to cognitive, emotional, and social growth, as well as how representation can lead to an increase in fear. Sleep disorders in the preschool years are discussed. Lastly, this chapter explores widening influences of peers, education, stories, and media.

KEYWORDS

- Imagination
- Cooperative play
- Fears in childhood
- Dreams and nightmares
- Night terrors
- Sleep disorders
- Early childhood education
- Stories, fairy tales
- Television and digital media

IMAGINATION AS A CORE MENTAL FUNCTION

Although the charm of a child's **imagination** is easily apparent to pediatricians and caregivers, adults may miss its significance and function. Imagination relies on the child's ability to let one thing stand for something else. This core mental function, called **representation**, is the foundation of imaginative play and of complex language. Although younger children imitate, it is in the late second to fifth years of life that neurotypical children create complex play with imagined scenarios, roles, costumes, voices,

Previous edition chapter by Suzanne D. Dixon.

and sequences of events. Play changes across this time frame in three ways:

- Play becomes more detached from real-life objects, for example, a 1-year-old pretends to drink from an empty toy cup.

  A 3-year-old makes a cup into a hat or a banana into a telephone.

- Play becomes less self-centered, for example, a 1-year-old dances like their mom.

  A 3-year-old makes their dolls dance and talk and take on roles.

- Play becomes more complex and prolonged, for example, a 1-year-old runs a car around a track. A 4-year-old plays "house" with dolls, little brother, and a friend, changing the story all afternoon.

Imagination and Cognitive Growth

> Maria and Esteban were playing firefighters with pretend hoses, running around and putting out imagined fires. Maria said, "Now we go to space. There's a fire on the moon!" They then sat down and "blasted off," hoses in hand.

The mental capacity to imagine emerges in toddlerhood and, like all new abilities, is exercised frequently. The active processes of imagination and fantasy open an entirely new world for a child. Previously, the world was limited to direct

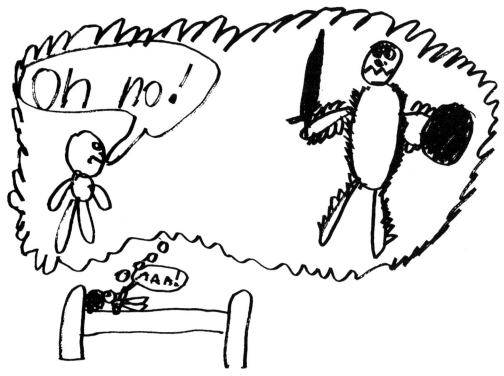

"A scary dream." By Ryan Hennessy.

experience. Now the child can imagine possibilities, causes, and sequences of events that go beyond the immediate or even the possible. The ability to imagine strengthens the ability to learn and in no way detracts from the skill of understanding "the real world." Imagination can serve, as well as define, a new level of cognitive growth throughout the preschool years.

> Ta'Sheena's grandmother took her and a cousin to the zoo last week. Since then, Ta'Sheena has played "zoo" every day, setting up enclosures and walking around with her dolls, talking about the animals and where to get snacks. When her dad tells Grandma about the play, they are pleasantly surprised by how specifically it matches parts of the earlier outing.

A child of this age can review, rework, and repetitively process the events of daily life through actions, language, and "mental movies." Events of the day may be overwhelming and incomprehensible as they occur, yet through imagination, the child can recall them, process them at their own rate, and set down memories. Children frequently recall and experiment with rules, limits, or behaviors in their play. Overall, imagination fuels the cognitive functions of attention, memory, reasoning, language, and creativity.

Imagination and Emotional and Social Growth

Imagination promotes emotional and social growth. Through imagination, children experiment with strong feelings, negotiate conflicts, conquer fears, and build resilience. They can pretend to be new characters in a safe, flexible way, including roles of a different sex, their parent, a superhero, or an animal.

At this age, expressive language abilities lag behind the child's cognitive capacities; children can think, want, and feel things that are much more complex than they can say out loud. Therefore nonverbal forms of communication, including play, are particularly important so the child can share feelings, frustrations, anxieties, and wishes. Observing a child at play is a valuable clue to what they are thinking and feeling.

> Sidra was heard talking to his stuffed animal, Stripey, in bed. "Now, just you stop this. I told you never to do it. That's bad. I'm mad." Stripey hits the wall. Sidra hugs Stripey and strokes its head. "OK, Stripey, you're all right now." Sidra may have been reworking a rough spot in his day.

Expressing negative feelings through imagination is less likely to draw rejection or punishment than expressing them in "real-world" interactions. When using imagination, the child has the time to process responses, the ability to repeat outcomes, and the power to end an interaction whenever they see fit, which allows them to vent frustrations and practice resolution. However, while aggression and negative emotions can be normal in imaginative play, they can still be challenging to observe and tolerate. It is important for clinicians to recognize and have empathy for the impact of daily stress, cultural norms, and the experience of trauma on parents' understanding and response to aggressive or negative play. For example, a parent with posttraumatic stress disorder may perceive aggressive play as a threat and react harshly. Clinicians must balance their advocacy for the child's imagination with empathy for parenting challenges and connecting families with needed resources.

As well as richer solitary play, taking on imaginative roles leads to more elaborate interaction play. One child can be caught up in another's imaginative world, be challenged while having fun, and learn from the interaction. Through scaffolding (discussed in detail in Chapter 2), play with older children allows preschoolers to function at a higher level, while play with younger playmates allows for the expression of nurture and leadership.

> Oliver, age 3, was playing house with his 5-year-old cousin, Henry. He was pouring the "tea" (water) into cups when Henry told him to "Be careful. Tea makes a big stain." Oliver asked, "What's a stain?" "A big mark you can't get out even if your mom washes it." Oliver was just settling in when Henry announced that they now had to do the washing. Oliver had not done that before. They turned over the step stool for a pretend basin. (Through this interaction with Henry, Oliver is participating in play that is much more complex than what he would do on his own.)

Cooperative play with age-mates teaches compromise, negotiation, assertiveness, and conflict resolution, each of which fuels the development of a sense of justice and fair play. Imaginative play with peers demands clear communication without relying on the shorthand and scaffolding that family members and adults can provide. Experiences with a variety of playmates offer the best opportunity to learn these important skills. Healthy imaginative play with others, in dramas, stories, and long sequences, is associated with enhanced social competency.

Parents playing with their child can increase the complexity and length of play episodes, provided that the caregiver does not take over, push too hard, or ignore signs of disengagement (e.g., the child leaving or playing with something else). Plus, it is fun! The joy and benefits of playing with the child are explored below. Parents, however, cannot always provide an exciting enough play experience by themselves. Children in the third year and beyond need other children, such as relatives, neighbors, a play group, or a preschool group. This need is challenged by community disasters that require social isolation, such as the COVID-19 pandemic, during which young children have fewer peer socialization opportunities. Families can be creative about seeking safe solutions and opportunities for play, and most children will demonstrate resilience. During and after periods of social isolation, however, parents and clinicians should anticipate that many children may demonstrate concurrent and later challenges with social situations, ranging from needing more practice with cooperative play, to greater than usual challenges with separation, to symptoms of anxiety. Therefore when the broader context allows, parents should seek peer group experience for their child by age 3 or earlier. This is not to be a substitute for social experiences at home, but rather a necessary supplement. This expanded world brings new challenges and opportunities, which will be discussed below.

The emergence of imagination is both a marker of cognitive function and a tool for cognitive, emotional, and social development. Imagination promotes interactive play, relationship building, and fun. Therefore all children, independent of sex or racial identity, should be encouraged to fully express themselves in imaginative play.

IMAGINATION AS A PATH TO CONNECTION

In addition to the direct and crucial benefits for the child, promoting and observing imaginative play also provides benefits for pediatric clinicians and caregivers. For clinicians, the level of complexity of a child's imaginative play is a sign of developmental health, while the content of imaginative play may illustrate their emotional well-being. For caregivers, engaging with their child's imagination can lead to insights into the child's thought processes and contexts for otherwise challenging behaviors. For all invested adults, imaginative play can ease a stressful situation, while allowing yourself to be pulled into a child's imaginative world is just plain fun.

Imagination in the Pediatric Office

Identifying where the child is on the continuum of play (imitative, symbolic, imaginative, cooperative) provides efficient insight into cognitive, language, and social development. The clinician should monitor children's play during all well-child visits from early infancy through middle childhood as part of developmental surveillance. In addition, the current American Academy of Pediatrics (AAP) guidelines recommend screening social development annually, using the Ages and Stages Questionnaire: Social Emotional or similar tools. Sample questions and prompts are provided at the end of this chapter.

Imaginative play, and especially play that is shifting from parallel play to cooperative play, is normative by age 3. Even from the second half of the first year of life, if a child is not demonstrating age-appropriate play, this can indicate cognitive delay, forms of anxiety, or atypical development, including autism spectrum disorder. Intervention and further evaluation are needed. Families should be connected with resources such as peer playgroups and Early Intervention. At the same time and in parallel, the child should be evaluated for additional delays and autism, with a low threshold for referral for subspecialist evaluations and specific interventions. The importance of timely evaluation and intervention is why clinicians should consider play and imagination at every early childhood visit.

Incorporating imagination into the pediatric visit has other benefits as well. Connecting with children around favorite toys and characters is a simple way to build trust and rapport, while elements of pretend can make stressful processes and procedures more tolerable. When incorporating imagination, it is important to adapt to the child's age and neurodiversity. Follow the child's lead and interests.

David is a 3-year-old boy with autism spectrum disorder at his well-child visit. He often struggles during the physical examination. He did not enjoy his pediatrician's tiger-shaped penlight and seemed confused and mildly distressed when Dr. Montoya tried to "look for monkeys" in his ears. Dr. Montoya regroups, stopping the examination to ask his mother how David likes to play at home. He is currently most interested in stacking and counting. Dr. Montoya provides David with a tin of small blocks and is able to finish her examination while mom and David sort, count, and stack happily.

Imagination at Home

Observing and engaging with a child's imaginative play is a window in their inner lives. At home, parents can foster imaginative play by protecting their child's unscheduled time and providing access to simple, open-ended toys like dolls, blocks, and art supplies. Parents who share imaginative play with their children are being supportive and nurturing. In short, playtime is bonding time. Yet, to be aware of and engage with their child's imagination, parents need to have mental space and flexibility. This mental space and flexibility are challenged by systemic stressors on caregivers and families, including levels of resources, experiences of trauma, and racism.

Parents of all income levels want their children to thrive. Many children live in families of lower income, in which the parents must focus first on day-to-day needs. It is difficult to prioritize imaginative play when food and shelter are precarious. Lower-income families are also more likely to live in neighborhoods with fewer outdoor spaces like playgrounds and fewer still perceived as safe.

Individual and systemic racism also impacts play. Black children are often perceived as older than they are, and their imaginative play is more likely to be described as negative or aggressive. Parents of Black children may fear how their child will be perceived and disciplined and so place stricter boundaries on imaginary play.

Overlapping with yet distinct from the above stressors is the parents' experience of trauma. A parent's experience of traumatic stress when they were a child may lead to a more reactive, harsh parenting style. Varied experiences of significant trauma are common, and trauma/stressor-related disorders are underdiagnosed. Parents with these experiences of trauma perceive themselves to be less effective parents and enjoy parenting less. Parents with experiences of trauma may be less able to distance themselves from negative emotions expressed in play and are more likely to be intrusive or controlling during cooperative play with their children.

Julie and her mom are in the office. Julie is throwing her bear on the floor and stomping on it, and you witness her mother speaking to her sharply. Dr. Liu redirects Julie to play with the bear on the examination table and then asks mom about how she is feeling. Mom reports that it is the anniversary of an experience of interpersonal violence; she becomes tearful. She acknowledges that it is hard for her to be patient when Julie is "aggressive" and worries about how Julie's play will be seen at school. Dr. Liu talks with the mom about her own therapeutic support, places a referral for parent-child interaction therapy (PCIT), gives her a prepared document about community resources related to interpersonal violence, and connects the family with social work.

Clinicians should work on behalf of children's right to imaginative play by advocating for their families on multiple levels. First, they can join with other leaders to support antipoverty policies, promote antiracism efforts within schools and communities, and create safe and pleasing family-friendly spaces outdoors. Within pediatric clinics, primary prevention

programs like Family Check Up and Video Interaction Project help parents gain confidence in playing with their children and practicing imaginative play in a trusted setting. In patient encounters, clinicians should be aware of systemic stressors and help parents to identify their strengths. Clinicians should be prepared to connect families with social workers and mental health professionals. For example, PCIT is an intervention structured around cooperative play that helps parents build self-efficacy and the skills of responsiveness and reciprocity. Clinicians should have at hand information about economic resources, safe community spaces that support play (e.g., community centers, play gyms, libraries), and information about low-cost, simple toys.

The challenges can be steep, but when imaginative, cooperative play takes place, it can be a source of pleasure, joy, and fun for parent and child. The fun of play should not be overlooked within science and policy. When adults, including parents, have fun, it leads to improved self-efficacy (including in parenting!), less burnout, and more meaningful relationships, including with their children. It is the ultimate feedback loop of positive reinforcement.

IMAGINATION AND FEAR

Every child, beginning in infancy, has fearful responses to some things, but at this age, fears become more complex. The child can imagine fearful things that *might* happen and can imagine other meanings for things that have happened in the past or are occurring in the present. Current and future events can be feared not just for their immediate danger but for what is perceived as an anticipated or ongoing threat. The ability to imagine can enlarge and modify these real or perceived dangers, as well as help the child manage them better.

Fears in childhood have their own expected developmental course linked to cognitive development and are presented in Table 16.1. Although subject to both individual and environmental features, the objects of fear are remarkably consistent across children. Emerging fears that appear where none have been may raise concerns for regression but really are due to an expanding imagination. For example, a previously fearless 5-year-old may become afraid of a monster in the closet while age 6.

In addition to an expanding imagination, as children grow they are often exposed to frightening real events. Fears related to political upheaval, interpersonal violence, natural disasters, and climate change can appear at very young ages, expressed through the child's developmental capacity. Since indirect exposure through the media or overheard conversations can be very impactful, these types of fears affect many children beyond those with direct experiences of events.

TABLE 16.1   Fears in Childhood

Age	Fears
0–7 months	Change in stimulus level, loss of support; loud, sudden noises
8–18 months	Separation, strangers, loud events, sudden movements toward, touching, physical restraints, large crowds, water, being bathed
2 years	Loud sounds, large objects, large moving things, changes in location of physical things, going down the drain or toilet, wind and rain, animals
2½ years	Movement, familiar objects moved, moving objects, unexpected events linked to the otherwise familiar (e.g., Grandma in mom's hat)
3 years	Visual fears, masks, old people, unexpected physical differences, the dark, parents going out at night, animals, burglars
4 years	Auditory fears, the dark, wild animals, parent's departure, imaginary creatures, recalled past events, aggressive actions, threats
5 years	Injury, falls, dogs; overall, a decrease in fears
6 years	Supernatural events, hidden people, being left or lost, small bodily injuries (e.g., splinters, small cuts), being left alone, death of loved ones, the elements, fire, thunder; a more fearful age
7 years	Spaces (cellars), shadows, ideas suggested by media, being late for school, missing answers in school
8–9 years	School failure, personal failure, ridicule by peers, illness, unanticipated events
10–11 years	Wild animals, high places, criminals, older kids, loss of possessions, parental anger, possibilities of catastrophe (e.g., earthquake), school failure, climate change, gun violence
12–17 years	Physical changes in one's own body, isolation, sexual fears, loss of respect or acceptance by peer group, political events, gun violence, climate change

Modified from Jersild AT, Holmes FB: *Child Dev Monogr* 20:358, 1935; Ilg FL, Ames L, Baker SM: *Child behavior*, New York, 1981, Harper & Row.

After practicing lockdown drills at school, Luke told Dr. Rogers that he was worried that a bad guy in a mask was coming to "get" him and his family in their house. Note: Children do not understand causal complexity, so identifying one person or one specific action is the way a child expresses complex fears.

No child can be fully protected from the task of working through these fears. Children's fears, especially in early childhood, seem to cross cultural barriers, although the intensity of the child's response and the *specific* circumstances that intensify fears vary from child to child and across cultural or subcultural groups. The expression of fear is individual yet is often summarized as "fight, flight, or freeze"; behaviors include irritability, aggression, fleeing, calling for help, rigidity, shyness, and withdrawal.

Management of Fears

Fears cannot be avoided. In fact, fears serve to keep us safe, restrain our behavior, and cause us to seek help and support from our environment. The goal in managing fear is not elimination but rather adaptive coping and protection from anxiety.

It is normative for toddlers to be afraid of strangers, dogs, noisy environments, and separation from care providers. Children should not be scolded for crying at the approach of a stranger or dog, nor coerced to happily greet or hug new arrivals. Stranger anxiety peaks from 8 to 18 months; new adults should approach a toddler slowly after talking to a familiar adult and should be prepared to back off if the child resists their approach. Separation anxiety is expected in the second year of life. Predictable patterns of parental leave taking and return rituals help toddlers cope with necessary separations and the fears they may incite.

Preschoolers' imaginary fears should be respected. Parents should acknowledge the fearful feeling without validating the existence of the imaginary creature or events. Demonstration of support and safety and giving a child a sense of control of part of the situation will restore some equanimity. Drawings and pretend play with dolls or with other children can be used to cope. Minimizing overwhelming or frightening media or situations may help decrease episodes of fearfulness. Attempting to use logic to argue kids out of imaginary fears is almost always futile.

School-age children continue to have imaginary fears, with the addition of fears around interpersonal and practical experiences. Unmentionable events or topics often become sources of fear. School-age children need opportunities to identify their fears, discuss possible outcomes, and practice coping skills. They can use words and logic to cope with fears, tools not available to a younger child. Factual information generally reduces the fears of a school-age child, whereas it may overwhelm a preschooler. Reminders of the normalcy of fears are usually helpful, along with parental models for identifying and coping with fears. Children, particularly those older than 5, often like to mentally rehearse or talk through their plans about fearful things.

Jackson's family was moving to a new house. He asked his mom over and over where his bed was going and where would he take his bath. His mom reassured him that his bed would be moved to his new room, which was painted blue, and that his room was right next to the bathroom, which had yellow walls and white tile. He drew a picture of his new house and showed it to everyone in the neighborhood, being careful to show the address. He calmed down considerably after taking a "walk through" with his family.

Fears are distinct from anxiousness or **anxiety**. In children, for whom imaginary fears and fears of the unknown are common, the most important distinguishing factor is the impact of a worry on the child's functioning. Is a fear leading the child to avoid certain activities or impacting their sleep? Is a desire to avoid the *feeling* of fear driving behavior change? This is more accurately considered anxiety and requires a different coping approach. Though treatment of anxiety is beyond the scope of this chapter, it is important for the clinician to help children, and indeed families, to be familiar with the concepts of treatment. In early childhood, therapy usually is dyadic, meaning it includes caregiver and child working with a therapist on play, helping the child self-regulate, and helping the caregiver understand and respond to the child's negative behaviors. Parent management training and behavioral modification therapy are used for more disruptive or hyperactive behaviors. A summary of early childhood therapy components is provided in Table 16.2.

For anxiety in school-aged children, therapy approaches include cognitive behavioral therapy (CBT) and exposure. CBT helps children and their families identify how thoughts, behaviors, and feelings are interconnected; work on changing their thoughts to change their feelings (anxiousness); and unlearn behaviors that avoid rather than acknowledge and tolerate anxiety. For example, a child may learn self-talk about being brave and ways to "be in charge" rather than allowing the bully who is anxious to make decisions. Families may learn and practice how to allow their children to take risks and not rely on overprotection.

Exposure involves children identifying what makes them anxious and then purposefully experiencing mild forms of the trigger in a controlled environment, gradually moving to experiences of moderate and significant forms of the trigger. For example, if a child is afraid of butterflies, they may schedule a few times per week to sit with a cartoon drawing of a butterfly, noticing how they feel. When this becomes tolerable, they may move on to a photograph of a butterfly, then a stuffed animal, then a realistic toy, until they are going to a butterfly exhibit and letting them land on their hands. CBT and exposure should be practiced with a licensed and experienced therapist; clinicians should be comfortable discussing and endorsing its principles.

Most days in clinical practice offer opportunities to learn about children's fears and their coping styles. It is also a chance to model support for a child when fearful events come up. Empathy, minimal discussion, and providing some aspect of control will help. A child's fears should never be dismissed as trivial. The fear is real, even if the object of the fear is not. They offer clear testimony to a child's affective, cognitive, and social level. Fears are the other side of imagination, and both are to be respected as sources of and testimony to mental growth.

Nightmares and Night Terrors

The emergence of imagination means that **dreams and nightmares** will also make their appearance. Nightmares and dreams are the product of rapid eye movement (REM) sleep, a mentally active part of the sleep cycle. Not every REM period has dreams; they are more likely to emerge in the early morning, particularly as the child grows. Children may or may not be able to discuss the content of these dreams, depending on their cognitive level and linguistic skills. Dream content is a jumble of things and events and cannot be taken literally. However, dreams may increase during times of stress because they serve as a strong coping mechanism. Firm and consistent bedtime rituals help all kids cope with nighttime fears and awakenings. Avoidance of overly intense media may decrease some nighttime fears.

Night terrors, on the other hand, are abrupt partial awakenings from deep sleep (non-REM) and are accompanied by dramatic physiological arousal with no wakefulness or awareness of surroundings. They usually occur in the second sleep cycle (about 3 hours after initial sleep onset), increase at times of fatigue and stress, and run in

TABLE 16.2　Approaches to Therapy in Early Childhood

Therapy	Description/Goals of Therapy
Parent-child relational support (i.e., infant mental health, home visiting)	• Help caregiver read child's social-emotional cues and understand child's emotional states • Increase parenting sensitivity • Support caregiver self-regulation and mental health, social support, self-efficacy
Parent-child trauma-informed therapy	• Same as infant mental health approaches, but involves approaches that help caregiver deal with trauma symptoms and understand child behaviors that stem from trauma exposure
Parent-child interaction therapy	• Often used for children with hyperactivity, defiance, dysregulation, or withdrawal • Caregiver is coached on play interactions via "bug in the ear" support from a therapist • Starts with child-directed interaction, in which caregiver practices following the child's lead, reducing controlling or avoidant behaviors, and increasing engagement that provides autonomy support/scaffolding • Once this is mastered, moves to parent-directed interaction, in which the caregiver is coached on delivering effective instructions and builds reciprocity/engagement from the child in following their lead
Behavioral modification therapy/parent management training	• For early attention-deficit/hyperactivity disorder, dysregulated or aggressive behavior • Uses principles of behavioral reinforcement to teach and reward desired behaviors while attempting to extinguish negative behaviors • Includes natural consequences or withdrawing privileges for negative behaviors (rather than harsh discipline) • Caregivers coached on how to provide specific praise, use token economies (e.g., behavior charts, stickers) to provide concrete reinforcement for positive behaviors, and not unintentionally reinforce negative behaviors • Consistency and routines encouraged
Applied behavior analysis	• For autism spectrum disorder • Usually implemented in an intensive manner (15–40 h/week) in early childhood to build communication, social, cognitive, and play skills • Involves breaking down desired behaviors (e.g., hand washing, waving hello) into smaller steps and reinforcing when these occur, while tracking response to intervention over time • Most effective when caregivers are involved in training and apply the same approaches at home and in community settings through play and everyday activities

families. During night terrors, children appear flushed and wide-eyed and may cry or yell, but they are unresponsive to comfort. They will not remember the event later. Though very frightening to parents, night terrors are not harmful, and specific events resolve without intervention. During an event, parents should be soothing and calm, while making sure the environment is safe from any movements. Night terrors rarely occur past late childhood.

ENTERING A WIDER WORLD

While imagination deepens the child's inner world, at age 3 the child is expanding knowledge and relationships beyond the family home, especially through experiences of early childhood education (ECE), reading, and media. This section is not meant to imply that ECE or the love of story only begins or becomes important at age 3. Indeed, from infancy, many children have connected with their broader community through childcare, playgroups, gatherings of extended family, and community or religious celebrations; similarly, many children and their parents enjoy reading together from a very young age. Rather, it is at around age 3 that the child takes a personal interest in these experiences, building independent relationships outside the home, developing and pursuing interests at preschool, picking stories based on their interest, and flipping through picture books on their own. The emergence of cooperative play, improving memory, and the development of personal preferences combine at this age to expand the knowledge and relationships in the child's world.

EARLY CHILDHOOD EDUCATION

While a child may attend childcare from an early age, at this age most children are eligible to transition to an "ECE" setting within their community. While states and municipalities have different guidelines and requirements, all **high-quality ECEs** seek to provide children with a safe, healthy, and supervised space to play and learn with their peers. Ideal ECE environments are nurturing spaces that support the development of all young children. They may include classrooms, play spaces, areas for caregiving routines, and outdoor areas. ECEs should be well organized, with developmentally appropriate schedules and opportunities for choice, play, exploration, and experimentation using age-appropriate equipment, materials, and supplies.

Children who attend ECEs will experience improved development in social, emotional, language, and cognitive domains. They gain self-efficacy as they learn to interact with trusted adults, to engage in cooperative play and solve problems with their peers, and to identify, express, and manage a broad range of emotions. If, like Early Head Start, the ECE also has an academic focus, the child will also learn literacy, mathematics, and scientific reasoning skills.

The benefits of ECEs are broad, yet many children will need time and support to embrace this expanded world.

Ha-Yoon started a 3-year-old preschool 2 weeks ago. Parents report that after school, she is having frequent meltdowns—crying, yelling, throwing toys, etc. She can become upset over "the smallest things," like the color of her cup or if her 9-month-old brother crawls near her chair. Days where she is able to have a snack on the drive home from school have been better.

It is common for children to experience separation anxiety at drop-off times, especially if it is the beginning of time in a new space or with new adults. Parents can be empathic and calm, working with the ECE staff to make the transition relatively quick and drama free. There may also be emotional dysregulation after the child returns home at the end of the day; children's reserves are often depleted by the increased cognitive, social, and even physical demands of an ECE setting. A child who has held it together all day is likely to need an outlet for emotional frustration and personal demands, which, from the

parents' perspective, may seem out of proportion and out of context. Again, empathy and calm are the parents' best strategies. It can also be helpful to anticipate the child's dysregulation by meeting core needs (food, rest) and promoting low energy, preferred activities.

Within the ECE setting, children may face a variety of challenges. Unfortunately, neurodiversity, including hyperactivity/inattention, autism spectrum disorder, and disruptive behavior, is not always well supported within ECEs. Some children will enter with preexisting diagnoses, while for other children, exposure to novel or increased structure and group expectations can newly highlight differences and needs. This can be a significant source of stress for the child and family. Clinicians should ask about these concerns during office visits and pursue evaluation as needed. ECE educators and staff should be trained in observing and assessing children to identify unique learning and developmental needs and should use their knowledge to create a learning environment that is accessible and responsive to each child. This should include close cooperation with families to set individual goals and identify specific resources and supports for the child, which may include a formal school evaluation and an Individualized Educational Program.

When a child's needs are not well supported or when child's behaviors are misunderstood, it may result in **preschool expulsion**. About 5000 children per year are expelled from ECE settings, with many downstream consequences. Black children are expelled at the highest rates, and boys are more than 4.5 times more likely than girls to be expelled. Large classroom sizes, individual bias, systemic racism, and lack of behavioral support for ECE educators all contribute to expulsion rates. Parents and clinicians should advocate for ECE policies that eliminate expulsion for behavioral problems. The AAP recommends that all children who are expelled or are at risk for expulsion should be assessed for developmental, behavioral, and medical problems to identify underlying concerns that might be targeted through intervention services. Children with severe behavior problems that cannot be safely maintained in a typical ECE program may require specialized services, such as special education or therapeutic ECE programs.

STORIES AND BOOKS

Stories are a delight to kids and are useful as well. They assist kids in working through their own imagination, fears, interests, and experiences. Parents and children reading together is a source of connection and cognitive development, building language, literacy, and social-emotional skills that last a lifetime. Pediatric providers have a unique opportunity to encourage parents to engage in this important and pleasant activity with their children early and often.

Literacy starts early and follows a predictable course:

- In the first year, children should become familiar with books as objects, turn pages, and learn to look at the pictures.
- Between ages 1 and 2, children can name objects or actions of one picture at a time.
- At ages 3 to 4, children learn how the pictures are connected in a story and can then tell the story with no book present.
- The ability to guess "what will happen next?" is really evident at age 5 to 6, about the same time that the child appreciates motivations of the book's characters.

The AAP recommends families read with children every day. It is okay for this time to be brief and to follow the child's lead. Parents should let the child pick stories, even if it is the same story over and over again. It is great to use expressive voices, to ask the child questions about the story, and to talk about the illustrations. Parents need not feel intimidated though; a simple read-through in their natural voice is just as effective. All print media counts as reading! This includes comic books, graphic novels, and magazines. Audiobooks are also a great way for parents and children to share stories if there is limited parental literacy or just to add story time to experiences like riding in the car. The local library is a great source of free and diverse books and audiobooks.

In the office, clinicians can listen to how parents read to their child; this will provide insight into the child's development and about parent-child interactions. Simple books in the examination room allow this observation to be made incidentally. Direct clinician involvement in encouraging reading (e.g., Reach Out and Read Program) is highly effective in improving language skills and parent-child interactions. A clinician who actively encourages reading really does make a difference.

SCREENS AND DIGITAL MEDIA

Digital media have changed significantly since the time when most parents were children themselves. With the advent of mobile devices, apps, streaming video, online games, and social media over the past 2 decades, children have options beyond broadcast and Cable TV. Most infants have interacted with a mobile device by the time they turn 1, and many 3-year-olds will have their own tablet or mobile device that they share with family members. Young children's viewing is now dominated both by TV programs and online videos such as YouTube. Parents, too, spend several hours per day on their smartphones—for work, entertainment, and social support.

Families' individual patterns of media use vary based on preferences, household structure, and access to other opportunities (e.g., childcare, after-school programs, safe neighborhood parks), so guidance about media cannot use a one-size-fits-all approach.

Several concepts should guide the thinking of pediatric clinicians when it comes to early childhood media use.

- Content quality: Studies show that the quality of content is key to shaping whether media has a negative or positive effect on young children. Viewing well-designed educational programming such as PBS KIDS or Sesame Street, which have developmental psychologists on their design teams and evaluate that children actually learn from their products, is associated with better language, early academic, and some social-emotional skills. Exposure to adult-appropriate or violent programming is linked with worse sleep, externalizing behavior, and developmental delays. With the vast amount of low-quality videos on YouTube and falsely labeled "educational" apps on app stores, one of the best things pediatric clinicians can do is encourage quality content—choosing media that is worth a child's time and attention.
- Pacing and design: Young children have a harder time processing fast-paced, jerky, fantastical, and confusing content. In a classic study, preschool-aged children who watched 9 minutes of *Spongebob Squarepants* showed worse executive functioning immediately afterward, compared to children who had watched the slow-paced, realistic show *Caillou* or colored with crayons for 9 minutes. As videos become shorter and try harder to capture young children's attention—for example, through gimmicks like including branded toys, candy, fast food, or luxury items—it is important to encourage caregivers to have their child watch higher quality programs or movies that tell meaningful stories.
- Parasocial relationships: Because of young children's imaginations and magical thinking, they form strong parasocial relationships with book and media characters. This can facilitate learning, but caregivers should be wary of characters who try to persuade children to make purchases or ask for certain brands.
- Coviewing between caregivers and children cannot only help young children transfer what they learn on media to their everyday lives, but it also helps them identify advertising (which they cannot do on their own).
- Displacement: The reason prolonged screen time is associated with developmental delays and behavioral issues is not only related to age-inappropriate content but also due to what it displaces. This includes a good night's sleep, language exposure from conversations and play with caregivers and siblings, and solo play in

BOX 16.1   Components of A Family Media Plan in Early Childhood

From infancy through adolescence, clinicians should encourage caregivers to have a plan for how digital media (e.g., television, video-streaming platforms, devices, apps, and social media) will be used in their homes. Because much of media use is habitual, and the design of media itself reinforces repeated and prolonged use throughout the day, caregivers may need help being intentional about what, when, where, and how media are used in their family.

What

- Discuss expectations of content quality, including wanting prosocial and educational shows, good role modeling, and limited violence or rude behavior.
- Caregivers may find it easiest to limit their child's media use to only nonprofit or evidence-based groups such as PBS KIDS, Sesame Workshop, Noggin, CBeebies, or similar. These groups develop and test their shows and games with developmental psychologists and families.
- Understand the limitations of YouTube content, which usually has low educational values, has lots of commercial product placement, and is created by people with no child development background.
- Many children are interested in funny videos on social media platforms, but this should be limited and always viewed with an adult.

When

- Avoid screen media in the hour before bedtime because it is arousing and the blue light from screens can decrease melatonin. If children are used to having screens playing videos at bedtime, suggest audio-only books or meditation instead.
- Talk about the other times when families do not want media interrupting their day—either from children or parents' use—such as playtime, reading/snuggling at night, or mealtime.

Where

- Options include designating screen-free rooms in a family's home, such as bedrooms and dinner tables.
- In cars, use hands-free options so that children do not learn that it is OK to text and drive.

How

- Make consistent routines so that use is not on-demand every time a child asks for their device or favorite show.
- Time limits will vary from family to family, but in early childhood suggest only 1 to 2 hours per day. Some families will want to keep certain days of the week screen-free and have other days where children indulge more.
- Transitions away from media can be challenging; help a child with a visual timer, verbal or visual schedule or warning, and having an activity to transition to.
- Coview and discuss programs with kids, including advertising, influencers, and why different characters behave or think the way they do.

Based on AAP Family Media Plan. www.healthychildren.org/mediaplan

which the child plans and carries out their own ideas and imagination. Therefore having time-limit boundaries around media use, keeping devices out of bedrooms, and making time for other enriching and social activities is crucial in the early years.

Parent media use is also important to address. "Technoference" (defined as parent technology use that interrupts parent-child activities) is associated with more internalizing and externalizing early childhood behaviors, more parenting stress, and attachment difficulties. Encourage parents to create their own tech boundaries during time with their children, from infancy through the teen years, because it is much easier to respond to child needs and behaviors when parent attention is not pulled in several different directions. Other strengths-based approaches to helping families make a Media Plan are described in Box 16.1. Addressing screen use during visit encounters is described in Chapter 4.

DURING THE VISIT

What to Observe

The clinician should observe and make note of the following:

- The child's use of toys in the office. Having a bin with puppets, small doll figures, blocks, small cars, and toy food can facilitate this.
- The child's ability to fill in downtime within the visit (e.g., while the clinician is interviewing the parent) with imaginative play.
- Interest in books. Do they look at the pictures, point, name, or tell a story?

- General response to the office environment/examination and any manifestations of fear, or wariness. How does the child cope?
- Ask the child about any costume, special clothing, or toy from home to assess interest in "pretend."

What to Ask

The clinician should ask the following questions during the examination:

- How does the child play at home?
- Does the child approach and play with other kids? How do these interactions go?
- What are the child's favorite toys? How are they used?
- Does the child have imaginary friends or an interest in costumes or role-playing?
- How do the caregivers choose what the child watches?
- What things make the child fearful?
- Is the child having dreams or nightmares?
- What is the parents' response to nightmares and fearful situations?
- Does a child have regular social experiences with other children?
- Does the child attend a daycare or preschool? Is the family satisfied with this experience? Has the child had behavioral challenges at school?
- How often does the family read together?
- What types of books does the child like? How do they read them?
- Do they have their own tablet? What is the plan for how much time they spend with screen media?
- How do the caregivers decide what the child can watch?

ASSESSMENT

The following factors should be assessed during the examination:

- Quality of eye contact.
- Frequency of joint attention and social referencing between the clinician and caregiver.
- How the child explores the examination room—level of activity, level of focus, presence of sensory-seeking behaviors, etc.
- How easily does the child transition from one activity to another?
- Does the child move easily into imaginative play with provided toys?
- Can the child accept and build on the clinician's own imaginative suggestion (e.g., tongue blade becomes a car)?
- What does the child do with open-ended objects (e.g., several tongue blades, paper clips, paper cups)?
- Does the child make simple shapes with a crayon on paper?

- How easily can the child engage in back-and-forth conversation?
- Is the child fearful? If so, how is fear handled?

ANTICIPATORY GUIDANCE

The following are some guidelines for clinicians to help guide parents of toddlers:

- Encourage families to make a media plan that includes the number of hours the child will use media (if at all) and the other activities young children need in a given day; the content or programs the child can watch (emphasizing trusted educational programming like PBS KIDS or Sesame Street); the importance of coviewing; keeping technology out of bedrooms, cars, and mealtimes; and helping parents set their own technology boundaries. Recommend families make a Family Media Plan at www.healthychildren.org/mediaplan. See Table 16.1 for components of a Family Media Plan.
- Encourage play with open-ended toys that the child can imagine as multiple things (e.g., blocks, balls, toy buildings, dolls, puppets, crayons and papers, and simple vehicles). Old clothes and simple costumes are also fun props. Parents can learn so much from observing their children's play. The child's inner life and personhood are demonstrated, as well as their individual preferences, fears, and interests.
- Reflect on the emergence of dreams and nightmares as markers of this new phase of cognitive and affective development. Welcome them as indicators of healthy mental development. Caregivers should respond to the child's reaction to the nightmare rather than the content of it. A brief demonstration of the caregivers' presence and safety should be central to this response.
- Encourage parents to read every day. The office can provide tip sheets and books for the families to take home. Discuss ways of obtaining books and stories for the home, depending on parents' resources, including libraries, book swaps, and story podcasts. Emphasize that it is the practice of reading and not the sheer number of books that is most important.
- Encourage parents to enroll the child in childcare or preschool. The clinic should have resources to connect low-income families with high-quality preschool or childcare within the local community.
- Parents should never force the child to meet the object of fear. The child should not be ridiculed or threatened for being afraid. If a child appears excessively fearful or nightmares are very frequent, look at the child's daily experience for evidence of overstimulation and exposure to emotions or situations that are overwhelming.

QUICK CHECK—TYPICAL DEVELOPMENT AT 3 YEARS

✓ Tells **3** things about themselves: first name, last name, and age

✓ Imitates **3** figures: line, circle, and cross

✓ Builds **3** cube structures: a tower of 8 to 10 cubes, a train, and a bridge

✓ Uses **3** types of utensils: spoon, fork, and cup/pitcher (i.e., can pour liquids)

✓ Speaks in **3**-word (or more) phrases or sentences

✓ Carries out **3**-step commands

✓ Can be understood **three** fourths of the time by a stranger

✓ Understands **3** prepositions (e.g., on, under, next to)

✓ Counts **3** objects

✓ Rides a **3**-wheel vehicle using the pedals

✓ Does simple puzzles of **3** or more pieces

✓ Dresses with supervision

✓ Alternates feet on stairs, at least going up

✓ Walks on tiptoe, a few steps at least, on request

✓ Does make-believe play

✓ Understands (but may not like) turn-taking

HEADS UP—3 YEARS

Identifying where the child is on the continuum of play (imitative, symbolic, imaginative, cooperative) provides efficient insight into cognitive, language, and social development. Clinicians should surveil children's play during all well-child visits from early infancy and screen social-emotional development annually.

If a child is not demonstrating age-appropriate play, this can indicate cognitive delay, mood disorder, or atypical development, including autism spectrum disorder. Timely evaluation and intervention are essential.

Fears are common and normative. Anxiety occurs when fears impact a child's function, and the child and family change behaviors to avoid feared experiences and the feeling of anxiety itself. Children with anxiety will benefit from evidence-based therapies involving parent and child

that focus on self-regulation and coping skills, especially PCIT, CBT approaches for parents, and exposure.

Encourage peer interaction through daycare, play group, community celebrations, or ECE program.

ECE provides many long-lasting benefits for children, but not every ECE setting is supportive of every child, especially minoritized children and children with neurodiversity. These children are at higher risk of preschool expulsion and its downstream impacts. Clinicians should advocate for behavioral health support in all ECE settings and a moratorium on preschool expulsions.

Emotional dysregulation at this age due to fears, fatigue, or stress is characterized by frequent periods of irritability, whininess, aggression, or meltdowns. Empathy, calm, and meeting concrete needs are the most helpful approach.

RECOMMENDED READINGS

Imagination

Christie H, Hamilton-Giachritsis C, Alves-Costa F, Tomlinson M, Halligan SL. The impact of parental posttraumatic stress disorder on parenting: a systematic review. *Eur J Psychotraumatol*. 2019;10(1):1550345.

Committee on Communications. Committee on Psychosocial Aspects of Child and Family Health The importance of play in promoting healthy child development and maintaining strong parent-child bonds. *Pediatrics*. 2007;119(1):182–191.

Council on Communications and Media Committee on Psychosocial Aspects of Child and Family Health. The importance of play in promoting healthy child development and maintaining strong parent-child bond: focus on children in poverty. *Pediatrics*. 2012;129(1):e204–e213.

Family Check Up. Available from https://cpc.pitt.edu/intervention-models/the-family-check-up/

Lieneman CC, Brabson LA, Highlander A, Wallace NM, McNeil CB. Parent–child interaction therapy: current perspectives. *Psychol Res Behav Manag*. 2017;10:239–256.

Video Interaction Project. Available from https://www.videointeractionproject.org

Early Childhood Education

Alanís I, Sturdivant T, eds. *Focus on developmentally appropriate practice: equitable and joyful learning in preschool*. Washington: NAEYC; 2023.

Council on Early Childhood. Quality early education and child care from birth to kindergarten. *Pediatrics*. 2017;140(2):e20171488.

Gilliam WS: *Implementing policies to reduce the likelihood of preschool expulsion*, 2010, Foundation for Child Development.

Head Start Programs. Available from https://eclkc.ohs.acf.hhs.gov/programs/article/head-start-programs

Literacy

Council on Early Childhood. Literacy promotion: an essential component of primary care pediatric practice. *Pediatrics*. 2014;134(2):404–409. https://doi.org/10.1542/peds.2014-1384.

Media

AAP Center of Excellence on Social Media and Youth Mental Health. Available from www.aap.org/socialmedia

ZERO TO THREE Resources on Screen Use in Young Children. Available from www.zerotothree.org/screensense/

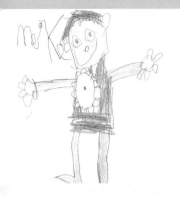

17

Four Years: Clearer Sense of Self

Lauren K. O'Connell

The 4-year-old health supervision visit should be efficient and quite entertaining if the clinician focuses on what kind of person this child is becoming, how they define themself, and how they interact with outside world. The 4-year-old child is an active and usually cooperative participant in the encounter. Information is easy to obtain; they will usually reveal everything by word or action. Typically developing children can converse about past and future events, ask and answer questions, and are often curious about and eager to discuss themselves. This growing sense of and interest in the self is explored in this chapter, including the progression of understanding one's gender, racial-ethnic identity, and moral self. This is an age of accomplishments and taking great pride in the developmental milestones achieved; this chapter provides an overview of milestones in language, motor, social, and emotional domains. As the child becomes more self-aware, challenges with school and behavior are frequent, particularly for children with developmental differences. Interventions related to behavioral self-regulation and emotional awareness can be very effective at this age and may serve as a foundation for discipline. In this chapter, common challenges, including lying, aggression, and preschool expulsion, are placed within the context of the establishment of identity and considered over the course of childhood and adolescence.

KEYWORDS

- Self-concept
- Gender identity
- Racial identity
- Autonomy/autonomy support
- Emotional regulation
- Lying
- Aggression
- Preschool expulsion

Previous edition by Suzanne D. Dixon.

CONCEPTS OF IDENTITY

Evolution of Self-Concept

The 4-year health supervision visit often brings into sharp focus the important process of self-development. At this age, children are just beginning the shift from the concrete, behaviorally grounded sense of the very young child's self to the more comparative, social self of middle childhood. The preschooler is growing in self-awareness, self-agency, and self-continuity: they are able to describe themselves, recognize that they can impact the environment and can control themselves, and are starting to project themselves into the future.

The preschooler's self-assessments are concrete statements ("I am 4 and a half. I have brown eyes."), possessive ("I have two cats."), and overwhelmingly positive ("I know all the dinosaurs! I can draw my mom! I can kick this ball to the moon!"). The 4-year-old is just beginning to compare themselves to others; the first comparisons will be temporal, to younger versions of themselves, and inevitably reveal that they are faster, taller, and better at all kinds of skills than they were when they were "little." They may compare themselves to age-mates to determine what is fair but are less likely to think in terms of who is better or worse at a given skill or attribute; those comparisons will emerge in middle childhood. Four-year-olds' positive self-assessments are adaptive, contributing to self-efficacy and likely serving as emotional buffers. There is no need for clinicians or caregivers to correct a child's self-assessment; on the contrary, adults should reframe the meaning of success and scaffold difficult tasks (see Chapter 2 for more about scaffolding) to help preschool children attain their goals.

The positive self-assessments of 4-year-olds contribute to high degrees of confidence. As the 4-year-old gains experience of and evidence for their impact on the world around them, they gain belief in their agency and generic confidence begins to shift to specific competencies. The

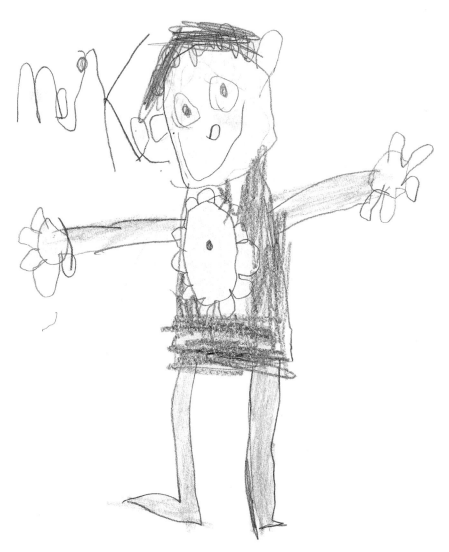

A 5-year-old girl draws a picture of herself. By Meike Messick.

4-year-old is, therefore, seeking autonomy and opportunities to take initiative. Parents can provide these opportunities in many concrete ways, including providing choices when possible (what to wear to school), engaging the child in family decision-making and household tasks (helping set the weekly meal plan, having simple chores), asking for their opinion, and sharing power when possible (parent decides what to serve for dinner and child decides how much they eat).

Four-year-olds have the beginning of self-continuity—the ability to project themselves into the past or future and to wonder how it may differ from the present. This ability includes perspective taking (understanding the mind of others), modeling/matching to others, and noticing others' reactions as they regulate behavior. Self-continuity is just beginning in a 4-year-old and is often hampered by the 4-year-old's cognitive shortcuts, especially all-or-none thinking. All-or-none thinking makes it difficult, for example, for a child to recognize that they are great at climbing but less great at tying their shoes (they are great at everything!) or that their classmate is both generally a nice person but shoved them in line before story time (they are mean!) or that they can be happy and nervous at the same time (they do not want to go!). The family can build the child's sense of continuity through telling autobiographical family stories, creating and noting family rituals, and documenting family life by posting artwork and photos.

During the clinic visit, it is valuable to ask the child to describe themselves ("What do you like to do?"). Parents describe the child's strengths and the new things they are learning. A 4-year-old should be able to define some aspect of themselves that is positive and satisfying, even if other dimensions are concerning to self or others. Parents should be able to describe the child's abilities and interests in positive terms. A negative self-concept or persistently negative parent-child interactions at this age are concerning and require more evaluation of the parent-child relationship and screening for trauma and stressors. As the child grows into an adolescent, their self-concept grows more complex, as outlined in Table 17.1.

TABLE 17.1   The Emergence of Self-Concept: How Children Describe Themselves at Different Ages

Level	Physical	Activity Based	Social	Psychological
Categorical identification (4–7 years) Basic descriptive features: concrete, often external	I have green eyes. I am 5 years old.	I play soccer. I play on the computer.	I am in Mrs. Smith's class. I am Jake's friend.	I think about Power Rangers. I am happy.
Comparative assessments (8–11 years) The lineup of self with peers Linear, often rigid and rule based	I am stronger than most kids. I have the longest hair of anyone in my class.	I am not very good at school. I am good at math, but I am not so good at reading. I am the best kicker on the team.	I am the second most popular girl in my class. I do well in school because I do more book reports than anyone.	I am calmer than a lot of kids. I cry more than the other kids.
Interpersonal implications (12–15 years) Sense of self based on relationships Personal characteristics as the basis and reasons for relationships Often, lack of flexibility	I have blonde hair, which is good because folks like blondes. No one sits near me because my pimples are so bad.	I play basketball, which is good because athletes are cool at my school. I treat people well so I will have friends when I need them. I like to join things so I can do things with people.	I can keep a secret, so people trust me. I am very shy, so I do not have many friends. I can almost always get the rebound, so people pick me for their teams.	I understand people, so they come to me with their problems. I am the kind of person who loves being with my friends. We can talk about anything.

Modified from Damon W, Hart D: *Self understanding in childhood and adolescence*, New York, 1988, Cambridge University Press.

Gender Identity

Concepts of gender have varied across cultures and history. While most children are assigned a sex at birth based on external sex characteristics and/or chromosomes, this may or may not match their gender identity. **Gender identity** is defined by the American Academy of Pediatrics as "A person's deep internal sense of being female, male, a combination of both, somewhere in between, or neither, resulting from a multifaceted interaction of biological traits, environmental factors, self-understanding, and cultural expectations." The 4-year-old child likely has a consistent sense of gender identity that they clearly articulate; moreover, young children who identify differently than their sex assigned at birth know their gender as clearly and as consistently as their developmentally equivalent peers who identify as cisgender. While research varies on the stability of gender identity from early childhood to adulthood, what is clear is that, rather than focusing on who they may become, valuing the child for who they are, even at a young age, fosters secure attachment and resilience, not only for the child but also for the whole family.

During the preschool years, many children begin to observe different aspects of gender expression around them, including clothing, hair, mannerisms, activities, or social roles. It is very common for 4-year-olds to play with gender expression, independent of their gender identity. Dressing up, taking on different types of household tasks, and imaginative play as differently gendered characters are all normal, fun aspects of this age. Variations in gender identity and expression are normal aspects of human diversity.

Independent of gender identity and expression, 4-year-olds are increasingly aware of their external sex organs and bodies more generally. Self-stimulation of the sex organs is normal and reflects physical pleasantness rather than a sexual drive or attraction to others. Many families may use self-stimulation as an opportunity to teach their expectations around private versus public behaviors. Remaining calm and matter-of-fact is important, like when discussing bathroom or other hygiene behaviors. There is no place for shame or punishment when discussing any part of the body.

Parents and clinicians should use accurate terms for body parts. Four-year-olds are likely to start having questions about how the body, including sex organs, works. Children should be allowed to ask questions early and often. Parents and clinicians should provide straightforward and accurate answers, following the child's lead. Clear, open, and frequent discussion of bodies, affection, and setting limits help children develop healthy concepts of body autonomy and consent, increasing the child's safety.

Clinicians are an important model and advocate for this approach. It is recommended that clinics have age-appropriate materials available for families to explore. Potential books are listed in the bibliography. Parents and the clinician should be aware of what types of sexual interests or play are concerning for children and possibly indicative of inappropriate sexual experience (Table 17.2).

Racial Identity

As discussed throughout the text, there is clear evidence that racism continues to impact the health and well-being of children and their families. Racism can be present through implicit and explicit biases, institutional structures, and interpersonal relationships. Clinicians must themselves proactively oppose all forms of racism and its impacts, as well as empower parents to promote positive racial identity in their children.

Race itself is a social construct rooted in history and culture; it is a mechanism that has been used to disempower groups of people and maintain caste status and control. There are no biological underpinnings for racial categories.

TABLE 17.2 Sexual Behavior in Childhood—When to be Concerned

- Masturbation begins in infancy and is nearly universal from toddlerhood. It is normal unless:
  It is compulsive and takes a child away from other activities
  It is consistently done in public in spite of feedback to do otherwise
  It is done in groups
  It is done with objects
- Observation and exploration of other children's external sex organs is very common. It is worrisome if one of the following is true:
  It is forceful, not mutual
  The participants are more than 2 years apart in age
  Penetration is attempted
  Behavior is accompanied by aggressive themes or activities
- Always concerning:
  Chronic interest in pornography
  Simulated intercourse or penetration with objects
  Explicit sexual conversations
  Preoccupation with sexual themes in play or conversation
  Sexual activities or exploration with animals
  Violent sexual ideas, themes in play or actions

However, the social construct of race infuses the environment in which children are raised.

Children distinguish phenotypic differences during infancy, including those associated with race. It is therefore important for parents of toddlers and preschoolers to proactively shape conversations around race. All families should discuss stereotypes and racism directly. Parents of minoritized children are likely to have little choice in the timing, as unfortunately, experiences of racism will require discussion, empathy, and problem solving.

In addition to preventing and processing experiences of racism, clinicians should also help parents to promote positive racial identity in preschool children. A positive racial identity decreases the impact of experiences of discrimination. Dimensions of racial identity include awareness of the child's racial affiliation, as well as having knowledge about, feeling positively toward, and engaging in positive behaviors relative to child's race. Essentially, it is feeling proud and comfortable in their own skin, exemplified by such social media trends as "Black Boy Joy" or "Black Girl Magic." Building positive racial identity in preschoolers is aided by relationships with family, friends, and community and by exposure to diverse portrayals in media and toys.

Preschoolers benefit from toys, screen media experiences, and books that are both mirrors and windows—that both reflect their own identity and experience and also provide insight into children with different experiences. It is especially important for minoritized children to have access to dolls, superheroes, and characters in books, videos, and games who look like them and have a variety of personalities, roles, and experiences. Resources for books and other media are listed in the bibliography.

BEGINNINGS OF A MORAL SELF

A preschool-aged child is faced with learning not only who they are, but also how they are expected to behave: the foundation for **moral development** is laid down. A 4-year-old shows increasing reasoning ability and can apply this ability to some moral issues, but they still apply many cognitive shortcuts. For example, for a preschooler, what they *want* to be true is *essentially* true. Because of this, they can understand rules but still bend them to accommodate immediate circumstances. Property rights are often a little vague; the child may really believe that they're "just borrowing" a toy. In addition, perspective taking is just beginning, as discussed earlier, which makes empathy, and especially retrospective or prospective empathy, very difficult.

On the other hand, all-or-nothing thinking gives the 4-year-old an acute sense of justice ("That's not fair; Jason never gets to be first."), and they can show unselfish sympathy and concern for others when directly confronted with some unfairness or sadness on the face of another. The child likes consistency, clear expectations, and instances in which the same judgment is applied to everyone. The 4-year-old wants approval and avoids negative outcomes; direct, specific feedback on both correct and incorrect choices, as well as the experience of natural consequences being closely linked to actions (e.g., "Give Sarah's book back. She did not say you could borrow it," *not* "Don't take other people's stuff") is the most effective way to build the child's moral sense over time.

PRESCHOOLER DEVELOPMENTAL DOMAINS

Language and Cognitive Development

Enhanced skills in the areas of language and cognitive development at this late preschool period give the child new ways to figure out who they are (Table 17.3). Language skills blossom during this period, which enables complex social interactions that go beyond the family. They also help the child get more specific information from all aspects of the environment. The child's vocabulary increases, and speech begins to contain all the elements of adult speech with regard to syntax and grammar. The "w" words—who, what, when, and so on—enable children to probe every event in detail. The use of conditional phrases, qualifiers, and subordinate clauses means that their narratives, arguments, and negotiations are much more complex. Although speech may be slightly imperfect in articulation (e.g., "r's" and "l's" may still be confused), the child is, for the most part, intelligible to strangers (e.g., the health care provider) virtually 100% of the time. Children may have a whole host of "facts" ready for recitation. You should be able to have an entertaining, though brief, conversation with a typically developing 4-year-old. The length, complexity, and content will vary by temperament and context.

The 4-year-old engages in extensive imaginative and cooperative play. Their growing sense of self, as outlined earlier, allows for creative role-play, acting out narratives, and world building with their peers. They are increasingly able to recognize colors, letters, numbers, and shapes. The 4-year-old is able to think about the whole, the parts, and their related functions; this influences problem solving and their ability to draw more complex figures. Many are starting to write letters, especially those in their names.

Four-year-old children with language delays may experience significant frustration. These children's understanding and cognition outpace their ability to communicate, leading to misunderstandings. Frustration over language can lead to tantrums, intrusive behaviors, and occasional aggression. In addition to delays in identification of colors, letters, and so on, the 4-year-old children with a delay

TABLE 17.3 Language and Cognitive Skills in Preschoolers

Language Area	Ability Level
Production	Hundreds to thousands of words; parents cannot even begin to count
	100% intelligible to strangers
	A few errors in articulation ("r" and "l" confusion)
	Extensive prosody (emotional expressiveness)
Grammar	Uses plural nouns, including some but not all irregulars ("mice" but also "feets")
	Uses verb suffixes, helper verbs (have, had) to indicate past, ongoing, and future
	Many adjectives and adverbs
Content	Asks questions using "w" words
	Uses clauses and phrases
	Understands conditionals; for example, "If it rains tomorrow, we will …"
	Can give full name, gender, and age of self and siblings; name of the teacher; and the name of at least one friend and can describe that friend
	Identify colors, perhaps some letters and numbers.
	Can identify composition of object and function ("What's a car made of?"; "What does your heart do?")
	Can follow a story, anticipate events, and ascribe feelings and motivation ("What will happen next?"; "How does he feel?")
	May write name or a few letters Copies a "+"
	Draws a person with two to five parts
	Sustained cooperative play

TABLE 17.4 Motor Skills in Preschoolers

- Walks up and down stairs, alternating feet
- Skips on one foot
- Can broad jump
- Climbs up jungle gym
- Throws overhand and catches a large ball
- Stands on one foot for longer than 10 seconds
- Holds a crayon well
- Uses scissors
- Can use a computer mouse
- Uses table utensils well except a knife
- Pours reliably
- Dresses self (mostly, most of the time)

in cognitive development are likely to play like a younger child: engaging in cause and effect, physical play, or simple pretend rather than world building and cooperative play.

Motor Development

Large motor skills have improved, and elaborate play and outside activities are available to the 4-year-old (Table 17.4). Fine motor skills have also matured, so working with pencils, scissors, and other tools is fun and produces more skilled creations. Although many basic sports activities are enjoyed and can be encouraged, competence in activities that demand accuracy, careful timing, or complex planning of multiple steps is still several years in the future. Team sports, choreographed dance, and other complex activities will be most enjoyed when the child is older and when the child is able to engage in: motor planning of several actions at once, sustained attention and anticipation of actions, and memory for several steps. For the 4-year-old, it is best to focus on learning specific skills, cooperative group games, and movement for fun.

Social and Emotional Development

Four-year-old children are trying to take initiative. Taking the lead, standing up for oneself, and making needs clear are big parts of the work at this age. The 4-year-old child's generally positive self-concept, increasing language and cognitive abilities, and improved motor skills combine to make autonomy both more desirable and more possible. When misunderstood or denied by parents, a 4-year-old's push for independence can lead to power struggles. On the contrary, parental **autonomy support**—scaffolding independence and sharing power—during the preschool years is associated with improved child behaviors, both in preschool and in later childhood. For example, many 4-year-olds want more control over dressing themselves and personal hygiene. If the parent tries to maintain total control over what the child wears, that 4-year-old is going to resist. Beware, tantrums ahead! Instead, the parent might choose to fill the child's drawers or shelves with clothes that are "preapproved" for weather, cleanliness, and family norms; then on any given morning, the child can be given free range to assemble an outfit from those clothes. Preschoolers also love to feel valuable to the family, through engagement in household tasks and decisions.

Encouraging the child to dust some low shelves or helping them measure out ingredients for cookies is going to take longer than the parent doing it themselves, but this practice builds responsibility and efficacy in addition to the skills themselves.

It should also be acknowledged that when children try to do things on their own, they will make mistakes. Parents should strive to respond with patience to accidents and mishaps, recognizing and labeling the desire and effort behind the action and working together to fix the problem. For example, the 4-year-old attempting to wash the cat is likely to cause a huge mess and chaos. Parents are likely to feel quite exasperated! But rather than respond with anger, it is best if the parent can take a breath and a moment and then describe what the child wanted to do, what happened, and how to restore order: "You were trying to give Socks a bath like you saw on that video! But Socks didn't like it and now there is water all over. Let's use this towel to wipe up the floor while Daddy finds Socks and gives her a treat."

Much of the emotional work of this age is self-regulation. Emotional regulation is not achieved once and for all during the preschool years, but there is a huge progression from the reactivity of toddlers. A 4-year-old child can identify and label emotional states. With coaching and modeling, they can learn to (1) pause, (2) identify an emotion, and (3) use strategies like mindful breathing, asking for help, movement, or taking a time out to calm down. Emotional regulation is possible for the preschooler, but it is not intuitive. Parents and preschoolers are often trying to regulate at the same time, which creates its own challenges and opportunities. Practicing strategies and skills together at times when neither parent nor child is upset and connecting them to shared interests or activities (loved characters from media, family jokes, or rituals) will build regulation and the parent-child relationship.

COMMON CHALLENGES

Lying

Parents may report that their child is "telling lies"—however, "inaccurate talk" is a better term than "lies" at this age. Premeditated plans to deceive are not possible until the child reaches school age, around 6 or 7 years. Children at this age do not (indeed cannot) intentionally plan to deceive others. However, their reports of events, particularly under pressure, most often reflect how they perceive things to be, how they creatively process these impressions, how they wish things were, or how they think things should be to please. These perceptions are real, even if the reported events are not. They should be seen as "creative coping" with a situation that may be stressful for the child. Parents should reflect on the underlying issue rather than struggle

TABLE 17.5   **Responding to Common Misbehaviors of Preschoolers**
Developmentally Appropriate
• "I wish those crayon marks weren't on the wall. Let's clean it together." • "You and Joaquín must have had a fight. Tell him you are sorry for hitting, and let's go out to swing." • "Give Clara's truck back to her now. The rule is: don't take anyone's toys unless you ask them. No borrowing." • "I see that my vase is broken. Oh, that makes me sad. Let's clean it up." • "I found my pack of gum in your room. Put it back in my purse, please. Ask me if you want gum."

with the content of the story. Untruths should not be supported, but it does no good to press a child to retract back a story. The parent should label and reflect on the reality of the situation and formulate a specific action plan to address it. See Table 17.5 for examples of specific situations and potential responses.

Aggressive Behavior

Aggressive behaviors are common in the preschool years. These behaviors include actions that are destructive to property (throwing, ripping), physically hurtful to others (hitting, biting, kicking), or hurtful to oneself (scratching, hair pulling). Verbal or relational aggression is not covered in this section.

Aggressive behaviors typically begin early in the child's second year, as a way to explore the world and get needs met. These acts often decline as language and problem-solving skills increase but may increase again with the increased cognitive and emotional demands of the preschool years. During the 4-year-old well-child visit, and any time aggressive behaviors are a concern, the clinician should obtain a detailed history. The clinician should ask:

- How often do these aggressive behaviors occur?
- Has the parent noticed any patterns of when they occur? Time of day, type of activity or transition, location?
- What types of behaviors occur?
- Who or what is targeted? Is it usually family members? Other adults or children? Pets?
- Has the parent been able to intervene to stop aggressive behaviors from happening? What works to calm the child down or stop the behaviors?

Aggressive behaviors may have many antecedents, and differentiating between different sources will help guide management. For example, a child with poor impulse control may act aggressively in frustration or attention-seeking behavior. Another child may have significant sadness, worry, or anger, and these big emotions spill over into aggression. Still another child may have irritability or sensory-seeking behaviors, and aggressive behaviors are a form of self-soothing. Children with developmental differences are at increased risk for aggressive behaviors for a number of reasons, ranging from difficulties with communication and executive function to neuroirritability. The presence of significant aggressive behavior that is impacting the child's ability to make friends, learn, or function in their family system requires evaluation for additional diagnoses, ranging from trauma exposure to delayed or atypical development to mood disorders and attention deficit hyperactivity disorder. If an underlying diagnosis is identified, treating this condition will almost always decrease the impact of aggressive behaviors.

Aggressive behaviors can be treated directly with therapeutic approaches. When the source of aggression seems to be impulse control or low frustration tolerance, behavior therapy and parent management training may be helpful (see Recommended Readings and Chapter 16). For mood- and anger-related behaviors, cognitive behavioral therapy is recommended, and a trauma-informed approach is best. Occupational therapy can help with sensory-seeking behaviors and emotional regulation. Clinicians should identify local providers of these therapies and be ready to direct families to local resources.

Preschool Expulsion

Preschool expulsions are unfortunately common. The actions of some children, particularly those with disruptive behavior, present a challenge within childcare and preschool settings. Behaviors cited as the reasons for suspension and expulsion include physical impulsiveness, aggression, biting, throwing chairs, disruptive behavior, defiance, constant tantrums, running away, and inability to function independently. Preschool teachers may not have the expertise or the consultative backup to provide optimal care for children with these behaviors.

There are significant disparities in who is expelled from preschool and childcare. Risk factors for expulsion include being Black or Hispanic, being male, and having a disability. Black preschoolers are 3.6 times more likely to be expelled than white preschoolers. Preschool children with developmental differences are 14.5 times more likely to be expelled than their neurotypical peers. It is children with challenging behaviors, often exacerbated by developmental difference, traumatic experiences, and systemic racism, who can most benefit from the opportunities offered in early education settings. (These benefits are discussed in

Chapter 16.) It is all the more frustrating than when these children are expelled or suspended.

Preschool teachers need to be trained to recognize that behavior is a symptom and try to understand the child's underlying emotions and thoughts. Preschool teachers also need training in trauma-informed practices and recognizing and combating implicit biases. Beyond individual teachers, preschools need to have access to consultative early childhood mental health services. Such access has been shown to reduce behaviors leading to expulsion.

Pediatric clinicians have a significant role to play in preventing preschool expulsion. With individual patients and families, clinicians can encourage positive parent-child interactions from an early age, guide families toward positive discipline strategies, and encourage collaboration between parents and educators. For children with developmental differences, clinicians can provide guidance in interpreting the child's behavior in the context of the child's communication and adaptive abilities and address any physical concerns that may be contributing to negative behaviors. Clinicians should advocate for all children with developmental differences to be evaluated for special education, as obtaining an Individualized Family Service Plan in Early Intervention, followed by an Individual Education Plan in school, provides both necessary support and services and legal protections for the child. On a practice level, integrated behavioral health and medical-legal partnerships in primary care settings can be effective in developing strategies that prevent early childhood expulsion.

AT THE VISIT

What to Observe

- What is the child's relationship with caregivers? Do they enjoy each other? Is there evidence of harsh discipline?
- What signs are present of growing independence?
- How emotionally regulated or dysregulated is the child? Are they seem sad, angry, worried, or distressed? Are they easily soothed by you or their parents? Are they demonstrating aggressive behaviors?
- How active is the child in the room? Can they climb on the examination table without difficulty? Are they demonstrating hyperactive or repetitive behaviors?
- Does the child make eye contact with you? Share enjoyment or other emotions? Do they initiate an interaction with you? Do they carry on a conversation?
- What kind of pictures do they draw? How do they hold the crayon?
- Do they separate from the parent easily, such as for weighing or another nonstressful event?

- Can they dress and undress by themselves? Does the parent intervene, and if so why?
- Can they follow a three-step command and get up on the examination table without difficulty?

What to Ask

Questions for the child:

- How are you? Why did you come today? Tell me about your (cool shirt, toy that you brought). Who is this in the room with you?
- Do you have anything you want checked? Is there anything you want to ask me?
- How do you like your school/daycare? What do you like about your teacher?
- What is your favorite thing to do there? What do you not like about (school, daycare)?
- Tell me your friend's name? What do you do together? What do you play?

Continue with open-ended questions, following the child's interests. Reflect on local and seasonal events. Additional possible questions are presented in Table 17.6. Use this time to explore how this child sees themself in their world and who is important in it. You are also listening for language, in line with the skills outlined in Table 17.3. You should be able to understand all of the child's speech.

Questions for the Parent:

Parent concerns should be elicited. Some exploration of these issues should be done with the child present, but some sensitive or negative concerns may be discussed without the child. Children should not be shamed or embarrassed, although their own views of difficulties should be elicited.

Ask caregivers for several details about the child's life, such as the following:

- Child's favorite type of play
- Child's favorite toys
- Child's preferred playmates
- Child's preferred shows, videos, or games
- How the child engage in self-care (e.g., brushing teeth, getting dressed)
- How does the child engage with family chores and decision-making?

Additional questions are listed in Table 17.7.

ANTICIPATORY GUIDANCE

- Four-year-olds are growing in self-awareness, self-agency, and self-continuity. Positive self-assessments are adaptive, and there is no need for clinicians or caregivers to correct a child's self-assessment. Instead, adults should scaffold difficult tasks to help preschool children attain their goals.

TABLE 17.6   Questions to Ask the Child During the 4-Year-Old Well-Child Visit
Do you have any pets? Tell me about them.
What do you do when you want something and mommy/daddy says you cannot have it?
How do you like your preschool/daycare center, etc. (by name if possible)?
What do you like to play?
What is your favorite book/show?
What do you do when you are angry? How do you calm down?

- The family can build the child's sense of self through telling family stories (their birth or adoption story, favorite trips), creating and noting family rituals, and documenting family life by posting artwork and photos.
- Four-year-old children will often clearly state their gender identity and will play with gender expression. Variations in gender identity and expression are normal aspects of human diversity, and caregivers should not force the child to express themselves or play in a particular way.
- Discuss the normalcy of interest in body parts and how the body works, including sex organs. Model and encourage accurate labels for body parts. Parents should answer the child's questions but not overload them with too much information at one time. Clinicians and parents should counsel the child about body autonomy, that is, no one should touch the child's private parts, except parents and clinicians if necessary, and no one should touch the child's body without their permission.
- Clinicians should model and encourage support for children and families to (1) recognize racism in all forms, from subversive to blatant displays of racism; (2) differentiate racism from other forms of unfair treatment and/or routine developmental stressors; (3) safely oppose the negative messages and/or behaviors of others; and (4) counter or replace those messages and experiences with something positive.
- Encourage families to seek out toys, media, and books that are both mirrors and windows—that both reflect their own identity and experience and also provide insight into children with different experiences.
- Encourage parents to read every day. The office can provide tip sheets and books for the families to take home. Discuss ways of obtaining books and stories for the home, depending on parents' resources, including libraries, book swaps, and story podcasts. Emphasize that it is the practice of reading and not the sheer number of books that is most important.

TABLE 17.7   Questions to Ask the Parent During the 4-Year-Old Well-Child Visit

What kinds of play activity does your child enjoy?	
What does the child's preschool teacher (babysitter, grandparent, etc.) say about them	Obtain additional information about the child's personality and behavior while separated from parents, and at the same time assess parents' openness to feedback about their child from outside the home; some parents find it difficult to accept any negative feedback about their child, whereas other parents seem surprised at favorable reports from outsiders about a child with whom they are experiencing difficulty.
What do you like most about your child?	Determine the parents' capacity to identify and articulate the child's positive and negative qualities; an inability to report some highly positive quality is unusual for parents and should be a sign for further evaluation by the clinician.
How often do they misbehave? What kind of things does your child do? What do you usually do when this happens?	An assessment of discipline practices at this age is absolutely essential; the clinician should be alert to the presence of inappropriately high or low behavioral expectations during this period; disciplinary techniques may be inconsistently applied, too harsh, or otherwise ineffective.
Do you take your child out to dinner at a friend's house or a restaurant?	Assesses the parents' comfort with their efforts to help the child meet social expectations outside the home; regardless of the parents' standard of behavior, parents should have a degree of confidence in their child's behavior by age 4 or 5.
How does your child act when angry?	Allows the parents to discuss concerns regarding the child's aggressive behavior or lack of aggressive behavior.
How has your child expressed an interest in their body (by asking questions, examining themself, or other people)?	Allows the parents to discuss evidence of sexual curiosity in the child while defining this as a normative process.

- Encourage families to make a media plan that includes the number of hours the child will use media (if at all) and the other activities young children need in a given day; the content or programs the child can watch (emphasizing trusted educational programming like PBS KIDS or Sesame Street); the importance of coviewing; keeping technology out of bedrooms, car rides, and mealtimes; and helping parents set their own technology boundaries.
- Encourage play with open-ended toys that the child can imagine as multiple things (e.g., blocks, balls, toy buildings, dolls, puppets, crayons and paper, and simple vehicles). Old clothes and simple costumes are also fun props. Explain the importance of playing with peers and help a family orchestrate playmates if this does not occur naturally.
- Parents can provide **autonomy support** in many concrete ways, including providing choices when possible (what to wear to school), engaging the child in family decision-making and household tasks (helping set the weekly meal plan, having simple chores), asking for their opinion, and sharing power when possible (the parent decides what to serve for dinner and the child decides how much they eat).
- Discuss with the family appropriate limit setting, management, and the importance of consistency in family expectations.
- With coaching and modeling, the 4-year-old can learn emotional regulation: (1) pause, (2) identify an emotion, and (3) use strategies like mindful breathing, asking for help, movement, or taking a time out to calm down.
- Caution parents about the differences between "inaccurate talk" and "lies."
- Aggressive behavior should be carefully evaluated to determine its source and direct its management. Therapy—ranging from behavioral management to parent-child interaction therapy—is almost always helpful.
- Assess the appropriateness of the child's preschool setting. Encourage the parent to collaborate with teachers

on the child's behalf. If the child is at risk for preschool expulsion, advocate for mental health consultation within the school system, evaluation for special education, and legal support if needed.

RECOMMENDED READINGS

Harter S. *The construction of the self: developmental and sociocultural foundations.* United Kingdom: Guilford Publications; 2015.

MR Hill: *The GENDER book*, Houston, 2014, Marshall House Press.

Rafferty J, Committee on Psychosocial Aspects of Child and Family Health, Committee on Adolescence, Section on Lesbian, Gay, Bisexual, and Transgender Health and Wellness: Ensuring comprehensive care and support for transgender and gender-diverse children and adolescents, *Pediatrics* 142(4): e20182162, 2018 (Reaffirmed August 2023).

It's not the stork!: a book about girls, boys, babies, bodies, families, and friends. Cambridge, 2006, Candlewick Press.

Trent M, Dooley DG, Dougé J, Section on Adolescent Health, Council on Community Pediatrics, Committee on Adolescence: The impact of racism on child and adolescent health, *Pediatrics* 144(2): e20191765, 2019.

The inclusion imperative: why media representation matters for kids' ethnic-racial development, San Francisco, 2021, Common Sense.

We Need Diverse Books. Available from diversebooks.org

PBS Kids for Parents. Available from www.pbs.org/parents/thrive

Williams PG, Yogman M, Council on Early Childhood, Committee on Psychosocial Aspects of Child and Family Health: Addressing early education and child care expulsion, *Pediatrics* 152(5):e2023064049, 2023.

Books for parents/teachers about early childhood behavior management

- *Good inside: a guide to becoming the parent you want to be* by Dr. Becky Kennedy.
- *No-drama discipline: the whole-brain way to calm the chaos and nurture your child's developing mind* by Daniel J.J. Siegel and Tina Payne Bryson.
- *How to talk so little kids will listen: a survival guide to life with children ages 2-7 (the how to talk series)* by Joanna Faber.
- *Positive discipline: the classic guide to helping children develop self-discipline, responsibility, cooperation, and problem-solving skills* by Jane Nelsen Ed.D.
- *Conscious discipline building resilient classrooms* by Dr. Becky A. Bailey
- *Raising confident black kids: a comprehensive guide for empowering parents and teachers of Black children (teaching resource, gift for parents, adolescent psychology)* by M.J. Fievre.

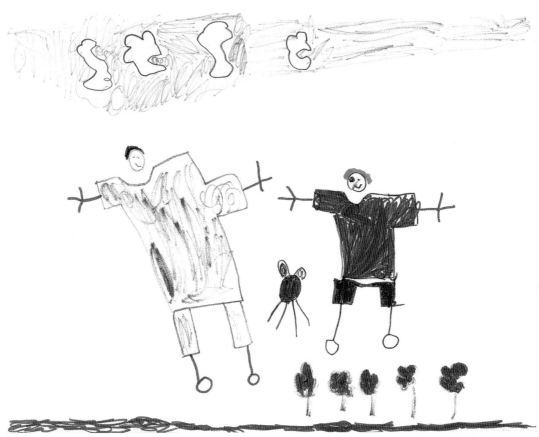

A 6-year-old aligns himself with his dad, with a dog in between. Identification with the same-sex parent often sets the stage for defining oneself. By Johnathan Zuidema, age 6. (Note the landscape).

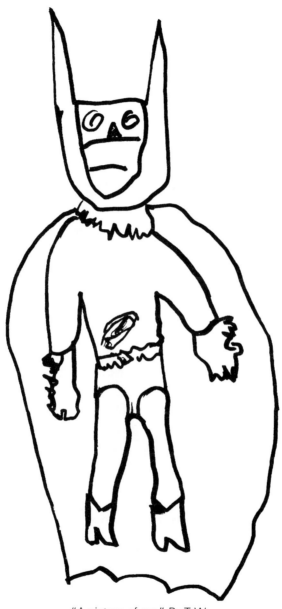

"A picture of me." By T. W.

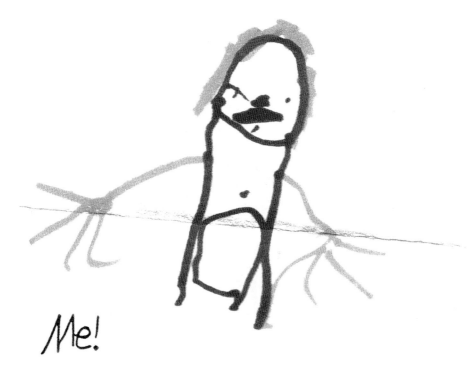

Me!

"Me." A boy depicts himself. By Logan Henderson, age 5.

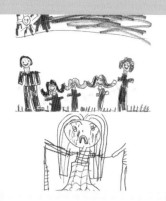

18

Five Years: Opening the School Door

Anna Klunk and Shaquita Bell

Kindergarten represents a significant change in a child's life. Social-emotional readiness, preschool learning, and interactions with peers and family members are some of the elements that can be assessed at this visit. Understanding a child's educational and social strengths and vulnerabilities can assist both caregivers and pediatric clinicians in planning for school entry.

KEYWORDS

- Assessing strengths and vulnerabilities
- Individual variation
- Language
- Communication skills
- Attention-deficit/hyperactivity disorder
- Prereading skills
- Separation and socialization

IMPORTANT DEVELOPMENTAL THEORIES AT THIS AGE

Entry into kindergarten or "kinder-ready/Young Fives" program between 5 and 6 years of age is a time of significant developmental expectations and achievements. It is a moment when multiple biological events and psychosocial tasks find a common ground focused on educational and social achievements: sustained attention for classroom learning, emotion regulation when facing new challenges, prolonged separation from family, comprehension and expression of language, and interactive and cooperative play (Box 18.1). It is a time when children develop a sense of mastery through achievements in cognitive, motor, and particularly social-emotional skills (Box 18.2). Schooling at

this age represents a shift, in most cases, from a more play-based preschool experience to more curriculum-driven classrooms with more focus on early academic skills.

Entering kindergarten is a qualitative change in cognitive and psychosocial tasks compared with preschool experiences. Children are still in the preoperational ("prelogical") stage of cognitive development. Their responses to the environment are guided by egocentric, animistic (giving living status to inanimate objects), and idiosyncratic thinking processes (see Chapter 2). Imagination and fantasy run high, and for most children, emotions start to feel under more control. It is also a time when sex identification is explored in interactive games and dress. Simultaneous with these cognitive and psychological growth characteristics is an acceleration of language (both expressive and receptive) and articulation. For children who are not meeting developmental expectations, it is also an important opportunity to help caregivers learn to work with their school system to advocate for educational supports.

The conceptual framework of cognitive social learning theory is a valuable clinical tool in understanding the reciprocal interactions that shape an individual's sense of competence (see Chapter 2). Bandura's model of social learning emphasizes the important influences of modeled and observed behavior on learning. Typically developing children in kindergarten spend considerable effort observing their teacher, peers, and the flow of the classroom to internalize new academic concepts and social norms. Cognitive social learning theory takes into account the mutual influences of the individual, the physical, and psychosocial environment—for example, how a child with impulsivity or dysregulated behavior might interact with a structured, responsive classroom versus an understaffed, chaotic classroom with an exhausted teacher. It is important to remember all of these factors that shape how a child learns and adapts to the school environment so that the focus is not only on the child's "problems."

Original chapter author by Martin T. Stein.

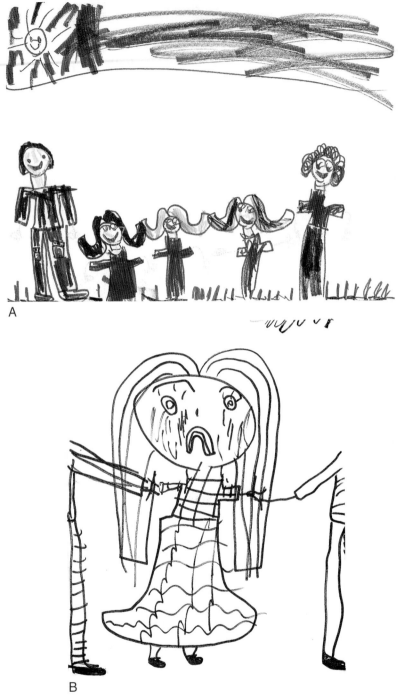

(A) A 5-year-old shows her upbeat spirit in this drawing of family and friends. (B) The same 5-year-old shows herself holding her caregivers' hands, reluctant to separate for a school event. School entry has its ups and downs. By Katherine Auerswald.

Factors That Shape School Readiness in Children

Understanding the family's own experiences with the educational system (either from their own schooling experiences or older children) is an important piece of information that a clinician should ask about at this time, because it shapes the concerns and goals that families have toward schooling. Some caregivers will have positive memories of their school years, more often if they had no learning challenges, attended well-funded schools, and did not face any systemic discrimination. However, it is important to explore any distrust caregivers may have regarding the educational system, to both validate their concerns and discuss strategies for advocating for their child's needs if and when concerns arise. For example, generations of Native American, First Nation, and Indigenous children attended residential or boarding schools in which they were forcibly removed from their parents, their culture and language were suppressed, children experienced physical and sexual abuse, and thousands died from neglect and disease. Black families aware of systemic racism in special education programs also may mistrust a school's evaluation of their child's learning needs, worrying about their child being labeled as "disabled" and removed from the regular education setting. The state of Georgia's special education system has been specifically criticized for practices like disproportionately giving Black children disability designations that lead to placement in substantially separate schools—leading to *de facto* segregation. In addition, Black parents and grandparents around the United States can recall difficult experiences of school desegregation, such as the Boston busing crisis in the 1970s. It is important to let families tell these stories to understand their perspectives on the educational system—the quality of which is a strong determinant of child success (see Chapters 20 and 24 for further discussion).

Even if caregivers are not feeling optimistic about their school system, it can help to highlight strengths-based protective factors, such as positive parenting or connection to culture, which they can leverage in helping the child cope and adapt to a new school. Encourage caregivers to be proactive in meeting teachers, other students' parents, and members of the parent-teacher organization, so that if concerns are identified, they have a support system to contact and discuss possible solutions.

BOX 18.1   Developmental Tasks Facing Children at School Entry

- Separation
- Increasing individualization
- Integration of cognitive skills required to learn to read
- Ability to form relationships with other children and adults
- Ability to participate in group activities and follow rules and directions
- Gradual formation of a sense of self or identity, both inside and outside the family environment

---

BOX 18.2   Social-Emotional Readiness Skills at School Entry and Example School Accommodations to Support Them

Social-Emotional Skills	School Support Approaches
Self-regulation: ability to control impulses, modulate attention and activity level, and regulate emotional reactivity for at least short periods	Social-emotional curricula that teach children breathing, stretching, or other self-regulation skills. Visual supports such as color zones, break cards, or places in the classroom to "rest and reset."
Executive function: planning and organizing skills, following directions, ability to demonstrate sequences, and taking turns	Teaching children to use checklists, visual organizers, or a daily schedule. Adult support to provide gentle reminders to take turns or follow multiple steps.
Capacity to tolerate separations from primary caregiver; to be responsive to the teacher	Plan for daily separations, such as a goodbye routine, a teacher or aide meeting the child at the door, or child being able to keep a photo of caregivers in their cubby.
Ability to master new experiences	For children resistant to trying new experiences, using visual supports (e.g., "first-then" boards), token rewards for trying new activity, or placement next to model peers who self-initiate new activities well.
Play skills, including taking turns and sharing	Adult support on the playground to provide gentle prompts on how to greet others, ask to play, take turns, resolve disagreements, or find collaborative activities.

One focus of well child visits around the age of school entry should be to discover a child's **strengths and vulnerabilities** that will have an impact on school function. Through a review of how the child has fared in prior classroom or childcare environments, presence of any developmental delays, attainment of preacademic skills (e.g., ABCs, counting), and social-emotional development, the primary care provider can help a family feel ready to partner with their child's school and intervene if challenges occur. Additionally, by helping demystify aspects of education such as behavior intervention plans and special education supports (see Chapter 19), clinicians can help caregivers communicate with schools about their child's needs.

It is unlikely that moderate-to-severe developmental problems, disabilities, or illnesses will have gone undetected up to this time when the child has received previous comprehensive pediatric care. The exception is a child who has not received comprehensive medical care in the past—for example, a child who has recently immigrated, is in the care of a foster family, or has had limited follow-up by developmental providers such as early intervention. When a clinician discovers a significant delay in development (e.g., in language, visual-perceptual, or social skills) or emotional/behavioral regulation challenges, appropriate outpatient and school-based assessments can be planned. It is important that this is followed by communication and coordination with the child's school, so that teachers, parents, and clinicians can be "on the same page" about the child's needs and supports. Sometimes appropriate supports are available through the child's school, but it is often the case that outpatient therapies and resources are needed as well, to which the pediatric clinician should refer. The special education system can feel intimidating and convoluted to families, so it can help to demystify the steps involved in obtaining special education supports, including (1) requesting a psychoeducational evaluation in writing and bringing it to the main office, (2) signing a consent form for school evaluations to take place, (3) understanding what tests will be performed and what they mean, (4) what to discuss at an Individualized Educational Program [IEP] meeting, (5) how to advocate if services are denied (see Chapter 19 for more detail). Information should be provided on protections offered through the Individuals with Disabilities Education Act (see Resources) and, if possible, have a list of local resources—such as educational advocates—for families.

Helping Families Choose a School

It is common that caregivers will choose the preassigned or neighborhood school for their child, due to ease of transportation and communication with the school. However, caregivers may have a choice between several kindergarten programs in their community and may seek help in choosing the best fit for their child. Some may wish to pursue homeschooling out of a concern for child safety (i.e., due to gun violence), wanting to pursue a unique curriculum, or worrying that the child will not "fit in" or be able to handle the classroom experience. In this case, it is important for the clinician to explore the reasons for wanting to homeschool, how these might be addressed through special education supports or outpatient therapies, and making sure that homeschooled children have adequate opportunities for social interaction and friendship development.

It is often useful to know about the educational philosophy and cultural differences of local schools. For example, caregivers may describe an "active, inquisitive, independent and creative" 5-year-old who is later described by a teacher as "restless, stubborn, resistant and rebellious." This more negative interpretation of the child's temperament or learning style can be internalized by the child and lead to a more negative mindset toward school and learning later on. It is important to understand that Black, Indigenous, and People of Color children are more likely to be labeled or perceived as disruptive and punished for their behavior due to implicit or explicit bias that exists in the classroom. If these concerns are brought up by the caregiver or child, clinicians can provide resources on how to discuss these issues with the child and educators. Caregivers are usually quite upset if they perceive their child is being discriminated against, so validate their emotional experience while providing concrete steps they can take to arrange appropriate behavioral supports at the school. This might include asking for a *functional behavior analysis*, obtaining a 504 plan or IEP for attention-deficit/hyperactivity disorder (ADHD), autism, or other developmental differences, or having outpatient therapists (e.g., psychologist and family therapist) attend school meetings.

There are several other variables to consider when helping a family choose a school for their child. Would they like a highly structured curriculum or one that is child-led? Do they think the child will do better with a larger or smaller class size? Does the school have a high rate of teacher turnover? Is the school known to foster an environment of cultural support and inclusivity? Schools can also be evaluated through ratings on US Department of Education websites, word of mouth, or prior sibling attendance. Many families will not have the option to choose a school other than the public school for their neighborhood, but it is still important to discuss these factors, so potential areas of support can be identified prior to the child entering school.

A visit to a prospective school should be advised. This is desirable even if no choice is anticipated, because all children do better if caregivers are visible and involved from the start. A classroom environment that is able to adapt to the needs of a wide variety of developmental levels would be the most ideal. Public schools, for the most part, have access to a greater range of specialized services for children with special needs than do private or parochial schools. In some public school systems, a cluster of schools focus on a specific area of interest (e.g., science, math, drama, music, history) that may be more suitable to a particular child. Caregivers can also be encouraged to inquire about classroom size, which may vary within schools and between school districts. Smaller class size may enhance learning in children with learning disabilities, inattention, or behavioral problems.

"Should We Delay Kindergarten for a Year?"

Frequently, caregivers may ask whether the clinician thinks their child should be kept back at home, in preschool, or a "Young 5's" or "Kinder-ready"-type program for another year. Caregivers who perceive their child as excessively shy and slow to warm up in new situations, clingy, or impulsive and hyperactive may raise this issue. You can reassure caregivers that a supportive school environment will actually help address and improve these issues. Through social learning, children internalize the classroom structure, teacher feedback, and peer role modeling and therefore develop skills that they might not have demonstrated at home. Therefore a child should almost never be kept home or out of school.

The discussion of whether to delay kindergarten entry depends on multiple factors. First, the child's age matters. Children with summer or early fall birthdays often benefit from a "Young 5's" program where they can learn early academic skills while still being in a smaller classroom with a more play-based curriculum. Second, the child's peer group might factor in; if children have formed strong bonds with other children who are progressing onto kindergarten, the child might benefit from this added peer support in a more advanced curriculum. Research studies suggest that both old-for-grade and young-for-grade students may have behavioral challenges, with young-for-grade students being more likely to be given an ADHD diagnosis. Therefore it is appropriate to guide parents that there is no "perfect" choice at this age. No matter what the family chooses, they should be guided to continue to communicate with the teachers and support staff regularly about how the child is doing. If concerns about communication, academics, or behavior are identified as the year progresses, caregivers can request a psychoeducational evaluation as well as accommodations (like sitting next to a peer role model or getting more movement breaks, see Box 18.2) that will help the child regulate their attention and behavior. In general, proactive collaboration with a school is much more effective and less stressful for the student and caregivers than reactive solutions once a child has been struggling for months to years.

SOURCES OF CHALLENGES AT KINDERGARTEN ENTRY

Prematurity and Low Birth Weight

School readiness, specifically development of the skills that help children thrive in kindergarten, starts at birth. It has been found that children born preterm or with a low birth weight can have difficulties with the transition to kindergarten. Children born premature who were assessed by their teachers using the Early Development Instrument showed increased vulnerability with the transition compared to their siblings and nonpreterm peers. Similar findings have been noted in many studies evaluating different aspects of school readiness involving completing tasks, reading, spelling, and math. As a clinician, it is important to review protective factors and interventions with families that have a preterm or low birth-weight child to help ease the transition to school. Resources such as preschool/early intervention programs, access to nutrition through WIC or SNAP, and caregiver smoking cessation are all topics to review with families to promote development of premature infants. Additionally, access to pediatric primary care has been shown to increase school readiness through identification of already existing difficulties by a provider so they can be addressed before school entry.

Early Stress, Trauma, and Racism

It is well documented that early childhood stress impacts child development and the ability of a child to respond to change, such as school entry. Children at the highest risk for not being ready for school are those living in poverty. This is often multifocal and can be attributed to many factors, such as access to quality early childhood education programs, parental education level, and systemic racism. It is important to note that the concept of "school readiness" in the United States is socially constructed around norms and expectations in White, middle-class families in Western society. This emphasizes individualism and performative Western, task-based activities as indicative of the child's readiness rather than broader aspects of development. This can pose an additional challenge to children who recently immigrated or grew up in cultures that emphasize community-based learning and engagement. However, it is recognized that poverty affects school readiness across racial and ethnic divisions.

Clinical interventions to promote school readiness in poor and marginalized communities usually involve more than just referring families for therapy or supports, as there are multiple structural barriers to families engaging in these services (e.g., copays, transportation, concern that Early Intervention may represent governmental services that might report immigrants). Effective interventions involve multiple levels with culturally responsive components. A recent study showed promising results for strategies that can mitigate the effects of poverty on school readiness through the *Smart Beginnings Integrative Model*. This cross-disciplinary model takes advantage of the already existing structure of pediatric primary care and builds prevention strategies through a multiplatform approach of video interaction projects and family check-ins. In addition to these factors, child self-regulation has been noted as a key component of school readiness, and it is often not effectively developed in children growing up in poverty. The transition to kindergarten for children experiencing poverty can be mitigated through educational programs that focus on developing child self-regulation skills alongside the normal academic curriculum.

Chronic Illness

Children with recurrent hospitalizations, surgical procedures, or other medical conditions that influence any developmental streams, caregiver/child stress, or activities of daily living are more likely to have challenges with school entry. Clinicians should be more vigilant about monitoring the school progress in any patients with medical conditions. More information on children's adaptation to illness is reviewed in Chapter 25.

Language-Related Delays

An early delay in language development has been shown to be the best single predictor of later learning problems. *Particular attention should be given to a child who has a history of early language delay, even if the current language competency falls within the expected range.* We should also be alert to how the child's language developed. Were there problems in fluency, comprehension, and the naming of objects? Expected language milestones leading up to school entry are shown in Table 18.1 and discussed in greater detail in Chapter 15. These language developmental tasks are associated with other areas of cognitive functioning that are important to the tasks of new learning that will be expected in school.

It is now recognized that children with **dyslexia** (a problem in reading associated with average intelligence, not responding to targeted reading intervention) have a neurobiological defect in a specific component of language development (see Chapter 19). These children, who constitute up to 7% of a school population, have a deficit in their ability to break down the smallest segment of speech in a word. This deficit in phonological awareness can be detected during a pediatric evaluation. Interacting with a child around a book allows assessment of many of these **prereading skills**, such as letter identification, letter-sound association, and word retrieval, may identify children who have a problem with phonological awareness and are at risk for dyslexia. Letter recognition, naming (objects, letters, numbers, and colors), and visual matching (identifying words that begin with the same letter from a list) are among the best predictors of reading readiness. A family history may be helpful here because classic dyslexia and some other types of learning difficulties do run in families.

Bilingual or non–English-speaking families may present special challenges in the assessment of children's language development for a clinician who does not speak the same

TABLE 18.1	**Selected Language Guideposts**			
Skill	**Age 2 Years**	**Age 3 Years**	**Age 4 Years**	**Age 5 Years**
Comprehension	Follows simple commands; identifies body parts; points to common objects	Understands spatial relationships (in, on, and under); knows functions of common objects	Follows two-part commands; understands concepts of same and different	Recalls parts of a story; understands number concepts (3, 4, 5, 6); follows three-part commands
Expression	Labels common objects; uses two- or three-word sentences; uses minimal jargon	Uses three- to four-word sentences; uses regular plurals; uses pronouns (I, me, you); can tell age, sex, and full name	Speaks four- to five-word sentences; can tell story; uses past tense; names one color; can count four objects	Speaks sentences of five words; uses future tense; names four colors; can count 10 or more objects
Speech	Intelligible to strangers 25% of the time	Intelligible to strangers 75% of the time	Normal dysfluency (stuttering)	Dysfluencies resolved

language. The clinician should be wary of ascribing learning and language problems entirely to bilingualism, however. It is often noted that true language delay is present in both English and the heritage language by school age. By age 5, confusion in use of the two languages should be gone, and the child should not have language dysfunction because of bilingualism. If a child's school is attributing their language delay to bilingualism, and therefore denying services, it is important to obtain an outside speech-language assessment (ideally in both languages) to demonstrate the extent of the delay and help advocate for supports.

Attention Problems

At or before the age of 3 to 4 years, a cluster of behaviors that have been associated with a high risk for school learning problems is identifiable; such behavior include a high degree of motoric activity, lack of ability to sustain attention and impulsivity with limited ability to delay gratification. These should be red flags in the preschool history and indicate a need for more vigilance of the child at school entry. The progressive improvement in a child's ability to focus and to differentiate between what is important to a task and what is not is often a key factor in how well the child can master early learning skills in the standard school environment (see Chapter 19). A child of 5 who can sustain attention only when information is given in a certain mode (e.g., a teacher or caregiver sitting next to a child and mentoring the learning process) or when all distractions are eliminated will have difficulty when faced with the complexities of the usual classroom with multiple forms of stimulation and sensory input. Other early signs of attention problems include a child:

- Not remembering or retaining taught material despite seeming to comprehend it at the time of instruction.
- Difficulty with transitions, as if the child's thinking were "stuck" on an activity, resulting in behavioral refusals or outbursts.
- High degree of sensory-seeking or sensory-averse behavior, such as craving hugs, crashing into furniture, stuffing food in their mouth, or being sensitive to food textures.
- Not seeming to understand or remember rules, plan their behavior, or inhibit impulses. Behavior may be described as going "from 0 to 60" very fast, without the child being able to pause and think.

Attention problems are difficult to evaluate in a pediatric office setting, an environment that may lack excessive visual and auditory stimulation. As described below, the clinician can ask about behavior at home, difficulty transitioning or following instructions, large behavioral reactions to frustration, or teacher concerns. ADHD and its management are described in greater detail in Chapter 19.

Socialization and Separation Difficulties

By this age, most children have had experiences leaving the comfort zones of their home environments and interacting with other members of their community; however, social isolation during early childhood became more common during the COVID-19 pandemic, when children spent much more time home with their primary caregivers. While some caregivers felt increased time at home helped to strengthen familial bonds, it also led to increased child tantrums, anxiety, and clinginess when they returned to school. Many families across the United States delayed kindergarten entry in an attempt to ease the transition. Keeping all of these factors in mind, the clinician can obtain information from both the preschool teacher and caregiver about a child's behavior after separating from a caregiver and a child's experiences with new adults and other children in a preschool environment. For some kindergarten children, riding a bus to school is a new experience that may challenge social skills and modify the response to separation.

The relationship between a child and a caregiver is modified by a developmental leap at the time of entering school. Not only is the child learning to successfully negotiate a period of separation from the caregiver, but caregivers themselves must also be able to separate from the child. A child with a shy or timid temperament may be challenged when separated from a caregiver at the start of school, and sometimes this is due to the parent themselves struggling with separation (since shy temperament and anxiety are genetically linked). The caregiver's views on their child's vulnerability and the pattern of child rearing up to this time will have an impact on this process. As in other areas of medicine, a focused history will help the clinician identify problems on which to work and strengths to reinforce.

Assessing a child's social-emotional readiness for kindergarten is one of the main components of a pre-K teacher's evaluation. Teacher perceptions of preparedness are often based on high child cognitive ability and direction following. This may pose challenges for students who have difficulty with emotional and behavioral control, including aggression and low frustration tolerance. These children are more likely to struggle with the development of social skills and externalizing problems; however, early identification and intervention can help prevent continued difficulty in development of emotional behavioral control skills. This can take the form of outpatient therapy (behavioral modification, trauma-informed, or play-based) or school-based positive behavioral intervention.

Children who use elopement (i.e., running out of the classroom, sometimes out of the building) as a form of coping can also face difficulties adjusting to the classroom. If elopement is mentioned by a teacher, it should be further assessed as it can be an indication of autism spectrum disorder or ADHD. Resources are available to help the child adjust to the classroom setting.

When assessing a child's readiness for school, a holistic approach should be used. In predominantly White communities, preschool teachers' written observations, when rated on such characteristics as peer relationships, teacher-pupil relationships, independence, participation in group activities, leadership characteristics, task orientation, attention span and persistence, self-confidence, and immaturity, were found to be relatively good predictors of school achievement and behavior in later elementary school. However, it is important to recognize that when serving communities of color that place less emphasis on individualistic, Western ideals, it may be useful to evaluate self-regulation, initiation/task persistence, and flexible problem solving as individual components of social-emotional readiness skills. Recognizing differences in cultural norms, and the fact that "desired" student behaviors may be defined by Western society, can help to prevent implicit bias and misinterpreting certain behaviors of children of color as "bad."

DURING THE VISIT

The assessment before **kindergarten entry** should include a complete update and review of the child's medical history and the family's medical and social history. Previous childcare or preschool experience should be reviewed. Rocky past experiences may suggest additional considerations.

The examination and formal assessment procedure should include a general physical examination with a growth assessment if one has not recently been completed. It should include a neurological screening and documentation of visual and auditory acuity. Finally, some paper-and-pencil tasks could be informally administered, such as asking the child to draw their family or copy shapes or letters. At this age, the child should be at least moderately comfortable with the examination as long as the caregiver is present, should be able to answer simple, concrete questions with clear and intelligible speech, and should follow requests. The child should be an active part of the assessment process. Early in the interview, questions should be directed to the child with the message, "You are the patient, I am your doctor and your thoughts and responses to questions are important to me." Cultural awareness can be key for the development of this physician-child relationship. For example, if the patient comes from a culture that emphasizes respect for elders, the previous message may be confusing for the patient as speaking directly to the physician may seem in opposition to this principle. Instead, the physician can engage the child through asking for an introduction or incorporating a story-telling motif.

What to Observe

The clinician should observe the child carefully during the interview and examination and during even brief separations from caregivers to make assessments regarding development. Table 18.2 outlines age-appropriate observations of development, temperament, and curiosity.

What to Ask

Table 18.3 presents questions that can be asked during the examination. Questions can be directed to the child, to the caregiver, or to both participants as the clinician engages child and caregiver during the encounter.

Examination and Assessment

Observing and talking with the child during the process of obtaining a careful history will help the child feel "known" and understood by the clinician, as well as provide insight into language and social skills. Careful attention to the child's social responses, language comprehension and expression, body language, attentiveness, eye contact, and motor skills adds to your understanding of the child's individual strengths and challenges. Drawing and/or paper-and-pencil tasks can be accomplished before the physical examination as a way to develop rapport and give the child the message that she will enjoy the office visit.

Tables 18.4 and 18.5 show age-appropriate abilities. Familiarity with these behaviors, drawn from the most popular tests for young children, will assist the pediatrician in the assessment process. Special attention should be paid to children who were born prematurely, exposed prenatally to alcohol or other drugs, or experienced a difficult perinatal course with children who have postnatal risk factors that may affect development (e.g., head trauma, meningitis, physical abuse, emotional abuse, witnessing violence). Family history of learning disabilities or school problems is important to ask about because many learning differences run in families.

Observation of how the child approaches various tasks, including those to facilitate the physical examination, can be revealing:

- Can the child follow auditory directions with no visual clues (e.g., "Take off your shoes, get up on the examination table and sit back")?
- Can these be one-, two-, or three-step directions?
- How attentive to the task is the child (e.g., can the child complete a drawing)?
- How facile is the child with pencil tasks (e.g., holding a pencil with a mature grasp, steady lines that are connected, clear hand dominance)?
- Is the task easy or slow and pressured (e.g., what does the child's face look like while doing the tasks)?

TABLE 18.2   Observations to Be Included in Examination

Observation	Assessment
Is the child quiet and reserved, outgoing, verbal, inquisitive, at ease, or frightened? Does the child initiate questions or comments?	Child's social interaction during the interview and examination. How does the child handle interactions with adults, caregivers, and nonfamily members?
Is the child active, passive, slow to warm? Do they communicate by nonverbal means (e.g., eye contact, gestures) in addition to language?	Child's language and verbal skills (see Appendix and Table 18.1).
Can the child be completely understood? Is language appropriate for the age? Are sentences clear, compound, and complex? Is the articulation clear? Does the child modulate speech well?	Child's language and verbal skills (see Appendix and Table 18.1).
Does the child show excessive dependence or independence? Observe the separation effect(s) if the occasion arises. What does the caregiver allow the child to do?	Caregiver-child interactions.
Can the child follow 1- to 3-step instructions and assist with the examination by holding still, looking at a specific point, cooperating on the neurological examination? Is the child moving around the office constantly and easily distracted by environmental stimuli?	Ability to attend and cooperate.
Does the child show evidence of the ability to solve hypothetical problems, ask questions, and draw interesting pictures?	Curiosity, creativity, problem-solving ability.

TABLE 18.3   Questions to Be Asked During Examination[a]

Question	Objective
Tell me about [child]. What words would you use to describe [child]?	Determine the caregivers' views of the child; what characteristics they mention first. It shows more sensitivity when caregivers describe behavior rather than make judgments about it ("he gets along well with other children").
How does [child] do with friends or classmates? Who in the family is [child] most like? How do you expect [child] to do in school? Why? **To the child:** Do you have friends? What are their names? What do you do with your friends? How are you the same/different than your friends? What are you really good at?	Follow-up of this line of questioning can open up areas of caregiver concern, expectations, and their own experiences with the education system.
Tell me what you know about the school where [child] will be starting?	Reveals how much work caregivers have done in learning about the school, visiting, it, and setting up special education supports if needed. Also reveals any negative perceptions of the school system.
Describe how they use crayons, pencils, and scissors	One child may laboriously use scissors to cut out a doll, whereas another will be engaged in a task, use the scissors, lay them down, and proceed with the next task. Indicates possible fine motor needs.
What do they like to do? Dislike? **To the child:** What do you like to do?	This may help in determining leisure time use, amount of television viewing or video gaming, interest in reading or being read to.

[a]Some questions are for both child and caregivers. They can be used when the clinician is interviewing them together or separately.

TABLE 18.4   Appropriate Abilities at Preschool and Kindergarten Entry Ages

Year	Abilities
3	Picks longer of two lines
	Can point to chin and teeth on request
	Cuts with scissors
	Makes three-cube pyramid in about 15 s
	Copies a circle
	Jumps with both feet together
4	Goes upstairs and downstairs one foot per step
	Copies cross (+)
	Washes hands
	Can tell "how many" when shown two circles
	Completes "A hat goes on your head, shoes on your ..."
5	Dresses self (except tying shoelaces)
	Copies square
	Can count six objects
	Can answer: "Why do we have houses, books, clocks, eyes, ears?"
	Can tell: "What is a chair made of? A dress?"
	Knows (or can be taught): address, phone number, where mother, and father work
	Finger counting (how it is done, pointing to or not) and finger identification
	Digit span—should be able to repeat four digits forward
6	Tells how a crayon and a pencil are the same and different
	Can tell differences between common objects: dog and bird, milk, and water
	Can complete "A lemon is sour, sugar is ..."
	Can tell what a forest is made of

From Hoeckelman R, Blatman S, Brunell PA: *Principles of pediatrics*, New York, 1978, McGraw-Hill.

TABLE 18.5   Neuromotor Abilities in the Years up to Kindergarten Entry

Age (years)	Gross Motor Skills	Fine Motor Skills
2	Runs well	Builds tower of 6 cubes
	Kicks ball	Imitates vertical crayon stroke
	Goes upstairs and downstairs (one step at a time)	Turns book pages singly
3	Goes upstairs (alternating feet)	Copies circle
	Jumps from bottom step	Copies cross (+)
	Pedals tricycle	
	Stands on 1 foot momentarily	
4	Hops on 1 foot	Copies square
	Goes downstairs (alternating feet)	Draws person with 2 to 4 parts
	Stands on 1 foot (5 s)	Uses scissors
	Throws ball overhand	
5	Stands on 1 foot (10 s)	Copies triangle
	May be able to skip	Draws person with body
		Prints some letters

Adapted from Levine MD, Carey WB, Crocker AC: *Developmental and behavioral pediatrics*, ed 3, Philadelphia, 1999, Saunders, p 39.

Children at risk for learning disabilities can and should be identified at school entry. This is especially important because most 5-year-old children with a learning disability have not been recognized at the beginning of kindergarten. A conservative estimate of the prevalence of learning disabilities is 7% of school-age children. Since the most common learning disability is a specific problem in reading (dyslexia), targeted questions and developmental tasks—such as looking at a book together—that assess early reading skills should be a routine part of the examination.

For a child in whom problems with attention or learning are suspected from historical data or observations in the office, administration of caregiver and teacher ADHD Scales (e.g., Vanderbilt scale) is warranted. Because children with ADHD can have sensory processing and motor coordination deficits, it can be helpful to evaluate motor tasks (e.g., standing on one foot for 5–10 seconds, hopping on one foot, climbing up onto an exam table, throwing a ball) and visual-perceptual tasks (e.g., drawing a person with at least six to eight body parts and copying standard geometrical shapes). If a child struggles with fine motor or gross motor coordination, a referral to outpatient occupational therapy should be considered.

Many healthcare providers find it valuable to ask a 5-year-old: "Draw a picture of your family doing something". The neuromaturational skills (e.g., visual-motor integration and fine motor coordination) and psychosocial characteristics of the child and family are revealed in often remarkable and surprising ways in these drawings. Clinical interpretation of the drawing should be cautious, however. The drawings also provide an opportunity to enhance the content and quality of communication with children and caregivers (see Chapter 4 for how to use family drawings in pediatric practice).

No child should enter school without the benefit of formal vision and hearing acuity tests. Many schools have such screening programs in place as well.

STANDARDIZED EVALUATIONS FOR SCHOOL READINESS

Although school readiness tests are routinely offered by school districts in the United States before preschool or kindergarten placement, not all families will have opted into these assessments—which can proactively identify children struggling in certain preacademic areas. This testing, sometimes performed as what is called a "Child Find" assessment, is generally used to help guide classroom instruction in children who may have an unidentified learning disability, but this information is not used to delay school entry. A distinction must be made between tests of academic readiness, which evaluate the child's ability to perform basic learning skills, and developmental screening tests, which attempt to evaluate a child's level of gross motor, fine motor, language and personal-social development in comparison to the performance of age-mates.

To complement school assessments, an important role for the pediatric provider to play is screening for behavioral and emotional challenges at school entry. The AAP has developed a Screening Technical Assistance Resource center for developmental screening tools that can be used by clinicians who wish to do a brief assessment themselves, such as the Pediatric Symptom Checklist (12–18 items, takes less than 3 minutes for parents to complete, see Appendix).

ANTICIPATORY GUIDANCE

The 5-year-old visit is an opportunity to help the caregiver reflect on the child's strengths, challenges, and curiosities that will shape their experience in Young 5's or Kindergarten. It is an opportunity to support caregivers in advocating for their child's unique needs, communicating with educational teams, and responding to developmental or behavioral challenges with patience and autonomy support (see Chapter 17). At the same time, it is important to clearly identify areas of concern that warrant therapy or school evaluation. Caregivers can respond with considerable guilt when their child experiences challenges in school, so clear and pragmatic communication is crucial, emphasizing that earlier intervention will help improve the child's long-term outlook in school. It is helpful to let caregivers know that children who struggle one year may thrive the next, and vice versa, all depending on how well the child is matched with teachers and peers, supports available, and how well the child feels included and understood in the school setting.

Pediatric clinicians in these situations can be optimistic and encourage the caregivers to be regularly involved in visits at school open houses, parent-teacher conferences, and by email/electronic communication—as well as listening to the child's descriptions of the school experience. Ongoing monitoring of each child's progress and fit with the school is indicated. Clinicians can advise and encourage interest in increased child school involvement, such as joining sports teams, clubs, or other community activities—and encourage a healthy relationship with digital media (Box 18.3) so that this doesn't displace sleep, homework, or play time.

Ideally, caregivers come to see their child's pediatric provider as a trusted source of advice and help regarding school issues. Discussing school progress early and regularly sets the stage for ongoing monitoring of family and school behavior and achievement. In this way, the clinician can be alert to early signs of a lack of fit between what the child brings to the situation and what the caregivers and school expect. The physician can assist the caregiver in responding if the school has concerns for their child or management for disciplinary action or outbursts. In addition, the clinician can share in the joy and excitement of a young school-age child's successful social and intellectual growth.

BOX 18.3 Supporting Healthy Digital Media Use at School Entry

Although conversations about digital media use should start in infancy, school entry is an important time to devote extra time to discussing healthy, balanced usage patterns. At age 5, some children have daily media routines that are predictable and follow the American Academy of Pediatrics (AAP) guidelines—consuming an hour or less per day, using age-appropriate programs and movies, with predictable access to devices such as iPads and handheld gaming devices. Other children spend several hours per day with media, have less oversight from their caregivers, and therefore start to use more mature or age-inappropriate games or videos. Children from lower income households and minoritized racial/ethnic groups are more likely to fall into the latter pattern, but heavy or inappropriate media use patterns occur across the socioeconomic spectrum, as media become more mobile, ubiquitous, and have designs such as autoplay and gamification that encourage prolonged use. Household factors such as number of caregivers, those needing to work multiple jobs at various hours of the day, lack of access to reliable childcare or after-school programs, and high caregiver stress also reduce families' capacity to create boundaries around media use. Therefore guidance should be tailored to the family's unique situation, what they feel is feasible, and aligned with caregiver goals (e.g., improved behavior, sleep, or learning). Some families seek guidance about ways to reduce arguments about media and devices, while others may not see it as a problem, since it keeps their child occupied. Therefore starting with general questions such as "do you have a plan for media and device use in your home?" and asking about sleep, mealtime, and play routines will give you an idea of how much media is involved. When giving guidance about physical activity, diet, shared book reading, or other health-promoting behaviors, it can become apparent that heavy media use is a barrier—this also presents an opportunity to provide strengths-based guidance. Avoid only talking about "screen time rules," since families have reported this induces a sense of guilt or obligation rather than agency. Rather, involve the caregiver in problem solving about (1) where media time could be reduced to make space for other activities the family enjoys, (2) which content (e.g., violent video games) could be shifted to more age-appropriate, and/or (3) finding other ways to help the child calm down, pay attention, or get to sleep.

- Specific points of guidance include:
- Encourage the family to make a media plan, including when, where, and how they want to use media, what times of day or spaces they want to be screen-free, and what types of shows, games, or movies are off limits. A guide is available at www.healthychildren.org/mediaplan
- If children use video games, this is an important age for preventing problematic or excessive use. Encourage families to have predictable times of day that their child can play games, not let it take up the whole afternoon or weekend, and avoid violent games. It is important for children to establish other activities that they enjoy and feel mastery over, such as sports, nondigital games, music, or art.
- Encourage caregivers to use media together with children, talk about what they see on the screen, and monitor the types of apps or games the child is playing. This is especially important if the child has their own tablet/iPad or watches YouTube, since app stores and video-sharing apps like YouTube can introduce children to age-inappropriate content with violence, hypercommercialism, or rude behavior.
- Have settings on child devices (e.g., Google Family Link, Apple Family Sharing) to restrict downloads and purchases and that allow caregivers to set time limits and filter inappropriate content.
- Discuss the activities that families enjoy doing together, such as cooking, playing board games, or playing with pets and encourage putting devices away so the time is undistracted.
- Talk about why media is hard to disengage from, because it has features like autoplay and recommendation feeds—so that caregivers do not feel as frustrated or guilty that setting limits is challenging.
- Advise families that the most educational activities are book reading and playing things like puzzles and games. Apps and video games marketed as "educational" usually have low quality, unless they are from trusted creators like PBS KIDS or Khan Academy.
- Young children may be curious about social media—especially platforms with funny videos, but these apps show lots of age-inappropriate content. Social media should be avoided and close caregiver supervision should be provided in times of use.
- If children rely on screens to fall asleep, recommend audiobooks or child-friendly meditation audiorecordings instead.
- If families are worried their child will react behaviorally when they start to set limits, provide ideas for positive behavioral supports (see Chapters 14 and 16) so caregivers do not give up when trying to implement new media plans.

⚠ HEADS UP—5 YEARS

- "Immature" is not a pediatric diagnosis. It is a sign that the child has been labeled and requires further evaluation. Many children with ADHD start to declare themselves in prekindergarten and kindergarten, a time when classroom accommodations can be effective in teaching self-regulation skills.
- Assess past separation experiences (preschool and childcare) and temperament to recognize a child who is especially shy and slow to warm up. Use the opportunity to guide caregivers in ways to modify the transition to kindergarten.

TEST	FUNCTION
Ask the child to tell you about a movie or video seen recently	Oral expression, memory, sequencing
Read the child a paragraph, followed by a few questions	Auditory processing and oral expression
Ask the child to copy a square and a triangle; to draw a person or the child's family	Fine motor and visual-spatial skills
Ask the child to tell you about the picture	Oral expression and affect
Ask the child to repeat a series of random and sequencing numbers (age minus one)	Short-term memory
Ask the child to complete a four- to five-step task in the order given	Auditory processing and motor skills
Ask the child to make up a sentence from three to four words	Expressive fluency and imagination

- The school entry visit is an optimal time to screen for developmental disabilities—visual impairment (refractive error and strabismus), hearing loss, mild cerebral palsy, language or speech delay, dyslexia, and visual-spatial dysfunction.
- A child who is a year or more delayed in motor milestones should be assessed for previously unrecognized cerebral palsy (e.g., cannot skip, delayed in figure drawing, difficulty holding a pencil or crayon) or developmental coordination disorder. A neurological exam will help inform need for subspecialty and therapy referrals.
- Assess the mental health of the child and family—evidence of depression, anxiety, and oppositional behavior.

ACKNOWLEDGMENT

Dr. Philip Nader contributed to this chapter in previous editions.

RECOMMENDED READINGS

For Children and Caregivers

Berenstein S. *Berenstein bears go to school.* New York: Random House; 1978.

Berenstein S. *Berenstein bears trouble at school.* New York: Random House; 1987.

Zeifert H. *Harry gets ready for school.* New York: Puffin Books; 1991.

Bertin M. *Mindful Parenting for ADHD: a Guide to Cultivating Calm, Reducing Stress, and Helping Children Thrive (a New Harbinger Self-Help Workbook).*

Services for Children With Disabilities: *Information about early childhood/kindergarten services.* Childcare.gov

Understanding the Child Find program: what is child find? understood.org)

NEA Center for Social Justice. 10 Principles for Talking About Race in School. National Education Association. Nov. 2020. https://www.nea.org/professional-excellence/student-engagement/tools-tips/10-principles-talking-about-race-school

For Professionals

Williams PG, Lerner MA, Sells J, Alderman SL, Hashikawa A, Mendelsohn A, McFadden T, Navsaria D, Peacock G, Scholer S, Takagishi J. School readiness. *Pediatrics.* 2019;144(2).

Scharf RJ. School readiness. *Pediatr Rev.* 2016;37(11):501–503.

Ricciardi C, Manfra L, Hartman S, Bleiker C, Dineheart L, Winsler A. School readiness skills at age four predict academic achievement through 5th grade. *Early Childhood Res Q.* 2021;57:110–120.

Anderson AT, Jackson A, Jones L, Kennedy DP, Wells K, Chung PJ. Minority parents' perspectives on racial socialization and school readiness in the early childhood period. *Acad Pediatr.* 2015;15(4):405–411.

Shaw DS, Mendelsohn AL, Morris PA. Reducing poverty-related disparities in child development and school readiness: the Smart Beginnings tiered prevention strategy that combines pediatric primary care with home visiting. *Clin Child Fam Psychol Rev.* 2021:1–5.

Accommodations to help students with ADD and ADHD. www.understood.org.

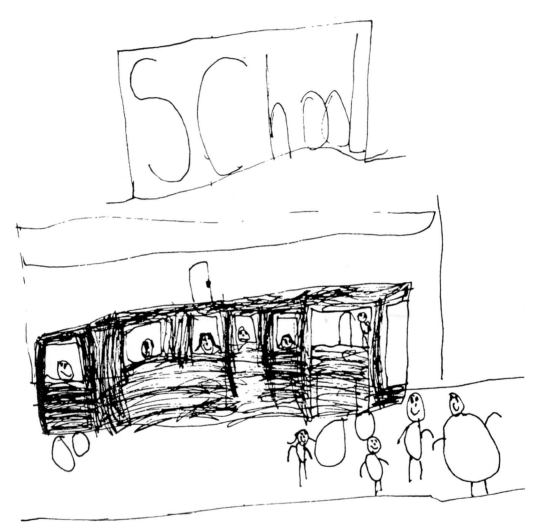

"A girl and a boy get on the bus. Their parents are watching."

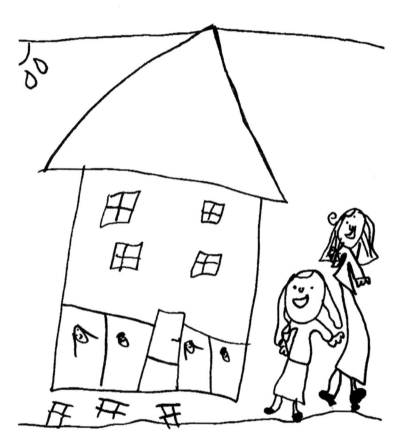

Siena and her teacher at school. This 6-year-old shows herself proudly standing next to her teacher; these personal relationship are vital at this age.

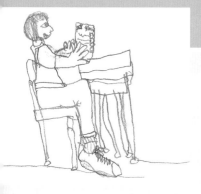

19

Six to Seven Years: Reading, Relationships, and Playing by the Rules

Jenny S. Radesky

The first grade is a time of cognitive challenge coupled with the requirement for sustained attention for learning. Educational strengths and weakness start to emerge during this time. It is an opportunity for pediatricians to provide early recognition of problems with attention and specific learning disabilities and help families navigate the educational system.

KEYWORDS

- Cognitive changes
- Concrete operations
- Attention and learning
- Executive functions
- Learning disabilities
- School refusal
- Special education
- Separation anxiety

A 6-year-old child stands on a threshold of exciting new cognitive and social capabilities. Compared to kindergarten experiences that include more play-based approaches, entry into first grade creates new challenges for many children. It is the first time they are expected to sit and attend to classwork, follow a schedule determined by their teacher, and delay gratification until recess and the end of the day. For all children, this provides an opportunity for rapid cognitive, social, and emotional growth.

For the pediatric clinician, this is an important window for helping caregivers monitor their child's adjustment to more structured classroom environments, including reading and math skills, friendship development, and response to nonpreferred demands that frequently occur in school. At the same time, it is an opportunity to support parents in being strong communicators with their child's educational team, advocates for the child's progress, and problem solvers when challenges arise. Parents can feel embarrassed and demoralized when they receive negative reports home from school, and pediatric clinicians can help demystify what a child might be struggling with and how to provide targeted help.

DEVELOPMENTAL CONCEPTS IMPORTANT AT THIS AGE

Educational Opportunity and Inequities

Before we cover children's cognitive development at the early grade-school ages, it is important to contextualize these experiences within the larger structures that shape children's school outcomes. A child with significant impairment from developmental delays, autism, or learning problems may make excellent progress in a well-funded school district with specially trained teachers. Conversely, a child with mild attention deficits may struggle and wind up several grade levels behind their peers in an underfunded school with high teacher turnover and stress, and low special education support, staffing shortages, or harsh disciplinary practices. A school's climate, funding, and personnel are factors that influence the larger concept of **educational opportunity**, which includes:

- Rigorous academics (e.g., offering advanced math and Advanced Placement courses).
- Effective teaching (e.g., low turnover, high number of teachers with 2+ years of experience).

Previous edition chapter by Martin T. Stein.

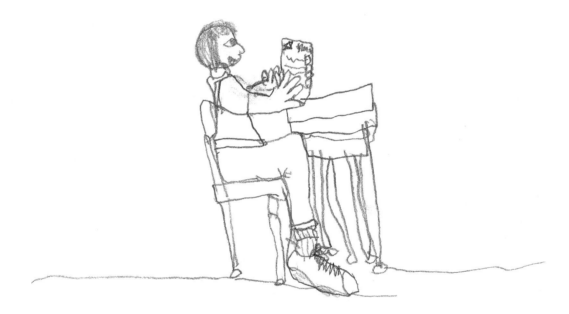

A girl shows her interest in reading and her considerable skill in drawing in this self-portrait. By a girl, age 8.

- Supportive conditions for learning (e.g., low rate of out-of-school suspensions, low chronic absenteeism).
- Nonacademic supports (e.g., low ratio of number of students for each school nurse, counselor, psychologist, or social worker).

A child's educational opportunity correlates with their life expectancy—likely through multiple mechanisms such as having strong relationships with teachers and trusted adults, better curriculum, educational support leading to higher high school graduation rates and college readiness, and higher lifetime earning potential. Educational opportunity metrics are consistently higher in zip codes where there is a higher proportion of higher-income White families, with a major contributor to these disparities being historical redlining that kept Black families and other families of minority race/ethnicity in underresourced and segregated neighborhoods in the United States. Educational opportunity is a structural determinant of health that clinicians should be aware of and address through advocacy for better funding and support for struggling school districts.

Such structural inequities in educational opportunity were brought to light during the COVID-19 pandemic. Over 55 million US school children were impacted by school closures in Spring 2020, during which time studies documented increasing rates of child depression, anxiety, disruptive behavior, sleep problems, and parent stress and depression while families adjusted to lockdowns and social isolation. When some schools reopened for in-person learning the following school year, data from the Centers for Disease Control and Prevention showed that non-Hispanic White children were more likely to have access to full-time, in-person school (75%) compared to non-Hispanic Black (63%) or Hispanic (59%) students. Several studies showed that children receiving in-person schooling had better academic readiness and fewer behavior problems than children in remote or hybrid school environments. Years into the pandemic, math and reading scores were estimated to be significantly more behind in Black, Hispanic, poor, and city-dwelling children. Thus identifying and remediating learning delays—and coaching families on educational advocacy—is especially important in current pediatric practice.

Brain and Cognitive Development at Ages 6 to 7

The accelerated physical growth of preschoolers begins to slow as children enter the years of middle childhood. By the age of 5 years, the brain has attained approximately 90% of its adult weight and size, and over the next 2 years, final myelinization of the central nervous system will be completed. Brain maturation, however, continues through the school-age period as new neuronal connections (synaptogenesis)

are formed. This process coincides with qualitative advances in cognitive capacities. Simultaneously, the child may participate in activities requiring the integration of fine and gross motor skills, such as dance, sports, and, in the classroom, handwriting and arts and crafts projects.

A 6-year-old begins to show less magical thinking and more concrete thinking, meaning that reasoning and understanding are tied to actual situations and objects. Six- and seven-year-old children focus on concrete aspects of the world, while hypothetical reasoning and abstract thought will have to await adolescence or later to emerge (see Chapters 21 and 22). Concrete explanations are unifaceted, sometimes literal, and do not take into account complex interactions between variables. Instead, they may adopt a single, simple explanation and continue to focus on one aspect of a situation; for example, a 6-year-old might think that as long as they stay out of their bedroom, it will not be bedtime. Likewise, a child may be able to make their way from home to school with great accuracy but may be unable to mentally reverse the directions to appropriately plan the trip home. (It is important to note that these cognitive changes have been documented in neurotypical children, while neurodiverse children may develop at a different pace or show precocious skills in some areas. For example, some children with autism spectrum disorder have remarkable ways of remembering driving routes but may get frustrated when their caregivers take a new route home.)

Piaget conducted tests with children to understand their judgments and thinking. These included playing with everyday objects such as clay to see how children understand visual-spatial concepts such as mass. When children could reason that the different shapes formed from a piece of clay split in half had the same amount of clay, Piaget said they showed "conversation of mass." As typically developing children age, they can reason about conservation of length and volume as well. While these Piagetian stages only capture part of how children develop visual-spatial reasoning (which is important for math success), they help us understand how children are increasingly logical and internalize rules about the world.

These abilities translate into the typical academic tasks presented to children in early elementary school. Children can now perform mental operations related to concrete objects (e.g., adding or subtracting objects, creating maps), understand serial relationships (e.g., ordering pictures or events, identifying patterns, number concepts), and identify similarities and categories. Children with cognitive delays will struggle with mastering these concepts in first and second grades.

Learning to read develops at varying times between ages 5 and 7 years and is a main component of any early elementary curriculum. Children with a history of language delays and attention problems are often on the later end of this spectrum and often need reading intervention in school (see later). Children who are even modestly delayed in the development of reading abilities may become stressed or feel negative about themselves, so understanding reading intervention systems in schools is important for pediatric clinicians.

The games that children play at 6 and 7 years old start to change as well. Children are now able to play simple board games, make up playground games with teams, or carry out more complex activities, such as having a lemonade stand. Magical thinking remains active at this age, so imaginative games and role playing remain some children's favorite ways to play. All games are an opportunity for children to release stress, express emotions, feel mastery, or practice tolerating frustration. Persistent magical thinking is also evidenced by the inaccurate conclusions some 6- to 7-year-olds may draw; they may feel sorry for a car that is heavily loaded with passengers as if the car had feelings. Similarly, they may interact with robot toys or virtual assistants like *Alexa* or *Siri* as if they were alive.

SCHOOL-RELATED CHALLENGES

Problems With Sustained Attention and Learning

First grade requires children to sustain their attention for periods of 20 to 40 minutes at a time, shift between activities, and persist in learning even when it feels challenging. While many children adapt to these demands, children with attention-deficit/hyperactivity disorder (ADHD) often struggle in first or second grade, even if their ADHD was previously diagnosed and managed with classroom accommodations. Approximately 7% of children have ADHD globally, although estimates are higher (up to 15%) in some community samples. Children with ADHD have weaknesses in one or several **executive functions** (EFs), the higher order cognitive processes that have been colloquially called the "air traffic controller of the brain."

- These functions include the following:
- Planning and reflection.
- Vigilance and processing of salient information while filtering out unimportant information.
- Inhibition of impulses or responses to distraction.
- Initiation of new activities by activating attention and sustaining that mental effort.
- Switching mentally between two or more different tasks.
- Working memory, which involves holding information in mind while working on new, incoming information.
- An ongoing monitoring capability to detect errors and make corrections.

Weaknesses in EF occur in many neurodevelopmental conditions but are a core feature of ADHD. They need to be addressed through medication, skill building, parenting

supports, and school accommodations to help children function well within increasingly demanding academic environments.

ADHD—whether inattentive subtype, hyperactive/impulsive subtype, or combined subtype—is often brought to light by a concerned caregiver or teacher. Children with a more surgent, intense, and impulsive temperament are at higher risk of developing ADHD, as are children born prematurely, with intrauterine alcohol or substance exposure, or with a family history of ADHD. Alternatively, the presenting complaint in a young child with ADHD might be problems falling or staying asleep; aggression at home or school; or eloping or disruptive behavior in school when demands are placed on the child. Children with more inattentive symptoms may come to clinical attention when they are having trouble retaining taught information, such as remembering sight words or math facts. Finally, children with autism spectrum disorder may have co-occurring ADHD that impedes their ability to focus on therapies or academic tasks.

Sometimes these symptoms are apparent in the office setting, such as an impulsive child who wants to grab all of the blood pressure cuffs or otoscope specula, but clinical observations are not sufficient for an ADHD diagnosis. Children may be dysregulated or sensory-seeking in office settings due to anxiety or may be calm because they are watching videos on a smartphone. Therefore the American Academy of Pediatrics' evidence-based guidelines for primary care clinicians in the evaluation and diagnosis of a child with ADHD (Wolraich et al., 2019) include the following specific recommendations:

1. The pediatrician or other primary care clinician should initiate an evaluation for ADHD for any child or adolescent age 4 years to the 18th birthday who presents with academic or behavioral problems and symptoms of inattention, hyperactivity, or impulsivity. Core symptoms are listed in Box 19.1. The following general screening questions are useful:
   - How is your child doing in school?
   - Are there any problems with learning that you or the teacher have seen?
   - Does your child like going to school?
   - Are you concerned with any behavioral problems in school, at home, or when your child is playing with friends?
   - Does their teacher have any concerns about completing classwork? Does your child seem to understand their homework, or have any problems completing it?

2. To make a diagnosis of ADHD, the clinician should determine that *DSM-5* (Diagnostic and Statistical Manual of Mental Disorders, Fifth Edition) criteria (Box 19.1) have been met, including documentation of symptoms and

BOX 19.1 DSM-5 Diagnostic Criteria for Attention-Deficit/Hyperactivity Disorder

Categories of ADHD

- **Attention-Deficit/Hyperactivity Disorder, Combined Type:** This subtype should be used if six (or more) symptoms of inattention and six (or more) symptoms of hyperactivity-impulsivity have persisted for at least 6 months. Most children and adolescents with the disorder have the combined type.
- **Attention-Deficit/Hyperactivity Disorder, Predominantly Inattentive Type:** This subtype should be used if six (or more) symptoms of inattention (but fewer than six symptoms of hyperactivity-impulsivity) have persisted for at least 6 months.
- **Attention-Deficit/Hyperactivity Disorder, Predominantly Hyperactive-Impulsive Type:** This subtype should be used if six (or more) symptoms of hyperactivity-impulsivity (but fewer than six symptoms of inattention) have persisted for at least 6 months. Inattention may often still be a significant clinical feature in such cases.

Inattention

- Often fails to give close attention to details or makes careless mistakes in schoolwork, at work, or during other activities (e.g., overlooks or misses details, work is inaccurate).
- Often has difficulty sustaining attention in tasks or play activities (e.g., has difficulty remaining focused during lectures, conversations, or lengthy reading).
- Often does not seem to listen when spoken to directly (e.g., mind seems elsewhere, even in the absence of any obvious distraction).
- Often does not follow through on instructions and fails to finish schoolwork, chores, or duties in the workplace (e.g., starts tasks but quickly loses focus and is easily sidetracked).
- Often has difficulty organizing tasks and activities (e.g., difficulty managing sequential tasks; difficulty keeping materials and belongings in order; messy, disorganized work; poor time management; fails to meet deadlines).
- Often avoids, dislikes, or is reluctant to engage in tasks that require sustained mental effort (e.g., schoolwork or homework; for older adolescents and adults, preparing reports, completing forms, reviewing lengthy papers).
- Often loses things necessary for tasks or activities (e.g., school materials, pencils, books, tools, wallets, keys, paperwork, eyeglasses, mobile telephones).
- Is often easily distracted by extraneous stimuli (for older adolescents and adults, this may include unrelated thoughts).
- Is often forgetful in daily activities (e.g., doing chores, running errands; for older adolescents and adults, returning calls, paying bills, keeping appointments).

Hyperactivity

- Often fidgets with or taps hands or feet or squirms in the seat.
- Often leaves seat in situations when remaining seated is expected (e.g., leaves his or her place in the classroom, in the office or other workplace, or in other situations that require remaining in place).
- Often runs about or climbs in situations where it is inappropriate (note: in adolescents or adults, it may be limited to feeling restless).
- Often unable to play or take part in leisure activities quietly.
- Is often "on the go" acting as if "driven by a motor" (e.g., is unable to be or uncomfortable being still for extended time, as in restaurants, meetings; may be experienced by others as being restless or difficult to keep up with).
- Often talks excessively.

Impulsivity

- Often blurts out an answer before a question has been completed (e.g., completes people's sentences; cannot wait for a turn in conversation).
- Often has trouble waiting his/her turn (e.g., while waiting in line).
- Often interrupts or intrudes on others (e.g., butts into conversations, games, or activities; may start using other people's things without asking or receiving permission; for adolescents and adults, may intrude into or take over what others are doing).
- Several inattentive or hyperactive-impulsive symptoms were present **before the age of 12 years**.
- Several inattentive or hyperactive-impulsive symptoms are present in **two or more settings** (e.g., at home, school, or work; with friends or relatives; in other activities).
- There is clear evidence that the **symptoms interfere with, or reduce the quality of, social, school, or work functioning**.

DSM-5, Diagnostic and Statistical Manual of Mental Disorders, Fifth Edition.
From American Psychiatric Association: *Diagnostic and statistical manual of mental disorders*, ed 5, Washington, 2013, American Psychiatric Association.

impairment in more than one major setting (i.e., social, academic, or occupational), with information obtained primarily from reports from parents or guardians, teachers, other school personnel, and mental health clinicians who are involved in the child or adolescent's care. The clinician should also rule out any alternative cause.

3. In the evaluation of a child or adolescent for ADHD, the clinician should include a process to at least screen for comorbid conditions, including emotional or behavioral conditions (e.g., anxiety, depression, oppositional defiant disorder, conduct disorders, posttraumatic stress disorder, substance use), developmental conditions (e.g., learning and language disorders, autism spectrum disorders), and physical conditions (e.g., tics, sleep apnea).

4. ADHD is a chronic condition; therefore the clinician should manage children and adolescents with ADHD in the same manner that they would treat children and youth with special health care needs, following the principles of the chronic care model and the medical home.

Other diagnostic tests are not routinely indicated to establish the diagnosis of ADHD. Current evidence does not support the routine use of other diagnostic tests, including blood lead, thyroid hormone levels, brain imaging studies, or electroencephalography.

It is important that parents and teachers understand that this diagnosis is largely descriptive of the child's behavior and does not reveal the etiology of the problem or predict an individual child's prognosis. Caregivers may be worried about the child being "labeled" or "put in a box" when they receive a diagnosis like ADHD, and many parents have questions and concerns about trying medication. However, evidence shows that children whose ADHD is adequately treated with behavioral supports, educational accommodations, and psychopharmaceutical intervention have lower risk of school and disciplinary problems. In fact, rates of substance use disorder and other risky behaviors in adolescence are lower when ADHD is adequately treated. Caregivers should be provided this information when discussing treatment approaches, to help them understand the longer term benefits of addressing ADHD symptoms and helping children learn the "lagging skills" that do not come easily to them (see Chapter 20).

To assist pediatric clinicians in the process of recognition, evaluation, and management of ADHD in an office practice, the American Academy of Pediatrics has developed toolkit and process of care algorithm that helps implement the steps above. Publications and websites for parents are listed at the end of this chapter.

Setting Intervention Goals

Treatment begins with providing parents and the child with information about the condition—the biological basis for ADHD and the effects of the school, home, and community environments. The clinician can help by guiding the parents in their work with the child's school, ensuring coordination of health and other services, and helping families set specific goals.

Initially, identifying three to six target outcomes (improvement in symptoms associated with ADHD), agreed on by the parents, child, and teacher, can be of enormous help after the diagnosis of ADHD in a child. Target outcomes bring precision to the setting of treatment goals with the parents and child and direct the follow-up process. Examples of target outcomes include improving academic performance (e.g., completing homework, retaining information, improvement in reading scores, needing less adult support to initiate and complete work), decreasing disruptive behavior (e.g., less elopement from the classroom; fewer incidents of aggression or destruction of property; less blurting out or chatting with peers during lessons), following instructions and daily routines more easily (e.g., getting out of the house for school; fewer arguments about bedtime or video games), improving self-esteem, and enhanced safety, such as in crossing streets or riding bicycles. The goals should be realistic, attainable, and measurable. It can help to write them in an after-visit summary and the encounter note so that caregivers, child, and clinician are on the same page about what the goals are.

Treatment of Attention-Deficit/Hyperactivity Disorder

It helps families to understand that treating ADHD is not just about "fixing" the child's behavior; it also involves modifying the home and school environments to help set the child up for success. At the point that ADHD is diagnosed, many caregivers feel exhausted and blame themselves for the child's struggles; therefore an empathic approach that builds on the families' strengths and love for the child—rather than pathologizing the behavior—will help build a therapeutic rapport. ADHD treatment includes behavioral intervention or psychoeducation aimed at improving the quality and effectiveness of caregiver-child interactions and household routines, as well as changes to the classroom environment and instructional approaches so that the child can better engage with social and academic tasks.

In younger children with ADHD (4–6 years), the American Academy of Pediatrics recommends evidence-based behavioral modification therapy and classroom accommodations as a first line of treatment. Evidence-based behavioral modification therapies (see Chapter 17) include Triple P and Incredible Years among others. These approaches all include praising/reinforcing positive behavior, ignoring or providing natural consequences (not harsh reactions) for negative behaviors, having clear limits and predictable structure to the day, and "special time" in which the caregiver plays with the child and follows their lead (see Chapter 17 for more detail). Parent-child interaction therapy is also effective for children with oppositional and defiant symptoms. Because access to behavioral therapy may be limited due to insurance coverage or geography, it is important for pediatric clinicians to know the local mental health agencies that may provide in-clinic or in-home behavioral therapy. Directing families to online written and video resources can be a helpful supplement to therapy (see Recommended Readings) but usually is not sufficient alone. When there has been trauma exposure, a trauma-focused therapy approach is important to help reduce child dysregulation and help caregivers understand the motivations and emotional states underlying their child's behavior.

In school, positive behavior modification strategies and classroom accommodations in the classroom will diminish many target behaviors. These include rewarding desired behaviors (e.g., staying in seat, completing an assignment, transitioning back from recess without difficulty) and having consistent responses to negative behaviors that help the child deescalate and learn alternate approaches. Practical accommodations that help a child with ADHD include things like preferential seating near the teacher or model peers, break to move their body, fidget objects, visual instructions, reteaching or "chunking" of material, assignments in written form, smaller volumes of work, and assistance in organization of classwork and homework (see Table 19.1).

Trauma-informed behavioral approaches are being increasingly practiced in schools, with the growing recognition of how traumatic and adverse experiences shape children's attention and behavior. Rather than punishment, trauma-informed approaches to school accommodations include a "rest and return" approach in which the child can take a break, "reset" their mindset and calm down, and rejoin the class activity. In essence, the goal is to change the adult response to children's difficult behavior from "What's wrong with you?" to "What happened to you?" or "how is life for you?" It is therapeutic for children with trauma and insecure attachment to realize that they can recover and repair after a challenging behavior—rather than be sent home from school, which sends the message that children's emotions and behaviors are "too much" for the school to handle. (School suspensions are discussed in more detail in Chapter 24.)

TABLE 19.1   Effective Behavioral Techniques for Children With Attention-Deficit/Hyperactivity Disorder

Technique	Description	Example
Delivering effective instructions	Adult gives instructions that are chunked for easier comprehension, provided in visual format, or delivered with other accommodation	Child is provided a personal visual schedule for the day, a 5-min transition timer, or teacher checks for student comprehension before moving on
Positive reinforcement	Providing rewards or privileges in response to desired behavior	Child completes an assignment and is permitted to go do a preferred activity
Reset/Rest and return	Taking a break from an activity that is contributing to dysregulation	Instead of being disciplined, a child is prompted to go to a designated calm-down area, which may have calming activities such as sensory tools, books, etc.
Natural consequences	Withdrawing rewards or privileges related to unwanted behavior	After disruptive episode, child may help clean up before going to recess
Token economy	Combining reward and consequence. The child earns rewards and privileges when performing desired behavior.	Child earns stars for completing assignments. Child cashes in the sum of her stars at the end of the week for a prize.
Trauma-informed social emotional learning practices	1. Create predictable routines 2. Build strong and supportive relationships 3. Empower students' agency 4. Support the development of self-regulation skills 5. Provide opportunities to explore individual and community identities	

Adapted from Reiff MI: *ADHD: a complete and authoritative guide.* Elk Grove Village, 2004, American Academy of Pediatrics, p 140. and Transforming Education (www.transformingeducation.org)

The use of medication improves inattentiveness, hyperactivity, and impulsivity in 70% to 80% of school-age children who have this disorder, often making them more ready to learn. Medication will not improve academic achievement directly but over time will allow children with ADHD to retain taught material and complete assignments. Hundreds of randomized controlled clinical trials of school-age children with ADHD support the benefit of stimulant medications (methylphenidate and amphetamine; their enantiomers dexmethylphenidate and lisdexamphetamine which have fewer side effects). In addition, nonstimulant medications such as guanfacine/clonidine (alpha-agonist class) and atomoxetine (selective norepinephrine reuptake inhibitor class) may be useful for treatment of ADHD behavior. Not only are documented benefits seen in core ADHD symptoms, but in many cases, medication also improves a child's ability to follow rules, improves relationships with peers and parents, and decreases oppositional behavior and anxiety. Children with autism or trauma may have less medication efficacy, more side effects, and need to trial several different medications before finding a good match.

The evaluation and management of children with chronic inattention involves ongoing contact with the school, as well as referral to educational and mental health specialists when indicated. Ongoing communication between caregivers and teachers is needed to monitor medication efficacy. This is often harder for families with low English proficiency, busy work schedules involving multiple jobs, financial strain, or those with low social support. Pediatric clinicians might therefore partner with clinical social workers, care coordinators, or educational advocates in the community to help provide wrap-around care. It is important for pediatric clinicians to understand the basics of school supports for ADHD (from 504 plans to Individualized Educational Programs [IEPs]—see Box 19.2) to demystify this process for families.

Learning Disabilities

A learning disability refers to a consistent difficulty in learning basic academic skills related to the acquisition and use of listening, speaking, reading, writing, reasoning, or mathematical abilities. ADHD and problems with social interactions may coexist with a learning disability, but they are considered separate conditions. Learning disabilities are neurologically based, a reflection of the "hard-wiring" network of the central nervous system. They are seen in approximately 5% to 10% of school-age children with a wide variation in aptitudes—from children with average intelligence to those with superior intellectual abilities. A learning disability is often suspected when the difference between aptitude (intelligence) and achievement (learning output) on standardized tests is wide—usually more than 15 to 20 points. School systems rely on the measurement of this discrepancy to determine which children require special services and adaptations. Most learning disabilities do not come to the attention of parents, educators, or clinicians until a child is challenged with cognitive work that requires the acquisition and use of reading, spelling, or math skills.

A clinically useful perspective on learning disabilities derives from the recognition that we learn either by visual or by auditory input of information. Assuming that a child has adequate visual acuity and hearing capacity, most learning disabilities can be conceptualized as a developmental variation in the sensory/perceptual-cognitive processing pathways of the brain that follow the sensory input. Visual-dependent learning problems may cause a delay in learning to read and manipulate numbers. Recognition and comprehension of the symbolic language represented by words or numbers are altered in a manner that may affect the development of reading skills (dyslexia) or mathematical abilities (dyscalculia). Children with auditory-dependent learning problems find it difficult to comprehend spoken language when presented with new information. These disabilities are associated with either a visual or an auditory processing disorder that may have a significant impact on the quality and quantity of learning.

Dyslexia, the most common learning disability, is a specific language-based learning disability that affects reading, spelling, and written expression. The major neuropsychological deficit is in phonological processing skills. This means difficulty learning the alphabet, lack of alphabet mastery, problems with letter-sound associations, and difficulty acquiring decoding skills and sight word vocabulary for reading. Intelligence is within the average range. Children with dyslexia often come to attention between ages 6 and 8 when they are struggling to learn to read and spell. Public schools use a system often called "Response to Intervention" or "Title I supports" to provide tiered supports for children struggling to read. This starts with small-group reading instruction a few times per week and increases in intensity to one-to-one daily reading instruction if the student is not showing progress with lighter tiers of intervention. Standardized reading scores should be collected by the teacher regularly. This allows families to monitor their child's progress and determine whether after-school tutoring or advocating for additional supports is needed. (Of note, schools will not provide a designation of "dyslexia," which is a medical diagnosis, but can provide a special educational eligibility of "learning disability in reading.")

The variety of other specific learning disabilities that come to the attention of pediatric clinicians during the early elementary years is presented in Table 19.2.

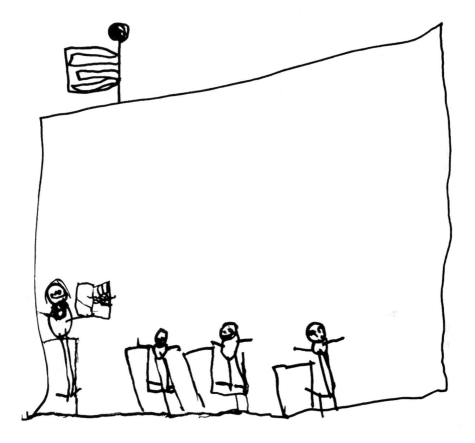

A 6½-year-old boy draws his classroom. The teacher holding the book illustrates the central focus on reading in the first years of school. By Ryan Hennessy.

BOX 19.2   Different Types of Special Educational Supports for Children With ADHD and Learning Disabilities

Definitions

- **504 Plan:** A plan for how the school will provide support and remove barriers for a student with a disability or health condition that is interfering with their ability to learn in a general education classroom. The name refers to Section 504 of the Rehabilitation Act of 1973. It includes accommodations, supports, and services, which are reviewed annually but do not have goals or benchmarks.
- **Individualized Educational Program (IEP):** A plan for a child's special education experience at school, based on assessments that have identified the child's unique needs. An IEP has goal related to each area of need, with measurable benchmarks that define how the special education team will know whether a child has met those goals. An IEP also describes accommodations; how the child will take tests; any modifications to curriculum; the type, frequency, and setting of different services; how much time is spent

in general versus special education settings; transportation; and whether an extended school year is provided. IEPs are revised annually, and an updated evaluation of the child's abilities is done every 3 years.

What services an IEP or 504 plan might provide

- Counseling/social work supports
- Positive behavioral support plan
- Social skills groups (to work on turn taking, perspective taking, conversation, problem solving, friendship building)
- Occupational therapy (fine motor, sensory integration, visual perception)
- Speech-language therapy (expressive, receptive, articulation, or pragmatic/social language)
- Resource room (for 1-1 or small-group special education instruction in reading, math, etc.)
- Classroom aide

The diagnostic assessment of a learning disability is based on more data than the physician can obtain during the interview with the family and examination of the child. It is established by means of standardized educational tests performed by a clinical or academic psychologist. However, critical clues to a learning disability can be identified by the use of screening questions in a primary care setting (Table 19.3). When a learning disability is suspected from the history, several neurodevelopmental procedures may reveal a specific type of disability (Table 19.4). Clinicians play an important role in suspecting learning disabilities early and helping refer children for assessment in the early elementary years, a time when educational interventions are more likely to be effective.

Schools are required by federal law to respond to a parent's request to assess learning or behavioral problems that affect school functioning. Clinicians can play an active role in educating parents about their rights and the referral process, as well as advocating for the child with the school. Two federal laws guarantee the rights of children with learning disabilities to receive timely and comprehensive evaluation and treatment services free of charge: the 1991 addendum to the 1990 Individuals with Disabilities Education Act (IDEA) and Section 504 of the 1973 Vocational Rehabilitation Act. A guide to these service for parents and pediatric clinicians is found in Box 19.3. It can

help to obtain the results of educational testing from the school or other source or to ask that such tests be performed if necessary. Parents can bring the documentation they receive from school evaluations to the medical visit to review with the clinician. Additional data on the child's learning patterns and output (grades, work completion), attention span, and social and behavioral adjustment can be obtained by contacting teachers directly with the parent's written permission. While it can be challenging for a clinician and teacher to find time when both are free to talk on the phone, meetings can be planned in advance and asynchronous updates over email or secure chat can be helpful as well.

Most specific learning disabilities typically become apparent during first grade, although other subtypes of academic difficulty may emerge initially in the fourth or fifth grade, and still others become apparent for the first time in junior high school when the expectations for planning and organization become more complex and challenging (see Chapter 21). The family history often provides an additional clue to a learning disability. Patterns of learning disabilities frequently surface during a clinical evaluation for school underachievement; specific questions about the educational performance of parents and other relatives are helpful.

It is essential that physicians routinely inquire about the progress of 6-year-olds in the first grade. Any concerns

TABLE 19.2   Definitions of Learning Disabilities

Term	Description
Visual perception deficit	Inability to differentiate between similar-looking letters, numbers, shapes, objects, symbols; may habitually skip over lines in the text.
Auditory discrimination deficit	Inability to distinguish similar sounds ("pig" and "big") or confusing the sequence of heard or spoken sounds ("ephelant").
Dyslexia	Difficulty sounding out letters and confusing words that sound similar resulting in problems acquiring basic reading skills. Dyslexia is a language-based learning disorder associated with difficulty in single word decoding and phonological awareness (the ability to translate letters and letter patterns into sound with precision and speed). Dyslexia affects reading, spelling, and written expression. A core deficit in phonological processing skills leads to difficulty learning the alphabet, lack of alphabet mastery, problems with letter-sound associations, and difficulty acquiring decoding skills and sight word vocabulary for reading. Prognosis is best if dyslexia is recognized and treated before grades 4–6.
Dysgraphia	Difficulty expressing thoughts on paper and with writing associated with unreadable penmanship and problems in gripping and manipulating a pencil. A history of difficulty with drawing (e.g., poorly structured drawings, distorted shapes or missing details) may give a clue to dysgraphia. It is often associated with problems in visual-motor control and fine motor abilities.
Dyscalculia	Problems with perception of shapes and confusion of arithmetic symbols leading to poor comprehension of simple mathematical functions. There are three neurological sources for dyscalculia: (1) difficulty with visual-spatial skills; these children often have intact reading and spelling skills; (2) difficulty with arithmetic fact retrieval associated with problems with memorization and retrieval from long-term memory; and (3) difficulties with use of arithmetic procedures such as counting, carrying and borrowing; associated with poor attention and lack of monitoring work when problem solving.
Dysnomia	Inability to recall names or words for common objects.
Pragmatic language disorder	Difficulty with the use of language in social contexts, including nonverbal aspects of tone, rate of speech and turn taking. Lacking observations skills of nonverbal cues results in impulsive social interchange.

TABLE 19.3   Screening Questions for Learning Disorders

These questions can be asked to parents, based on teacher reports of child learning, or to a child in elementary school

Reading
What is the hardest thing about reading?
Is it hard to sound out words?
Do you know words by just looking at them (sight word vocabulary)?
Do you forget things that you read at the beginning of a paragraph when you reach the end of the paragraph?
Do you understand what you read?

Mathematics
Do you understand the teacher when he/she is explaining something in math class?
Do you prefer to learn math by having the teacher explain it to you, or would you prefer to see how a math problem is solved correctly?
Do you have trouble remembering things in math? (If yes) What kinds of things do you have trouble remembering?
When you have a word problem, can you figure out what operation you should use (i.e., addition, subtraction)?
Do you make a lot of careless mistakes in math?

From: Lindsay RL: School failure/disorders of learning. In Bergman AB, editor: *20 Common problems in pediatrics*, New York, 2001, McGraw-Hill, p 328.

TABLE 19.4   Neurodevelopmental Screening Activities for Learning and Attention Problems

Pediatric clinicians can include neurodevelopmental tasks as a part of the physical examination. These tasks assess a variety of components of neurological function that are associated with learning and attention. They are helpful in at least two ways. They may give clinicians a clue to a specific learning disability. In addition, as a result of the mild stress induced by the task, often behavior consistent with hyperactivity (fidgetiness, getting up from seat, constant motion, etc.) and inattentiveness (distractibility, off-task, daydreaming) will emerge in the office only during this part of the examination. Examples of neurodevelopmental tests include the following:

Test	Function
Ask child to write a sentence	Written expression and dysgraphia
Ask child to tell you about a movie or video seen recently	Oral expression, memory, sequencing
Ask child to read a paragraph appropriate for age	Reading fluency and comprehension
Ask child to copy a geometrical figure or do a Draw-a-Person test (see Chapter 4)	Fine motor and visual-spatial skills
Ask child to repeat a series of random numbers (at least age minus one from 5 to 10 years old)	Short-term memory and sequencing
Ask child a multiple-step task to complete in order given (age minus one task from 5 to 10 years old)	Auditory processing

From Reiff MI, Stein MT: Attention-deficit/hyperactivity disorder evaluation and diagnosis: a practical approach in office practice. *Pediatr Clin North Am* 50:1020–1048, 2003.

BOX 19.3   Special Education Rights: How to Guide Families Through A Special Education Evaluation

The federal law, outlined in the Individuals with Disabilities Education Act (IDEA) and its amendments, states that a "free appropriate public education is available for all children with disabilities between the ages of 3 and 21.… " The difficulties that many parents face in accessing assessment and services for their children within our public education system make it critically important that pediatricians understand how to help parents. Pediatricians can play an important role as advocates for educational services for children with learning, emotional, or health conditions.

Information about special education procedures, including the full text of the IDEA amendments, is available from the US Department of Education. Each state's department of education has additional information relevant to your state. The initial assessment consists of procedures to "determine whether a child is a child with a disability and to determine the educational needs of such child." The basic procedures are listed below:

Step 1: Identification

When a child is identified as possibly needing special education and related services, states are required to conduct "Child Find" activities to identify and evaluate all children with disabilities who need special education

whether the child is in private, parochial, or public school. A request for assessment can be made by the parent or school personnel. The request can be verbal or in writing (e.g., a dated letter addressed to the principal of the local school and/or the district's Director of Special Education). Parental consent is needed before a child can be evaluated. Parents should keep copies of any correspondence, formal and informal, between themselves and the school; using a notebook format helps keep records in chronological order.

Some schools recommend a Student Study Team (SST) or similar group meeting before considering an assessment for special education. An SST meeting is not a substitute for the special education assessment process. It can be appropriate as a quick look and plan for children with their first school difficulty.

There are some children who are at high risk for persistent and significant problems in school but who have not fallen far enough behind to meet the formal criteria for a disabling condition under IDEA. Children with dyslexia may fall into this category because we can often predict the children who are going to have school difficulties at a young age, yet there may not be a significant discrepancy between achievement and intelligence, which is required to qualify a student as learning disabled. A parent or

BOX 19.3   Special education rights: how to guide families through a special education evaluation—cont'd

physician may need to ask for reassessment if school difficulties persist or worsen. Consider also that many of our patients have dual diagnoses and may qualify for and need services because of other health impairments such as ADHD, asthma, or anxiety disorders.

Step 2: Evaluation

After a written request is made and received by the school, the school has 15 calendar days to give the parents an assessment or evaluation plan that indicates the areas to be assessed and usually includes specific tests to be administered. Districts vary in the comprehensiveness of their initial assessments. At a minimum, districts will usually assess academic achievement. It is appropriate for a pediatrician or other specialist to ask for assessments in other areas of probable need, such as intelligence, executive functioning, language (expressive, receptive, or social skills related), motor, sensory processing, and social/emotional.

The parent reviews, modifies if necessary, signs the Evaluation Plan and returns it to the school as quickly as possible. The school then has 50 calendar days (with extensions for longer school holidays) to complete the testing and hold a team meeting to go over the child's evaluation results and together decide whether the child is eligible for special education services as defined by IDEA.

Step 3: Eligibility Is Decided

The team meets to determine whether the child meets eligibility criteria, whether special education services are needed, and what specific services are recommended. Parents should not sign special education documents that they do not agree with. Federal and state laws outline procedures to handle disagreements between schools and parents in areas such as eligibility, placement, and level of services. Parents or schools can request mediation or due process to challenge team decisions.

Step 4: If Child Is Eligible for Services

If the child is found to be eligible for special education and related services, the Individual Educational Plan (IEP) team must meet again within 30 calendar days to write the IEP. Parents and, when appropriate, the students are part of the IEP team. Services are to be provided "as soon as possible after the meeting." The IEP document must include current levels of performance, annual goals with interim short-term objectives, measurable goals, a list of the specific services provided to the child (e.g., supplementary aids, speech therapy, adaptive physical education, modifications, staff training, or supports), extent of participation in the general education versus special education classroom, transition service needs, and how progress will be measured. An IEP must also state when services begin, where, how often, and for how long services will last. Door-to-door transportation may be provided by districts, and some children qualify for extended-year programs that include summer services.

Step 5: IEP Reviews Are Scheduled

The specifics of the IEP are required to be reviewed once a year. Parents or the school can request a review of the IEP at any time, and a meeting must be held within 30 days of a written request for a review. A major review, usually including retesting in the areas of concern, must be held every 3 years but may be done more frequently if needed. Although the criteria for qualifying for special education are fairly specific, there are no specific criteria for exiting special education services. At times, a parent may be told that their child no longer qualifies for special education services; this may not be accurate. Decisions to end special education services need to be carefully examined.

From Stein MT, Lounsbury B: A child with a learning disability: navigating school-based services. *J Dev Behav Pediatr* 22:188–191, 191–192, 2001.

raised should not be dismissed as "adjustment" problems or entirely maturational in origin (i.e., "She will grow out of it" or "He's just immature"). Clinical attention to educational concerns from the start and all along will head off the establishment of a cycle of negative child behaviors, avoidance, or work refusal patterns. Children with a primary learning disability can experience academic difficulties without having behavioral or emotional problems if evaluated and addressed early on. However, without diagnosis and intervention, such children may subsequently develop low self-esteem and have disturbances in emotional well-being and conduct as a result of academic frustration. These secondary effects of academic problems will make accurate diagnosis much more difficult later. Because the best medicine is preventive medicine, it is important that learning disabilities be recognized early so that specific remedial measures may be undertaken to lessen the occurrence of secondary psychosocial problems.

Psychosocial Challenges That Affect Learning

A child's emotional life, family environment, school setting, and community resources are other important factors to consider when problems with learning occur in the first and second grades. Among children with mental health conditions (e.g., depression, anxiety, trauma exposure, or oppositional behavior), 30% to 80% have problems with academic achievement and classroom behavior. The low self-esteem and poor self-image in these children affect learning, especially in those with an associated learning disability.

Chronic family stress or even a temporary change in the family may cause or exacerbate school difficulties. A history of separation, divorce, an illness in the child or a family member, substance use, or child abuse or neglect is seen in many young school-age children with learning problems. Poverty negatively impacts readiness to learn and school attainment in multiple ways. Children who live in crowded or substandard housing often have poor sleep, due to the noise and light pollution that are more common in marginalized neighborhoods. Hunger impacts attention and focus, unreliable transportation contributes to poor attendance, and children in households where caregivers work "third shift"—including nights and weekends—may have less support with homework. Clinicians should advocate for school and community-based initiatives that serve low-income families, such as universal free breakfast and lunch programs, and should be prepared to connect individual patients and caregivers to necessary supports.

School Avoidance

All clinicians who work with children sooner or later will evaluate a child who refuses to attend school. Unexcused absences from school follow a bimodal pattern of incidence, with peaks in the early primary grades in about 5% of children, particularly first grade, and a second peak again in junior high school in 2% of youth. Some children are kept home from school by parents, although most unexcused absences from school are attributable to school refusal by the child.

First graders who spend the school day at home may have a variety of physical complaints, including stomachaches, headaches, dizziness, and fatigue, that often subside as the day progresses. Although a few of these children may be suffering from an actual phobia of school itself or some particular aspect of the school experience such as travel on the bus, most first graders who refuse to attend school appear to be suffering from separation anxiety.

These children are experiencing stress in response to leaving their parents and familiar surroundings for a full day of school. The pediatric clinician may diagnose separation anxiety, which often responds to simple behavioral measures combined with supportive counseling of the parents (e.g., caregiver works with the school to arrange a supporting hand-off at dropoff; takes the child to the school playground on a weekend when other students are not present; arranges a play date with another child after school). Such children may have unusually high levels of anxiety. Some anxiety is normal in all children as they begin their grade-school experience. Many children with school-related separation anxiety have a history of difficult separations as toddlers and preschoolers (see Chapter 17). Selective mutism, or refusal to speak to any person outside the home, is a less frequent condition associated with separation anxiety. Some parents may transmit their anxiety about separating to the child and thereby exacerbate the problem. Such families need to be reminded that separation from family at this time is a healthy and predictable stage of maturation.

The child's clinician should be sympathetic to the physical complaints and initiate a reasonable medical evaluation. Excessive medical attention to the physical complaints, however, which may occur when a large number of laboratory tests or specialty referrals are ordered, should be avoided when a functional condition is suspected (see Chapter 25). The clinician must make it clear to the family that the child is to attend school on a daily basis unless the symptoms are severe enough to require a visit to the physician's office. Returning to school will be both diagnostic and therapeutic. Children with separation anxiety disorder become rapidly asymptomatic as their school attendance becomes more regular. When school refusal does not respond to these measures or when pediatric evaluation of the child or family suggests a serious physical or emotional disorder, a further mental health or subspecialty referral may be indicated.

DURING THE VISIT

Children at the age of 6 may not be as candid in providing information to the physician as they once were. Obtaining information with the child and parent present is the most productive technique for 6-year-olds. As with preschool children, it is important to communicate to the child that you value the information they provide about their health and feelings. Asking the child first to describe any physical complaints and beliefs about the reasons for the medical examination may provide an opportunity to deal directly with the 6-year-old's lingering misconceptions about the reasons for the medical encounter. In the course of evaluating the child's physical health, the clinician may gather data about the child's development in the areas shown in Table 19.5.

TABLE 19.5 Gathering Data

Cognitive Development

Questions for Children	Objective
Where do you go to school? What grade are you in? What are you learning in school? Are there some things you do at school that you really like? Are there things about school that you do not like?	To assess whether a 6-year-old can provide acceptable answers to nearly all these questions. Answers may suggest that the child is having difficulty in particular areas. When the child is reluctant to talk about school or provides very little information, the clinician should then invite the parent to enter the discussion.
What town do you live in? On what street? Do you know your address? Do you know your telephone number?	To assess the child's attention to basic information important to well-being as they spend increasing amounts of time away from their family; to assess visual or auditory memory skills.
Ask the child to copy a cross (4-year-old), a square (5-year-old), a triangle (6-year-old), and a diamond (7-year-old).	To observe the child's handedness, ability to grasp and control a writing instrument, and competence in increasingly difficult fine motor and visual-perceptual tasks.
Ask the child to draw a person while you are interviewing the parent.	Can reveal information about the child's attentiveness, following instructions, and ability to work independently. You can then ask the child about the drawing as part of your interview (see Chapter 4).
Have you seen a recent movie? Tell me about the story.	To assess the child's capacity for sequencing events, memory, and content of a story.
Do you ever have dreams? Do the dreams ever really happen? Where do the dreams take place?	To assess the child's capacity for distinguishing between reality and fantasy, which should be well developed at this age.

Questions for Parents	Objective
Does (name) have a problem concentrating or paying attention? Do you think that (name) is more active, less attentive than other children his age?	To assess the parent's perception of the child's ability to attend to a classroom learning environment.
Do you frequently find yourself repeating directions or instructions?	To assess auditory processing maturation.
How is school going? Have you had a conference with the teacher? How does (name) fit in with the classroom? What are the teacher's expectations for (name)?	To assess the parent's understanding and involvement with the school; to model the expected close interaction between parents and school personnel.

Social and Emotional Development

Questions for Children	Objective
Do you know the name of the team that plays baseball or football for your city? What is your favorite movie? What is your favorite television show? Where did you go on your vacation?	To assess the child's general fund of information and the child's interest in and retention of information about events that occur outside the home.
Who are your good friends?	To assess the child's relationships outside the home. By this time, a child should have formed several close relationships outside the home. The child should name one and, preferably, more friends close to their age. A child who does not name anybody or who names an adult, a family member, or a much younger child requires further evaluation. The parent may be asked to comment on the child's response.
What games do you like to play?	To assess the child's preferences for solitary versus peer activities. Are they comfortable with the give-and-take of peer group activities? Do they understand the necessity for and nature of rules? Are they involved in organized community-wide activities, such as team sports?

Continued

TABLE 19.5 Gathering Data—cont'd

Cognitive Development

Questions for Children	Objective
Who lives at your house? What do you think about your brother/sister/the new baby?	To assess the child's capacity to express both positive and negative feelings relating to family members and the degree of sibling rivalry that may be present.

Questions for Parents	Objective
How long has (name) been in school? What does (name) do after school? What chores does (name) do around the house? What are your rules for TV, video games, and media after school and on weekends?	To assess the demands on the child's and family's circumstances and arrangements. To assess family responsibilities that the child shares.

QUICK CHECK—6 TO 7 YEARS

- Six to seven years begins the shift in cognitive function from preoperational ("magical") thinking to concrete operations (reasoning and understanding connect to actual situations and objects).
- Most typically developing children acquire reading skills between ages 5 and 7.
- Academic success in the first grade occurs when decoding letters leads to reading, simple addition and subtraction problems are solved, and simple words in short sentences are spelled correctly.
- ADHD occurs in about 7% of school-age children. Diagnostic criteria are specific, including documentation of behavior that reflects hyperactivity, impulsivity, and inattention at school and home, persistence of such behavior for at least 6 months (beginning before 12 years old) and an association between ADHD behavior and impairment in either educational output or social functioning.
- Coexisting conditions (e.g., oppositional behavior, anxiety, depression, and learning disabilities) occur in many children with ADHD.
- Medication improves core ADHD behavior in 70% to 80% of school-age children. Behavior management and classroom accommodations are also effective.
- A learning disability occurs in at least 5% of school-age children. It may affect the acquisition and use of reading, spelling, mathematical, listening, writing, or speaking skills.
- Dyslexia, a neurologically based deficit in phonological processing skills, is the most common learning disability. It may impair reading, spelling, and written expression.
- School avoidance (refusal to attend school) occurs in 5% of elementary school children and 2% of adolescents. It is often associated with separation anxiety in younger children.

! HEADS UP—6 TO 7 YEARS

- Not all school-age children who are wiggly, fidgety, and inattentive have ADHD. An assessment of social development, family structure, trauma history, learning strengths and weakness, and consideration of physical causes for the behavior are required before making a diagnosis of ADHD.
- Specific learning disabilities are common and early recognition is critical to a good outcome. Focused questions about learning progress during a health supervision visit will generate clues to a learning disability; further testing through school is then needed to clarify a child's unique learning needs.
- Behavior modification for ADHD and disruptive behavior is powerful when applied appropriately. Knowing the principles of behavior management, trauma-informed approaches, and referral sources in your community should be a part of every pediatric practice.
- School refusal in early elementary school is usually due to separation anxiety. It is often associated with physical symptoms in the morning, such as abdominal pain, headache, or sore throat. Go further with each case by exploring symptoms of generalized anxiety, depression, an emerging and undetected learning disability, or a history of persistent bullying. Primary depression and/or anxiety disorder must be considered.

ACKNOWLEDGMENT

Nicholas Putnam, MD, contributed to this chapter in previous editions.

RECOMMENDED READINGS

For Parents

Barkley R. *12 Principles for raising a child with ADHD*. The Guilford Press; 2020.

Bass R:. *A Beginner's guide on parenting children with ADHD: a modern approach to understand and lead your hyperactive child to success*, 2021 Independently published.

Dawson P, Guare R. *Smart but scattered: the revolutionary "executive skills" approach to helping kids reach their potential*. The Guilford Press; 2009.

Franklin D, Cozolino L. *Helping your child with language-based learning disabilities: strategies to succeed in school and life with dyslexia, dysgraphia, dyscalculia, ADHD, and processing disorders*. New Harbinger Publications; 2018.

Shaywitz S. *Overcoming dyslexia*. Vintage; 2005.

U.S. Dept of Education: Educational advocates: a guide for parents. https://files.eric.ed.gov/fulltext/ED592770.pdf

Wolraich M. *ADHD: what every parent needs to know*. American Academy of Pediatrics; 2019.

For Pediatricians

American Academy of Pediatrics/National Initiative for Children's Healthcare Quality (NICHQ): *ADHD: caring for children with ADHD: a practical resource toolkit for clinicians*, ed 3, Chicago, 2019, American Academy of Pediatrics.https://www.aap.org/en/catalog/categories/mental-health-resources/adhd---caring-for-children-with-adhd-a-practical-resource-toolkit-for-clinicians-3rd-edition/

Dworkin PH:. School failure. In: Parker SJ, Zuckerman BS, Augustyn MC, eds. *Developmental and behavioral pediatrics: a handbook for primary care*. ed 2. Philadelphia: Lippincott Williams & Wilkins; 2004:281–1284.

Ryberg R, et al: *Mapping the link between life expectancy and educational opportunity*, Child Trends. https://www.childtrends.org/publications/mapping-the-link-between-life-expectancy-and-educational-opportunity

Wolraich ML, et al: AAP Clinical Practice Guideline for the diagnosis, evaluation, and treatment of attention-deficit/hyperactivity disorder in children and adolescents, *Pediatrics* 144(4):e20192528, 2019. https://publications.aap.org/pediatrics/article/144/4/e20192528/81590/Clinical-Practice-Guideline-for-the-Diagnosis?autologincheck=redirected

AAP Mental Health Initiatives Web site (https://www.aap.org/en-us/advocacy-and-policy/aap-health-initiatives/Mental-Health/Pages/Tips-For-Pediatricians.aspx).

WEBSITES

Children and Adults with Attention-Deficit/Hyperactivity Disorder (CHADD). http://www.chadd.org

Child Mind Institute Complete Guide to Dyslexia. https://childmind.org/guide/parents-guide-to-dyslexia/

Child Mind Institute Complete Guide to ADHD. https://childmind.org/guide/parents-guide-to-adhd/

Child Mind Institute Complete Guide to Dyslexia. https://childmind.org/guide/parents-guide-to-dyslexia/

National Center for Learning Disabilities. http://www.ncld.org

ADHD parenting resources from ADDitude Magazine. https://www.additudemag.com/category/parenting-adhd-kids/behavior-discipline/

Understood.org—website with resources for families raising neurodiverse children. Includes IEP/special education guidance and parenting tips: www.understood.org

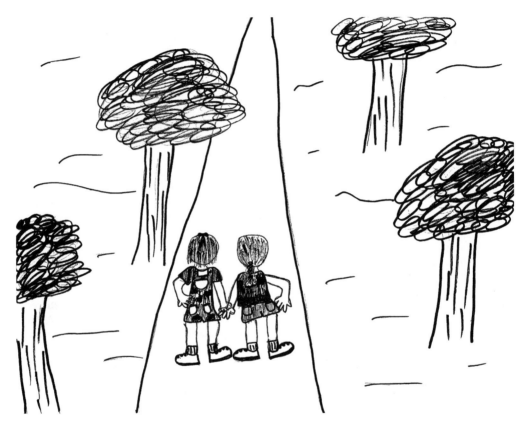

"Friends Forever." A precocious 10-year-old shows herself walking with a friend. A clear-distance perspective usually emerges at an older age. By Kaitlin Thomas, age 10.

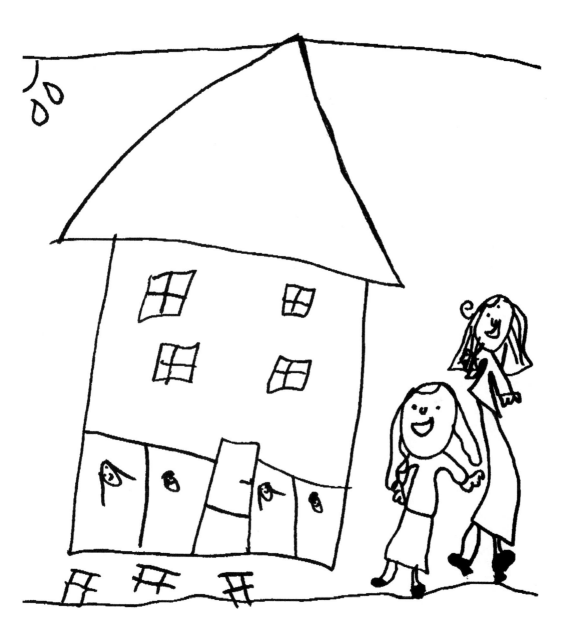

This school-age child with William syndrome demonstrates with her drawing the visual/spatial difficulties that can occur with that disorder.

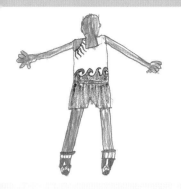

20

Seven to 10 Years: The World of Middle Childhood

Jenny S. Radesky and Caroline J. Kistin

This chapter describes the cognitive, social, and motor skills that are necessary for learning in school and during play. Developmental growth in emotional regulation and thinking brings new opportunities and challenges. The concepts of social competencies and lagging skills are discussed.

KEYWORDS

- Mastery of cognitive skills
- Moral development
- Motivation
- Mindset
- Socialization and independence
- Academic skills and learning disabilities
- Coping skills
- Friendships
- Stress
- Social skills
- Lagging skills
- Video games
- Smartphones

Middle childhood is a period of significant changes in cognitive, social, and motor development. Developmental tasks include expansion of a child's intellectual, moral, and social reasoning, as well as increased engagement in social activities guided by rules of conduct. The ability to access previously gained knowledge, organize it, and express it verbally and in writing reflects maturation of the central nervous system in the areas of perception, memory, reasoning, reflection, and insight. The quest for social involvement and social acceptance is a key characteristic of middle childhood. Relationships with family members, peers, and others in the community influence this period of growth.

Original chapter by Robert D. Wells and Martin T. Stein.

Understanding a child in this period requires consideration of these complex threads of developmental change.

The middle childhood years are, for most children, a time when physical growth and development is relatively minor compared to the surges of competencies in behavioral and developmental areas. Self-awareness, control over new feelings and desires, and making a wider net of friendships deepen and evolve. Despite being called the Latency Period by Erik Erikson (see Chapter 2), this is not really a "latent" period at all but one of consolidating and building skills. Routine health care visits become less frequent at this time, even though many behavior and learning problems may appear. Clinicians should take the opportunity to check in about these developmental gains whenever children present for care, including visits for annual physicals, acute illnesses, or minor injuries.

A significant number of school-aged children face obstacles to developing these competencies. Approximately 30% of all children have a chronic condition, of which asthma, obesity, attention-deficit/hyperactivity disorder (ADHD), and learning disabilities are the most common. About 1 in 15 has multiple chronic conditions, which can limit usual activities, including missing school, limiting physical activities, or needing to attend therapies frequently. The tension between requiring additional care from their family and school during a period of growing independence and self-responsibility may lead to frustration in children.

Since the COVID-19 pandemic, an increasing number of children in elementary school struggle with academics such as reading comprehension and mathematical concepts—learning loss was especially pronounced in low-income and rural communities and Black or Hispanic

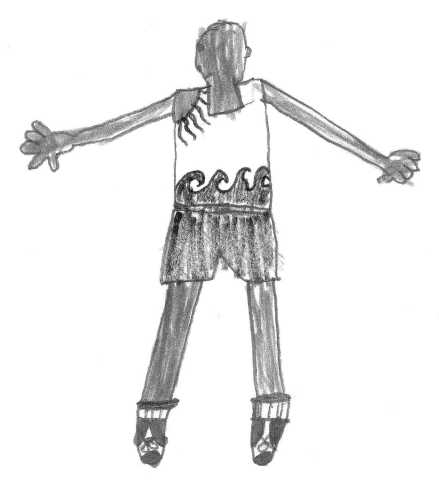

A 9-year old shows himself ready to take on the world. Details of his clothes and the profile show advanced skills.

children. Children on remote schooling had less practice in social problem solving and cooperation with peers in educational and extracurricular environments. Suspension rates in elementary school-aged children also increased in parts of the country after return from COVID-19 schooling, often resulting from a combination of children's dysregulated behavior and shortages in school staffing with social workers and psychologists. Rates of suicidality in 9- to 10-year olds have been rising over the past decade as well, reflecting the greater mental health burden in this age group—as well as the continued insufficient access to mental health treatment in most communities. Therefore surveillance for both school problems and emotional/behavioral challenges has become increasingly crucial at these ages—not only during adolescence.

DEVELOPMENTAL TASKS OF THE MIDDLE YEARS OF CHILDHOOD

New Cognitive Skills

Mastery, in a developmental context, refers to an internalized awareness of achievement. Although it is a part of each developmental stage, mastery takes on special meaning during the school-age years as a result of the child's increased capacity for making independent decisions, and therefore feeling independent pride in their successes. This also means that children will be increasingly self-conscious of their failures—which can be a trigger for externalizing or internalizing behavior at home or school.

At this stage, a school-aged child is able to consider two or more aspects of a situation simultaneously. In making comparisons, they can take into account more than one variable. For example, a typically developing school-aged child appreciates that a tall, narrow lump of clay can be made short and wide without any net gain or loss of clay (see Chapter 2 for more discussion of these Piagetian cognitive development concepts). Such reasoning extends to the child's capacity for making a variety of judgments. They may appreciate for the first time another child who is clumsy but bright, a teacher who is strict but fair, or medicine that is difficult to swallow but brings down a fever.

Compared to 5- to 7-year olds, who tend to understand rules in a concrete manner, older school-aged children begin to understand that rules in games and in life are the product of mutual consent and that rules may be changed under certain circumstances. They are also starting to show more complex **moral development**. While many 7-to 10-year-olds behave well to earn some tangible rewards or avoid punishment, some are beginning to conform to greater behavioral expectations of their community. They also can start to see the universality and value of a rule system.

Motivation

Motivation is a person's underlying reasons for a behavior and is characterized by drive and volition to complete a task. Intrinsic motivation refers to a drive that comes from within the child—from interest, enjoyment, or sense of satisfaction—while extrinsic motivation relies on reinforcement or rewards from external contingencies. Intrinsic motivation and sensitivity to extrinsic motivation vary significantly between children and vary by different activities and subject areas. For example, one child may be very driven to climb and explore outdoors, but less motivated to settle down with a book. Differences in intrinsic motivation may stem from children's unique strengths and challenges, as a child with language delay or weaker reading skills may avoid language-based academic tasks, or a child with motor incoordination may not be motivated to participate in gym class. Motivation in children tends to correlate with motivation later in life, so finding ways to help children engage and persist through less preferred activities can help with longer term academic success. Children with ADHD often have lower levels of intrinsic motivation.

Use of external motivators is typically more pronounced in early childhood, when sticker charts and verbal praise are recommended as ways to reinforce positive behaviors. Teachers may use token systems, with treats such as a "treasure box" of small toys for children who accrue enough tokens by the end of the week. Such use of rewards may either increase or decrease motivation, depending on the specific type of rewards: meaningful rewards that relate to the challenge (e.g., being line leader in class as a reward for persisting at a difficult academic task) tend to be more effective than irrelevant rewards (e.g., stickers for completing a session of speech-language therapy). Caregivers and educators are encouraged to provide autonomy support (see Chapter 2 for more detail) to help support intrinsic motivation, give children more control over their own learning, while providing clear goals and structure.

Many educators now encourage a **growth mindset** in which children are praised for the process of their hard work ("You thought very hard about that!") rather than praising the outcome ("You got that right!") or the child ("You're so smart!"). Research shows that when children receive support related to their work *process and effort*—rather than the *outcome*—they persist longer in challenging tasks and score higher on standardized tests.

Identification and Socialization

During this time, the child continues to consolidate their identification with important adults in their life. In addition to primary caregivers, other people inside and outside the child's family—such as teachers and coaches—also serve as role models and mentors for the child and help support their growing sense of self. Emotional growth and cognitive growth interact and result in the early development of a more personal conscience and ability to self-reflect on emotions and behavior. Norms of behavior are developed within the context of the family (including formal and informal learning from caregivers and siblings), culture (including online culture, such as favorite influencers or characters), community (including school and peers), and society as a whole. Therefore it is important for late school-aged children to have role models and positive relationships beyond their immediate family, including aunts/uncles, coaches, and teammates; this is associated with resilience in children growing up in underresourced communities or with traumatic stressors.

According to Erikson, children at this age are negotiating a stage of *contrasting industry and inferiority* in which achievement is linked with self-concept and the development of the belief in their relative ability to master a given situation to achieve their goals. In contrast, children who feel ineffective, are repeatedly shamed or belittled by adults, or are not provided sufficient supports to achieve in school often feel a very inferior sense of self. This can manifest as internalizing or externalizing behavior (see Table 20.3).

Self-efficacy at this age is related in large part to prior success meeting challenges in academic, extracurricular, social, and family realms, having role models who demonstrate overcoming challenge, receiving individualized encouragement or coaching, and by a child's personal response to stress. Self-efficacy is not a fixed or innate characteristic, but a trait that is influenced by the environment and can be cultivated. Low self-efficacy at this age may reflect a child's prior experience with racism, bias, discrimination, or a lack of opportunity to approach challenges in a supportive environment.

Children of this age, now that they are more self-reflective and aware of their differences from other children, often measure themselves and their achievements against others. This may be exaggerated in families or schools that push competition and competitiveness, or by unrealistic social comparison that occurs on social media. Because social media artificially measures children's "worth" through quantification of likes, followers, and comments, it can become the focus of a child's developing identity, compared to the more dynamic and nuanced feedback that they receive from others in their family, school, or community.

Children must experience some success to build a strong sense of themselves and a feeling of control over their world. For this reason, we recommend that all children take part in activities that foster areas of relative strength. This is particularly important for children whose skills and interests may not naturally align with the characteristics that are commonly praised and rewarded in the school setting, including children with ADHD, learning disabilities, a history of trauma, or other differences that decrease their sense of self-efficacy. For example, a child with ADHD and learning disability may feel ineffective within the classroom setting, but their unique skills with dancing, animals, or art can be supported through in-school or extracurricular activities that give them a sense of self-worth and belonging.

Although earlier explorations into separation have already been experienced, the school-age years are filled with a need to start separating from caregivers. This occurs in a physical sense (e.g., sleepovers, camp) and an emotional sense (e.g., using independent **coping skills** rather than being told how to feel/what to do by an adult). This becomes a time of increased arguments between caregivers and children if caregivers are still "micromanaging" too much of the child's daily tasks (e.g., morning routine, homework). With the child's increased cognitive and verbal sophistication, arguments between parent and child can take on the appearance of a courtroom as each side argues passionately over the logic and illogic of the case. Stepping back from the particulars allows parents and the clinician to see the larger issues here related to the tasks of psychological separation and emerging independence.

Academic Skills and School Performance

Achievement at school becomes more demanding at this stage, and distinct *learning disabilities and learning styles* may become more obvious as the cognitive operations required in class become increasingly complex, sequential, and reading based.

By the third grade, it is said that children shift from "learning to read" to "reading to learn." Up to this point, much of their education has focused on *decoding* basic symbols; reading, sounding out words, and understanding what a number means. Academic demands change qualitatively midway through elementary school and require a new set of skills, *encoding*. During the *encoding* process, the child may now be asked to access previously gained knowledge, organize it, and express it verbally or in writing. Writing an essay and solving a numerical word problem are examples of encoding tasks.

Mussen and colleagues have pointed out five related aspects of learning abilities at this age that are the results of central nervous system maturation:

- Perception—detection, organization, and interpretation of information from both the outside world and the internal environment. A child notices more details, more similarities, and more differences.
- Memory—storage and later retrieval of information. A child can recall more and more and bring information of greater diversity to solving a problem or understanding a situation.

- Reasoning—use of information to make inferences and draw conclusions. The child learns to assemble facts to explain things in increasingly complex ways.
- Reflection—evaluation of the quality of ideas and solutions. The child can compare ideas or consider a proposal before accepting or rejecting it.
- Insight—recognition of new relationships between two or more bits of information.

Children with disabilities that limit their capacity for learning are at twice the risk for school avoidance, disruptive behavior problems, depression, and psychosomatic reactions. Caregivers may raise concerns about academic performance directly to a clinician; at other times, it is the child's emotional or psychosomatic symptoms that raise parental concern. Stress-related symptoms (e.g., headaches, stomach aches) that appear during school days but either lessen or resolve during holidays and weekends may be important clues to discovering developmental disorders and behavioral concerns.

A frustrated child will show frustrating behaviors, which parents will often describe through a very negative lens: "he's driving me crazy; she has anger issues; he knows how to do this, he just refuses"). The clinician serves such children by helping families, teachers, and the children themselves understand their challenges in terms of underlying neurodevelopmental issues—"lagging skills" that do not come naturally to them—rather than problems with character (e.g., "He's just lazy.") or morality (e.g., "She's not making good choices."). By helping families identify the child's specific lagging skills (Table 20.1), sometimes through referral for a neuropsychology evaluation or by interpreting school testing, clinicians can help advocate for services that help build these skills. Tips on helping a family navigatess and understand an Individualized Educational Program and related school testing are provided in Chapter 19.

Due to new standardized testing mandates around the country, many children, particularly in underfunded school districts, are faced with the request of being retained in the third grade because of low reading scores. This happens more frequently to Black, Hispanic, and Indigenous children and should not be allowed; instead, pediatric providers should help families advocate for the reading, academic, and socioemotional supports their child needs to succeed in the next grade.

Family functioning is a strong predictor of child school success at this age, including the extent to which parents can model coping skills and provide both predictable structure and opportunities for emerging child independence at home. Clinicians can screen for common stressors that may be impacting family wellness, such as food insecurity and housing instability (see Appendix), and connect families with community-based resources. Parents may also benefit from assistance navigating their own physical and mental health needs and connecting with adult clinicians.

Expansion of Activities With Peers

School-aged children commonly immerse themselves in sports, clubs, crafts, organizations, music, and a variety of other activities. These pursuits reflect a drive to master specific motor, social, and artistic skills that are shaped by individual experiences, skills, and cultural expectations. Some children spend hours drawing, whereas others play basketball, read books, or play video games.

Participation in organized athletic and artistic **activities** becomes a part of the life of most school-aged children. By the age of 6 years, children become aware of their abilities in various areas and in comparison with other children. At this age, they may participate in team sports competitively, although they rely on adults to structure the activity. At times, they may have difficulty maintaining interest throughout the game. They may even be unclear about the outcome of a game in which they were involved. Nevertheless, by 10 years of age, most children have participated in sports and other performance activities in school or outside of it. These activities allow a child to follow rules, control their body, build relationships with a coach and peers, and build social skills such as adapting their behavior in response to what teammates are doing.

For a child who is resistant to participation in a team sport, an individual sport (e.g., tennis or swimming), a martial arts program, or other structured artistic activities may be an important outlet. Every child would benefit from an activity beyond school work and family at this age. Accessibility of these types of activities varies based on family socioeconomic status, zip code, or district special education funding for after-school programs. Therefore it can be helpful to know your community's local activities that offer scholarships or reduced price for families who qualify financially.

Perhaps most central to the school-age years is the *quest for social involvement and social acceptance*. Most children seek to find a place for themselves among a cohesive group of (often, but not always) same-sex friends. Their success in maintaining a positive sense of self during the day-to-day process of making and breaking friendships is in part dependent on the resilience of their coping and social skills. Children with positive peer relationships tend to give and receive positive attention, follow classroom rules (often due to peers being positive role models), and have more confidence in school—and therefore are more likely to perform well academically. Maintaining friendships allows practice in many of the social-emotional skills that are important to develop at this age, including perspective taking, flexible problem solving, and self-advocacy. Children with ADHD, autism spectrum disorder, and other developmental differences usually require specific support in making and sustaining friendships—from their families or schools—to give them a regular venue for practicing these skills.

TABLE 20.1   Lagging Skills and Related Problems With School, Home, or Friendships

Lagging Skills	Related Problems in School, Home, or with Friends
Difficulty in maintaining focus	Not processing what is going on around them, what other people are saying, following instructions, or quickly losing interest in activities
Difficulty in handling transitions, shifting from one mindset task to another	Problems with transitioning between activities, particularly preferred to nonpreferred activities, leading to refusals or dysregulation
Difficulty in considering the likely outcomes or consequences of actions	Impulsive behavior; seeming to have "poor judgment," often with remorse afterward
Difficulty in persisting on challenging or tedious tasks	Giving up quickly; rushing through mentally challenging activities; avoiding new challenges
Difficulty in considering a range of solutions to a problem	"Stuck" thinking; repeating the same negative behavior despite consequences; wanting to be "right" all the time
Difficulty in expressing concerns, needs, or thoughts in words	Explosive or rude behavior; unintentionally insulting others
Difficulty in managing emotional response to frustration so as to think rationally	Explosive behavior, aggression, or withdrawal when upset
Chronic irritability and/or anxiety significantly impede capacity for problem solving or heighten frustration	Baseline state is irritable or mildly dysregulated so that minor frustrations lead to big emotional reactions
Sensory/motor difficulties	Physical aggression from sensory-seeking behavior without realizing how much force they are using; unawareness of body position leads to invading other's personal space
Difficulty in seeing "grays"/concrete, literal, black & white thinking	"Stuck" thinking; snap judgments; seeing problems in an all-or-nothing way
Difficulty in taking into account situational factors that would suggest the need to adjust a plan of action	Inflexible behavior
Inflexible, inaccurate interpretations/cognitive distortions or biases (e.g., "Everyone's out to get me," "Nobody likes me.")	Difficulty in making friends or responding to peer feedback; overreaction to perceived slights from others; may form fixed negative opinions of others
Difficulty attending to or accurately interpreting social cues/poor perception of social nuances	Over— or underreaction to teacher, peer, sibling, or parent behavior
Difficulty in shifting from original idea, plan, or solution	"Stuck" or rigid thinking that can only see things one way
Difficulty in appreciating how their behavior is affecting others	Rude, insensitive, bossy behavior
Difficulty in starting conversations, entering groups, connecting with people/lacking other basic social skills	Avoidance or scripted approaches to social interaction
Difficulty in empathizing with others, appreciating another person's perspective or point of view	Insensitive behavior
Difficulty in handling unpredictability, ambiguity, uncertainty, and novelty	Avoidance or dysregulated behavior in new/unexpected situations

Adapted from Ross Greene's list of lagging skills from *The Explosive Child* and www.LivesintheBalance.org

Social skills may include a good sense of humor, an ability to make others feel wanted, a willingness to share, a positive mood, creativity, leadership, and negotiation skills (see Table 20.2). These abilities are influenced by a child's innate temperament and are also developed through observation of others (e.g., peers, parents, siblings, teachers) and role models in media (e.g., books, graphic novels, movies, television). For most children, friendships develop naturally as social involvement is pursued. At the same time, if the social environment is competitive, involves mockery or degrading behavior, as is common with social media "influencers" or on multiplayer video games, a child at this age will learn that these social behaviors hold power.

Social Skill Challenges

There are many reasons that neurotypical and neurodiverse children may struggle with **social competencies** (Table 20.2) that help them build friendships, resolve conflicts, and handle new social situations:

- A slow-to-warm-up child may be inhibited at school because of the large number of people, frequent demands for verbal interaction with the teacher and peers, and because they are away from their "comfort zone" of home. Inhibited children may have anxiety about separating from their caregivers at drop off, being called on by the teacher, getting up in front of the class, or approaching other children on the playground.

- Impulsive children may appear "immature" as a result of unpredictable, disruptive behavior in class and on the playground. A child with low persistence, a short attention span, high distractibility, and a high activity level is at risk for early unfavorable judgments by peers. Children with ADHD may experience significant problems in social skills because they may be more controlling of peers, more inflexible when peers want to play differently, or may impulsively insult other children to try to control the situation.

- Children with a history of trauma or neglect may have had insecure early relationships and missed opportunities to learn reciprocal, serve-and-return interactions. They may therefore have a lower sense of trust in others or may be more aloof, overreactive, or controlling in interactions with others.

- Children with autism spectrum disorder (including the symptom constellation previously called "Asperger Syndrome") may have a constellation of different lagging skills that make social skills more challenging. These include lower social interest/motivation, decreased perspective taking or how others are feeling, difficulty reading nonverbal social cues, limitations in their own expression of social cues, rigid or repetitive play behaviors, pragmatic communication challenges that lead to difficulties with conversation, and sensory sensitivities that may lead them to feel overwhelmed in social settings.

TABLE 20.2   Social Skills and Related Challenges

Social Skills	Difficulties With Relating to Others
Greeting skills	Initiating social contact with a peer in a way that is expected for the social context
Social predicting	Estimating peer reactions before acting or talking
Conflict resolution	Settling social disputes without name calling, threats, or aggression
Affective matching	Sensing and fitting in with others' moods
Social self-monitoring	Knowing when one is having a social difficulty, has hurt someone else's feelings, others are not interested, etc.
Social reciprocity	Sharing and supporting, reinforcing others, enjoying give-and-take with others
Verbalization of feelings	Using language to communicate true feelings
Inference of feelings	Reading others' feelings through language and nonverbal cues
Code switching	Matching language style and behavior to current audience
Topic choice and maintenance	Knowing what to talk about and for how long
Requesting skills	Knowing how to ask for something tactfully
Social memory	Learning from previous social experience; remembering details about another person
Assertiveness	Exerting the right level of influence over group actions without being bossy or controlling
Social comfort	Feeling relaxed while relating to peers

Modified from Levine MD, Unpopular child. In Parker S, Zuckerman B, editors: *Behavioral and developmental pediatrics: a handbook for primary care*, ed 2, Philadelphia, Lippincott Williams and Wilkins, p 359.

- Nonverbal learning disability often overlaps with autism spectrum disorder but children have particular deficits in visual-spatial organization (so they struggle with invading others' "personal space"), motor planning (therefore sports are more challenging), reading nonverbal cues, and self-regulation.
- Children with a language-based learning disability or specific language impairment may struggle with language-rich play and conversation.
- Children with physical illnesses or motor disabilities may have movement limitations that impact their access to sports, playground equipment, or other socializing opportunities.
- Adjustment disorder or reaction to a stressful event can impact social skills. Divorce, domestic violence, child abuse, natural disasters, or a serious accident or illness of a family member—all can have significant emotional effects on the developmental work of school-aged children.

In each of these cases, 504 plan accommodations, social skills groups, or targeted therapy or supports in school will help the child make friends and reduce altercations. Importantly, research has demonstrated that Black, Latino, and Native American children, as well as children with disabilities of all races and ethnicities, are more likely than other children to be punished for externalizing behaviors and arguments at school, more likely to be removed from the classroom, and more likely to be sent from school to the emergency room for assessment for "out-of-control" behavior. Clinicians should be aware of these inequities in school response and be prepared to advocate for children and families affected by harmful practices.

Bullies. Scapegoating, teasing, bullying, and self-isolation become social dynamics that can seriously hinder children, especially those with poor social skills. Approximately 20% of school-aged children are involved in bullying—as perpetrator, victim, or both. Physical aggression is more common with boys, increases in elementary school, peaks in middle school, and declines in high school; verbal abuse remains constant. Social isolation practices, such as ignoring and ostracism, are more commonly seen among girls. Bullying can occur in person or online (e.g., through text or social media), often both. Children and teens who are bullies and bullied by others have higher incidence of depression, anxiety, and suicidality. As they approach adolescence, a child with a persistent lack of regard for others can be at significant risk for more serious problems, such as bringing a weapon to school. Bully victims are typically socially isolated and may lack the social skills to self-advocate. Children with physical and emotional disabilities are bullied more frequently. See Recommended Readings for resources to address bullying.

When social and behavioral challenges come to light in a pediatric visit, it is often with a nonspecific complaint: *My child …. Keeps getting bullied; … keeps getting suspended or I have to pick them up early because they were acting up; … got in a physical fight at school; …. has a stomachache/headache when they come home from school frequently; …. says they have no friends.* It is helpful to delineate the specific social skill areas that the child might be struggling with, as described in Table 20.2 and provide supports as summarized in Box 20.1.

Structural Factors That Influence Social-Emotional Well-being in School

It is important to understand that it is not only *child-level factors* that influence child well-being and social competence in the school setting but also *structural factors* that matter as well. These include:

- School district funding. Districts in historically disinvested or racially segregated communities often have lower real estate values, and therefore lower tax revenue. Therefore these schools may not have the funding for robust after-school programs, social work or psychologist staffing, social-emotional curricula, paraprofessionals to help during playground and other unstructured times, or safe school buildings and drinking water. Families in financially disinvested districts will need to advocate more strongly for their child to get adequate supports, or find neighboring school districts that allow transfers.
- Staff and teachers in better funded districts may receive higher salaries, more time for in-service training (e.g., in topics like social-emotional learning), more support from administrators, and therefore may have lower turnover rate than in underfunded districts. Lack of training in behavior management is one reason that neurodiverse children are disciplined for behaviors related to their underlying disabilities (e.g., aggression in a child with autism who is frustrated due to communication challenges).
- Racial/ethnic discordance of teachers and students has been linked with more discordant reporting of problematic behavior in Black and Hispanic children.
- Parent involvement in school activities leads to better parent-teacher communication and relationships but is harder for parents who are not proficient in English or who have multiple jobs and do not have time to volunteer at school.

BOX 20.1	Social Skills Challenges—Management Strategies

- **Explain the social skill problems sensitively to the child**. This should avoid shame and blame, and rather help improve the child's insight into what feels challenging to them.
- **Have the parent gently debrief with the child after mistakes**. Do not overreact when the child makes a social mistake; during a calm and private interlude afterwards, the parent can discuss the social interactions and help the child think of solutions.
- **Help the child locate one or two companions with whom to relate and begin to build skills**. It can be helpful if such peers share interests and sense of humor.
- **Inform the classroom teacher or building principal if a child is victimized by peer abuse in school**. It is the school's responsibility to make every effort to contain this activity. A strongly worded note from a primary health care provider may be vital in such cases.
- **Help a rejected child develop skills, hobbies, or areas of expertise that can enhance self-esteem and be impressive to other children**. Ideally, such pursuits should have the potential for generating collaborative activities with other children.
- **Never force these children into potentially embarrassing situations before their peers**. For example, an unpopular child with poor gross motor skills needs some protection from humiliation in physical education classes.
- **Manage any family problems or medical conditions** through counseling, specific therapies (e.g., language intervention or help with motor skills) and/or medication (e.g., for attention deficits or depression).
- **Identify social skills training programs within schools and in clinical settings**. Clinicians should be aware of local resources that offer social skills training. Most commonly, this training makes use of specific curricula that are used in small group settings in a school or in the community.
- **Reassure these children that it is appropriate for them to be themselves, that they need not act and talk like everyone else in school, and that there is true heroism in individuality**. Clinicians, teachers, and parents must tread a fine line between helping with social skills and coercing a child into blind conformity with peer pressures, expectations, and models.

From Levine MD: Unpopular child. In Parker S, Zuckerman B, editors: *Behavioral and developmental pediatrics: a handbook for primary care*, ed 2, Philadelphia, Lippincott Williams and Wilkins, pp 359–360.

MENTAL HEALTH IN MIDDLE CHILDHOOD

When **stress** exceeds coping resources, maladaptation results. Some children will respond to stress overload by becoming depressed, anxious, or preoccupied with body functions, whereas others may become provocative, angry, and demanding. The array of psychological disorders has been conceptualized as fitting into two broad groupings of disorders—internalizing and externalizing responses (Table 20.3). Rates of mood and behavioral disorders in school-aged children have been increasing both before and since the COVID-19 pandemic, as have rates of eating disorders and suicidality. These are discussed in more detail in Chapter 23, but surveillance and screening tools are available to help clinicians identify children who would benefit from therapy and possible medication.

Recurrent symptoms of pain, especially head, abdominal, and limb pain, are frequent during the school-age years and in some cases may lead to difficulties in functioning in several areas. Although most of these recurrent pains are idiopathic with negative physical examination findings,

many parents of these children have higher rates of depression and somatic preoccupation, thus suggesting a familial pattern of underlying stress (see Chapter 25).

DURING THE VISIT

In recognition of the child's concerns about competency, the interview should first focus on abilities and strengths. Such an approach will allow the child to present themselves in a controlled fashion, thereby furthering the development of trust. Early questions about stressful events or feelings should be avoided until the child appears comfortable in the interview. Consequently, questions about the three arenas (family, school, and social functioning) can be ordered such that the least stressful area is discussed first and the most worrisome is left for the last. Predictions about this order can be made from the information gained from parents and your own observations.

Developmental and behavioral assessments of a school-aged child should broadly assess the child's functioning at home, in school, with friends, and in the community. The

TABLE 20.3   Free Screening Tools for Internalizing, Externalizing, and Behavior Disorders in Middle Childhood

Internalizing and Externalizing Disorders	PSC	Vanderbilt Scale	SDQ	SCARED
Age range (years)	4–17	6–12	4–17	8–18
Internalizing disorders				
Psychosomatic complaints	X			X
Depression	X	X	X	
Withdrawal/school avoidance				X
Anxiety	X	X	X	X
Externalizing disorders				
Disruptive behavior		X	X	
Hyperactivity		X	X	
Conduct disorders		X	X	

PSC, Pediatric Symptom Checklist; *SCARED*, Screen for Child Anxiety and Related Disorders; *SDQ*, Strengths and Difficulties Questionnaire.

child and parents can be interviewed together, but some time with the child alone will be important to communicate your sense of them as an independent and competent individual.

OBSERVATIONS

While the clinician is engaged in developing rapport, observations of the child and family will be helpful.
- What are the child's and parent's general mood and level of interaction?
- Is the child's behavior appropriate for age?
- How well does the parent allow the child to answer questions?
- Are there indications of underlying irritability, distrust, or worry?
- How are the child's skills of speech, concentration, attention, and compliance?
- How do the parents respond if their child seems anxious, irritable, or embarrassed?
- How much do the parents control the child's behavior during the visit?

Questions regarding the child's functioning should focus on strengths and successes, as well as concerns and weaknesses. The terms such as *problems* and *failures* should be avoided. It may be more helpful to inquire about difficult or challenging situations they have had to cope with. Helping the family keep a balanced perspective while discussing the child is extremely important to avoid belittling the child in a disrespectful and potentially harmful fashion.

The Child Interview

The clinician should gather information from the child about all aspects of their life—family, school, and social. Some questions are listed below that can help engage an older school-aged child in telling you their story. Showing curiosity about the child's experience is also helpful role modeling to caregivers who may be reacting to the child's increasing independence with more strict or harsh responses.

Family Functioning

Tell me about what the family enjoys doing together.
What are you allowed to do now that you could not do when you were younger?
What chores do you have at home? How easy is it to do them? What happens if you forget?
If you have a problem at school or with a friend, whom do you talk to about it?
How much fighting goes on between you and your brother or sister?
What are the most important rules at home? What type of consequences do your parents use?
What are the rules about technology and media at home?
Tell me about a usual day after school. What happens?
What do your parents argue about with you?
What are your parents most proud of about you?
What do you worry about at home?
What would you change about your family if you could?

School Functioning

What do you like about school the most?
What do you dislike about school?

What would you change about school if you could?

What subjects are easy? Which ones are hard?

What kind of grades are you getting this year? How about the last year? Are you happy with them?

What is your teacher like this year?

Do you ever worry that it is extra hard for you to do something the teacher asks?

Have you ever gotten into trouble for the way you behave at school? What happened?

How much school have you missed recently?

Do you ever visit the nurse's office or feel sick in school?

How do you get along with the other children at school? Do you have friends? Do you have enemies or people who pick on you?

If you were the principal or teacher, what rules would you change?

What jobs or careers do you think you would enjoy?

Do you like to read? Do you read for fun?

What is your favorite subject? Which one do you dislike?

Social Functioning

What kinds of things do you like to do on weekends?

What are you good at? What types of things do you enjoy and do well?

Who is your best friend? How long have you known him or her? How often do you get together?

What do you like about him or her? What are some of the things that your best friend likes to do?

Whom did you eat lunch with yesterday (at school)?

Can you talk about worries and problems with your friends?

Have you ever lost a friend? What happened? How did you cope with it?

Do you and your friends ever fight or have misunderstandings? How do you settle it?

Do you have a phone or social media? Have you ever experienced drama with friends?

Do you play video games where you can chat with other people? Who do you talk to?

Have you slept over at friends' homes? Have they stayed with you?

What types of things do you wish you could do or learn?

Have your friends become interested in boys or girls? What kind of grades do they get? Are they experimenting with cigarettes, alcohol, or drugs?

Do you belong to any teams, groups, or clubs?

Has anyone ever hurt you or made you do something you did not want to do?

What are some of the harder things you have had to deal with?

Projection/Insight

If you could have three wishes, any wishes, what would they be?

If you were the captain of a spaceship, which three people would you take along?

What would you change about yourself if you could make any change?

What are you best at doing?

What is your biggest problem?

If you could be any age, what age would you pick?

Is this year going better, worse, or about the same as the last year? How come?

ANTICIPATORY GUIDANCE

The child's clinician can offer specific guidance to the child and family directed toward the development of responsible, increasingly independent behavior.

- Counseling about *accident prevention* recognizes the school-aged child's cognitive ability to connect an event with an outcome and focuses on the innate interest in controlling one's environment. Thus the need for seat belts and responsible helmet use during bike riding, skating, rollerblading, skiing, and snowboarding should be mentioned because these activities continue to be a leading cause of death and injury in children. Safe storage of guns and ammunition should be reviewed with caregivers.
- Counseling children about *smoking and drinking alcohol* should begin at this age. By encouraging the child's active involvement in these discussions, responsibility and self-control are promoted at an early age. Parents who smoke are more likely to stop when the impact of their smoking on the health of their children is emphasized (e.g., ear infections, allergies, asthma, other respiratory infections, and behavior problems).
- Parents can enhance the child's feeling of *responsibility* by having clear expectations of the child for initiating and completing chores and homework.
- Gradual increases in *independent activities* can be an encouragement for child behavior that demonstrates trustworthiness and competence.
- Reading for fun should be encouraged at this age; ideally children will be able to read chapter books, but for reluctant readers, there are a wide variety of graphic novels, e-books (with or without accompanying audio), and audiobooks to help children be more engaged with literature and their imagination.

Boundaries and Expectations

Parents may be encouraged to maintain reasonable, predictable, and observable boundaries and rules so that the child can accurately predict the parents' positive and negative responses to behavior. Children need to learn a variety of skills, including delay of gratification and tolerance of frustration, which can be developed when negative events are experienced. Parents may consult with the child about their concerns, but they are wise to avoid premature suggestions or advice in favor of supporting the child's own problem-solving efforts. The clinician can identify areas of stress for the child and invite family-initiated solutions. Changes in the school and social environments that will support positive growth should be encouraged. Parents must get involved in these environments and understand their impact on the child to affect such positive changes.

Managing Digital Media

Counseling about a first phone, social media, and video gaming is needed for most children at this age (Boxes 20.2 and 20.3)

The average age of getting a first smartphone is 8–10 years in US children—an age when children are not developmentally ready to access all that a smartphone provides (such as the whole Internet, apps and games, and social media). Most families get their child a smartphone for convenience of communication, logistics such as school pickups, and to allow the child to socialize with friends. Clinicians should coach parents on (1) deciding if a smartphone is truly necessary, or whether a flip phone or other "starter" device (such as a smartwatch) would meet the child's needs; (2) setting filters, privacy controls, and download controls on the smartphone so that the child does not access inappropriate content; (3) keep boundaries around phone use such as bedrooms/overnight, mealtimes, and during homework; (4) regular open-minded conversations about how the phone and social interactions are going so that children and teens know they can come to caregivers if problems arise. Box 20.3 provides more details on guidance about the first phone.

Social media accounts should be avoided in children under 13. First, these platforms' policies do not allow users under 13. Although these policies were created due to data privacy law, there is research showing that younger age of social media use is linked with worse outcomes. One study demonstrated that children who started social media accounts young—at ages 8, 9, or 10—had more problematic media use (e.g., spending long amounts of time, getting in arguments, displacing sleep, and other activities) and more online contacts from strangers (see Chapter 21 for more information on social media and tweens/teens).

Social media is one venue through which tweens and teens are exposed to negative media content. This ranges from upsetting news, images of war or racial violence on TV or YouTube, to misogynist and White supremacist hate speech on social media platforms. Unfortunately, even with a lot of oversight and Internet filters, most

---

BOX 20.2   Signs of Problematic Video Gaming

The World Health Organization included gaming disorder in the 11th revision of the International Classification of Diseases, defining it as "a pattern of gaming behavior ("digital gaming" or "video gaming") characterized by impaired control over gaming, increasing priority given to gaming over other activities to the extent that gaming takes precedence over other interests and daily activities, and continuation or escalation of gaming despite the occurrence of negative consequences." The gaming behavior must exist for at least 12 months and result in significant impairment to a person's functioning in personal, family, social, educational, occupational, or other important areas.

In pediatric clinic, parents may endorse several of the following when children's video gaming habits have become problematic:

- Child plays video games for prolonged period every day, interfering with other essential activities (e.g., sleep, completing homework)

- Child frequently asks or argues for more time and does not want to take part in other activities they used to like (e.g., seeing friends, playing outside, sports)
- Child makes excessive purchases on video games
- Child shows compulsive symptoms such as thinking about video games through the school day, waking up at night to use the game
- Chatting/talking online to other players they do not know, which can lead to harassment, rude behavior, and grooming
- Video games become the only way a child calms down or relaxes
- Aggressive or explosive behavior when video gaming stops

From *Gaming disorder*, who.int.

BOX 20.3 First Phone: How to Guide Families on Responsibility Milestones and Alternate Approaches

What does research say is the right age for a phone? When do kids feel ready?

Most experts agree that there is no one magic age when kids should get a phone. When teens were interviewed to see what they think is the right age for a phone, they said:

- There is not an ideal age when a phone should be obtained.
- Phones are helpful when kids start being more independent from parents and need to contact them.
- There should be conversations between parents and kids, and kids should be showing responsibility first (e.g., follow rules around other technology, when they make a mistake, try to make it better).
- Kids need to be able to take care of and maintain a phone—so if they are frequently losing mittens, hats, backpacks, an expensive phone is not a good idea.
- Parents need to be ready to enforce rules around use (e.g., checking phone, plugging it in at night).

Parents should consider:

1. Why is the phone needed?
   - Many parents want it to communicate with kids moving between houses, safety coming home from school when parents cannot be home.
   - It is socially normative for tweens/teens to want to chat and be in touch with each other.
   - Remember that getting a phone does not automatically equal getting social media.
2. Are there alternate models you could get through your carrier?
   - Flip phone (cannot group text or videochat)
   - Smartwatch or other phone models with GPS, texting, maps but limited app store or browser access
3. Are there alternative ways to communicate with friends, such as a tablet with a messenger app?
4. With any new device:
   - Set privacy, content, contact, download, and downtime settings and explain to kids why this is important.
   - Set phone-free locations and times, such as bedroom, dinner table, homework time, family time, car rides, etc.
   - Establish expectations that the child needs to respond to texts and calls from caregivers.
   - Make a plan for whether caregiver has password and can check child's phone.
   - Talk about how it is going every few weeks—expand or cut down access accordingly

---

teenagers have encountered such content, as well as pornography (intentionally or unintentionally). Although these topics can be hard to talk about, encourage families to have open-minded and understanding conversations about media so that kids know they can come to their caregivers when they have negative experiences online. Some children and teens avoid telling their caregivers about bullying or negative experiences—for fear that their device will be taken away—so caregivers need to proactively create a space where media can be discussed.

Playing video games is a common pastime for school-aged children, and research shows that a modest amount of video gaming per day (1–2 hours) is not associated with any developmental, behavioral, or academic problems. However, because video games are designed to be very engaging—to keep players moving from level to level—it can be hard to get kids to transition off of them. This is a good reason for having predictable times of day or the week when children are allowed access to video games, ideally once homework, chores, and responsibilities are done. Parents should check video game ratings to avoid overly violent, gory, or sexualized game design. Playing online with other players at this age should be kept to only players the child knows in real life—not strangers on the Internet—since this can be a source of inappropriate behavior or grooming. Parents should be encouraged to play along or have their children shown them their video games, so they understand what the child likes about it. Video console and app store settings should be set to private and not allow purchases without caregiver approval. The signs of problematic gaming are described in Table 20.2.

The main way media—whether smartphones, video games, or TV/movies—get in the way of developmental tasks at this age is through *displacement*. Media and games are pleasurable, so it is tempting to fill any downtime, boredom, or moment of negative emotions with a video, app, or social media feed. However, this can easily displace sleep, learning emotion regulation strategies, or building internal motivation to complete challenging tasks like homework. There should also be boundaries around media for *parents* so that mealtimes, car rides, and other family activities open for connection and conversation.

! HEADS UP—7 TO 10 YEARS

- A quiet, reserved school-aged child may reflect an individual temperament, depression, or psychosocial stress. A focused history usually provides the needed information.
- Consider the degree to which a child has emotionally separated from their family through success in school, sports, and other activities.
- Digital media, smartphones, and video gaming may take up a significant proportion of the day and displace healthy activities like sleep, physical activity, and family connection. Many families need guidance on creating boundaries around digital media, keeping content age appropriate, and maintaining open, shame-free communication with children about online activities.
- Learning problems at this age may reflect a problem with a variety of different cognitive or attentional processes. A formal learning disability educational evaluation should be initiated. "He's lazy" is not a diagnosis.
- A school-aged child, who lacks a best friend is not invited to birthday parties or does not participate in any social play activities with peers, is at risk for social isolation. Look for individual strengths that can be encouraged and provide suggestions about structured activities that facilitate connections with like-minded peers.
- Physical complaints without an apparent cause may be associated with emotional and social stresses in the child's immediate environment—family, school, peers, and neighborhood. A focused history, often interviewing the child and parent separately, frequently provides clues to the etiology of the physical symptom. The interview process itself is often therapeutic.
- Ask about bullying—either being bullied or acting as the bully. A pediatric encounter may be the only opportunity for early recognition and intervention to enhance social competency and prevent isolation.

ACKNOWLEDGMENT

Nicholas Putnam, MD, contributed to portions of this chapter in previous editions.

RECOMMENDED READINGS

For Clinicians

Levine M. *A mind at a time: how every child can succeed.* Simon and Schuster; 2012.
Gresham FM. Social skills assessment and intervention for children and youth. *Cambridge J Educ.* 2016;46(3):319–332.
Silva JLD, Oliveira WAD, Mello FCMD, Andrade LSD, Bazon MR, Silva MAI. Anti-bullying interventions in schools: a systematic literature review. *Ciencia saude coletiva.* 2017;22:2329–2340.
Moscoviz L, Evans DK: *Learning loss and student dropouts during the covid-19 pandemic: a review of the evidence two years after schools shut down*, 2022. https://www.ungei.org/sites/default/files/2022-04/learning-loss-and-student-dropouts-during-covid-19-pandemic-review-evidence-two-years.pdf

Cyberbullying Resources

Fast Facts: Preventing Bullying |Violence Prevention|Injury Center|CDC. www.stopbullying.gov
Lives in the Balance: Ross Greene's website about lagging skills and related resources. https://livesinthebalance.org/
Mental Health Screening Tools for Grades K–12 (https://safesupportivelearning.ed.gov/sites/default/files/10-MntlHlthScrn-TlsGrK-12-508.pdf).

For Parents

Greene RW. *The explosive child.* HarperCollins World; 1999.
Smart but scattered: the revolutionary "executive skills" approach to helping kids reach their potential by Peg Dawson.
Screenwise: helping kids thrive (and survive) in their digital world by Devorah Heitner.
Raising humans in a digital world: helping kids build a healthy relationship with technology by Diana Graber.

For Children

First Phone: A Child's Guide to Digital Responsibility, Safety, and Etiquette by Catherine Pearlman.
The Asperkid's (secret) book of social rules, 10th anniversary edition by Jennifer Cook.
Me and my feelings: a kids' guide to understanding and expressing themselves by Vanessa Green Allen, MEd.
Putting on the brakes: understanding and taking control of your add or ADHD by Patricia O. Quinn and Judith M. Stern.
Learning to slow down & pay attention: a book for kids about ADHD by Kathleen G Nadeau.
What to Do When You Worry Too Much: A Kid's Guide to Overcoming Anxiety (What-to-Do Guides for Kids Series) by Dawn Huebner and Bonnie Matthews.
What to do when you feel too shy: a kid's guide to overcoming social anxiety (what-to-do guides for kids series) by Claire A.B. Freeland, Jacqueline B Toner, et al.
What to do when your brain gets stuck: a kid's guide to overcoming ocd (what-to-do guides for kids series) by Dawn Huebner and Bonnie Matthews.
What to do when your temper flares: a kid's guide to overcoming problems with anger (what-to-do guides for kids series) by Dawn Huebner and Bonnie Matthews.

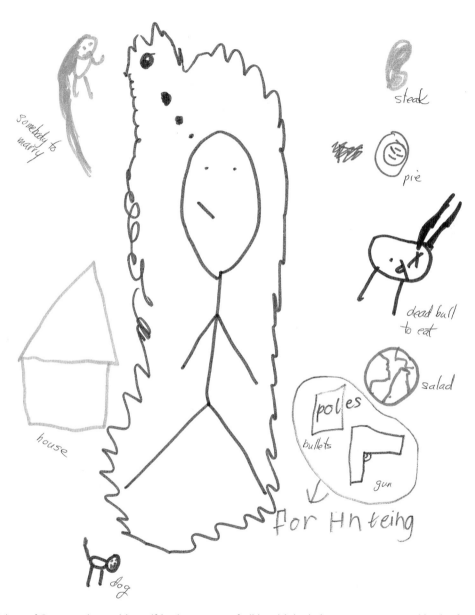

A boy of 9 years shows himself in the center of all he thinks is important, now and in the future.

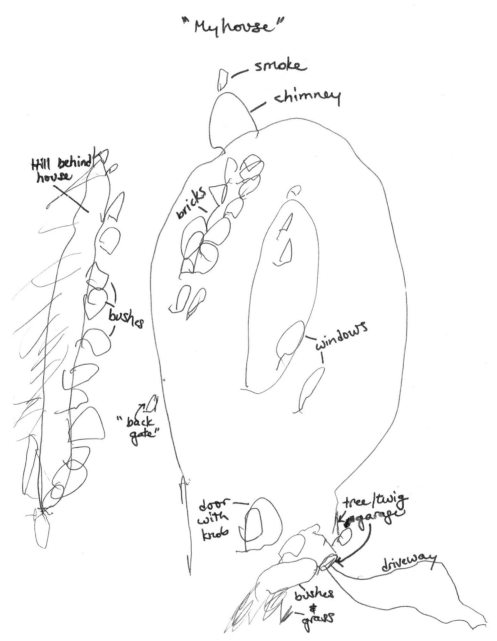

A 7-year old with Tourette syndrome and a nonverbal learning disability draws his house. By Ryan, age 7.

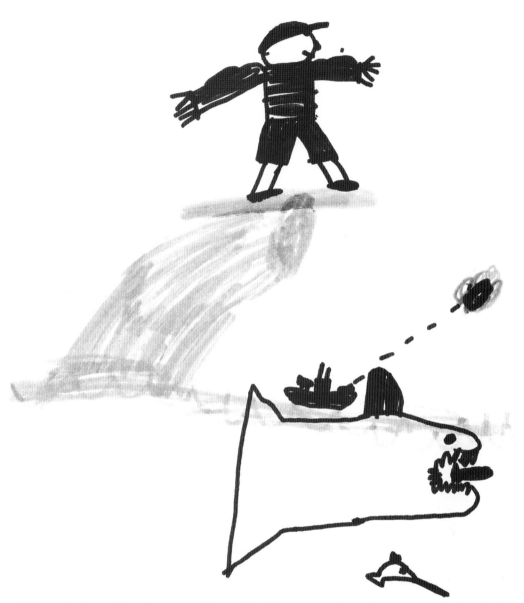

Neil, age 9, shows himself on top of the world, riding a wave above the monster whale, missile-launching ships, and swordfish. A good sense of confidence is conveyed.

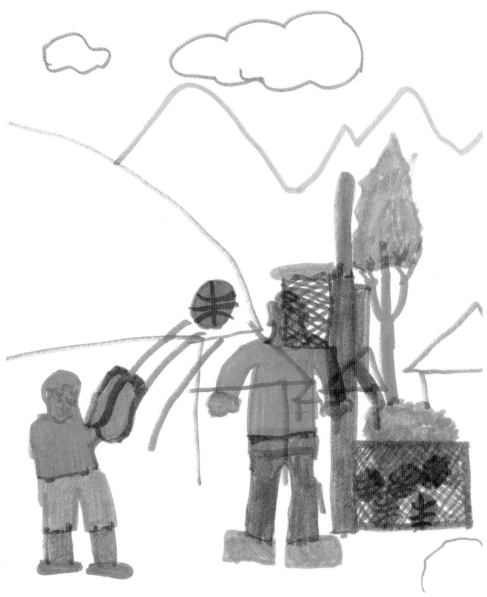

Playing with my Dad. Motor activities can be the forum for rich family interactions if coaching is sensitive to the child's ability to learn complex tasks, understand directions, and alter his actions from the instruction. By HH, a boy aged 8 years.

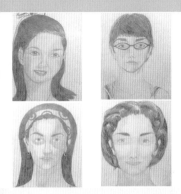

21

Eleven to 14 Years: Early Adolescence—Age of Rapid Changes

Jenny S. Radesky and Caroline J. Kistin

This chapter explores the behavioral, social-emotional, and physical changes characteristic of early adolescence. The significance of emerging gender and sexual identity development, importance of peer relationships, and technology/social media are described.

KEYWORDS

- Adolescence
- Puberty
- Identity
- Gender identity
- Gender dysphoria
- Social media
- Independence
- Substance use
- School transition
- Confidentiality
- Exercise

OVERVIEW OF ADOLESCENCE

Adolescence is the developmental phase between childhood and adulthood and is marked by rapid changes in physical, psychosocial, sexual, moral, and cognitive growth. This developmental phase consists of three substages: early, middle, and late adolescence. Early adolescence generally occurs between the ages of 11 and 14 years and mid-adolescence, between 15 and 17 years. Youth 18 years or older are typically in late adolescence, a substage

---

Previous edition authors are Jennifer Maehr and Marianne E. Felice.

also called emerging adulthood. These age ranges are simply guidelines; many other factors contribute to the adolescent's placement in early, middle, or late adolescence, including sex, neurodiversity, early childhood experiences, and socioeconomic status.

Certain psychosocial growth tasks are specific to adolescence in general and to each substage of adolescence, as summarized in Table 21.1. *The key issues are separation and independence, gender identity, sexual identity, cognitive expansion, moral maturation, and preparation for an adult role in society.* In other words, during adolescence, the individual must ask themselves, "Who am I, where am I going, and what is important to me?" Adolescents' use of technology and social media often acts as an important environment in which these key issues are explored.

Although the stage of adolescence can feel tumultuous for some families, it also is accompanied by a remarkable increase in the child's way of seeing the world, forming opinions, discovering themselves, and figuring out how to be a citizen of the world. Building relationships with adolescents and hearing their perspectives is an important step in helping them trust the medical system, feel understood, and engage with their health care into adulthood.

EARLY ADOLESCENT PHYSICAL DEVELOPMENT

Early adolescence is characterized by the physical onset and continuation of **puberty** and the gradual emergence of independence from the family. As physical changes occur in the body, many early adolescents develop sexual curiosity and heightened body consciousness. It is an important transition time that calls for developmental work by both parents and their growing teens. With anticipatory

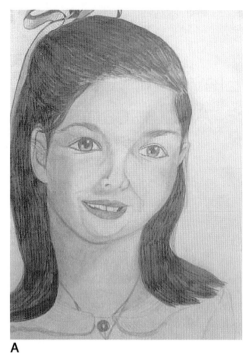

A

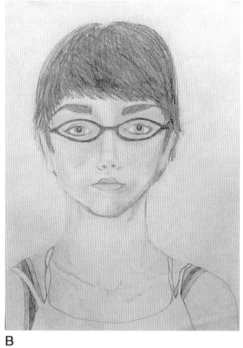

B

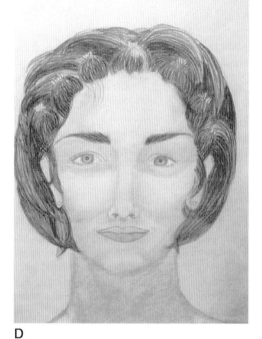

C

D

(A–D) A series of four self-portraits "Myself at Different Ages." She draws herself as she goes through adolescence and beyond. By Shala Abdi, age 16.

TABLE 21.1	Growth Tasks by Developmental Phase		
Task	Early: 11–14 Years	Mid: 15–17 Years	Late: 18 Years+
Independence	Emotional break from parents; prefers friends to family	Ambivalence about separation	Integration of independence issues
Body image	Adjustment to pubescent changes	"Trying on" different images to find real self	Integration of satisfying body image
Sexual interests	Sexual curiosity; occasional masturbation	Sexual experimentation	Beginning of intimacy/caring
Relationships	Tend to have more unisex peer group	Multiple sexes in the peer group; multiple adult role models	Individual relationships more important than peer group
Career plans	Vague and unrealistic plans	Vague and unrealistic plans	Specific goals/specific steps to implement them
Conceptualization	Concrete thinking dominates, with some self-reflection and abstraction	Concrete thinking and developing more introspection and abstract thought	Abstract thinking

Adapted from Felice ME: Adolescence. In Levine MD, Carey WB, Crocker AC, editor: *Developmental-behavioral pediatrics*, ed 2, Philadelphia, 1992, WB Saunders.

guidance, the healthcare provider can prepare and support the parent and adolescent for these changes.

Puberty

For children assigned female at birth, puberty typically begins between the ages 8 and 13 years with the development of breast buds (thelarche). It is normal, however, for some adolescents to have the onset of pubic hair development (adrenarche) before breast development. The onset of menarche occurs on average between 2 and 3 years after thelarche. Pubescence starts later for children assigned male at birth, beginning with testicular enlargement followed by lengthening of the penis and pubic hair development. The majority of children assigned male at birth have entered puberty, by evidence of increased testicular volume, by or before age 14; some start puberty as early as 8 or 9 years. Puberty is typically completed within 4 to 5 years.

There has been a trend over the past century toward earlier puberty onset, which is largely attributed to better health and nutrition. There are differences in the average age of puberty onset by child race, however, and it is also hypothesized that structural racism and related environmental factors—such as disproportionate exposure to endocrine-disrupting pollutants or access to calorie-dense processed foods—may be contributing to an earlier onset of pubertal development in Black and Latinx children.

PHYSICAL DEVELOPMENT

Before puberty, children typically grow in height and weight at a steady pace. During puberty, physical changes become more dramatic and rapid. For instance, height increases suddenly compared to earlier growth. The physical changes are also qualitatively different from previous years. Children adapt to having hair that is coarser and distributed differently; changes in body odor; oiler skin that is acne prone; and changes in distribution of body fat and musculature.

Young adolescents have variable insight into their changing bodies. Some may appear to be unaware of changes, such as the development of body odor, while others may be acutely sensitive and self-conscious. Furthermore, the physical changes that occur may be asynchronous; that is, body organs and subsystems may appear to grow at different rates, so the arms, legs, nose, or chin may seem to enlarge with no apparent respect for overall body harmony, which can make teens feel out of control. Families also have different cultural practices regarding pubertal changes, so these physical changes might be celebrated, ridiculed, or dismissed more in some families than in others.

Sometimes the physical changes that are observed are worrisome to young adolescents, who may harbor their own "explanatory models" for these events. For example, a pubertal child assigned male at birth who has gynecomastia (a normal occurrence in many boys during puberty) may be alarmed that he is developing breasts like a girl or may fear that he has breast cancer. Transgender youth often start to feel more dysphoric as pubertal changes start but may not know how to express their discomfort (see later). Clinicians can provide an important space for normalization and discussion of these topics.

BODY IMAGE AND WEIGHT

Early adolescence is an important window for developing a healthy body image and relationship to both food and physical activity. Puberty is accompanied by weight gain and changes in body shape and composition, at a time when teens are increasingly exposed to advertising and other body images in the media. Young adolescents are often acutely aware of how their physical changes compare with those of their friends, and they may harbor some anxiety about comparisons of who is growing too soon or too late. Consistent with the typical self-absorption or egocentrism expected at this age, they may become more critical or embarrassed of their bodies and imagine that the world is as focused on these changes as they are. Distorted body image and eating disorders, which can affect teens of all backgrounds, are discussed in detail in Chapter 22.

In general, young adolescents often start to have more responsibility for, and control over, what they eat, especially when they are not at home. Medical visits at this age are a good opportunity to learn more about current likes and dislikes, as well as the mealtime environments at home, school, and other settings. Understanding how, when, and with whom a teen eats during the day can provide insight into their family and peer relationships as well. Guidance at this age should include education around eating a balanced diet with a variety of nutrients, as well as the social and psychological benefits of eating together with family and friends.

On average, adolescents get significantly less daily exercise compared to younger children, and very few meet the World Health Organization's recommendation of at least 60 minutes of physical activity per day. Young adolescents may find themselves with less time for daily physical activity as their schoolwork and other responsibilities intensify. Many face additional barriers related to the cost of playing organized sports and the lack of safe and welcoming outdoor space where they live; still others may feel like they are not athletic or coordinated and cannot participate, based on the games and sports they have been required to play at school in the past. Guidance at this age should focus on broadening young adolescents' concept of physical activity with a focus on finding activities they enjoy and can work into their routines, as well as connecting families with low-cost or free teen-oriented community organizations and clubs. Some young teens with autism, attention-deficit/hyperactivity disorder (ADHD), or other developmental conditions will benefit from occupational or physical therapy to build motor coordination, stamina, and core strength.

The number of youth who are overweight or obese continues to increase. In the 2017–18 National Health and Nutrition Examination Survey, over 21% of adolescents 12 to 19 years of age were overweight (body mass index at or above the 95% percentile), a 43% increase from the 1999–2000 survey. Obesity is multifactorial in its etiology and is associated with factors including low socioeconomic status and food insecurity. Genetics, psychosocial stressors, mood disorders, pubertal changes, and other medical conditions can also contribute. Obesity is associated with significant stigma, including within the healthcare system, which has negative impact on self-esteem, mental health, and overall well-being.

Clinicians should follow recommended screening guidelines for youth with overweight and obesity while at the same time identifying and eliminating sources of weight bias during the healthcare encounter. Studies have shown that patients with obesity are more likely to be treated by healthcare workers as "lazy" or "undisciplined," which often stems from a simplistic and erroneous mental model of the causes of obesity. Clinicians should consider recommendations and evaluations targeted toward the etiologies of obesity: for example, assessing and addressing food insecurity that may lead to patients consuming cheaper but more calorie-dense foods or a lack of access to safe outdoor space for physical activity that contributes to a more sedentary lifestyle. Clinicians can also partner with patients and their families to identify strategies of incorporating healthy foods and movement without a focus on weight loss in particular.

IDENTITY AND INDEPENDENCE

During the school-age stage of development (6–10 years), children generally identify strongly with their own families and model their actions after the adults they are around. In adolescence, youth have an appropriate psychological need to separate from their caregivers and establish their own identities as individuals. In most young adolescents, this task is generally accomplished quietly, without open rebellion, through the choice of clothes, hair, jewelry, music, and the increased importance of close friends. In some families, especially those that are close-knit, this process may still pose difficulties.

This struggle recalls that of an earlier era, the second year of life. As toddlers, the bids for independence heralded the transition from infancy to childhood; now these bids are renewed as the child begins the journey from childhood to adulthood. Most parents need that perspective clearly laid out. A teen's choice in clothing is a concrete way for them to express individuality and peer-group identification. Symbols of that identification take on new importance that may not be apparent to adults. The more dramatic those symbols—for example, use of disrespectful language—the greater the tensions between parent and child. Sensitive limit setting by parents is still necessary, such as boundaries around when, where, and how much the teen can use their phone, or expectations for completing chores or homework. Compromises can often be found and this is an important time for parents to learn collaborative problem solving (see Recommended Readings).

As adolescents separate from parents, a peer group helps provide a safe psychological space in which to grow outside the family. The peer group provides a sounding board against which a young teen can test ideas, and it serves as a barometer of their own physical and psychological growth. In other words, the peer group provides an important supportive structure to an adolescent's psychosocial development. An adolescent must often juggle the differences between what friends want and what family rules dictate and navigate the tension between these forces. Families can be advised to provide a loving, open, and supportive space for teens to seek communication, affection, or learning from their caregivers. What this looks like will differ by family, so it can help to ask adolescents and caregivers what they like doing best together, where they feel the most connection and meaning, and how they carve out time for each other.

Gender Identity Development

Gender identity is defined as how people appraise their compatibility with, and motivation to fit in with, a gender collective. It is a multidimensional construct that includes gender self-categorization in early childhood (see Chapter 17), how children perceive their own similarity to peers of their own gender or other genders, and gender satisfaction/contentedness. In adolescence, the estimated prevalence of adolescents reporting a gender identity different from than assigned at birth is 1.2% to 4.1%. Many of these adolescents identify as nonbinary.

Primary care clinicians may see young adolescents who overtly report that they are transgender, but others may not feel comfortable disclosing or discussing it. Instead, they may present with mood difficulties, bullying, decline in academic performance, missed school, or parent-child relationship dysfunction. Depression symptoms impact about one-third of adolescents with gender dysphoria, although estimates vary between studies; anxiety affects up to 25%; up to 15% have an eating disorder diagnosis, up to 50% have self-harmed, and up to 30% have attempted suicide. Rates of bullying and family rejection are higher among transgender teens, which contributes to higher rates of homelessness.

Not all youth who report gender identities different from their gender assigned at birth will experience persistent **gender dysphoria**. A diagnosis of gender dysphoria requires children to have substantial distress or problems with functioning for at least 6 months, which young teens who have been living in their affirmed gender may not experience. It is important to note that transgender youth and adults report bias from the healthcare system adding to their stress, so it helps to have an approach that is sensitive to a patient's sex/pronouns and demonstrates acceptance of gender diversity (e.g., through flyers or posters).

Clinical approaches for transgender children and teens should include validation of the patient's experience regarding their sex, using an affirming approach that allows the child's voice to be heard and avoids influencing them to choose a path they would not have chosen for themselves. Seeing a primary care provider affirm a teen's gender identity can help caregivers as well, especially those who are struggling to provide support. Research shows that children and teens who feel socially affirmed by their communities and have a collaborative decision-making style with their caregivers and clinicians have better mental health outcomes.

Definitions of important concepts in transgender care are listed in Table 21.2. Although gender-affirming treatment is typically performed within a multidisciplinary clinic, there are geographic, legal, and family-level barriers to many children accessing such care. Therefore primary care clinicians play an important role in initial guidance and should know about the steps in gender-affirming care. These include:

- Social transition: Social transitioning may include changing a name, choosing a preferred pronoun, altering clothing or hairstyle, and adopting new activities and mannerisms. Each adolescent's social transition will be different and timing of transitioning varies, but it is important for families to know that children who feel affirmed through social transitioning have significantly lower rates of mental health problems.
- Puberty suppression: Once puberty begins, young teens may experience discomfort due to discordance of their gender identity and sex assigned at birth. For example, breast development or vaginal bleeding may be upsetting to a teen assigned female at birth; erections and facial hair may be distressing to teens assigned male at birth. Hormonal suppression of puberty usually can start around ages 10 to 12 (Tanner II stage) and allows youth time to explore their gender identity without having to worry about undesired body changes. During this time, the family can also access resources.
- Hormonal therapy: Hormonal therapy to induce secondary sex changes that are concordant with the teen's gender identity can start at age 16 based on treatment recommendations from most professional societies.

TABLE 21.2 Definitions of Commonly Used Terms in Gender Identity Care

- **Gender assigned at birth:** A person's initial assignment as male or female at birth. It is based on the child's genitalia and other visible physical sex characteristics.
- **Cisgender:** Individuals whose affirmed gender matches their gender assigned at birth and their physical sex characteristics.
- **Gender dysphoria:** Distress that is caused by a discrepancy between a person's gender identity and that person's gender assigned at birth. Not all gender-variant individuals experience gender dysphoria. It is more specifically defined by the *Diagnostic and Statistical Manual of Mental Disorders, Fifth Edition* (DSM-5; American Psychiatric Association) as a diagnosis.
- **Gender expression:** The way a person communicates about gender to others through external means such as clothing, appearance, or mannerisms. This communication may be conscious or subconscious and may or may not reflect gender identity or sexual orientation.
- **Gender identity (or affirmed gender):** A person's intrinsic sense of self as male, female, or an alternate gender, reflecting a complex interplay of biological, genetic, environmental, and cultural factors. It does not always correspond to biological or anatomic sex.
- **Female-to-male (FTM):** Persons assigned female gender at birth who identify as male.
- **Male-to-female (MTF):** Persons assigned male gender at birth who identify as female.
- **Transgender:** Used to describe individuals with an affirmed gender identity different from their gender assigned at birth and physical sex characteristics. Transgender persons are not necessarily female to male or male to female, as "transgender" can also be used to describe people whose gender identity, expression, or behaviors cross or transcend culturally defined categories of gender.
- **Transitioning:** A process whereby individuals change their social or physical characteristics or both for the purpose of living according to their affirmed gender. Transitioning may or may not include hormonal or surgical procedures.
- **Sexual orientation:** The personal quality inclining persons to be romantically or physically attracted to persons of the same sex, opposite sex, both sexes, or neither sex. Sexual orientation is distinct from gender identity and gender expression.
- **Social transitioning:** Change in social role to one's affirmed gender and may include a change of name, pronoun, clothing, appearance, mannerisms, and use of gender-affirming devices such as chest binders or packers.
- **Top surgery:** Mastectomy or chest contouring in FTM or breast implants in MTF.
- **Bottom surgery:** Usually metoidioplasty or phalloplasty in FTM or vaginoplasty in MTF. Bottom surgery does not necessarily involve gonadectomy.

Adapted from Bonifacio C, Maser K, Palmert SM: Management of gender dysphoria in adolescents in primary care, *CMAJ* 191(3):E69–E75, 2019.

Sexual Identity Development

Sexual interest and drive start to develop in early adolescence. It is expected that young teens will start to have crushes or an interest in dating, and parents should be supported in not overreacting to their child's interests. It is important for young teens and their parents to have access to accurate information about sex, sexuality, and relationships. Some adolescents formulate concepts regarding sexuality (authentic or unrealistic) from what they can glean from television, movies, pornography, and social media. On the other hand, television, movies, and social media can sometimes serve as an opportunity for conversation between caregivers and their children on topics such as sex, gender stereotypes, violence, and relationship safety. Not all children have access to safe adults at home to talk about sexuality, so clinicians, teachers, and other community members play an important role. The HEADS/SSHADESS assessment includes several questions about emerging sexual identity and activity (Table 21.3).

Social Development and Peer Relationships

In early adolescence, the peer group generally consists of people who share similar interests and spend a considerable amount of time together. An adolescent may belong to several different groups of friends whose members may or may not overlap, for example, one group of friends at school, another from the home neighborhood or extended family, and potentially others from various

TABLE 21.3   Components of the Early Adolescent Health Maintenance Visit and SSHADESS Interview

What to Observe	Objective
Interactions between adolescent and parent	To assess whether they communicate well or whether the caregiver answers all the questions for the adolescent or allows the teen to answer themself; these interactions may reveal the status of the separation process
The adolescent's willingness to be interviewed and/or examined alone without parental presence	To determine the adolescent's willingness to begin to act independently from their parents

What to Ask (SSHADESS Format)	Objective
Strengths: What would you say is your biggest strength? What are some things you're good at? What do you like most about yourself? What do you think other people like about you?	Assess the adolescent's self-esteem and skills. Adolescents who struggle to identify one or more personal strengths may benefit from more detailed screening for mental health conditions such as depression and/or anxiety
Supports: Who in your life is a source of support for you?	Assess for support in the teen's family, peer group, and/or community
Home: Where are you living now? Who else lives where you live? Questions about household violence should include: what happens when people in your household argue and does anyone ever get hurt during arguments? This should be followed by, do arguments ever happen when someone has been drinking or is using drugs? Ask whether there are firearms in the residence. Ask about meals served at home (quality and availability of food)	Determine where the patient lives and whether they live independently, at home with parents, with friends, or in cohabitation with a significant partner; determine the psychological and physical safety of the home environment
Activity: What do you do for fun? Are you involved in any clubs, organizations, religious groups, sports, or hobbies? What social media platforms do you use? Who do you follow or what do you post? How do you usually feel after using social media? Is it ever a problem? How do you feel about your body shape and size? Have you tried to change it? If so, how? What were/are your goals for your body?	Evaluate social interactions, interests, self-esteem, problematic video gaming/social media/Internet use, and eating disorder-related behaviors. Adolescents who participate only in solitary activities may have difficulty with social skills, feel alienated, or be depressed
Drugs: Are any of your friends smoking cigarettes or using tobacco or vaping? Does anyone in your family smoke? What about you? Do you or your friends ever drink alcohol? Use marijuana or other drugs? What about pills? Have you ever worried about someone in your family who used alcohol or drugs?	Determine personal, environmental, and genetic risks for substance use and assess current pattern of use. Identify those whose substance use is likely to interfere with their functioning, quality of life, and/or physical or mental health. Reinforce the behavior of those who have chosen not to use drugs or alcohol
Education: What do you like best/worst about school? What are your favorite and least favorite subjects? Do you have a favorite teacher? Why? Do you do any after-school activities? Who are your friends at school? What are your actual grades? Do you get any extra help in any classes? Have you ever been suspended/expelled? Do you feel safe at school? Have you ever brought a weapon to school?	Evaluate current achievements, strengths, and weaknesses and their realistic connection to future plans. Assess for unrecognized learning disabilities and stress or anxiety related to college, employment, or separation from family, school, and community

Continued

TABLE 21.3   Components of the Early Adolescent Health Maintenance Visit and SSHADESS Interview—cont'd

What to Ask (SSHADESS Format)	Objective
Sex/Sexuality: What is your gender identity? Are you or any of your friends dating or going out with someone? Have any of your friends started to have any sexual experiences, including kissing, oral sex, or sexual intercourse? What about you? (If sexually active): How do you protect yourself from sexually transmitted infections (STIs)?	Evaluate and counsel about sexuality; sexual practices; reproductive health, including family planning and STIs; and sexual abuse/exploitation
Suicide: How has your mood been recently? Have there been any times recently when you have felt stuck in feeling sad, down, or bad about yourself? Have you ever harmed yourself on purpose or thought about harming yourself? Do you think about death or suicide? (If the answer is yes): Ask how long the behavior has been going on, how frequently it occurs, which body parts are affected, and whether the patient has needed medical attention for intentional injuries. For patients who endorse suicidal ideation, inquire about plan(s), intent, access to means, and any preparatory steps	Assess for nonsuicidal self-injurious behavior, suicidal ideation, and any history of prior suicide attempt. Identify adolescents at risk for suicide and in need of intervention. Identify and address any immediate safety concerns (e.g., current active suicidal ideation with a plan)

social activities (e.g., sports, clubs, church). Membership in particular peer groups can be very important to the young teen and is a means by which they define or label themselves and others. Teens are often hyperaware of the social "pecking order" and where they fall in the hierarchy. Social media is often a source of accentuated social comparison or peer rejection that can negatively affect young teens' well-being; at the same time, it is a source of finding positive community and social affirmation in many teens. A few teens may not be accepted by any peer group, a condition that can eventually contribute to poor self-esteem, loneliness, and depression. Social isolation or alienation may indicate challenges with social skills or impulse control and warrants support in and out of school.

Social Media

Social media comprises a range of different online platforms where individuals interact with each other where users can post content (e.g., text, photos, videos) and react to each other's posts. Celebrities, corporations, brands, health organizations, governments, and other groups also use social media to spread information and attract followers. "Social media" should not be thought of as a monolith. Design features are constantly evolving, so it can be hard for clinicians or caregivers to feel that they can keep up. For example, early social media platforms such as MySpace were very different from the current billion-dollar multinational corporations such as Twitter, Meta (Facebook, Instagram, and WhatsApp), TikTok, Reddit, and YouTube that are currently competing for teens' attention.

It is important to address social media use in the early teen years for several reasons. First, although users must state that they are 13 years or older to make an account, many children use false ages to gain access to social media. Children in elementary school and middle school often make social media accounts to chat with friends, watch entertaining videos, or follow celebrities. Research has shown that starting a social media account young (e.g., 8–10 years) is associated with being contacted by unwanted strangers and having more problematic media use over time; therefore this should be avoided.

Wanting to use social media in the teen years is developmentally normal, since these platforms allow access to peer relationships, exploring identity, finding out information about the world, and planning with friends. Teens can have a healthy relationship with devices and social media, but it usually takes some effort—including having rules about not using overnight, trying to maintain positive communities and block/report people who are inappropriate, and talking with caregivers about their experiences, so caregivers can monitor and support them. However, some adolescents have mixed or negative experiences with social media, of which causes include:

- Unwanted contact or harassment (sexual or otherwise) from strangers is more likely to happen if teens set their accounts to "public." Young teens in particular should keep accounts "private" and know how to block and report others.
- Negative social comparison with others. Many people present a perfectly polished version of themselves online, and it is common for beauty or fitness content to be recommended to teens, which can lead to teens thinking less of themselves. Seeing more unrealistic beauty ideals on social media is linked with less satisfaction with ones' own body in teens. Despite attempts at removal from social media platforms, pro-anorexia "eating disorder bubbles" still exist and can be recommended to teens who search for diets or fitness content.
- Negative interactions such as bullying, harassment, and hate speech. While these also exist in the offline world, they can be accentuated online due to anonymity or norms about criticizing others online. Children from minoritized race/ethnicities or LGBT+ identities are more likely to be harassed online, but they also find important support through online social networks—so they may need additional help navigating this complex combination.
- What types of content they search for or are recommended. It is important to ask teens whether they are seeing content that is educational, inspirational, or helps them understand others' perspectives versus content that is dehumanizing, biased, dangerous, or violent.
- How compulsively they use it and whether it is interfering with other activities. Social media companies make more money if teens spend more time on their platforms; therefore companies use design tricks (e.g., autoplay, daily rewards, quantified popularity such as "likes," infinite scroll, notifications, and algorithmic recommendations) to keep them engaged. This can become problematic when it interferes with sleep, school, homework, or other activities important to the child. Children with preexisting mental health or emotion regulation challenges or attention deficits are more likely to develop problematic media use habits so may need extra monitoring and conversations with caregivers.

It is also important for caregivers to know that their own social media use factors into child's well-being. When teens see a parent on their own phone, this might be received as a signal of unavailability. Clinicians can encourage caregivers to create their own boundaries around phone and laptop use so that space is left open for conversations and connection with teens. It is also important to remind parents that relationships between media use and mental health are complex. In most cases, just taking away a phone, social media account, or gaming console is not likely to solve the whole problem (and could make things worse, as teens see their phones as their connection to peers and can get quite anxious when phones are taken away). Other supports such as psychotherapy/family therapy, special education, medication, opportunities for meaningful activities, and self-regulation skills will need to be needed in addition to modifying media use.

SCHOOL ENVIRONMENT

Early adolescents are usually in middle school (grades 6, 7, and 8) or just starting high school. For most teens, this is a new social experience with a different milieu from elementary school. The teen must adapt to changing classes, multiple teachers and teaching styles, varying homework loads and testing schedules, and a larger student population. Social dynamics become more complicated and intense. These new experiences may cause social discomfort and challenge executive functioning. Most young people make this transition with minimal anxiety, tempered by the comfort of knowing that their grade school companions are in the same predicament. Children who receive special education may feel more overwhelmed with the higher number of teachers and peers, and a shift in special education teams. Those who must attend a new school with all new classmates may be more anxious. This anxiety may be manifested as psychosomatic complaints (e.g., headaches, stomach cramps, chest pain, shortness of breath), school avoidance (e.g., unexcused absences, tardiness, skipped classes, missed homework assignments), and academic problems such as declining grade point average.

Youth with ADHD, autism, or executive dysfunction who were previously functioning well in elementary school may suddenly experience academic difficulties in this more challenging school environment. These students may require alterations in their medication; additional supervision or strategies with organization, self-management, and homework completion; as well as meetings between their parents and school staff to develop an individual education plan to meet their needs. This plan might include daily check-ins with a special education teacher or advisor, weekly meetings with a social worker who can help with problem solving, extra time in resource room, or an aide to help throughout the school day. In middle school, more independence and self-advocacy are expected by teachers from students, and disruptive behavior are less tolerated—so extra time with a speech-language pathologist to work on self-advocacy skills may be needed. Adaptation to a new school year usually takes 6 to 8 weeks, but more lasting difficulty warrants an evaluation. Caregivers should be encouraged to attend parent-teacher conferences, which usually occur in the mid-fall, to discuss any concerns with teachers and be proactive about addressing them.

BOX 21.1   Important Components of a Transition Plan for Young Adolescents with Developmental Disabilities

- At age 14, adolescents can start attending their own Individualized Educational Program (IEP) meetings and develop a postsecondary vision or plan for life after high school.
- Caregivers can ask for a pre-IEP transition planning meeting and ask what transition assessments are being done to develop IEP goals.
- Along with the teen, caregivers can start inviting agencies or individuals providing services to the teen to the IEP meetings, to allow continuity between school and community.
- IEP and vision goals and objectives can be revised as the adolescent's interests and goals change. A large decision when entering high school is whether to get a diploma

(has met the state's competency determination and local graduation requirements) or a certificate acknowledging attendance, course completion, achievement, and/or participation. Students may usually take part in a graduation ceremony even if they do not receive a diploma.
- At age 16, look for work and/or volunteer opportunities both inside and outside of school programming.
- If caregivers are planning to pursue guardianship, begin saving for the costs of legal fees and the documentation needed. Other options are shared decision-making (caregiver and child make decisions together and both sign off) and delegated decision-making (caregiver and child talk about choices, but the caregiver makes the decisions on the child's behalf).

Continuing school difficulty should be taken seriously and evaluated by the school and possibly outpatient evaluators (e.g., neuropsychologist, speech-language pathologist). If a caregiver feels that their concerns are not being addressed by the school, it helps to refer them to an educational advocacy group or provide resources on how to advocate on their child's behalf. Learning disabilities are underidentified in children from lower income families, so advocacy and demystifying the process (see Box 19.3) may be needed. For children with developmental disabilities (autism requiring significant support, cognitive delay), transition planning should start in the middle school years (Box 21.1).

AT THE VISIT

Adolescent health maintenance visits and physical examination should be performed yearly as recommended by the American Academy of Pediatrics. The annual well-child examination presents an opportunity to update immunizations and to screen as appropriate for medical conditions that may affect this age group, such as vision problems, hypertension, weight-related problems, scoliosis, anemia, hyperlipidemia, and sexually transmitted infections. The physical examination is also an ideal time to talk to teens about their bodies, act as a role model and offer support of their identity, and to answer any question that they may have. Some clinicians may find it useful to perform components of the risk assessment or anticipatory guidance while completing the physical examination, for example, discussing vaping and e-cigarette use after listening to the lungs or asking about physical activity after examining the

heart. The components of the early adolescent health maintenance interview are reviewed in Table 21.3.

COGNITIVE DEVELOPMENT: IMPLICATIONS FOR THE CLINICAL INTERVIEW

When evaluating a child in early adolescence, it is important to remember that 11-year-olds still think concretely; that is, most do not yet have the cognitive abilities to think abstractly, to develop contingency plans, or to conceptualize. Children with cognitive delay or autism spectrum disorder may retain concrete thinking for longer. Piaget classified this stage of cognitive development as *concrete operational thinking*; teens in this stage may experience difficulty organizing large bodies of data or inferential tasks. They may not relate present actions with future consequences. This inability has important implications for health counseling and the management and treatment of illnesses. Explicit linkages and short-term consequences must be spelled out clearly for a young adolescent.

Physicians who care for young adolescents frequently proclaim that they are difficult to interview, so it helps to use specific and positively framed questions or prompts if there are only limited responses to open-ended questions. For example, instead of saying, "Tell me about yourself," the clinician may be more successful in saying, "Tell me, what do you do after school?" Because of limitations in conceptualization, young adolescents may be unable to sustain lengthy verbal interviews. Others may view a physician's questions as a test and interpret the medical interview like an examination at school, with right or wrong answers. In those instances, the physician may glean more information by interacting with the patient through talking about current events or asking about a favorite game. This approach may be more successful in building rapport and getting to the core issues than more "standardized" interviews. Some children of age 11 or 12 may talk more freely in a relaxed, nonformal environment. In addition, a young adolescent may be more able to describe specific behaviors, beliefs, and attitudes in their peer group than in themselves. The clinician can even use these approaches in data gathering. For instance, "Some young people your age try vaping. Are any of your friends starting to vape?"

MENTAL HEALTH AND RISKY BEHAVIOR SCREENING

Depression, anxiety, and other mental health conditions often present in the early teen years. The US Preventive Services Task Force (USPSTF) recommends screening all teens aged 12 to 18 years for depression using tools such as the Patient Health Questionnaire 9 (see Box 22.1) or Beck Depression Inventory. Notably, these are not diagnostic instruments, and a positive screen does not necessarily mean a diagnosis of depression but indicates a need for further assessment. The USPSTF notes that it is important that systems be in place to ensure accurate diagnosis, connection to evidence-based therapy such as cognitive behavioral therapy, and ongoing follow-up. This also presents an opportunity to teach teens and parents about why we screen for mental health concerns, how we interpret tests, and what they can do with the information to help build insight and get needed help.

Bright Futures also recommends asking the teen-directed questions such as:
- Have you been feeling sad? Had difficulty sleeping? Frequently irritable?
- Do you worry a lot or feel overly stressed out?
- Do you find that you have lost interest in things you used to enjoy doing?
- What do you do when you feel really down and depressed?

See Chapter 22 for additional questions and screening for and managing suicidality.

The sources of depression, suicidality, and nonsuicidal self-harm in young teens are multifactorial. Children with underlying ADHD or learning differences, family history of mood disorders, or traumatic or adverse experiences are more likely to develop depression and anxiety. Teens report multiple sources of stress including climate change, gun violence in communities and schools, harassment or negative content on social media, and family discord. Therefore interventions may need to take into account the sources of stress individual teens are experiencing.

Some young teens also start using substances or engaging in risky behaviors that can be addressed through motivational interviewing (see Chapter 25 for a detailed description of this approach) or connection with services or social supports. Clinicians can use the CRAFFT screening tool (see Chapter 23) to systematically review the use of substances or gather information through the SSHADESS interview. The SSHADESS (previously known as HEADSS) inventory is an excellent tool for ensuring a thorough psychosocial interview (see Table 21.3). When using this inventory to interview a teen, a clinician starts with questions that a teen is used to answering, those about home and school, and then proceeds to more sensitive questions about substance use, sex, abuse, and suicide. The idea is that over the course of the interview, teens will develop some level of trust that enables them to share more personal information with the clinician.

Confidentiality

Clinicians seeing adolescent patients must develop policies and procedures regarding confidentiality and the delivery of adolescent care. These policies will depend on local state laws and are discussed in depth in Chapter 22. Briefly, these should address when an adolescent can give informed consent and receive confidential care for the counseling and treatment of family planning and reproductive health issues, sexually transmitted infections, substance use, and mental health concerns. They must also outline situations in which confidentiality will be broken, for example, when a teenager discloses a history of abuse or if the teen is at risk of harming themselves or someone else (e.g., suicidal or homicidal ideation or personal neglect of a serious medical condition).

It is helpful to review confidentiality policies with both the teen patient and the parent around the 11- to 12-year visit for established patients and at the first visit for an adolescent patient new to the practice. Let them know that the teenager will be interviewed separately from the parent for at least a portion of the visit, and electronic health record portals will limit the parent's access to some details of care. Some parents also benefit from an opportunity to discuss their concerns privately with the clinician. Separate interviews not only enable the clinician to obtain sensitive information from the adolescent and parents in private but also emphasize the emerging independence of the pre-teen and help establish rapport.

Helping Teens Feel Comfortable

It is important to try to make the teenager feel comfortable. Adolescent clinics and school-based health centers are particularly adept at customizing the setting to the adolescent patient. If the setting is in a general pediatric practice, it is helpful to have a separate room that is age appropriate in which to interview and examine the teen patient. Clinic staff should have indications of the patient's gender identity in the medical record, so this can be affirmed during the rooming process. Reading materials, such as pamphlets, magazines, and posters geared toward adolescent issues should be provided. These materials, along with waiting and exam room artwork, should depict teens with a diversity of racial and ethnic backgrounds, gender identities, and sexual orientations. In this way, the teen may be more inclined to bring up sensitive issues or may even find answers to questions that were not addressed during the visit.

Sensitivity in Examination

The examination must be done with sensitivity and awareness of the young adolescent's self-consciousness and possible prior experiences of trauma. For example, the clinician should give clear directions concerning disrobing and gowning in preparation for a physical examination. The examination should be performed behind a drape or in a closed room with a chaperone regardless of the gender of the provider or patient.

Provide advance description of what will happen during the exam, such as "I'm going to listen to your heart first, then your lungs"—particularly during sensitive parts of the exam, and recognize that there may need to be modifications to the exam for youth with a history of trauma, sexual assault, or those who are transgender or experiencing gender dysphoria. To help teens understand their bodies and what clinicians are looking for during the physical exam, it can help to narrate what you are seeing, but without value-laden wording (e.g., avoid words like "normal" or "good"). Concomitantly, the healthcare provider must use active listening skills to pick up on the patient's underlying concerns. Showing interest along with giving nonjudgmental counseling also lets the teenage patient know that they are taken seriously.

ANTICIPATORY GUIDANCE FOR THE EARLY ADOLESCENT

Physical Development

Young teenagers need reassurance and education about their bodies. Explain the patterns of physical and sexual maturation, what is expected to come next and when. Many teens will have completed health classes in school or will have looked on the Internet for the answers to some of their questions, but they may still have gaps in knowledge or misunderstandings about what they have learned. It can be helpful to start by asking what they know, what

their questions are, and where they look for information. Common topics to cover include menstruation, masturbation and nocturnal emissions, and pubertal development of the opposite sex.

Sexual Activity and Reproductive Health

In early adolescence, one of the most important concepts to review is consent. This includes how to provide consent, self-advocate or reject unwanted advances, and how to recognize consent in the other person. For young teens who are sexually active, it is important to inquire about the age of their sexual partner or partners and any history of nonconsensual sex, sexual assault, or abuse. Provide resources about pregnancy, contraception, and prevention of sexually transmitted infections (see Chapter 22 for additional detail).

Tobacco, Alcohol, and Drugs

Early adolescence is an important time to begin conversations about tobacco, alcohol, and drugs, since their use may start in middle school. In the 2023 National Youth Tobacco Survey, 6.6% of middle schoolers reported using any tobacco product, with e-cigarettes ("vaping") the most popular form. According to YouGov data, about 12% of Americans say they had their first alcoholic drink before the age of 13. Similar rates (13%) of early marijuana initiation have been reported, and the earlier young teens start using marijuana, the less likely they are to graduate from high school. Year 2023 statistics show that 9% of 8th graders reported using illicit substances in the past month, and 21% had tried illicit drugs at least once.

Substance use in early adolescence may be due to multiple different factors. The healthcare clinician can build on their trusted relationships with teens to explore their motivations and identify related supports to help them stop or slow the progression of substance use. Some young teens may be using substances as a means of coping with stress, anxiety, or other mental health conditions. In these cases, validating their symptoms and desire to feel better, coupled with connection to available mental health treatments and support, may decrease or eliminate the need for self-medication. Other young teens may be following the behaviors of their peers or experimenting with use without consideration of the potential risk. Developmentally, the limited future-thinking or abstract thinking common at this age may make it difficult for them to wrap their heads around health risks that will occur decades from now, such as cancer, heart disease, and emphysema from tobacco. Stressing the short-term effects on health and functioning may be more effective. This might include how vaping impacts sport performance, how marijuana impacts thinking and concentration, or how other drugs impact impulse control, which could lead to situations the teen did not intend. It may also be impactful to discuss strategies that can be used to disagree with friends and peers who are engaged in risky behaviors. It also helps to point teens to resources such as the Partnership to End Addiction (see Recommended Readings).

Safety

Safety in the early adolescent years relies on both individual choices (e.g., wearing a helmet while biking or skiing) and systems-level factors (e.g., being able to afford equipment, access to safe outdoor space, living in a neighborhood where gun violence is prevalent). Therefore, promoting safety depends on equipping teens and families with knowledge, helping them find safe and supportive community-based after-school programs and other experiences, and advocating for systemic neighborhood and town- or city-level improvements that benefit children and families.

For many Black and Latino teens in the United States, safety is also threatened by violence at the hands of the police. A disproportionate number of teens from minority race/ethnicity report being stopped by police and about half these interactions are described by teens to be negative and disrespectful. Incidence of arrest and excessive use of police force are also disproportionately high among Black and Latino teens compared to white teens for the same activities, and according to the National Center for Health Statistics, between 2003 and 2018, Black children (most of them boys) were six times more likely to be killed by police than white children. To address this risk, many Black families address the topic with their children in what colloquially is called "the talk." Mooney and Zuckerman recommend an approach pediatric clinicians can take to "the talk" that starts with asking a question such as:

- Have you had any negative police interactions? If yes, probe those experiences to offer support; if no, provide positive support.
- Ask if they have talked about this topic with their parents. If yes, ask what they discussed. Either way, the clinician can say something like: "The police are there to help all of us, including you. But sometimes, you might feel like they are trying to harass or hurt you. This comes up for a lot of kids, and I want to help keep you safe."
- Three points should then be discussed: (1) knowing your legal rights around police; (2) remembering that your main goal is to get home safely, so speak politely, do not run, and show the police you are cooperating; and (3) it is not fair that you have to worry about negative police interactions.

Pediatric clinicians play an important role in acknowledging the stress that many families feel about this topic, and being a voice for advocacy around equitable and community-responsive law enforcement.

ANTICIPATORY GUIDANCE FOR PARENTS

Quest for Independence

Parents must be reassured that their teenager's quest for independence is normal and should not be interpreted as rejection of the family by the child. Give examples of this situation. For instance, young teenagers may not want to join the family on every family outing or may not want the parents at school or social functions in a chaperone capacity. If possible, another authority figure may do better. Young teens may begin to confide in an adult outside the family rather than their parents, possibly a change from previous years.

It is difficult at times to avoid arguing about trivial things, but it is best to concentrate on physical safety, basic hygiene, and school attendance when deciding which specific behavior to address. Parents of a teenager must maintain a delicate balance of providing parental monitoring while allowing the teen to stride toward independence.

Managing Media Use

Media use should be discussed with both teens and caregivers at the same time (not including the more sensitive SSHADESS questions, which should be asked to the teen alone). Many families find media to be a guilt-ridden topic that makes them anxious. Talking about it during a visit provides role-modeling for the caregiver of ways to discuss media that are curious and practical, not panicky or judgmental. It also provides an opportunity for the teen to contribute to problem solving about any issues that are identified.

Conversations should go deeper than "screen time." Like any health-related behavior, it is important to understand the *drivers* and *function* of social media use, smartphones, and video gaming, as well as their costs and benefits from the teen's perspective. Does the child use media to relieve stress or escape family arguments? To try to fall asleep? To find emotional support or feel understood? Because they feel anxious about missing out on something? Is there a lot of "friend drama" or competitive video gaming? Once these drivers are understood by the caregiver, it is easier to meet the teen "where they are" and make subsequent conversations easier. Clinicians should recommend:

- Regular open-minded conversations about technology and life. This could include how the parent feels overloaded with emails or social media stress, what types of funny or inspirational things they are seeing online, and when tech use is feeling out of balance. Topics could also include privacy, safety, witnessing or responding to harassment, seeing misinformation or dehumanizing content, influencers, and unrealistic beauty standards.

- It is important for caregivers and teens to reflect on their *emotional drivers* of media use, and their *emotional reactions* to media use—whether positive or negative. This will help teens tease out what parts of their digital life are a net positive, and which ones they can get rid of or take a break from.
- In the early teen years, it helps to have more oversight and use of parental controls that filter out age-inappropriate content or contacts with strangers. Once teens demonstrate more responsibility and kindness online, oversight can be loosened—but conversations should continue.
- Set devices, video game consoles, and social media accounts to "do not disturb" at night and at other times the family agrees upon, such as mealtimes.
- To encourage more intentional use, set time limits so that media does not crowd out other activities. What is more important is *setting periods of non-tech-use*—for caregivers and children/teens—so that there are opportunities to get outside, play sports or a board game, and have conversations.
- When media use is becoming problematic (e.g., leading to lots of arguments, getting in the way of sleep or activities, the only way a teen calms down, compulsive use), tell the pediatrician. Iinterventions could include taking a break from a particular app or game, keeping devices out of room at night, and teens changing what content they see, games they play, or who they follow on social media.
- Overall, encourage conversations to stay nonjudgmental so that kids can feel comfortable coming to caregivers with negative online experiences.

Many parents wonder about the right age for a social media account. Research suggests that it is better to wait until children are teenagers and not be dishonest about age. Although the official age is 13, some teens may not need or not be emotionally ready for access to one or several social media accounts. Teen girls between 13 and 15 years of age in particular may struggle more with social comparison and body image on social media—therefore messaging and videochat apps may be better "starter" experiences for young teens. Whenever an account is made, caregivers should help teens with privacy, content, and do-not-disturb settings and check in regularly about how teens are feeling about their relationship with social media.

! HEADS UP—11 TO 14 YEARS

Chronic Illness

A teenager who has a chronic illness, such as immune deficiency, cystic fibrosis, diabetes, or sickle cell anemia, may have delayed or atypical psychosocial development because of dependence on parental support, medical personnel, and therapeutic regimens. Physical development, including puberty, may also be delayed secondary to the disease process. With the limitations imposed by the illness, either physically or mentally, adolescence can be a difficult time for a child with a chronic disease. Independence, a positive body image, and a supportive peer group may be difficult to obtain. As a result, some adolescents with a chronic illness may become depressed, angry with parents and medical staff, and less adherent with medical therapy. Teens with a mental health condition may experience similar problems with obtaining independence and healthy self-esteem. Adolescents with a serious, chronic health condition often require mental health counseling for support and assistance with adjustment.

Challenges With School Adjustment

Children who are adjusting poorly to middle school after 6 weeks often benefit from a psychological and/or educational assessment. Such assessment may lead to an individual education plan, tutoring, or counseling. Declining school performance should never be attributed to benign causes or be played down with a "let's just watch how things go" statement.

Social Challenges

Middle school can be a period of increased social demands that are difficult for some children to navigate—for example, those with autism spectrum disorder, ADHD, anxiety, or trauma history. Additional help is available through schools (e.g., social skills groups), outpatient therapy centers, or local clubs/groups where children can meet others with similar interests (e.g., robotics, role-playing games, and LEGOs). Chapter 20 provides additional details on challenges and supports of social skills.

Family Conflict

Families that have persistent conflict may need additional sessions to identify areas of disagreement and to develop strategies to improve mutual respect and functioning. Family counseling may be indicated and may bring significant insight and improvement in family function, collaborative problem solving, and boundaries. Some turbulence is expected in all families, but a decline in functioning or prolonged conflict is not to be expected.

ACKNOWLEDGMENTS

Caitlin Camfield contributed to the section on body image and obesity. Alessandra Angelino and Shaquita Bell provided an initial review and feedback on this chapter.

RECOMMENDED READINGS

For Clinicians

Bonifacio JH, Maser C, Stadelman K, Palmert M. Management of gender dysphoria in adolescents in primary care. *CMAJ*. 2019;191(3):E69–75.

Nesi J, Telzer A, Prinstein MJ. *Handbook of adolescent digital media and mental health*. Cambridge University Press; 2022. https://www.cambridge.org/core/books/handbook-of-adolescent-digital-media-use-and-mental-health/91853243C8B7900B46EA26C3570577B2.

American Psychological Association: *American Psychological Association Health Advisory on social media use in adolescence*. https://www.apa.org/topics/social-media-internet/health-advisory-adolescent-social-media-use

Goldenring JM, Rosen DS:. Getting into adolescent heads: an essential update. *Contemp Pediatr*. 2004;21:64.

Adolescent Health Initiative: https://umhs-adolescenthealth.org

The Gender Unicorn: https://transstudent.org/gender/

Cornell Research Program on Self-Injury and Recovery: Non-suicidal self-injury resources. https://www.selfinjury.bctr.cornell.edu/resources.html.

Substance Use and Mental Health Services Administration: *Prevention of substance use and mental disorders*. https://www.samhsa.gov/find-help/prevention#resources-publications.

American Academy of Child & Adolescent Psychiatry: *Resources for youth*. https://www.aacap.org/AACAP/Families_and_Youth/Resource_Centers/Depression_Resource_Center/Resources_for_Youth_Depression.aspx

National Eating Disorders Association: *Eating Disorders Helpline | Chat, Call, or Text*. NEDA. https://www.nationaleatingdisorders.org/get-help/.

Center for Excellence of Transgender Health: http://transhealth.ucsf.edu

For Parents and Teens

McCoy K, Wibbelsman C:. *Life happens: a teenager's guide to friends, failure, sexuality, love, rejection, addiction, peer pressure, families, loss, depression, change and other challenges of living*. New York, Berkeley; 1996.

McCoy K, Wibbelsman C:. *The teenage body book*. New York: Perigee; 2016.

Aggarwal S, Darpinian S, Sterling W. *No weigh! A teen's guide to positive body image, food, and emotional wisdom*. Jessica Kingsley Publishers; 2018.

Weinstein E, James C. *Behind their screens: what teens are facing (and adults are missing)*. Boston: MIT Press; 2022.

Green R. *The explosive child*. ed 6. New York: Harper; 2021.

Faber A, Mazlish E. *How to talk so your kids will listen and listen so your kids will talk*. New York: Avon Books; 1980.

Harris K. *Life skills for teens: how to cook, clean, manage money, fix your car, perform first aid, and just about everything in between*. Spotlight Media; 2021.

Harris RH. *It's perfectly normal: changing bodies, growing up, sex and sexual health*. Cambridge: Candlewick Press; 1996.

Madaras L, Madaras A. *My body, my self for boys*. Revised ed 2. New York: New Market Press; 2007.

Madaras L, Madaras A. Revised *My Body, My Self for Girls*. ed 2. New York: New Market Press; 2007.

Madaras L, Madaras A. Revised ed *The "What's happening to my body?" Book for boys: a growing-up guide for parents and sons*. New York: New Market Press; 2007.

Madaras L, Madaras A. Revised ed *The "what's happening to my body?" book for girls: a growing-up guide for parents and daughters*. New York: New Market Press; 2007.

Damour Lisa. *The emotional lives of teenagers: raising connected, capable, and compassionate adolescents*. New York: Ballantine Books; 2023.

Jensen F, Ellis.Nutt A. *The Teenage brain: a neuroscientist's survival guide to raising adolescents and young adults*. New York: HarperCollins; 2015.

Harris RH, Emberley M. *It's perfectly normal: a book about changing bodies, growing up, sex and sexual health*. ed 3. Somerville: Candlewick Press; 2009.

Natterson C, Masse J. *The care & keeping of you 2: the body book for older girls*. American Girl; 2012.

Websites

For Parents

Facts For Families. aacap.org. Excellent site that provides fact sheets on adolescent and mental health issues from the American Academy of Child and Adolescent Psychiatry. English/Spanish. https://www.aacap.org/AACAP/Families_Youth/Facts-for-Families/AACAP/Families_and_Youth/Facts_for_Families/Layout/FFF_Guide-01.aspx?hkey=fd45e409-3c3c-44ae-b5d4-39ba12e644b7

Resources & Tools—Advocates for Youth. An excellent site providing anticipatory guidance for parents on adolescents. https://www.advocatesforyouth.org/resources-tools/?_sft_type=fact-sheets

PFLAG—Parents, Families and Friends of Lesbians and Gays. https://pflag.org/

https://www.cdc.gov/parents/teens/

www.understood.org/en/articles/iep-transition-planning-preparing-for-young-adulthood

Center for Parent and Teen Communication: www.parentandteen.com

Society for Adolescent Health and Medicine, Resources for Parents and Adolescents https://adolescenthealth.org/resources/resources-for-adolescents-and-parents/

AAP Center of Excellence on Social Media and Youth Mental Health: www.aap.org/socialmedia

For Teens

https://youngwomenshealth.org/

https://youngmenshealthsite.org/

The Trevor Project: https://thetrevorproject.org

Bedsider (Birth control, sexual health and wellness): www.bedsider.org

This is Quitting: This is Quitting (https://truthinitiative.org/this is quitting)

www.drugfree.org—Partnership to End Addiction

http://www.iwannaknow.org—Information from the American Social Health Association for teens on sexuality, sexual transmitted infections and related topics with a parent's guide and great links.

http://www.kidshealth.org/ teen—A great site for teens on health with separate sections geared toward boys and girls. From the Nemours Foundation.

Suicidality and Non-Suicidal Self-Injury: https://www.crisistextline.org

Society for Adolescent Health and Medicine: Resources for Parents and Adolescents: https://adolescenthealth.org/resources/resources-for-adolescents-and-parents/

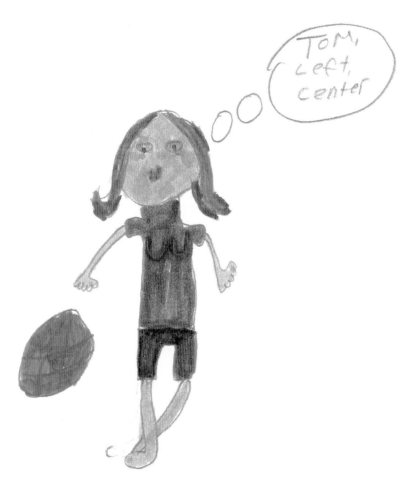

A middle schooler shows her sports competence. Her partner on the court is a boy. By a girl, age 12.

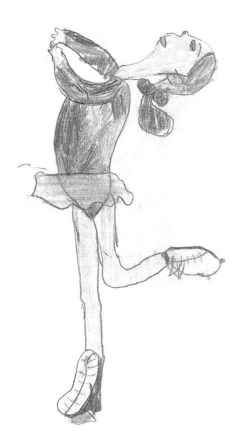

This artist is working on profiles, three dimensions, body movement, and a changing image of the age. By MD, age 11.

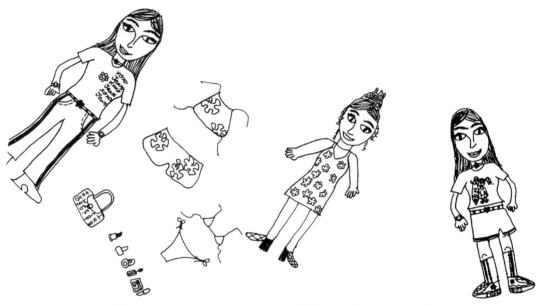

"Dressing for school, party and beach." By Sarah Stein, age 11.

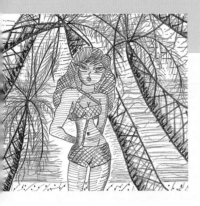

22

Fifteen to Seventeen Years: Mid-Adolescence—Redefining Self

Caitlin Camfield, Yolanda N. Evans, and Alana K. Otto

KEYWORDS

- Self-image
- Disordered eating
- Sexual activity
- Sexual orientation
- Sexual abuse, assault, exploitation, and trafficking
- Contraception
- Sexually transmitted infections
- Risky behavior
- Substance use
- Depression
- Anxiety
- Suicide
- Confidentiality

Mid-adolescence typically spans the ages of 15 to 17 years. The major developmental task of mid-adolescence is identity development, including the critical task of developing a sense of self as independent from one's caregiver(s). This chapter describes the cognitive, emotional, and social development experienced by young people in the heart of adolescence. Exploring one's values, establishing relationships with friends and romantic partners, and navigating changing relationships with caregivers are prominent themes during these years.

MID-ADOLESCENT DEVELOPMENTAL CONCEPTS

Cognitive and Moral Development

Mid-adolescence is characterized by marked cognitive development. Most neurotypical mid-adolescents develop the capacity for **abstract thinking** and introspection.

Previous edition authors: Jennifer Maehr and Marianne E. Felice.

In other words, they become capable of logical thinking, deduction, and conjecture and able to reflect on their own thought processes in an "objective" manner. This stage of cognitive development is known as **formal operational thinking** in the framework of Piaget (see Chapter 2) and is a giant step in mental development. At this age, adolescents are developing the ability to think about their own thoughts (e.g., notice when they are distracted; also called **metacognition**), build self-management skills at home and at school, reflect on their feelings (e.g., recognize when they might have overreacted), and adapt their behavior based on feedback. Some adolescents struggle with these self-regulatory processes and may need support from therapists, caregivers, and teachers to develop them.

With the development of abstract thinking, mid-adolescents have new capacities for moral decision-making. In the Kohlberg theory of moral development, young children (age 3–7) are in the first (or "preconventional") stage of moral development, in which good behavior results in reward and misbehavior results in punishment (see Chapter 2 regarding behavioral theories). Hence, "good" or "bad" behaviors are defined solely by their consequences. The second (or "conventional") stage of moral development, which occurs around age 8 to 13, is marked by the need to meet the expectations or follow the rules of one's family, peer group, or community. In fact, maintaining the rules of the group becomes a value in itself for a child in mid-childhood. The third and final stage of moral development is defined by the development of more autonomous moral principles that have validity apart from the authority of the group and are based on the individual's own beliefs and conclusions concerning what is right or wrong. This is called adult, or "postconventional," morality. This stage usually begins in mid-adolescence, but it is not completed until young adulthood, and the timing of its development varies between individuals.

A mid-adolescent may be capable of making moral judgments based on the principles of what they believe is

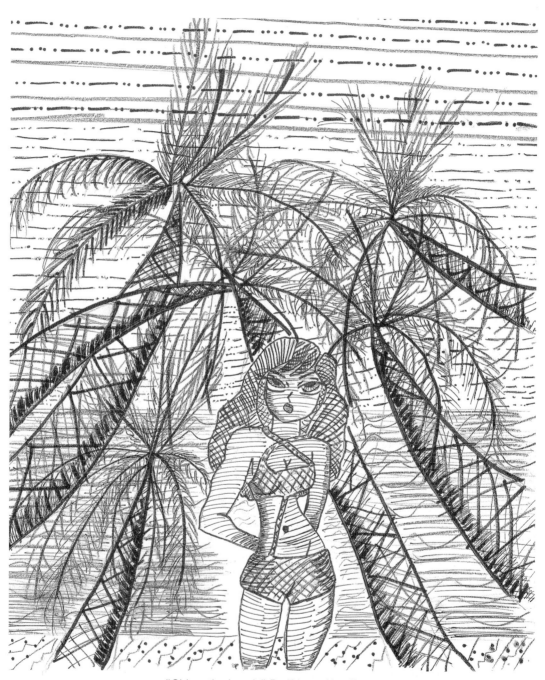

"Girl on the beach." By Kristen Hamilton.

"right" and "wrong," but they may continue to take part in **risky behaviors** due to their evolving impulse control. The prefrontal cortex, which is responsible for executive functions such as prioritizing tasks, planning, analyzing options and consequences, and controlling urges, is the last part of the brain to fully mature and continues to develop into young adulthood. It is hypothesized that teens may be more likely to engage in emotion-driven decision-making because of the relatively reduced maturity of the prefrontal cortex (which communicates closely with the amygdala, the emotion center of the brain) compared to other parts of the brain. As teens mature and approach adulthood, the prefrontal cortex becomes more involved in decision-making processes. Until then, the pediatrician can help guide families on establishing positive health routines (e.g., sleep, physical activity, healthy eating) from an earlier age, so that these behaviors are more internalized and automatic for the developing adolescent. In addition, it can be helpful for caregivers and mid-adolescents to discuss, and plan for, situations in which a teen might make an impulsive or emotional decision, such as those related to sexual relationships, substance use, or conflict with peers. Finally, establishing open, nonjudgmental communication patterns between caregivers and teens can help adolescents understand that they can come to the adults in their life to discuss difficult decisions or mistakes.

Social Development

Mid-adolescence is also marked by changing relationships with friends and other peers. During this time, friendships typically evolve from play- or activity-based relationships, as are common among younger children, into those based on shared values. As peer relationships become more important and meaningful in mid-adolescence, many teens spend less time with their families and more time with friends. For many mid-adolescents, maturing friendships provide support and connectedness in addition to that provided by family. During this period, one's social standing, for example, at school, may become intensely important to a teen. Interactions with friends and peers allow adolescents to develop communication, negotiation, problem-solving, and conflict resolution skills. Mid-adolescents may also develop romantic attraction and have romantic relationships with peers (see "Sexual Development and Sexuality").

Most mid-adolescents attend school; in the United States, adolescents in this age range are typically in high school (9th–12th grades). During this time, adolescents may discover new or heightened interests and talents in varying disciplines such as the arts or sports; these interests often support the development of a positive self-image and provide an outlet for personal expression. They also provide a means by which a teen can transfer internal feelings and struggles into something concrete and positive. Teachers and coaches can provide valuable insight into the important developmental work being done by teens as they participate in these activities and are often among the first adults to notice when a teen is struggling and in need of help. Mid-adolescents may find a particular teacher or coach to serve as an important mentor in their lives.

Many teens will obtain employment or volunteer for the first time during mid-adolescence. Some do so out of financial necessity, others as part of their education, and some by their own choice. Potential positive effects of employment or regular volunteering during adolescence include a sense of accomplishment and responsibility, job experience that enhances the probability of future employment, and social skills that come from working with others. Employment allows teens greater independence from parents, which fosters important developmental growth. However, employment during the mid-adolescent period may also have downsides. Excessive work hours during adolescence can have a negative impact on school performance and/or sleep. Adolescence is also an age when trafficking—for child labor or sexual exploitation—begins. Teens from minoritized communities, particularly Native American or refugee populations, are more likely to be exploited for labor or sex work purposes. It is crucial to recognize signs of potential trafficking (see Chapter 23, Box 23.1) during clinical encounters.

Adolescents may also become interested in civic or societal issues, including climate change, gun violence, and reproductive justice. This is an important aspect of identity development as teens develop their values, competence in helping others, and critical thinking about online information/debates.

Physical Development and Self-image

Nearly all mid-adolescents have begun puberty, and many have completed or nearly completed puberty by this stage; however, many mid-adolescents are still adjusting to the physical changes of puberty. As mid-adolescents embark on the key developmental task of identity formation, it is normative for them to explore and experiment with different aspects of their appearance, for example, hairstyles, makeup, body modifications (e.g., tattoos, piercings), and/or fashion, to express themselves. Identity exploration also occurs through social media platforms that allow expression of emotions, physical appearance, or skills (e.g., dancing, singing). This experimentation is expected and is evidence of developmental work; it is important for pediatric providers to help caregivers support their adolescent's autonomy and exploration and help teens reflect on their identity-related experiences, including which experiences feel authentic versus performative.

Unfortunately, society's preoccupation with physical perfection of the human body can derail adolescents from attaining a positive sense of self and acceptance of their recent physical changes. Youth are bombarded by images of thin, attractive, muscular people as well as advertisements for plastic surgery, cosmetic procedures, fad diets, and weight-loss drugs. Some social media influencers are very appearance focused, describing their experience with Botox, lip fillers, and other cosmetic procedures. Many content creators also use video filters or photo editing to portray a more idealized physical appearance. This leads to unrealistic beauty standards that young people describe as leading to significant body comparisons and feelings of inadequacy or contributing to **disordered eating** (see "Disordered Eating").

THE EVOLVING ROLE OF CAREGIVERS

As mid-adolescents develop their self-identity, they are characteristically ambivalent about their relationships with parents. Having already progressed through early adolescence, they have declared their need for independence in one way or another. Mid-adolescence may be a time in which the adolescent occasionally seeks closer engagement with their caregivers and at other times completely rejects offers of help and feels smothered by parental intrusiveness. This push and pull of the adolescent-caregiver relationship is normal but can be confusing and disheartening for caregivers.

Caregivers should be encouraged to remain a constant, consistent presence and source of support in their adolescent's life; to be willing to be a sounding board for their teenager's ideas; and to set and enforce consistent boundaries. Supportive communication, supervision, and availability from caregivers are associated with positive identity formation and the development of skills critical for the transition to adulthood.

SEXUAL DEVELOPMENT AND SEXUALITY

Sexual Activity and Consent

For many teens, mid-adolescence is marked by the emergence of sexual and romantic interests, and approximately half of mid-adolescents report they have dated or been in a romantic relationship. Although specific data vary, it is estimated that approximately one-quarter of 15-year-olds and one-half of 17-year-olds in the United States have had sexual intercourse. This may include vaginal, oral, or anal intercourse. Although sexual activity among adolescents is often viewed by medical providers—and society more broadly—as pathologic, sexuality is a fundamental part of being human, and romantic and sexual relationships can be an important part of an adolescent's development. Engaging in romantic and sexual relationships is one way in which adolescents explore their identities and build skills necessary for a successful adulthood, including communication, negotiation, and self-advocacy. Teens in this age group start to learn to manage sexual feelings in a healthy, responsible, and age- and culturally appropriate way. In addition, they are learning to define their own identity within romantic and sexual relationships, including defining their expectations surrounding healthy partnerships. Notably, while the emergence of sexual and romantic attraction—and exploration of romantic and sexual relationships—are common among mid-adolescents, not all teens experience sexual attraction, are interested in intimate interpersonal relationships, or engage in sexual activity.

As adolescents navigate new relationships, both romantic and sexual, they will be faced with opportunities to both obtain and give consent. Conversations around bodily autonomy and consent are ideally started early in childhood and reinforced in age-appropriate ways as children develop. These conversations should involve educating adolescents on how to give consent as well as the importance of obtaining enthusiastic consent from sexual partners. Caregivers and medical providers are important sources of information on these topics. Teens in mid-adolescence may feel pressured to engage in sexual contact and have had limited experience communicating their boundaries. For many adolescents, these challenges are compounded by the need to simultaneously navigate the additional developmental tasks of exploring new relationships, including navigating norms around sex and engaging in discussions about intimacy with others. It is important that teens have trusted adults with whom they can communicate in an open and nonjudgmental manner as they explore their own romantic relationships.

Conversations with, and anticipatory guidance from, pediatric providers can be particularly valuable as adolescents learn to face potential challenges in their relationships; for example, a provider might help a teen develop a "script" for responding to a partner who does not want to use condoms. Motivational interviewing (described in more detail in Chapter 25) can be a helpful tool for adolescents who wish to change sexual behaviors, for example, to increase the frequency of condom use or improve adherence to an oral contraceptive pill, by empowering teens to self-identify next steps that will be most effective for them. While many providers have been taught to focus solely on mitigating the negative consequences of sex instead of emphasizing the positive aspects of sexual relationships, by asking about sexual pleasure, providers can obtain important information about sexual dysfunction and relationship dynamics and gain an opportunity for additional counseling. Sexual intercourse should be a pleasurable experience for all partners involved, and educating adolescents about this expectation can help individuals advocate for themselves if sexual intercourse is ever associated with physical or emotional pain.

Conversations with providers about sexuality and sexual activity are important for teens who are not having sex as well. Providers can support choices that positively influence health and provide anticipatory guidance regarding relationships, which may encourage adolescents to reach out to their healthcare provider with questions or concerns if and when they become sexually active.

LGB+ Youth

As many as 15% of high schoolers identify as lesbian, gay, or bisexual (LGB), and an additional 9% identify as something other than straight or LGB or are unsure of their sexual orientation. The word(s) a teen uses to describe their sexual orientation may change over time, and sexual orientation may not always reflect one's sexual practices. For example, a teen may identify as bisexual but only have experience with romantic or sexual partners of one sex. Alternatively, one may identify as "straight" or heterosexual but have a sexual history involving same-sex partners. Teens may also identify as asexual or "ace," meaning they experience minimal sexual attraction, or experience attraction but have low or no desire to engage in sexual contact. However, it is important to note that even those who identify as asexual may still engage in sexual activity or be in intimate relationships.

Teens who are LGB+ are more likely than their heterosexual peers to experience mental health challenges, substance use, and disordered eating and to attempt suicide. These risks are primarily related to stigma and discrimination against LGB+ people, and consistent evidence has shown that LGB+ teens in supportive environments have mental health outcomes comparable to heterosexual youth. Unsupportive caregiving environments are also associated with increased rates of homelessness, which may leave youth desperate to obtain resources necessary to survive. Indeed, LGB+ youth are more likely to be involved in human trafficking than their heterosexual peers. This further emphasizes the importance of love and acceptance as adolescents develop their sexual identities.

Unfortunately, many LGB+ youth may be afraid to trust their healthcare provider because of fears about judgment, rejection, and breach of confidentiality. Teens may receive signals directly from the clinician or indirectly from the atmosphere in the office that—rightly or erroneously—tell them the provider would not be supportive of their identities or behaviors. It is critical to create clinical environments that positively support, and foster discussion about, topics related to sex and sexuality, including LGB+ sexual orientations. Signage, posters, visible brochures, and the availability of referral resources that support LGB+ youth can indicate to adolescents they are welcome and supported in the clinical space. Pediatricians should also ask questions regarding sex and sexuality because the topics may not be broached by mid-adolescents themselves. The clinician should be ready to discuss these topics with the adolescent patient in a nonjudgmental fashion. This means the provider must be comfortable with their own sexuality, as well as comfortable with and knowledgeable about the subject of sex. Clinicians must be aware of their own limitations and biases in this area and not impose their viewpoints on an adolescent patient. Pediatricians should also be aware of local, national, and online resources to support LGB+ youth and their families.

Sexual and Reproductive Health

Adolescent reproductive health is often defined in negative terms, for example, the absence of sexually transmitted infections (STIs) or the avoidance of pregnancy. There is also generally a focus on reproduction, that is, pregnancy (or, more commonly for adolescents, the prevention of pregnancy), while sexual health topics such as sexual function and pleasure are minimized or intentionally avoided. A more holistic view frames adolescent sexual and reproductive health as a positive state of physical and emotional well-being versus simply the absence of disease and acknowledges the importance of sexual satisfaction. Conceptualizing sexual and reproductive health in this way lends itself to a strengths-based approach to care, which frames adolescent sexuality as normal and normative and focuses on supporting adolescents in exploring and working toward their own goals related to health, sexuality, relationships, and family planning.

Preventing pregnancy is an important goal for some, but not all, adolescents. Pediatric providers should not assume all sexually active adolescents want or need contraception, or that all pregnancies are unintended or unwanted. All adolescents—not just those with uteruses—may be interested in, and benefit from, information about contraception. Conversations about birth control and pregnancy should be approached in a spirit of humble inquiry and start by exploring the individual adolescent's values, priorities, and goals. Preferences regarding contraception vary widely, and there is no single method, or class of methods, that is "best" for all adolescents. Contraceptive counseling (for adolescents who want it) should therefore be a collaborative process, with the pediatrician acknowledging the patient's expertise regarding their own body, experiences, preferences, and goals; providing medical information about each method; and supporting the patient in choosing the method that best meets their needs. The Centers for Disease Control (CDC) publishes Medical Eligibility Criteria for Contraceptive Use as guidance for providers to determine which methods are safe for a particular patient. Patient-facing information about contraceptive options may be found at bedsider.org.

Providers must be mindful of the ways their implicit and explicit biases about adolescent sexuality, pregnancy, and parenting influence their practices around contraception. Adolescents and young adults of color have described feeling pressured by providers to use birth control and to choose certain methods, particularly long-acting reversible contraceptives such as intrauterine devices and implants. Patients who feel pressured are less likely to trust their providers or to return for future care. Also of note is that adolescents with disabilities are often infantilized by their families and healthcare providers, who may erroneously assume they are asexual and/or aromantic and do not need information or care related to sexual and reproductive health. Providers must be prepared to provide developmentally appropriate anticipatory guidance, advice, and care related to sexual and reproductive health for adolescents with disabilities. For all adolescents, providers should strive to maximize sexual well-being and autonomy with a goal of achieving reproductive justice—that is, the full realization of the rights to decide if, when, how, and with whom to have children, or not to have children, the dismantling of systems and policies that either intentionally or unintentionally limit or devalue the reproduction of certain people, and the promotion of equity and justice.

Adolescents who become pregnant may present to healthcare providers to learn about options, including parenting, adoption, and abortion. Providers should be prepared to counsel adolescents about these options and provide referrals, for example, to prenatal care or termination services, as needed. Pediatricians may also be an important source of support, as well as connections to concrete resources, for pregnant and parenting adolescents. Again, providers must be mindful of their biases around adolescent pregnancy and parenting and approach the care of these patients in a supportive, nonjudgmental way.

Sexually active adolescents should be informed that barrier methods, such as condoms, are the only method (other than abstinence) that can prevent bacterial STIs and can be used in conjunction with other contraceptives. Adolescents are disproportionately affected by STIs, and many STIs are asymptomatic, especially in males. For these reasons, routine screening for STIs, including HIV, is recommended for all sexually active adolescents and young adults. Both adolescents and providers may erroneously believe LGB+ teens are at low risk for STIs. For all adolescents, a careful history, inquiring about an individual's partners and practices, will guide the provider to order the appropriate tests, obtained from the appropriate sites (e.g., genitourinary tract, rectum, pharynx). Providers should take care

to ask open-ended questions and avoid assumptions about an adolescent's sexuality or sexual practices—for example, asking "who are you attracted to?" instead of "are you attracted to men or women?" (see SSHADESS/HEADSS Assessment below for more information).

Some adolescents are candidates for HIV preexposure prophylaxis, commonly called PrEP, which can significantly reduce the risk of HIV. Indications for use, and detailed guidance on the use of these medications, have been published by the US CDC.

Sexual Abuse and Assault

Not all sexual activity in adolescence is consensual. Teens may be victims or perpetrators of **sexual violence**, including **abuse** and **assault**. Child sexual abuse is a type of child abuse (i.e., intentional harm to a child) that includes any type of sexual activity, which may or may not involve direct sexual contact. Healthcare providers are mandated by law to report cases of actual or suspected child sexual abuse, including any contact or conduct of a sexual nature between a minor and a person responsible for the child's welfare, such as a relative, caregiver, teacher, or coach. Providers must be aware of the specific reporting requirements of their state.

The term sexual assault refers to any sexual contact or behavior that occurs without explicit consent, including sexual activity with a person who is legally unable to consent, such as a mentally or physically impaired person, intoxicated or drugged person, or a child/adolescent under the age of consent as specified by state law. Legal definitions of specific crimes differ by state. Statutory rape refers to sexual contact where there is an age discrepancy between two partners, typically when an adult has sex with an adolescent who is younger than a specified age as set by state law or who is more than a specific number of years younger than the older partner. The rationale behind statutory rape laws is that until a certain age, adolescents are unable to consent to sex and need to be protected from predatory adults. In some states, healthcare providers must report statutory rape; again, providers must be familiar with reporting requirements in their state.

Adolescents have the highest rates of sexual assault victimization of any age group. When compared with their adult counterparts, adolescent rape victims are more likely to have used or been given alcohol or drugs before the assault. Adolescents are also more likely than adults to delay medical care after an assault. Sexual abuse and assault are associated with significant morbidity, including depressive symptoms, anxiety, and substance use, and therefore identification by and support from the clinical team are essential. Pediatricians should be familiar with local, national, and online resources for victims and survivors of sexual violence and able to provide, or refer to, appropriate medical services, that is, emergency contraception or testing for STIs.

MENTAL HEALTH

Disordered Eating

Up to one-third of adolescents report being self-conscious about their weight, even if they are not overweight. As a result, teens may exercise, restrict dietary intake, use medications and herbal remedies, and/or purge to try to change their weight. Social media content and "pro-anorexia" websites may further promote negative body image and provide strategies for restricting food and calories as well as hiding these behaviors from others. These dietary practices and attempts to lose weight can result in inadequate intake of the calories and nutrients required during adolescence. While some focus on body shape and its modification is expected during this developmental stage, an **eating disorder** is characterized by behaviors related to eating that result in malnutrition or other negative health consequences, significant psychological distress, and/or functional impairment. Despite common stereotypes about eating disorders, these disorders affect people of all socioeconomic statuses, races/ethnicities, and sexes.

Perhaps the most well known—although not most common—eating disorder is anorexia nervosa, which is characterized by intentional dietary restriction leading to significant weight loss, an intense fear of weight gain, and distorted body image (i.e., a perception of one's self as "fat" or overweight despite one's weight loss or underweight status). Anorexia nervosa may be categorized into restricting or binge-eating/purging subtypes; individuals with the latter engage in self-induced vomiting or misuse of diuretics, laxatives, or enemas in addition to restriction. Notably, some patients with anorexia nervosa have weights or body mass indices (BMI) in the normal, overweight, or obese ranges by population standards despite significant weight loss; the term "atypical anorexia nervosa" is used in the *Diagnostic and Statistical Manual of Mental Disorders, Fifth Edition* (DSM-5) to refer to these patients. Atypical anorexia nervosa is often missed or dismissed by providers, both because providers may be unaware that eating disorders—and their sequelae—can affect individuals in larger bodies, and because of biases and stereotypes about how eating disorders present. Diagnosis is critical, as atypical anorexia nervosa can lead to the same medical and psychological consequences as anorexia nervosa.

Eating disorders that do not lead to weight loss or are not associated with intense fear of gaining weight include binge-eating disorder and bulimia nervosa. With binge eating disorder, individuals eat more food than would be expected for a typical person during a distinct period of time, cannot control how much is eaten, and experience marked distress regarding the binge eating. Bulimia nervosa is defined by binge-eating episodes followed by compensatory behaviors such as purging, misuse of medications such as laxatives, or exercise.

Not all eating disorders leading to weight loss are associated with distorted body image; for example, avoidant/restrictive food intake disorder (ARFID) involves food avoidance based on the sensory qualities of food or fear of adverse consequences of eating (e.g., choking or vomiting). The restriction of intake in ARFID leads to significant weight loss, malnutrition, and/or reliance on nutrition supplements to meet one's caloric needs. ARFID is more likely than anorexia nervosa, binge-eating disorder, or bulimia nervosa to present in young or prepubertal children but may present in adolescents as well.

Estimates vary by study, but the lifetime prevalence of anorexia nervosa is estimated to be between 0.5% and 2%, and the lifetime prevalence of bulimia nervosa is estimated to be between 0.9% and 3%. The incidences of both disorders peak during middle adolescence, and both have high mortality rates compared to other psychiatric disorders. Eating disorders are multifactorial, with no single cause; risk factors for the development of an eating disorder include female sex, puberty (particularly early pubertal development), LGB+ or gender-diverse identity, perfectionism, chronic health conditions requiring dietary control (e.g., diabetes), and a family history of eating disorder. It can be easy to overlook eating disorders in males, who represent between 10% and 25% of eating disorder cases. Certain sports are associated with an increased risk of developing eating disorders, including dance, gymnastics, figure skating, swimming, diving, running, cycling, and those with weight requirements such as wrestling, crew, and weightlifting. Teens with eating disorders commonly have other coexisting mental health problems such as depression, anxiety disorders, and obsessive-compulsive disorder. Because of this complexity, adolescents with eating disorders should be referred to an interdisciplinary treatment team with experience and expertise treating adolescents with eating disorders. Caregivers are particularly important allies in the treatment of eating disorders, and evidence strongly supports a family-based model of care with support from the interdisciplinary professional team.

Anxiety and Mood Disorders

A significant proportion of adolescents will meet diagnostic criteria for an **anxiety disorder** and/or **major depressive disorder** at some point during high school. Anxiety disorders are the most prevalent psychiatric diagnoses among children and adolescents, occurring in approximately one-quarter of adolescents. The most common anxiety disorders among adolescents include generalized anxiety disorder and social anxiety disorder. Anxiety disorders are associated with poor educational achievement and school absenteeism. Additionally, many adolescents with anxiety disorders experience physical symptoms (e.g., abdominal pain, nausea, headaches), which may compound school absenteeism and lead to frequent medical visits. The treatment of adolescent anxiety disorders involves psychotherapy and/or medications (e.g., selective serotonin reuptake inhibitors, or SSRIs). Patients and families should also be educated that avoidance of anxiety-provoking situations (e.g., school, social situations) only perpetuates the anxiety and that exposure is a critical part of treatment.

Symptoms of depression include sad or depressed mood; anhedonia (decreased interest or pleasure in activities); apathy; lack of motivation; feelings of guilt, worthlessness, hopelessness, and/or thoughts of death; poor sleep; poor or increased appetite; and difficulty concentrating. In adolescents, particularly adolescent boys, a sad or depressed mood may present as irritability or anger. Parents of adolescents with depression commonly report that their teens have become isolated and/or quit activities (e.g., sports) that were previously important to them. A decline in school performance may occur. Many people with depression experience physical symptoms, such as fatigue. Some patients with depression also experience suicidal ideation and/or nonsuicidal self-injury (NSSI; see below). A diagnosis of major depressive disorder requires the presence of five or more of the above symptoms (one of which must be depressed mood or anhedonia) for a period of at least 2 weeks.

Several self-reported depression screening tools have been developed and can be used with adolescents, including the Patient Health Questionnaire-2 (PHQ-2, a two-question tool) and the Patient Health Questionnaire-9 (PHQ-9, an expanded version of the PHQ-2 with nine questions—Box 22.1). Notably, these are not diagnostic instruments, and a positive screen does not necessarily mean a diagnosis of depression but indicates a need for further assessment.

The treatment of major depressive disorder in adolescents typically involves psychotherapy and/or medication. Data indicate both can be effective, but symptom relief occurs most quickly when treatment involves a combination of both therapy and medication. SSRIs are generally recommended as first line when medication is indicated. There appears to be a significant placebo effect with all medications used to treat depression. Patients and families should be counseled that it may take several weeks for an SSRI to take effect. As with any medication, providers should discuss all potential risks of SSRIs, which includes a black box warning in adolescents due to evidence of increased suicidality amongst young people taking these medications. The presence of this warning remains controversial, however, and must be weighed against risks of not starting a medication for depression.

Suicidal Behavior and Self-Harm

The phrase "suicidal behavior" describes a spectrum of thoughts and behaviors ranging from thoughts of death or suicide ("suicidal ideation") without intent or action to completed suicide. Rates of death by suicide among children and adolescents have increased dramatically over the last several decades, and suicide is now a leading cause of death among adolescents in the United States. Hypotheses as to the reason(s) for this increase include increased rates of depressive and substance use disorders and increased access to firearms. Suicide attempts are even more common than deaths by suicide and may lead to significant morbidity. Risk factors for suicidal behavior include psychiatric disorders (particularly depression), previous suicide attempt(s), LGB+ or gender-diverse identity, low self-esteem, impulsivity, exposure to violence, and a history of abuse. Additionally, precipitating factors (i.e., those that increase the likelihood of suicide attempt or death among adolescents at risk) include substance use, access to means (e.g., firearms, medications for overdose), significant stressors, and isolation. Adolescent girls are more likely than boys to experience suicidal ideation and to attempt suicide, while adolescent boys are more likely than girls to die by suicide.

The American Academy of Pediatrics and *Bright Futures* recommend universal screening for suicide risk beginning at age 12. Screening should be performed at least annually and more often for teens at risk. Several strategies for screening are available. Adolescents may be asked directly about suicidal behavior; notably, asking about suicide, including the use of the word "suicide," does not provoke suicidal ideation or increase the risk of suicide. In fact, it is important for providers to ask directly and clearly about suicide, as patients may not understand more vague attempts to broach the topic. Possible questions include "Do you ever feel like you don't want to be alive anymore?", "Have you ever had thoughts about killing yourself, or suicide?", "Have you ever tried to kill yourself?", and "Have you ever attempted suicide?" As an alternative, or in addition, to verbal questions, validated screening instruments such as the Ask Suicide-Screening Questions and the Suicide Behavior Questionnaire-Revised, both of which are publicly available, may be used. Positive screening should immediately prompt further questioning about the frequency, intensity, and specificity of the thoughts or behaviors, the presence or absence of a plan, the presence or absence of intent to act on a plan, access to means (e.g., a firearm), and any preparatory steps (e.g., writing a suicide note, stockpiling pills to overdose). For adolescents with passive suicidal ideation (i.e., thoughts of suicide with no plan or intent to act on these thoughts) assessed to be at low risk for attempt, completing a safety plan may be appropriate. Patients with active suicidal ideation (i.e., suicidal ideation with a plan) generally require emergent evaluation and intervention, for example, psychiatric hospitalization. For further information on assessing for and responding

BOX 22.1   Patient Health Questionnaire (2-item and 9-item) Depression Screening Instruments

PHQ-2 inquires about the frequency of depressed mood and anhedonia over the past 2 weeks. The PHQ-2 includes the first two items of the PHQ-9:

- The purpose of the PHQ-2 is to screen for depression in a "first-step" approach.
- Patients who screen positive should be further evaluated with the PHQ-9 to determine whether they meet criteria for a depressive disorder.

Over the **last 2 weeks**, how often have you been bothered by the following problems? (Not at all = 0, several days = 1, more than half the days = 2, nearly every day = 3)
1. Little interest or pleasure in doing things
2. Feeling down, depressed, or hopeless

Interpretation:
- A PHQ-2 score ranges from 0 to 6. The authors identified a score of 3 as the optimal cutpoint when using the PHQ-2 to screen for depression.
- If the score is 3 or greater, major depressive disorder is likely.
- Patients who screen positive should be further evaluated with the PHQ-9, other diagnostic instruments, or direct interview to determine whether they meet criteria for a depressive disorder.

PHQ-9

Over the **last 2 weeks**, how often have you been bothered by any of the following problems? (not at all = 0, several days = 1, more than half the days = 2, nearly every day = 3)
1. Little interest or pleasure in doing things
2. Feeling down, depressed, or hopeless
3. Trouble falling or staying asleep, or sleeping too much
4. Feeling tired or having little energy
5. Poor appetite or overeating
6. Feeling bad about yourself—or that you are a failure or have let yourself or your family down
7. Trouble concentrating on things, such as reading the newspaper or watching television
8. Moving or speaking so slowly that other people could have noticed? Or the opposite—being so fidgety or restless that you have been moving around a lot more than usual
9. Thoughts that you would be better off dead or hurting yourself in some way

If you checked off any problems, how difficult have these problems made it for you to do your work, take care of things at home, or get along with other people?
- Not at all difficult
- Somewhat difficult
- Very difficult
- Extremely difficult

Interpretation:
- Total score of 0–4 is none to minimal depression; no treatment indicated
- Total score of 5–9 is mild depression; treat with watchful waiting; repeat PHQ-9 at follow-up
- Total score of 10–14 is moderate depression; create a treatment plan, considering counseling, follow-up, and/or pharmacotherapy
- Total score of 15–19 is moderately severe depression; warrants active treatment with pharmacotherapy and/or psychotherapy
- Total score of 20–27 is severe depression; warrants immediate initiation of pharmacotherapy and, if severe impairment or poor response to therapy, expedited referral to a mental health specialist for psychotherapy and/or collaborative management
- Note: Question 9 is a single screening question on suicide risk. A patient who answers yes to question 9 needs further assessment for suicide risk by an individual who is competent to assess this risk

Kroenke K, Spitzer RL: The PHQ-9: a new depression diagnostic and severity measure, *Psychiatr Ann* 32:509–521, 2002; Kroenke K, Spitzer RL, Williams JB: The PHQ-9: validity of a brief depression severity measure, *J Gen Intern Med* 16:606–613, 2001; Kroenke K, Spitzer RL, Williams JB: The Patient Health Questionnaire-2: validity of a two-item depression screener, *Med Care* 41:1284–1292, 2003.

to suicidal behavior, see "Suicide" under "Taking a Medical History" below.

Although adolescents should be asked about suicide privately, in many cases, the presence of suicidal ideation and/or a history of suicide attempt needs to be disclosed to the adolescent's caregiver(s). See "Taking a Medical History" below for more information about strategies for partnering with adolescents to share confidential information with their caregivers.

NSSI, also called nonsuicidal self-injurious behavior, may be considered a phenomenon distinct from suicidal behavior; notably, however, patients with NSSI are at increased risk of suicide attempts and suicide. Individuals with NSSI engage in intentional harm to or destruction of bodily tissue(s) without an intent to die. The most common forms of NSSI include cutting, burning, and scratching the skin. Adolescents who engage in NSSI commonly describe the behavior as a means to relieve distress or as a way to punish themselves; adolescents who are depressed may report feeling numb and engaging in NSSI in an attempt to feel "something." The mainstay of treatment for NSSI is psychotherapy. Additionally, limiting access to means (e.g., razor blades, knives) is of critical importance, as are assessing any injuries or wounds and providing necessary medical care. Partnering with caregivers to develop and employ a safety plan is often indicated. The decision whether to inform parents about NSSI disclosed by an adolescent in confidence depends on the severity, frequency, and method(s) of injury, the risk of serious injury and/or other harm, and the presence or absence of concurring suicidal ideation.

Substance Use

Mid-adolescents may use substances for a variety of reasons, including coping with emotions, stress, or trauma; a desire to fit in with their peer group; or out of curiosity. Alcohol, nicotine (via vaping), and marijuana are the substances most commonly used by adolescents. Risk factors for substance use—and substance use disorders—include male sex, a family history of substance use disorder(s), parental substance use (or acceptance of use), and untreated psychiatric conditions. Among middle- and high-school students, signs that a young person may be struggling with substance use include declining grades, disengagement from activities, and increased anger, irritability, and/or family conflict.

Strategies for discussing substance use and assessing for substance use disorders are included in the section "Drugs" under "Taking a Medical History" (see below), and substance use disorders are discussed in more detail in Chapter 23.

DURING THE VISIT

The American Academy of Pediatrics' *Bright Futures* recommends annual health maintenance visits for all mid-adolescents. Health maintenance examinations are important opportunities to perform screening and to provide preventive care (e.g., immunizations) and anticipatory guidance. As noted above, all teens should be screened annually for depression and suicide risk, as well as for substance use. Sexually active adolescents should be screened for STIs. Immunizations should be given according to the CDC schedule.

Taking a Medical History

During the mid-adolescent years, the physician may begin to see the adolescent patient without a caregiver present. Indeed, all US states and the District of Columbia allow adolescents to receive certain types of care confidentially, that is, without the involvement or consent of caregivers. Such encounters offer teens opportunities to begin to develop the skills needed to manage their own health as they transition toward adulthood. Providers should discuss confidentiality and its limits with adolescents and their caregiver(s) before beginning a confidential interview. While laws differ by state, in general, providers are required to breach confidentiality (i.e., to share information the adolescent shared in confidence and does not want to be shared) in cases of child abuse or if the provider believes the patient or another person is at significant risk of serious harm (e.g., if the patient has active suicidal ideation or is driving under the influence of alcohol) and disclosing the information to a caregiver will likely prevent the harm. If a provider determines confidentiality must be breached, they should inform the adolescent before making the disclosure and allow the teen to plan, and participate in, the process if they wish. It is important to use clear, precise, and authoritative language with patients—for example, "I need to tell your mother about your recent suicide attempt" instead of "I think I should tell your mother about your recent suicide attempt, okay?" to minimize arguments or attempts to negotiate. Clearly outline for the adolescent what specific information needs to be shared and why. Allowing the adolescent some control over this process, when appropriate (e.g., asking if she would prefer to share the information herself, with the provider present to fill in any necessary additional details, or to have the provider share the information), may increase their comfort and preserve trust.

The potential for confidential information to be disclosed to parents via the electronic health record, online patient portals, and/or insurance documents should be considered. It is often beneficial for providers to obtain and record an adolescent's personal cell phone number, so confidential information (e.g., results of testing for STIs) can be communicated to the teen directly.

Providers who care for adolescents often use a standardized template to assess psychosocial and sensitive topics called SSHADESS (also known as HEADSS, as it was originally called, and several other variations as the topics have evolved over time). The SSHADESS topics—Strengths, Supports, Home, Activities, Drugs, Education and Employment, Sexuality, and Suicide—are designed to progress from generally nonthreatening topics, such as who an adolescent lives with and what they do for fun, to more sensitive topics such as substance use and suicide. The goals of the SSHADESS assessment are to gather important psychosocial history, identify an adolescent's strengths and sources of support, promote health behaviors, and identify and address risks or concerns. This history is typically collected verbally; paper or electronic questionnaires (e.g., through the electronic medical record) may also be used to gather information, but such questionnaires are usually best utilized as a catalyst, rather than replacement, for discussion.

Strengths

GOAL: Assess the adolescent's self-esteem and skills. Most teens can identify several things they are good at, things they like about themselves, or things other people like about them. Adolescents who struggle to identify one or more personal strengths may benefit from more detailed screening for mental health conditions such as depression and/or anxiety.

QUESTIONS: "What would you say is your biggest strength?" Other options include "What are some things you're good at?", "What do you like most about yourself?", and "What do you think other people like about you?"

Supports

GOAL: Assess for support in the teen's family, peer group, and/or community. There is strong evidence that teenagers who feel closely connected to their families, schools, and communities are more resilient and less likely to engage in negative health behaviors than peers who are not well connected. Again, most adolescents can identify at least one adult who is a source of support for them; a teen who struggles to do so may benefit from more detailed questioning about depression, substance use, abuse, and/or neglect.

QUESTIONS: "Who in your life is a source of support for you?"

Home

GOAL: Determine where the patient lives and whether they live independently, at home with parents, with friends, or in cohabitation with a significant partner; determine the psychological and physical safety of the home environment.

QUESTIONS: "Where are you living now?" and "Who else lives where you live?" Ask whether the living situation is satisfactory and whether the patient feels safe. For instance, vaping by roommates may explain recurrent asthma exacerbations, or financial hardship may prevent proper diet and nutrition. Questions about household violence may include, "What happens when people in your household argue?" and "Does anyone ever get hurt during arguments?" This should be followed by "Do arguments ever happen when someone has been drinking or is using drugs?" Ask whether there are firearms in the residence. If there are, recommend that they be removed or stored safely. Ask about meals served at home (quality and availability of food).

Activity

GOAL: Evaluate social interactions, interests, self-esteem, problematic video gaming/social media/internet use, and eating disorder-related behaviors.

QUESTIONS: "What do you do for fun?" or "Are you involved in any clubs, organizations, religious groups, sports, or hobbies?" Because participation in such organizations is often linked to self-esteem, this may be a non-threatening way to assess social skills and peer group and community connections. Adolescents who participate only in solitary activities may have difficulty with social skills, feel alienated, or be depressed.

When asking about social media and video gaming, avoid only asking about "screen time." An adolescent may spend several hours per day in affirmative, positive social media interactions, or only a few minutes per day being bullied or seeing hate speech online, so time is not the best measure of how healthy a teen's relationship with media is. Providers can ask open-ended questions that explore online experiences, such as "What are some of the best things you've seen online? What are some of the most stressful? How do you wish social media were designed differently? How do you usually feel after using social media? Is it ever a problem?" Screening questions can also assess whether the teen thinks that media has become a problem for their sleep, friendships, or schoolwork—or whether they argue with caregivers frequently about media. Offer strength-based suggestions (Table 22.1) so that the adolescent can come up with their own plans for balancing media use with other life activities.

Depending on circumstances, the provider may also ask whether the patient belongs to a religious youth group or a gang. These activities, to varying degrees, provide a sense of community and belonging. In some situations, they may also be sources of extreme peer pressure and result in inappropriate drug and alcohol use, sexual behavior, or interpersonal violence. Gangs are a powerful source of identity for those who feel disempowered, disenfranchised, and alienated.

Conversations about peers and sports can be natural segues to questions about disordered eating behaviors, such as restriction, bingeing, purging, and excessive exercise. Providers may ask about the teen's body image and whether they are dieting or trying to change their weight, for example, "How do you feel about your body shape and size? Have you tried to change it? If so, how? What were/are your goals for your body?"

Drugs

GOAL: Determine personal, environmental, and genetic risks for substance use and assess current pattern of use. Identify those whose substance use is likely to interfere with their functioning, quality of life, and/or physical or mental health. Provide education on harm-reduction strategies and/or treatment for adolescents using substances. Reinforce the behavior of those who have chosen not to use drugs or alcohol.

QUESTIONS: Begin by acknowledging that it can be common for adolescents to have some experience with substances. Ask if the patient has ever tried any substances. It is often reasonable to inquire first about alcohol, nicotine (cigarettes and/or vaping), and marijuana (inhaled, including vaping, and/or edible), as these are the substances most commonly used by adolescents. Other substances to inquire about include over-the-counter medications (dextromethorphan, diphenhydramine, dimenhydrinate), stimulants (prescription attention-deficit/hypersensitivity disorder medications, cocaine, methamphetamine), opiates (prescription pills, heroin), and hallucinogens (inhalants, ecstasy, lysregic acid diethylamide). Most substances have numerous nicknames, which providers may be unfamiliar with; ask the patient to clarify if you are unsure which substance(s) they are referring to.

If the patient reports any use, assess the frequency of use (multiple times daily, daily, weekly, etc). Ask when they last used, how much they use at a time, and whether use is increasing (to determine whether tolerance is developing). Ask about the circumstances of use (at parties, with friends, alone). Ask where and how substances are obtained (from a friend, store or dispensary, the internet, a dealer, or unknown); the risk of contamination (e.g., with fentanyl) is higher with substances obtained online or from a dealer, or with an unknown source. Assess for safety risks (e.g., driving while intoxicated, blackouts, or loss of consciousness).

Determining the level of use and whether a substantial problem exists can challenge the most experienced clinician. Recognition of a problem depends on the patient's willingness to share and the clinician's willingness to receive information about the use of substances. Several questionnaires designed to detect problem substance use have been developed. The CRAFFT tool, which asks about driving or riding in a **C**ar while intoxicated, using substances to **R**elax, using substances **A**lone, **F**orgetting things as a result of substance use, concern from **F**amily or **F**riends regarding substance use, and getting into **T**rouble because of substances, is sensitive for problem substance use and has been validated for adolescents aged 12 to 21 years (see Box 23.3 for the CRAFFT tool and management for adolescents using substances).

Education and Employment

GOAL: Evaluate current achievements, strengths, and weaknesses and their realistic connection to future plans. Assess for unrecognized learning disabilities and stress or anxiety related to college, employment, or separation from family, school, and community.

QUESTIONS: For those in high school, ask "What classes are you taking? How are your grades? How do your grades compare with last year?" Without specific questioning

TABLE 22.1 Strengths-Based Recommendations for Healthy Social Media Use Practices in Adolescents
• Make a media plan that balances time with and without devices. Work together to set rules about media use so you and your caregivers agree on how devices fit into your lives. Talk about which tech-free activities you want to make time for on a regular basis.
• To preserve sleep and focus, keep devices out of bedrooms at night and set do-not-disturb on phones when you want undistracted time.
• Keep privacy settings more private so that you can spend time with friends online but not have to deal with strangers.
• Be savvy about what is real and what is edited, what misinformation looks like, when influencers are being authentic versus attention seeking, and how algorithms can elevate harmful content
• Curate your social media feed by following/unfollowing and giving feedback to train the algorithm toward the content that makes you feel good.
• Take breaks from social or gaming platforms that are causing you too much stress, to see how you feel after a few weeks.
• Use tools such as blocking, muting, and reporting when other users are being toxic.
• Think about how media and your emotions connect. We sometimes crave social media when we were stressed or want to share our joy, and this in turn shapes how we feel.
• Encourage your caregivers to put down their devices for family time or watch shows/movies with you. Try to have regular discussions as a family about online activities and social media, including positive and negative experiences.

Adapted with permission from American Academy of Pediatrics Center of Excellence on Social Media and Youth Mental Health.

about classes or grades, most adolescents will respond that everything is "fine." Falling grades may indicate a mental health condition, substance use, or trauma exposure.

For those not in school, ask "What is the last grade you completed? How did high school go for you? What were the hardest parts about it?" Answers to these questions may help uncover learning disabilities, family disruption, or abuse by family or peers. For instance, an unrecognized learning disability may result in school termination because of recurrent poor performance, low self-esteem, and expulsions related to negative behavior. Teens may leave home before completing high school because they have been sexually victimized or because LGB+ or sex-diverse youth have been ostracized by family, peers, and/or adults at school.

Inquire about employment, including whether an adolescent has a job and where and how many hours they work each week. If they are still in school, assess whether work hours interfere with schoolwork. Assess the motivation for working and the adolescent's degree of financial independence.

Sexuality

GOAL: Evaluate and counsel about sexuality; sexual practices; reproductive health, including family planning and STIs; and sexual abuse/exploitation. Reinforce behaviors that reduce the risk of undesired health outcomes, such as abstinence, condom use, and routine testing for STIs.

QUESTIONS: Ask open-ended questions, taking care not to make assumptions about gender identity, sexual orientation, or sexual practices—for example, "What is your gender identity?" (see Table 22.2 for a guide to terminology related to sex, sexual orientation, and gender). "Are you dating anyone?" is a generally nonthreatening question to begin a discussion about sexuality. Inquire about sexual partners (e.g., number of total and recent partners to assess

risk for STIs, partner(s)' sex assigned at birth to evaluate the potential for pregnancy) and practices (e.g., vaginal, oral, and/or anal sex, use of sex toys). Ask the patient about their thoughts around pregnancy and, if appropriate, whether they are using, or would like to use, anything to prevent pregnancy. Ask about condom use, for example, "How do you protect yourself from sexually transmitted infections?" People tend to overestimate or overreport how fastidiously they use condoms for a number of reasons, including fear of judgment by providers; normalize forgetting or neglecting to use condoms at times, for example, by asking "how often do you forget to use a condom?" instead of "do you use condoms every time?" Inquire about a history of STIs.

Although it is important to reinforce the decision of adolescents who have chosen sexual abstinence, they should be allowed to ask questions and be reassured that if their sexual behavior changes, they have a source of information, advice, and prevention resources.

Suicide

GOAL: Assess for nonsuicidal self-injurious behavior, suicidal ideation, and any history of prior suicide attempt. Identify adolescents at risk for suicide and in need of intervention. Identify and address any immediate safety concerns (e.g., current active suicidal ideation with a plan).

QUESTIONS: It is often helpful to begin by asking their patient about their mood more generally, for example, "How has your mood been recently?" or "Have there been any times recently when you've felt stuck in feeling sad, down, or bad about yourself?" Ask if the adolescent has ever intentionally harmed themself or thought about harming themself. If the answer is yes, ask how long the behavior has been going on, how frequently it occurs, which body part(s) are affected, and whether the patient has required medical attention for intentional injuries. Assess any acute injuries, if needed. Ask about thoughts of death or suicide. Evidence is clear that asking about suicide, including the use of the word *suicide*, with patients does not increase the risk of suicide. For patients who endorse suicidal ideation, inquire about plan(s), intent, access to means, and any preparatory steps (e.g., writing a suicide note, hoarding pills with an intent to overdose).

Physical Examination

Physical examination of mid-adolescents should include measurement of growth parameters (height, weight, BMI) and vital signs (including blood pressure). Growth charts should be monitored closely to assess for weight loss, which would be unexpected in a mid-adolescent and may be a sign of disease or disordered eating. Examine the skin, assessing for acne, the presence of acanthosis nigricans, and/or signs of self-injury. Complete cardiac, musculoskeletal, and

TABLE 22.2 **Terminology Related to Sex, Sexual Orientation, and Gender**	
Term	**Definition**
Sex	Classification of people as male, female, or intersex, based on anatomy, chromosomes, and/or hormones
Sexual orientation	Pattern of physical and/or romantic attraction (e.g., heterosexual, gay, lesbian, bisexual); may or may not align with sexual practices; distinct from gender identity
Gender	Social classification of people according to qualities of masculinity and femininity
Gender identity	An individual's innate sense of self as a male, female, or someone else along the gender spectrum
Gender expression	One's outward manifestation of gender through clothing, hairstyle, voice, mannerisms, etc; may or may not align with gender identity

neurologic examinations for patients presenting for sports preparticipation examinations. Assess pubertal status (testicular volume for patients assigned male at birth, breast development for patients assigned female at birth). Patients assigned male at birth should also be evaluated for the presence of hernia or testicular mass. Routine pelvic examination is not indicated for asymptomatic patients assigned female at birth, but an external genital exam and/or speculum exam may be indicated for patients with genitourinary symptoms.

Anticipatory Guidance

Discuss any further expected changes of puberty, if applicable. Discuss body image and nutrition. Encourage regular physical activity for enjoyment and socialization, not weight loss. Encourage oral hygiene and the use of sunscreen. Discuss screen use, including video games, and encourage caregivers and teens to establish and enforce limits on screens and gaming. Discuss social media use and encourage caregivers to set expectations regarding social media use with their teens (see Chapter 21). Provide adolescents information and resources on sexuality, condoms, contraception, and testing for STIs. Discuss seat belt and helmet use, safe driving (e.g., minimizing distractions such as texting), and firearm safety. Encourage teens and their families to communicate about, and plan for, potential unsafe situations (e.g., the teen [or their ride] becomes intoxicated and needs a ride home). Encourage graduated independence (e.g., chores or other family/household responsibilities, driving privileges, curfews) for adolescents.

QUICK CHECK—15 TO 17 YEARS

- Use the SSHEADSS format to gather psychosocial and sensitive histories.
- Understand your state confidentiality laws and explain them to patients and caregivers.
- Do not assume that all teens want contraception; use shared decision-making to help adolescents who want contraception choose a method.
- Screen sexually active adolescents for STIs at least annually.
- Assess body image and for the presence of disordered eating.
- Screen all adolescents 12 and older for suicide risk.
- Discuss social media use and encourage teens and their caregiver(s) to communicate about their social media use.
- Encourage age-appropriate independence and autonomy (e.g., curfews).

ANTICIPATORY GUIDANCE FOR CAREGIVERS

Limit Setting Versus Power Struggles

It is not unusual for mid-adolescents to "test" authority figures, including parents, but this does not mean they do not need or want rules or boundaries. Indeed, most mid-adolescents appreciate reasonable limit setting by parents as evidence of parental concern and as safe boundaries in which to function. However, there is a difference between limit setting and power struggles. Limit setting refers to rules and regulations concerning behavior; power struggles occur when authority itself is at stake, regardless of the issue being discussed. Limit setting is necessary; power struggles should be avoided, because someone always loses, and that person is inevitably resentful and bitter. One example of limit setting is the curfew. Teens and their parents should decide together on a reasonable curfew; the parent and teen should discuss in advance the consequences that will follow if the curfew is broken. In contrast, a power struggle may involve an argument over one person being "right" and the other person being "wrong." Usually, the subject matter is unimportant; being "right" or winning is all that counts. Because limit setting consists of rules, they may need to be modified as the adolescent matures or the situation changes. Adolescents and parents should be encouraged to communicate as these changing needs arise.

Effective Parenting of the Adolescent

It is not easy to be a parent, and the mid-adolescent years may be the most difficult for some parents. They should be prepared for the commonly experienced challenges involved in raising adolescents. For example, for the first time, parents may face unresolved issues from the adolescent's childhood and unresolved issues from their own adolescence, and they may find their authority as parents repeatedly challenged. Parents should be reassured that the best approach to their teenagers (and to themselves) is to keep the lines of communication open. Parental connectedness—that is, the adolescent's perception of warmth, love, and caring from parents—and parental availability to the adolescent are keys to the successful development and health of every adolescent. This includes caregivers limiting their own smartphone and media use so that they appear available to their adolescent when they want to talk. In most families, parents find themselves growing in wisdom as they struggle with the issues that teenage children force them to face.

ACKNOWLEDGMENTS

The authors thank Shaquita Bell and Alessandra Angelino for their high-level review in the chapter.

RECOMMENDED READINGS

For Teens

McCoy K, Wibbelsman C:. *Life happens: a teenager's guide to friends, failure, sexuality, love, rejection, addiction, peer pressure, families, loss, depression, change and other challenges of living.* Berkeley; 1996.

McCoy K, Wibbelsman C:. *The teenage body book.* New York: Perigee; 2016.

Aggarwal S, Darpinian S, Sterling W. *No weigh! A teen's guide to positive body image, food, and emotional wisdom.* Jessica Kingsley Publishers; 2018.

https://youngwomenshealth.org/

https://youngmenshealthsite.org/

The Trevor Project: https://thetrevorproject.org

Bedsider (Birth control, sexual health and wellness): www.bedsider.org

This is Quitting: This is Quitting: truthinitiative.org

Suicidality and Non-Suicidal Self-Injury: https://www.crisistextline.org

The Social Media Workbook for Teens: Skills to Help You Balance Screen Time, Manage Stress, and Take Charge of Your Life by Goali Saedi Bocci PhD and Gina M. Biegel MA LMFT.

The DBT Workbook for Teens: Mindfulness and Emotion Regulation Techniques for Overcoming Stress and Negative Thoughts (Successful Parenting) by Richard Bass.

Don't Let Your Emotions Run Your Life for Teens: Dialectical Behavior Therapy Skills for Helping You Manage Mood Swings, Control Angry Outbursts, and Get Along With Others by Sheri Van Dijk MSW.

For Parents

Damour Lisa. *The emotional lives of teenagers: raising connected, capable, and compassionate adolescents.* New York: Ballantine Books; 2023.

Jensen F, Ellis Nutt A. *The teenage brain: a neuroscientist's survival guide to raising adolescents and young adults.* New York: HarperCollins; 2015.

https://hr.mit.edu/static/worklife/raising-teens/five-basics.html

https://www.cdc.gov/parents/teens/

www.understood.org/en/articles/iep-transition-planning-preparing-for-young-adulthood

Center for Parent and Teen Communication: www.parentandteen.com

For Clinicians

CDC Youth Risk Behavior Survey: https://www.cdc.gov/healthyyouth/data/yrbs/index.htm

Summary Chart of U.S. Medical Eligibility Criteria for Contraceptive Use. cdc.gov.

Adolescent Health Initiative: https://umhs-adolescenthealth.org

The Gender Unicorn: https://transstudent.org/gender/

Non-suicidal self-injury resources: The Cornell Research Program on Self-Injury and Recovery

SAMHSA: Mood disorder and substance use resources. In *Prevention of substance use and mental disorders.*

AACAP Resources for Youth: Resources for youth. aacap.org.

National Eating Disorders Association: Eating Disorders Helpline | Chat, Call, or Text | NEDA. nationaleatingdisorders.org.

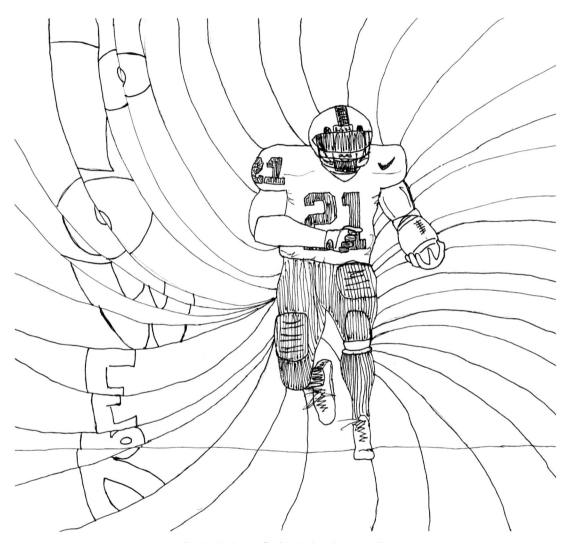

Football player. By Nasir Austin, age 15.

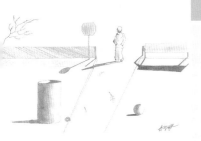

23

Seventeen to Twenty-One Years: Transition to Adulthood

Alana K. Otto and Yolanda N. Evans

This chapter covers key behavioral and developmental considerations for older adolescents during their transition to adulthood. Topics include supporting young adults in setting and pursuing goals, including those related to education, employment, and family planning; fostering healthy relationships with romantic partners and friends; and identifying adult role models, peers and other communities, and additional sources of support. The chapter focuses on identifying and leveraging adolescents' strengths, resilience, and supports during this critical period of transition; identifying and mitigating health risks is also important.

KEYWORDS

- Identity
- Resilience
- Critical life transitions
- Education
- Employment
- Community supports
- Relationships
- Sexuality
- Sexual exploitation
- Substance use
- Mental health

Late adolescence marks an important transition from childhood to early adulthood. Although autonomy, self-awareness, and critical thinking are more mature at this stage relative to earlier in childhood, these capacities are still evolving; development of these key skills is supported by positive adult role models. Because many adolescents continue to see pediatric medical providers through early adulthood, these providers may play important roles as positive adults and sources of support, stability, and trusted information. The transition to young adulthood is an important time for clinicians to partner with young people to help them manage their health and navigate the health-care system, increase independence as they embark on key life transitions, build healthy relationships and coping strategies, and become thriving members of their communities.

At this stage, adolescents are developing their sense of self as independent from their parent(s) (in this chapter, we use the term "parents" to refer to parents of all types as well as legal guardians and other caregivers); they are also developing an understanding of themselves in the contexts of their families, peers, communities, and society. Many older adolescents are less focused on comparing themselves to peers, relative to middle adolescence, and are developing the emotional and cognitive maturity to set educational and/or vocational goals, pursue meaningful interpersonal relationships, and define and examine their own values. Although the independent "self," defined by skills, passions, relationships, and values, becomes clearer during late adolescence, the process of identity formation continues throughout the lifetime.

As with earlier stages of development, not all adolescents progress, physically or emotionally, at the same time or rate. Opportunities for graduated independence and responsibility at home, school, and in the community are critical for positive developmental progress, as is the support of families, teachers, and other trusted adults. Neurodiverse adolescents, those with mental health conditions, and those who have experienced trauma, multiple adverse childhood events, or chronic stress may experience additional challenges during this time, including challenges developing a coherent sense of self, developing independent decision-making skills, and

---

Previous edition of this chapter by Lawrence S. Friedman.

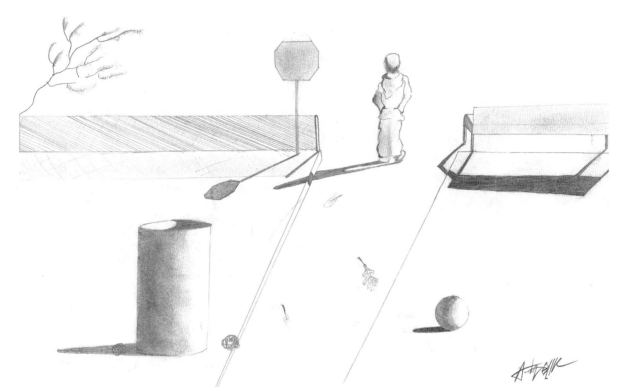

"Still Life." A young person is shown at a boundary, a transition. By Andre Bullock. *"You can't cross the sea merely by standing and staring at the water." – Rabindranath Tagore*

learning impulse inhibition and healthy forms of emotional regulation, and additional supports may be needed. For all adolescents, medical providers should strive to identify and leverage the unique strengths of the individual young person, their family, and their community and to partner with the adolescent to mitigate health risks.

CRITICAL LIFE TRANSITIONS OF EMERGING ADULTHOOD

Late adolescence is a time of profound emotional and cognitive transition; for many adolescents, it is also a time of significant life transitions (e.g., educational, vocational, financial) and increasing independence.

Vocation and Career Planning

As teenagers prepare to enter the adult world, career planning may become a focus. Vocational options usually depend on a combination of the adolescent's social environment, financial resources, educational achievement, individual strengths, cognitive ability, and interests. Options are strongly shaped by opportunities presented to them, privilege, and positive adult support. Superimposed on these factors may be other responsibilities, such as contributing to family housing, meeting basic needs, and caring for others in the family. Decisions about education and employment may also be heavily influenced by family expectations, so teens may appreciate a pediatric clinician as a neutral "third party" with whom to discuss their interests and goals. For all adolescents, discussions with a provider about future goals and "next steps" can be a catalyst to assess the teen's outlook and ability to set and pursue goals, as well as a way to assess risk behavior and provide anticipatory guidance. Motivational interviewing can be used to help align teens' health behaviors with their goals.

Educational Planning

As they enter late adolescence, most teenagers will be in the final stages of completing secondary education. While most adolescents in the United States graduate with a diploma, some do not complete high school. Some may pursue alternative education and/or complete a General Education Development (GED) test to earn a certificate of high school equivalency. Neurodiverse adolescents, those with cognitive or learning disabilities, and those with mental health conditions may have needs that are not met by traditional education programs. For teens (and their parents) who have had frustrating or alienating experiences with the traditional school system, identifying and drawing on teens' unique skills, sources of resilience, and community supports are important ways clinicians may help these adolescents define and reach their goals.

Many adolescents and young adults in the United States pursue higher education; in 2020, 40% of Americans between the ages of 18 and 24 were enrolled in a 2- or 4-year college program. For many adolescents, "going to college" means moving out of their family's home and taking on more responsibility for their housing, nutrition, day-to-day functioning, and finances. However, a significant proportion of adolescents attending higher education programs live with their families, particularly as costs have increased. Multiple factors influence young adults' social and psychological adjustment to college, including whether they have developed age-appropriate independence and emotional regulation skills, existence of mental health conditions (e.g., substance use disorders [SUD], anxiety, or depression), and whether they want to attend college (vs. it being a parent expectation). Performance and social pressures on young adults enrolled in college can also contribute to alcohol and/or substance use as a coping strategy for emotion regulation. For adolescents with a known learning difference (e.g., learning disability, attention-deficit/hyperactivity disorder [ADHD]) or mental health disorder, educational accommodations and/or access to a therapist or other mental health supports should be arranged before college starts.

Higher education is not the goal for all emerging adults. Some adolescents will enroll in vocational or trade schools, while others pursue certificate or apprenticeship programs (e.g., automotive repair, construction, medical assistant); still others may engage in less formal on-the-job training or enter the workforce immediately after graduating, or without finishing, high school. Some young adults pursue military service, either in the short or long term. Success is defined differently for each emerging adult; the most important thing is that one's education or employment provides a sense of fulfillment and purpose. Clinicians may play an important role in helping adolescents reflect on their interests, passions, skills, and motivations and in identifying educational and/or vocational opportunities in their communities. Such conversations are a foundational component of supporting adolescents' well-being; indeed, opportunities to discuss a young person's interests and talents are built into most pediatric providers' standard practice, for example, when taking a social history. In addition, pediatric practices can be valuable sources of information about local resources for alternative education (e.g., GED programs) and job training and employment opportunities. Providers may also be important sources of information and support for adolescents experiencing labor exploitation or trafficking and should be aware of both warning signs of exploitation and resources for affected teens.

Unique Needs of Young Adults With Neurodiversity or Mental Health Challenges

Many adolescents at this stage will be required to interview, for example, for a job or college application, for the first time. Job (or other) interviews are a source of anxiety for many adolescents and adults alike. In particular, emerging adults with autism spectrum disorder (ASD) may find the job interview process stressful, as interviews involve meeting a new person and answering novel questions in a nonscripted, flexible way; virtual interview training is a new resource available for teens with ASD to help them prepare via Zoom-based coaching and interviews (see Recommended Readings at the end of the chapter). Furthermore, any teen or young adult who struggles with information processing, emotion regulation, or flexible thinking (e.g., due to ADHD, trauma, or anxiety) may experience challenges with following instructions, responding to dynamic situations, or personality mismatches at work or school. For adolescents with ADHD or other mental health conditions, it is often helpful to optimize treatment, for example, with medication and/or therapy, prior to beginning a new job or education program. For all emerging adults, connections with positive adult role models who can help them problem solve during a time of transition can be valuable.

Foster Care Transitions

At this age, some adolescents also transition out of the foster care system. Notably, there are significant disproportionalities in the foster care system in the United States, primarily related to race and ethnicity, with people of color overrepresented relative to their representation in the general population. These disproportionalities result from the disparate treatment of youth and families across the spectrum of child welfare services, largely because of racism, bias, and discrimination. Bias, discrimination, and structural oppression also contribute to inequitable health and educational outcomes, including increased rates of unmet medical and mental healthcare needs, among youth in or previously in the foster care system. Fragmented and inconsistent access to medical and/or mental healthcare is common, as are trauma, adversity, and toxic stress. As discussed in Chapter 24, pediatric providers must be familiar with, and take care to utilize, principles of trauma-informed care when working with youth in or previously in the foster system.

Interactions With the Carceral System

Some young adults may also be transitioning to or from the carceral system, which, like the child welfare system, is marred by significant racial and ethnic disproportionalities: nearly 44,000 youth in the United States are incarcerated in juvenile carceral facilities; about 90% are male, and over 60% are youth of color. Indeed, the US carceral system has been built on a foundation of racism, with youth of color disproportionately affected by school and municipal disciplinary policies that result in what has been called the "school-to-prison pipeline." People of color, including adolescents, may also experience police violence, not only in association with criminal activity but, because of racism, bias, and discrimination, for simply existing in predominantly white spaces. This trauma can be experienced by the youth or may be in the setting of witnessing violence inflicted by law enforcement on family, friends, or community members. For many families of color, and Black families in particular, conversations with children and teens about racism, bias, police violence, and minimizing risk when interacting with law enforcement are both necessary and a source of distress and anxiety. While pediatricians may have a role in providing anticipatory guidance to adolescents of color and their families, ultimately, addressing racism in the carceral system and police violence is not the responsibility of the individuals affected, and anticipatory guidance about safety alone is insufficient   pediatricians must also advocate at the community, state, and federal levels for systemic changes that reduce bias and discrimination and promote equity and justice. Young adults transitioning from the juvenile carceral system may have unique healthcare needs. While adolescents who are incarcerated typically have access to basic healthcare services, many have unmet medical, mental health, and dental needs. Establishing a primary medical home on transition home is of critical importance. Several visits may be needed to address all of the youth's needs, especially if they have not had access to robust healthcare services while incarcerated.

Addressing Unstable Housing and Homelessness

Young adults who are unstably housed or experiencing homelessness may have healthcare needs similar to youth transitioning from the foster care or carceral systems, including unmet primary care needs (e.g., vaccination) as a result of inconsistent or missed medical care as well as mental health needs. Adolescents experiencing homelessness may be uninsured or underinsured and face significant barriers to accessing medical and mental healthcare, including barriers related to transportation and cost. In some communities, mobile healthcare resources may be available and more accessible than traditional healthcare settings. Pediatric practices can be an important source of information (e.g., recommendations for mental health and dental providers) and resources (e.g., for housing, food, transportation, and other concrete needs) for young adults who are unstably housed or unhoused, as well as those transitioning from the foster care or carceral systems.

Notably, pediatricians should remember that adolescents who have been systematically disadvantaged, including those who have been in the child welfare system, incarcerated, or experienced homelessness, have unique interests, skills, and strengths and the potential to be thriving members of their communities.

DEVELOPING INTIMATE INTERPERSONAL RELATIONSHIPS

The transition from adolescence to adulthood is also marked by the development of intimate interpersonal relationships. The development of emotional and sexual interpersonal relationships is inextricably intertwined with the development of one's sense of self, including one's gender identity and romantic or sexual attraction. By late adolescence the security found in activities that are group centered (see Chapters 21 and 22) gives way to activities that are individual centered. As with other developmental tasks, past experiences with family, peers, teachers, and community influence one's experiences with intimate relationships. Positive relationships with family and peers lay the foundation for the communication, self-advocacy, and negotiation skills that mark healthy romantic and sexual partnerships; additionally, the development and refinement of these skills in intimate partner relationships may strengthen them across contexts. Conversely, adolescents with a history of insecure or disorganized attachment to caregivers, poor self-esteem, depression, inadequate role models, low peer group acceptance, or ASDs may have difficulty developing mature intimate relationships. Adolescents who have experienced abuse, neglect, or other significant trauma and those with disabilities are at increased risk for sexual exploitation. Pediatric providers should be familiar with the signs of sexual exploitation and human trafficking and aware of resources available to affected youth. Consider incorporating screening into clinical practice using a question such as "Has anyone ever asked or forced you to do something (such as work, have sex, or take nude pictures) in exchange for something you wanted or needed (such as money, food, shelter, or other items)?"

Intimate partner violence (IPV) and sexual violence are also highly prevalent in the general population, including among adolescents and young adults, and providers should be familiar with best practices for screening for, and addressing, IPV and sexual violence. A common strategy is to frame questions for patients as standard, for example, "I've started asking all my patients about safety in their relationships, because violence is so common and can have so many effects on health." Some patients experiencing IPV or sexual violence will say "no" to screening questions for a variety of reasons, including fear, shame, and stigma. It may also therefore be useful to follow screening questions with brief information on resources for all patients, including those who screen negative—for example, "Thanks for answering my questions. I know you said violence is not affecting you right now, but I want to make sure you are aware of some resources and information in case anything like this ever comes up…" Notably, laws regarding confidentiality and reporting requirements for violence against adults vary by state, and providers must be familiar with local laws.

Individual adolescents develop interest in, and experience with, intimate partner relationships at different ages and rates; overall, however, most late adolescents have had some experience with romantic relationships, and data indicate a majority of high school seniors have had sex. For all intimate partner relationships, regardless of whether they involve sexual contact, consent, mutual respect, trust, and support are critical. School sexuality education curricula in the United States vary widely, and adolescents may or may not have received education on consent, communicating with partners, and negotiation and self-advocacy (e.g., around condom use). Pediatricians are therefore often important sources of this information.

It is estimated that one-quarter or more of adolescents identify as lesbian, gay, bisexual, questioning, or another nonheterosexual orientation (LGB+). These teens experience the same joys and struggles as they explore their identities, sexuality, and relationships as heterosexual teens. In addition, because of bias and stigma, they may experience unique challenges, including stigmatization and discrimination in healthcare settings. Like all adolescents, LGB+ teens benefit from seeing providers who are informed, supportive, and nonjudgmental. As reviewed in Chapter 22, pediatricians may be a source of support for LGB+ adolescents as they navigate "coming out" or sharing their identities with families, friends, schools, and communities, as well as a of important medical information and connections to community supports. Providers should be aware of local, regional, and online support organizations for both LGB+ teens and their families.

EMERGING ADULTS WITH DISABILITIES AND OTHER CHRONIC OR SPECIAL HEALTHCARE NEEDS

Because there are no standardized definitions for disability, chronic illness, or special healthcare needs, estimates of the number of adolescents and young adults with these conditions vary widely. The US Maternal and Child Health Bureau defines "children and youth with special health care needs" as those "who have or are at increased risk for a chronic physical, developmental, behavioral, or emotional condition and who also require health and related services of a type or amount beyond that required by children generally"; they estimate approximately 20% of children in the United States meet this definition. This includes adolescents with a wide variety of conditions, with impacts ranging from mild to severe. This diverse group enters adulthood with a variety of medical needs and concerns. Like other teenagers, they may also have concerns around physical, social, and sexual development. Care must be tailored to the individual adolescent's abilities and developmental stage.

For children with chronic illnesses, adolescence is a critical time to build skills and independence by allowing the teenager to take a progressively greater role in their medical care and decisions. As adolescents with disabilities and other chronic or special healthcare needs enter adulthood, it is especially important for healthcare providers to assess patients' understanding of their condition and ability to navigate the healthcare system and to assist patients and families with the transition to an adult healthcare provider(s). Adolescents with special healthcare needs and their families may have developed close relationships with pediatric providers, nurses, and other clinic staff, often over many years, and transitions of care may be difficult for all involved. This process is often most successful if completed intentionally, proactively, and over a period of time that allows for overlap between visits with the pediatric provider(s) and those with the new adult provider(s). Direct communication between the pediatric and adult providers helps to facilitate a smooth and safe transition of care.

Generally, adolescents assume the legal right to make medical, legal, and financial decisions for themselves when they reach the age of majority (18 years in the United States). Young adults with intellectual disability (i.e., intelligence quotient <70) or other neurodevelopmental conditions who are not able to make medical decisions independently may require guardianship, which allows a parent or other adult to make medical decisions on the young adult's behalf. Less restrictive options are available to allow the young adult to stay involved in decisions and advocate for their needs, such as power of attorney, healthcare proxy, or supported decision-making (in which an advisory group helps the young person make decisions—Box 23.1). It is important to start these conversations with families, and for them to seek input from the school and therapists, no later than age 16, since the process of establishing guardianship takes time and paperwork. Many families will benefit from having a case manager or advocate who helps them navigate issues around finances, education, services, and housing. Because disability services vary from state to state, it is important for providers to know their state and community's resources or at least whom to refer to for assistance.

ALCOHOL AND OTHER SUBSTANCE USE

By late adolescence, most American teenagers have seen their peers use or had some personal experience with vaping, alcohol, or other substances. While brief experimentation with substances during late adolescence may be normative, early initiation of substance use has been clearly linked to an increased risk of problematic use and SUD. In the United States, young adults have the highest rates of substance misuse and SUD. Risk factors for problematic substance use in this age group include male sex; a family history of SUD; parental substance use or acceptance of use; a history of childhood maltreatment, including abuse or neglect; substance use among friends; peer pressure and popularity; bullying (victimization or perpetration); lack of connectedness to family, peers, or community; and untreated or undertreated mental health diagnoses, including ADHD. Conversely, family support, positive connections with adults, community connectedness, engagement in athletics or other structured activities, and opportunities to develop one's skills and interests are associated with a decreased risk of substance use.

Historically, SUD have been viewed as character flaws or moral failings; these disorders are now understood to be chronic illnesses influenced by genetic, environmental, and social factors. The neurobiology of SUD is complex, with changes in the circuitry and function of areas of the brain involved in pleasure, reward, stress, decision-making, and self-control. Alcohol and other drugs produce a pleasurable sensation through the effects of dopamine in the basal ganglia; repeated substance use decreases sensitivity to dopamine, leading to tolerance, that is, the need to use more of a given substance to achieve the same pleasurable result. Repeated substance use also leads to increased activation of the amygdala, or stress center of the brain, in turn causing intense distress when one is not using the substance. Additionally, chronic substance use disrupts functioning in the prefrontal cortex, including judgment and impulse control. Together, these alterations lead to a vicious cycle of repeated use to avoid unpleasant physical and/or emotional symptoms that develop with cessation. The developing adolescent brain is thought to be particularly susceptible to these effects and thus to SUD. Adolescents are also highly susceptible to peer influence, and peer substance use is a risk factor for adolescent substance use. Notably, substances have also become more easily accessible, particularly to adolescents, in the age of the Internet.

Despite advances in the understanding of SUD as chronic medical illnesses, there is still tremendous stigma around substance use and substance use treatment, and many adolescents and their families may hesitate to seek treatment

BOX 23.1	**Components of a Transition Plan for Adolescents and Young Adults with Developmental Disabilities Before an Adolescent Turns 18**	
Housing	• Provide information on Section 8 housing vouchers or support services for caregivers of adults with disabilities
Educational	• Young persons and caregivers have worked on a postsecondary vision that has been incorporated into the IEP through high school
	• School and family have discussed whether student will have a high school diploma (in which case services end at age 18) or a certificate program and stay in young adult services until allowed by their state of residence (usually 21–26 years of age).
	• Vocational training and life skills training have been or are part of high school and young adult services curriculum
	• If adolescent has left school, help family look into postsecondary programs (higher education, vocational, or day programs)
Legal/Financial	• Apply for a nondriver ID card if the adolescent does not have a driver's license
	• Family decides if guardianship makes sense for their family. Other less restrictive options include (1) healthcare proxy for medical decisions, (2) power of attorney for legal/financial decisions, (3) representative payee for management of SSI benefits, (4) conservatorship for estate decision-making and management, and (5) supported decision-making (creates an advisory team for the adolescent, who retains legal rights to decision-making).
	• Family should apply for SSI for the adolescent if they are financially eligible (varies by state)
Services	• Make sure school has made a referral to the state for adult services or family should apply independently
	• Apply for Medicaid health insurance, even as secondary insurance to the family's private insurance

IEP, Individual Educational Plan; *SSI*, supplemental security income.
Adapted from Boston Medical Center Turning 18 Checklist: APTC-Turning-18-Checklist.pdf (bmc.org).

as a result. For adolescents with significant SUD, intensive treatment may be necessary. For others with less significant impairment, brief interventions by medical providers may be effective. Providers should utilize motivational interviewing techniques, tailored to the patient's current stage of change. This evidence-based approach involves identifying a patient's readiness to change a problem - from precontemplation, contemplation, preparation/determination, action, maintenance, to relapse - and adapting the tasks and treatment to their level of readiness. Screening, Brief Intervention, and Referral to Treatment is an evidence-based model aimed at identifying patients with or at risk for SUD and connecting them with treatment. Screening can be performed with a number of instruments including the Screening to Brief Intervention (S2BI) tool, the Brief Screener for Tobacco, Alcohol, and other Drugs (BSTAD) tool, and the Car, Relax, Alone, Forget, Friends, Trouble (CRAFFT) tool. If screening detects problematic or potentially problematic substance use, the provider engages in a brief intervention using principles of motivational interviewing (see Chapter 25 for more details). For patients for whom a brief intervention is insufficient or has not been successful, the provider should refer to more formal treatment services. Medication-assisted treatment, for

example, with a combination of buprenorphine and naloxone, may be indicated for adolescents with opioid and other SUD.

Providers should also be aware that experimental substance use, or other use that does not meet criteria for SUD, may also be dangerous and potentially life threatening. In particular, highly potent opioids such as fentanyl are increasingly found in substances such as counterfeit opioid pills, cocaine, methamphetamines, and heroin or in combination with synthetic substances or cannabis products. Those buying and/or taking these substances are often unaware they have been tainted with fentanyl, and a single dose may be deadly. Adolescents should be informed about the risk of unintentional overdose, particularly with oral opioids obtained on the street or ordered online. For adolescents using opioids and other substances, counseling on harm reduction strategies (e.g., only using in the presence of other people to reduce the risk of fatal overdose) and the provision of the opioid antagonist naloxone may be lifesaving.

DURING THE VISIT

There is some debate as to whether asymptomatic adolescents benefit from regular health maintenance visits. The

American Academy of Pediatrics' *Bright Futures* recommends annual visits for health supervision and emphasizes that anticipatory guidance is a critical component of these visits for adolescents and young adults. Health maintenance visits are also opportunities to perform recommended routine screening. All adolescents should be screened at least annually for depression and substance use. Sexually active teenagers should be routinely screened for sexually transmitted diseases; the Centers for Disease Control and Prevention (CDC) has published guidelines on which specific test(s) to use and how often. Nucleic acid amplification tests for *Neisseria gonorrhoeae* and *Chlamydia trachomatis* are highly sensitive and specific and, in many cases, may be performed on urine. The National Heart, Lung, and Blood Institute and the American Academy of Pediatrics recommend cholesterol screening twice during adolescence, although the benefit of such testing is unclear. Otherwise, routine laboratory evaluation (e.g., with chemistry panels, complete blood counts, or urinalysis) in an asymptomatic adolescent is usually unnecessary. Immunizations should be given when they are due. Asymptomatic adolescents may not present for annual health maintenance examinations. Clinic visits for other complaints should be used as opportunities to provide age-appropriate anticipatory guidance, perform routine screening (e.g., for sexually transmitted infections), and provide vaccinations (including catch-up vaccinations), regardless of the chief complaint.

Taking A Medical History

As with younger adolescents, clinicians working with late adolescents and young adults should discuss confidentiality and its limits with patients and families before beginning the interview. As noted above, young adults who have reached the age of majority have the right to make their own medical decisions, and medical information can generally not be shared with others without the patient's consent. Additionally, all states and the District of Columbia have minor consent laws allowing minors to consent to certain types of medical care (e.g., sexual and reproductive health, mental health, substance use treatment) without parental consent or notification. Specific laws vary by state, and providers must be familiar with the minor consent laws in their state. Providers—and adolescents—should also be mindful of the potential for health information to be inadvertently disclosed to parents or others via electronic health records (EHR) and/or online patient portals. Practice- or system-level interventions to optimize EHR confidentiality are critical.

For some adolescents the connection between their health and more sensitive parts of the history, such as sexual activity or substance use, may not be obvious. Prior to obtaining a history, the provider should set the stage by explaining to the adolescent that they are going to ask about some topics that may be personal, not to be nosy, but with a goal of assessing and supporting the young person's health. The adolescent should also be reassured that they can decline to answer any question(s) they are uncomfortable with or otherwise do not wish to answer. The provider should also ensure the adolescent (and their family, if applicable) understand the state's mandated reporting guidelines and the types of concerns (e.g., abuse, neglect, sexual assault) that must be reported. The HEADS/SSHADESS framework (described in detail in Chapter 22) remains an appropriate series of questions for assessing health behaviors in emerging adulthood. In addition to the questions outlined in Chapter 22, some additional topics to cover in young adults include:

- HOME: For college students, determine the living situation while at school and during vacations. If the patient is living with roommates, inquire about the household use of nicotine, alcohol, and other drugs.
- EDUCATION/EMPLOYMENT: Ask "Have you completed high school?" or "How did high school go for you?" This helps determine the barriers or learning challenges the patient may have had as an adolescent, as well as their motivation to return to school or obtain a GED.

Physical Examination

The physical examination of a late adolescent begins with vital signs (including blood pressure), height, and weight. The provider should pay attention to the adolescent's growth trajectory, noting any significant downward deviations in weight or body mass index percentiles, which would generally be unexpected and may be signs of illness or an eating disorder. Visual examination can offer insights about the teen's interests, social connections, and well-being; for example, adolescents may wear clothing with logos of their sports team, club, or favorite musician. Assess the skin for the presence of acne, acanthosis nigricans, and/or signs of self-injury. For patients assigned male at birth, assess sexual maturity rating of the testes and for abnormalities such as hernia, hydrocele, varicoceles, and testicular mass. For patients assigned female at birth, assess sexual maturity rating of the breasts. Routine pelvic examination (including speculum examination) is not indicated for asymptomatic patients, but an external genital and/or speculum examination may be indicated for specific symptoms or concerns.

ANTICIPATORY GUIDANCE

Discuss life transitions as described earlier. Provide resources, such as information on education programs, job training, food or other public benefits, and housing, as needed. Counsel about substance use and connect patients to treatment as indicated. Discuss conflict resolution, violence, and firearm safety. Encourage patients to eat regularly and engage in physical activity they enjoy. Assess sleep hygiene and provide guidance as needed. Encourage adolescents to make and/or maintain connections with family, peers, and community. For patients who have turned 18 or will turn 18 soon, discuss considerations related to medical decision-making and privacy. Assess for the potential for changes to health insurance coverage for patients turning 18, moving out of state, and/or beginning full-time employment. Discuss the process of transition to an adult healthcare provider and assess any particular needs related to transitioning.

QUICK CHECK — 17 TO 21 YEARS

✓ Developing sense of self; increasing independence
✓ Transitions to higher education, the workforce, or the military and/or other transitions
✓ Developing intimate interpersonal relationships and exploring sexuality
✓ Inquiring about and assessing substance use
✓ Taking a behavior-directed medical history
✓ Guidelines for physical examination and laboratory investigations
✓ Anticipatory guidance

! HEADS UP — 17 TO 21 YEARS

- Use the SSHEADSS format to interview.
- Understand the consent and confidentiality laws in your state—and explain them to your patient.
- Ask open-ended, nonjudgmental questions that facilitate honest discussion about gender identity, sexuality, substance use, history of abuse, and mental health concerns.
- Screen all adolescents for depression and substance use; screen sexually active teens for sexually transmitted infections according to the CDC guidelines.
- Alcohol, nicotine (increasingly via vaping), and marijuana are the substances most commonly used by adolescents.
- Adolescents with disabilities, chronic illnesses, or other special healthcare needs should gradually increase responsibility and autonomy related to medical care to facilitate a smooth and safe transition to the adult healthcare system.
- Assess each adolescent's unique skills and strengths; focus on leveraging their strengths, resilience, and supports to promote health and minimize risk.
- Motivational interviewing can be used to promote behavior change.
- Adolescents who feel connected to family, school, and community are far less likely to participate in risky behaviors than those who feel disconnected.

RECOMMENDED READINGS

For Youth

McCoy K, Wibbelsman C. *Life happens: a teenager's guide to friends, failure, sexuality, love, rejection, addiction, peer pressure, families, loss, depression, change and other challenges of living.* New York: Berkeley; 1996.
McCoy K, Wibbelsman C. *The teenage body book.* New York: Perigee; 2016.
https://youngwomenshealth.org/
https://youngmenshealthsite.org/

For Parents

Damour L. *The emotional lives of teenagers: raising connected, capable, and compassionate adolescents.* New York: Ballantine Books; 2023.
Jensen F, Ellis Nutt A. *The teenage brain: a neuroscientist's survival guide to raising adolescents and young adults.* New York: HarperCollins; 2015.
https://hr.mit.edu/static/worklife/raising-teens/five-basics.html
https://www.cdc.gov/parents/teens/
www.understood.org/en/articles/
    iep-transition-planning-preparing-for-young-adulthood
Autism Consortium: Transitioning teens with autism spectrum disorders. https://www.bmc.org/
    sites/default/files/Patient_Care/Specialty_Care/
    AutismConsortiumTransitiontoAdulthoodManual.pdf

For Clinicians

Incorporating health care transition services into preventive care for adolescents and young adults: a toolkit for clinicians. https://gottransition.org/
    resource/?clinician-toolkit-preventive-care
What is motivational interviewing? Child Mind Institute: https://
    childmind.org/article/what-is-motivational-interviewing/

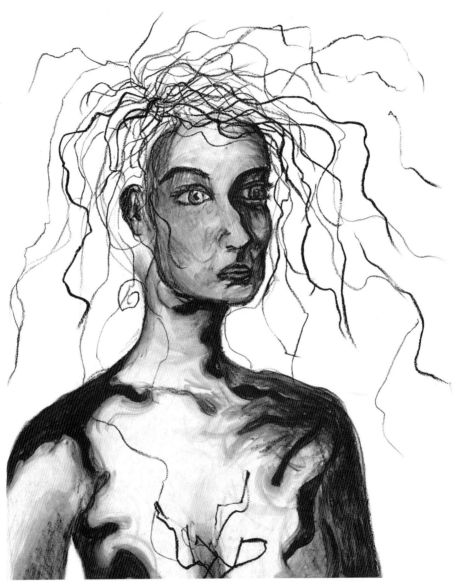

A 17-year-old's self-portrait. By Jessie Boilek (original 16 × 21 inches, charcoal).

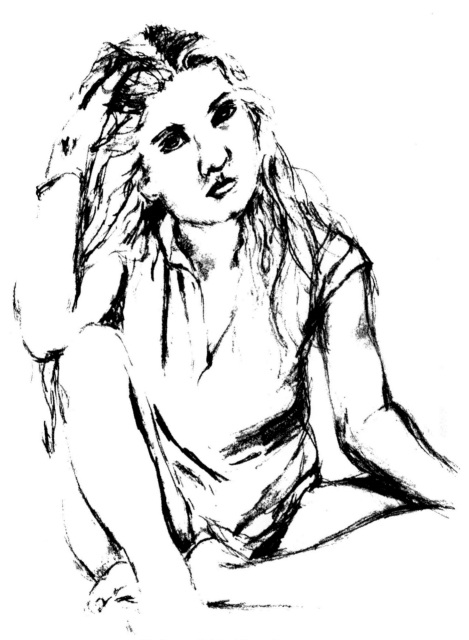

"Self-portrait." By Eileen Fitz, age 18.

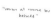
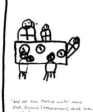

24

Specific Considerations: Families Impacted by Incarceration and the Criminal Legal System

Destiny G. Tolliver

This chapter describes the impact of incarceration on child health and development and the role of the pediatrician in supporting families and improving child outcomes.

KEYWORDS

- Family stress and child development
- Incarceration
- Stigma
- Criminal legal system
- Juvenile criminal legal system
- School-to-prison pipeline

Incarceration rates in the United States have increased substantially over the past several decades, peaking in 2007. It is estimated that 1 in 14, or more than 5 million, children in the United States have experienced the incarceration of a parent or close caregiver, which is a significant stressor. Incarceration disproportionally impacts Black, Latinx, and Indigenous families, which contributes to long-term inequities in child and family health. Pediatricians with knowledge of the impact of the criminal legal system on children and their parents are in a position to provide more attention to both the medical and psychosocial needs of this population and to advocate for structural change to support family well-being and prevent incarceration.

FAMILY STRESS AND CHILD DEVELOPMENT

Families play a critical role in child health and development across the different stages of childhood. Several family characteristics and functions are important for children, regardless of the specific makeup of the child's household:

- Regular provision of necessities, including food, housing, clothing, and medical care
- Demonstrated warmth, unconditional love, and constructive limit setting for the child
- Continuity and stability in caregiving for the child
- Stimulation of cognitive development and opportunities to enhance moral reasoning
- Capacity for meaningful interpersonal relationships, good communication, problem-solving capacity, and motivation to achieve
- Fostering of socialization by helping children function as cooperative members of society

These aspects of family functioning help children acquire a sense of security and self-esteem, learn to socialize, and develop long-term goals. Families provide concrete resources, expectations, modeling, and emotional support to their children.

When families face severe strain and acute or chronic loss, as in the case of incarceration of a family member, they commonly require additional support to continue to meet the needs of their children. Family stress may be experienced differently by families; clinicians should not make assumptions about how a family is coping but rather provide opportunities for caregivers and children to share their experiences and needs. In general, the impact of family stressors on children may be affected by several factors, including:

- The extent of loss experienced
- The duration of the loss and amount of time that has elapsed since the acute event
- The child's age and developmental stage
- The degree to which household stressors—including those that may have led to or been exacerbated by incarceration—are acute, chronic, or recurrent

- The adaptive capacity of the child
- The caregiver's ability to meet the needs of the child

The amount of time that has elapsed since the family change or loss is important in determining the nature of an individual child and family's adjustment. Acute changes can pose a profound challenge to the child and family, and there may be a period of initial shock, followed by adaptation. Age and developmental stage play an important role in determining the child's state of adjustment. For example, separations or changes in caregivers appear to be increasingly stressful to children between about 8 and 18 months of life, compared to early infancy, when the developmental stage of attachment is more prominent. Older children and other family members may experience a decrease in academic and occupational functioning, depressed mood, anxiety, and sleep disturbances in response to significant stress and loss. In the long term, child adaptation is influenced in large part by their caregiver's ability to model effective coping strategies while providing responsive and predictable care. When a child's clinician supports caregiver's well-being and recovery, they therefore encourage the child's adaptation and recovery as well.

FAMILIES IMPACTED BY INCARCERATION

In addition to common responses to loss and stress, families affected by incarceration may face specific challenges, including stigma, short- and long-term financial strain, and the stress of uncertainty.

The **stigma** associated with incarceration can isolate family members from their friends and communities and make it challenging for a parent to discuss their concerns during the pediatric visit. In general, during pediatric health supervision visits, clinicians should strive to create a welcoming, nonjudgmental space where caregivers can share family events and changes in the home and be connected with referrals or services which may be of assistance. Periodic focused questions about family function can both inform and deepen the relationship between the parents and the clinician (see Chapter 3). Clinicians should be prepared to offer age-specific resources about incarceration, including how to talk with children in developmentally appropriate ways. Attention can be focused on ways to support the child's coping skills and to maintain appropriate contact with parents, friends, and other family members. Helping parents distinguish their own needs and feelings from those of their child is also important, and referral to a trauma-informed behavioral health professional may be appropriate. Anticipatory guidance for a child can be guided by recognition of predictable stress responses at each developmental stage (as detailed in Chapter 26) (Table 24.1).

The incarceration of a family member is often accompanied by significant financial strain, which can amplify stress and further impact child and family well-being. In the short run, this may be due to loss of income of the incarcerated family member, increased need for paid childcare or other assistance, and costs related to incarceration, including payments for telephone calls or other services and travel for visitation. In the long term, financial strain may be exacerbated by challenges finding employment after incarceration and specific exclusions from many federal benefits for formerly incarcerated people.

In addition, incarceration is frequently accompanied by uncertainty, which can exacerbate the stress experienced by families. The duration and location of incarceration may change, with accompanying unpredictability in the opportunity to visit or stay in touch. This can be a challenge for children and other adults in the home; children in particular may show more behavioral dysregulation if they perceive the ambiguous loss of a parent and are unable to assure themselves of their parents' safety and well-being through scheduled visits and calls. Incarceration may also lead to short- or long-term placement of children with other relatives (which may be a formal or informal arrangement) or entry into the foster care system, depending on the circumstances. Clinicians can help identify opportunities to establish new family routines as well as ways to stay in touch with family members during challenging times. If the child has moved homes or has new caregivers, clinicians should focus on providing continuity of care, communicating frequently with all involved parties about the child's preexisting conditions and health needs, and advocating for services to support well-being during the time of loss and stress related to parental incarceration.

WHO IS IMPACTED BY INCARCERATION

Over 1.9 million people in the United States are incarcerated in prisons, jails, detention centers, and other facilities. An additional 3.7 million are on probation or parole, meaning that in total, the US criminal legal system supervises about 5.7 million people. It is estimated that about 113 million adults have had an immediate family member incarcerated. Approximately 5 million children younger than 18 years old have ever had a parent incarcerated, and approximately 2.7 million currently have an incarcerated parent.

Incarceration is remarkably concentrated among Black, Latinx, and Indigenous people, resulting in higher rates of caregiver incarceration for children within these groups as well. Incarceration is also more common among people who have experienced other forms of disadvantage, including poverty, child welfare system involvement, or lower

TABLE 24.1 Factors That May Impact a Child's Reaction to Caregiver Incarceration

Factor	Child Responses	Clinician and Caregiver Roles
Age at time of incarceration	• Younger children may not understand what is happening and where their caregiver is, leading to more disorganized feelings and behaviors. • Older children may be able to grasp the complexity of the situation and respond with externalizing and internalizing behaviors (such as disruptive behaviors or depression). • Older children may take on different roles in the household due to caregiver incarceration, such as caring for siblings or working to help provide financial resources.	• Support young children in understanding how their needs will be met by maintaining routines, including bedtime stories, meal times, and brushing teeth. • Tell young children things like who will take them to school, who will prepare meals, and so on so that they know they will be cared for. • Help children identify and express feelings. • Support youth in finding feelings of accomplishment and expressing feelings through activities, sports, and the arts.
Relationship between child and incarcerated caregiver	• Children with a more secure attachment to the incarcerated adult are more likely to experience disruption and sadness due to their absence. • Maintaining contact with an incarcerated parent may improve a child's response to incarceration, including improved emotional and behavioral health. Positive parent-child relationships during incarceration and reentry are associated with reduced recidivism, benefiting the child through improved stability after incarceration.	• Encourage families to maintain relationships with incarcerated caregivers as the child feels ready to do so and in developmentally appropriate manners (e.g., writing letters, visiting in person, making phone or video calls). • Encourage families to connect and communicate with incarcerated family members during events and achievements such as graduations and holidays.
Experiences with stigma	• Children whose parents are absent due to incarceration instead of other reasons (such as caregiver death) may face stigma rather than sympathy and care. Stigma may be internalized and lead to lower self-esteem, anger, or a desire for retaliation against people who reject or bully them. • Experiences with stigma may last for a child long after a caregiver is released.	• Remind children that a caregiver's incarceration is not their fault. • Screen children for bullying and provide appropriate resources. • Encourage children to discuss caregiver incarceration with supportive people, including friends and teachers.
Relationships with other family and community members	• Communication about a caregiver's incarceration: Some families may choose not to disclose to a child that their caregiver has been incarcerated. This desire to "protect" a child from the truth can lead to feelings of worry, uncertainty, fear, and distrust. Younger children may wonder if they too will disappear. Children who are misled learn to distrust close caregivers. Additionally, children who are not told about the location of their caregiver are thus unlikely to visit their parent, which raises barriers to maintaining a relationship with them. • In contrast, strong relationships with caregivers, other family members, and community members may reduce the trauma of incarceration.	• Encourage family members to have honest conversations about where the incarcerated caregiver is. • Encourage families to visit incarcerated loved ones, in particular by engaging in developmentally appropriate visiting programs where available. • Connect youth to mentorship programs or other programs that support prosocial development.

Adapted from La Vigne NG, Davies E, Brazzell D: The Urban Institute research report: "Broken bonds: understanding and addressing the needs of children with incarcerated parents", 2008. Available from https://www.urban.org/research/publication/broken-bonds-understanding-and-addressing-needs-children-incarcerated-parents educational attainment. People who are structurally marginalized in other ways, including LGBT+ (lesbian, gay, bisexual, transsexual/transgender, and queer) people and people with mental health or substance use disorders, also experience incarceration at higher rates than people who are not members of these groups. These differences in incarceration rates are driven by policies including stringent sentencing laws, the war on drugs, and discriminatory policing that together criminalized a wide swath of behaviors and people. Some quantitative studies indicate some short-term improvement in household status following incarceration of a family member—particularly for households in which the incarcerated family member struggled with substance use, mental health problems, or other sources of household conflict like abuse or neglect. However, qualitative investigation has indicated that the benefit felt by families may be due to them having some respite from household disruptions, leading researchers to believe that the "benefits" are not benefits of incarceration itself but instead the benefit of incarceration when other high-quality services for addiction, mental health needs, and other problems are absent.

IMPACT OF CAREGIVER INCARCERATION ON CHILD HEALTH

Caregiver incarceration is associated with worse child physical health, including worse overall health and higher odds of reporting physical health problems like asthma and migraines both during childhood and young adulthood. Caregiver incarceration is also associated with child learning disabilities, speech delays, attention-deficit disorder/attention-deficit hyperactivity disorder (ADHD), depression, anxiety, and other behavioral disorders. It is not known whether these associations are due to inherited propensity toward developmental-behavioral conditions (i.e., learning disabilities, ADHD, and language delays have a strong genetic component), the stress the child undergoes when a caregiver is incarcerated, or the cooccurrence of other forms of household disadvantage that are known to shape child outcomes. However, studies indicate that the associations between caregiver incarceration and child health are not solely due to preexisting hardships. Qualitative research highlights that caregiver incarceration generally worsens existing family hardship through mechanisms such as lowering paternal prosocial family engagement, increasing maternal depression, and worsening economic hardship.

It is also worth noting that some caregivers express hesitancy for giving their child a developmental or behavioral "label" or ADHD medication because of past negative experiences with a family member who, after receiving similar labels or medication, went on to be involved in the criminal legal system. It is important to recognize that, for marginalized families, the same labels and diagnoses we seek to give children to facilitate receipt of services or special education may be seen as the medical or educational system putting their child in a "box." This is an important opportunity to engage your own cultural humility, meet the caregiver where they are, and be transparent about the treatment goals and plan for your partnership in helping a child with a new developmental-behavioral diagnosis.

JUVENILE CRIMINAL LEGAL SYSTEM INVOLVEMENT

Youth may become involved in the criminal legal system and experience incarceration at a young age as well. The United Nations Convention on the Rights of the Child decreed that all nations should set a minimum age of criminal responsibility of at least 14 years old. The United States has not endorsed these recommendations. At the time of this writing, there are minimum ages of juvenile court jurisdiction of 7 to 13 years, although approximately half of US states do not have a minimum age at all. Because of this, children across the United States experience police stops, arrests, prosecution, and even incarceration at higher rates than any other country in the world.

As of this writing, there are approximately 48,000 youth confined in facilities as a result of juvenile or adult criminal legal system involvement. The majority are younger than 18 years old, but this number also includes some youth 18 to 20 years old who were charged as juveniles and remain incarcerated within the juvenile system. In 2020, over 400,000 youth were arrested in the United States. At each stage of the criminal legal system, Black children and Indigenous children are overrepresented compared to their share of the population. Many of these encounters with the criminal legal system are driven by similar factors as those that drive adult incarceration, including overpoliced communities and discriminatory treatment by the criminal legal system. Additionally, youth may be connected to the criminal legal system via the school-to-prison pipeline.

The school-to-prison pipeline is a set of practices and policies that decrease school engagement, increase the likelihood of school dropout (a risk factor for later criminal legal system involvement), and even directly cause juvenile criminal legal system contact. Manifestations of the school-to-prison pipeline include creating a more prison-like school environment (e.g., metal detectors at the doors, police dogs on campus), a reduction in supportive services on campus (e.g., social workers, psychologists), and an increased use of punitive responses to child behavior through exclusionary discipline (i.e., suspension and expulsion). In response to shootings and other violent events in schools across the United States, many school administrators have taken a "zero tolerance" policy that leads to the suspension or expulsion of children who have made threats or acted aggressively, even if these behaviors are explained by the child's underlying disability. After the COVID-19 pandemic, when children returned to school with heightened stress levels and behavior dysregulation, there were reports of increased rates of suspension and use of restraints or isolation to manage child behavior. This was likely due to schools having insufficient therapeutic/support staff to help create and implement positive behavioral support plans. Additionally, the presence of school resource officers can lead to an escalation of school behavioral problems to legal problems through the use of in-school arrests. Children who are Black, Indigenous, or have disabilities (including autism spectrum disorder and learning disabilities) are more commonly impacted by the school-to-prison pipeline and are similarly overrepresented among children who are involved in the juvenile criminal legal system.

Child involvement in the juvenile criminal legal system or the adult criminal legal system is associated with worse health, both in childhood and later in adulthood. Police stops, arrests, and incarceration have all been associated with worse behavioral and mental health needs among youth and later on in adulthood. In particular, involvement in the criminal legal system, both informal (e.g., police stops) and formal (e.g., incarceration), can have important impacts on the development of a child's sense of self, including creating a self-perceived "criminal identity" that can lead to cycles of system involvement, developing barriers to prosocial activities (e.g., hanging out in public spaces with friends) due to fears of arrest, and feeling resigned to injustices.

WHAT CLINICIANS CAN DO

Clinicians can support families impacted by the criminal legal system by helping them to connect to resources and through advocacy.

In the clinical setting, clinicians can work with families to identify and address physical, mental, behavioral, and educational problems. In particular, referral to mental health clinicians may be an important tool to address mental and behavioral health needs early on and before they are exacerbated by the stressor of criminal legal system contact. Additionally, helping to ensure youth have optimized educational services through individualized education plans and 504 plans may help to improve educational outcomes. Families from historically marginalized communities may not feel confident in engaging with the school around their child's special education evaluation results and supports, and it may help to provide coaching about the types of questions to ask (e.g., "What other approaches could be tried? What data will you collect to make sure my child is improving? How often can we meet or communicate so that I can keep updated on their progress?"), resources (see the "Recommended Readings" section), and educational advocate contact information.

Clinicians can also screen for household needs, such as housing, food security, and income security, and help connect families to state and federal benefit programs. Clinicians should become familiar with local and community-level programs such as support groups, after-school programs, and summer camps that may provide additional support and connection for families impacted by the criminal legal system. For children who have been placed with relatives or in foster care, clinicians should communicate frequently with all caregivers and involved agencies to ensure there is shared understanding of the children's needs and available resources.

Clinicians can also advocate for less punitive approaches to child behavior, such as incorporating social-emotional learning, responsive classroom approaches (i.e., where negative behavior results in a prompt to "rest and return," so the child can learn to self-regulate rather than be punished), or restorative justice into school practices. Such universal interventions help all students learn social-emotional skills but are even more likely to improve outcomes for youth who have experienced caregiver incarceration and reduce the effect of the school-to-prison pipeline for children themselves.

Additionally, clinicians can advocate for policies that reduce family separation and improve access to resources. For example, some states have passed laws that allow judges to consider a person's role as a caregiver at the time of sentencing to help divert caregivers to shorter sentences or more community resources rather than incarceration. Additionally, clinicians can advocate for policies that eliminate the costs of phone calls and reduce barriers to visitation for family members. Clinicians can also support policies that reduce the criminalization of mental health and substance use disorders to ensure that they are treated as public health problems and approached with resources rather than incarceration. For families that have experienced incarceration, clinicians can advocate for an end to policies that exclude people with certain felony convictions from participating in public benefits (e.g., Medicaid, the Supplemental Nutrition Assistance Program, Temporary Assistance for Needy Families) to ensure that eligible families are able to access necessary resources.

CONCLUSION

Children in the United States are commonly impacted by incarceration and family involvement in the criminal legal system. Pediatric clinicians should understand the challenges faced by families and be prepared to provide increased support during times of need, with the aim of supporting healthy child development and family wellness.

> **⚠ HEADS UP**
>
> - Sensitivity to family circumstances at each pediatric encounter enhances the quality of communication among clinicians, parents, and children.
> - An individual child or parent's response to stress is subjective; ask about their sense of the severity of loss or upheaval rather than rely on assumptions and impressions.
> - Do not underestimate the value of supportive care when working with families impacted by incarceration, including asking empathic questions about the family constellation, discovering and commenting on family and child developmental strengths, and connecting families to community resources that will support the family and child's developmental needs.
> - Continue to ask about the effects of change on the child's well-being, including development and behavior, over time.
> - Consider behavioral health referrals for children and care-givers coping with the incarceration of a family member.
> - Recognize the enormous stress placed on the caregiving parent and provide additional support, along with referrals to relevant community resources.
> - Be attentive to the strengths of children and families that promote educational, psychological, and social resiliency. Support parents with positive feedback.

> **QUICK CHECK**
>
> - Involvement in the criminal legl system impacts many children and their families and disproportionately impacts children who are marginalized by race or income.
> - Criminal legal system involvement is a stressor for children and their caregivers that can cause or worsen physical and mental health needs.
> - Investing in supportive systems for children, families, communities, and schools may improve the health of children impacted by the criminal legal system.

RECOMMENDED READINGS

For Parents

Sesame street family resources on incarceration. Available from https://sesamestreetincommunities.org/topics/incarceration/

HealthyChildren.org: Tips to support children when a parent is in prison. Available from https://www.healthychildren.org/English/healthy-living/emotional-wellness/Building-Resilience/Pages/Tips-to-Support-Children-When-a-Parent-is-in-Prison.aspx

Rutgers University Director of Programs serving children & families of the incarcerated. Available from https://nrccfi.camden.rutgers.edu/resources/directory/national-programs/

Children's Bureau Learning & Coordination Center: Families impacted by incarceration: resources for working with families. Available from https://cblcc.acf.hhs.gov/topic-areas/incarceration-old/families/

Children's Welfare Information Gateway: Organizations in support of children and families of the incarcerated. Available from https://www.childwelfare.gov/organizations/?CWIGFunctionsaction=rols:main.dspList&rolType=Custom&RS_ID=113&rList=ROL

For Clinicians

Prison Policy Institute: Mass incarceration: the whole pie 2023, 2023. Available from https://www.prisonpolicy.org/reports/pie2023.html

Annie E Casey Foundation: A shared sentence: the devastating toll of parental incarceration on kids, families and communities, 2016. http://www.aecf.org/resources/a-shared-sentence/

Enns PK, Yi Y, Comfort M, et al. What percentage of Americans have ever had a family member incarcerated? Evidence from the Family History of Incarceration Survey (FamHIS). *Socius Sociol Res Dyn World*. 2019;5. https://doi.org/10.1177/2378023119829332. 237802311982933.

Lee H, Wildeman C. Assessing mass incarceration's effects on families. *Science*. 2021;374(6565):277–281. https://doi.org/10.1126/science.abj7777.

Wildeman C, Goldman AW, Turney K. Parental incarceration and child health in the United States. *Epidemiol Rev.* 2018;40(1):146–156. https://doi.org/10.1093/epirev/mxx013.

Turney K. Stress proliferation across generations? Examining the relationship between parental incarceration and childhood health. *J Health Soc Behav.* 2014;55(3):302–319. https://doi.org/10.1177/0022146514544173.

Heard-Garris N, Sacotte KA, Winkelman TNA, Cohen A, Ekwueme PO, Barnert E: Association of childhood history of parental incarceration and juvenile justice involvement with mental health in early adulthood, *JAMA Netw Open* 2(9):e1910465, 2019. doi:10.1001/jamanetworkopen.2019.10465

National Juvenile Justice Network: NJJN policy platform: raise the minimum age for trying children in juvenile court, 2020.

Office of Juvenile Justice and Delinquency Prevention: OJJDP statistical briefing book, 2020. http://www.ojjdp.gov/ojstatbb/crime/JAR_Display.asp?ID=qa05200

National Juvenile Justice Network: NJJN policy platform: racial and ethnic disparities in juvenile justice systems, 2010.

Owen MC, Wallace SB. Advocacy and collaborative health care for justice-involved youth. *Pediatrics.* 2020;146(1). https://doi.org/10.1542/peds.2020-1755.

Tolliver DG, Abrams LS, Barnert ES. Setting a US national minimum age for juvenile justice jurisdiction. *JAMA Pediatr.* 2021. https://doi.org/10.1542/peds.2020-1755.

Mallett CA. The school-to-prison pipeline: a critical review of the punitive paradigm shift. *Child Adolesc Soc Work J.* 2016;33(1):15–24. https://doi.org/10.1007/s10560-015-0397-1.

Jackson DB, Fahmy C, Vaughn MG, Testa A. Police stops among at-risk youth: repercussions for mental health. *J Adolesc Health.* 2019;65(5):627–632. https://doi.org/10.1016/j.jadohealth.2019.05.027.

Jackson DB, Testa A, Fix RL, Mendelson T: Adolescent police stops, self-harm, and attempted suicide: findings from the UK Millennium Cohort Study, 201232019, *Am J Public Health* 111(10):1885–1893, 2021. doi:10.2105/AJPH.2021.306434

Jindal M, Mistry KB, Trent M, McRae A, Thornton RLJ: Police exposures and the health and well-being of Black youth in the US: a systematic review, *JAMA Pediatr* 176(1):78–88, 2022. doi:10.1001/jamapediatrics.2021.2929

Barnert ES, Perry R, Azzi VF, et al. Incarcerated youths' perspectives on protective factors and risk factors for juvenile offending: a qualitative analysis. *Am J Public Health.* 2015;105(7):1365–1371. https://doi.org/10.2105/AJPH.2014.302228.

Barnert ES, Abrams LS, Dudovitz R, et al. What is the relationship between incarceration of children and adult health outcomes? *Acad Pediatr.* 2019;19(3):342–350. https://doi.org/10.1016/j.acap.2018.06.005.

Tolliver DG, Abrams LS, Biely C, et al: United States youth arrest and health across the life course: a nationally representative longitudinal study, *Acad Pediatr* 23(4):722–730, 2023. doi:10.1016/j.acap.2022.08.009

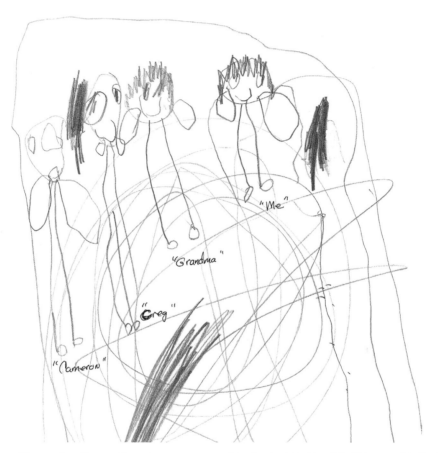

A home with grandmother as the primary care provider is depicted by this 5½-year-old. By Jared Mell.

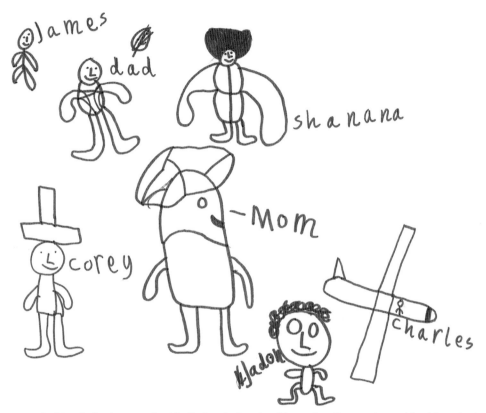

An extended family is shown, all with distinct hairstyles. The artist, Corey, shows his older adopted brother in the upper left; his uncle is seen departing in the plane. It seems that Mom is at the center of things, holding it all together.

25

Encounters With Illness: Coping and Growing

Cassie N. Ross

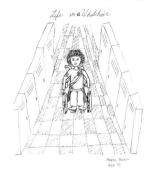

Pediatric clinicians can enhance quality of care with an understanding about the developmental and psychosocial significance of acute and chronic illness for both children and caregivers. An office visit offers an opportunity to enhance a child's understanding of their body, improve **coping**, and practice **self-advocacy**/communication as well as promote accurate caregiver perceptions of their child's health. The principles of chronic illness and developmentally specific responses to hospitalization and procedures are reviewed with recommendations for pediatric practice.

KEYWORDS

- Coping
- Functional symptoms or disorder
- Health belief model
- Illness, disorder, disease
- Motivational interviewing
- Self-advocacy
- Social determinants of health
- The pediatric psychosocial prevention health model
- Transtheoretical model
- Trauma-informed care

Pediatric clinicians pride themselves on accurate diagnosis of diseases and conditions. However, in addition to disease recognition and appropriate treatment, attention to the way a child and caregiver perceive an illness or disease as well as the behavior and feelings that are a result of their illness are important components of comprehensive care. By considering the biopsychosocial and socioecological frameworks of the child and family, the pediatric clinician

enhances their ability to provide comprehensive, family-centered, and culturally humble care.

The biopsychosocial framework postulates that biological, psychological, and social constructs are interrelated and impact an individual's overall health (Table 25.1). Biological factors may include genetics, physical symptoms, sleep, nutrition, and exercise. Psychological factors may include the emotional result of life stressors, how an individual thinks about their health and behaviors, diagnosis of mental health conditions, and so on. Finally, social factors can be expanded to the socioecological frameworks that play a major role in health (see Chapter 2 for more information on the socioecological model). The pediatric psychosocial preventive health model, based on Bronfenbrenner's Bioecological Systems Theory, describes the impact of social factors on child development by considering the various systems involved in every person's life (see Table 25.1). A pediatric clinician is well suited to explore the impact of biopsychosocial factors on a child's health as well as provide targeted interventions to reduce risk factors or other health disparities.

Acute and chronic illnesses can be viewed in the context of a particular child's development, as well as the family's experience, perceptions, and expectations with symptoms and disease, which vary greatly within family systems and cultures. Although an illness may interfere with normal developmental processes, it may also be an opportunity for mastery and enhancement of self-esteem. By helping caregivers and children build self-understanding of their perceptions and reactions to the diagnosis and treatments, how they cope in response to symptoms and/or stress, and how this impacts their overall well-being, clinicians can contribute to a trusting relationship with families and hopefully influence more positive long-term outcomes.

In primary care pediatric practice, about 50% of office visits are for an **acute illness**; 20% of visits are for **preventative care**; about 10% to 15% of visits are related to routine

Previous chapter author: Martin T. Stein.

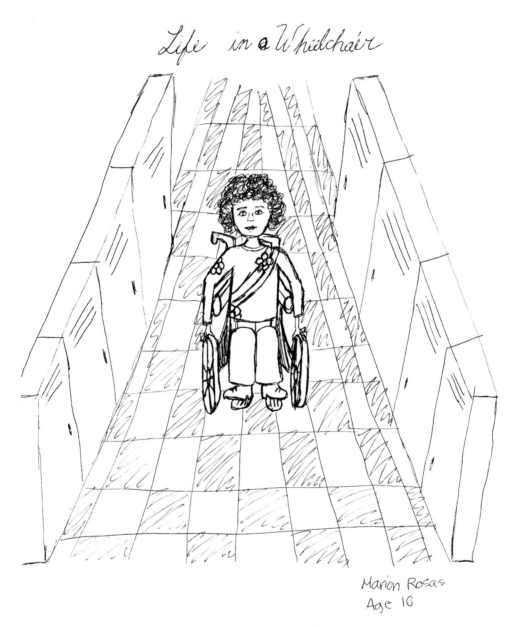

A 10-year-old girl portrays her life as she moves around her school in a wheelchair. By Marion Rosas, age 10.

TABLE 25.1   Biopsychosocial Approach to Evaluation and Intervention

Approach	Evaluation	Intervention
Biological	• Cognitive functioning • Developmental stage • Diet/nutrition • Genetics/family history • Known medical conditions or developmental disorder • Level of physical activity • Medications • Pain • Sleep	• Developmentally and cognitively appropriate education. Provide alternative educational methods (written, pictorial, videos, etc.) • Encourage optimal sleep, nutrition, and physical activity • Optimize pain control • Refer for neuropsychological evaluation • Simplify medication regimens. Limit drug interactions or side effects as much as possible
Psychological	• Anxiety/Fear • Coping style (avoidant versus active) • Externalizing or internalizing behaviors • Health beliefs: susceptibility, severity, and self-efficacy • Mood • Motivation • Previous traumatic experiences	• Developmentally and cognitively appropriate education. Provide alternative educational methods (written, pictorial, videos, etc.) • Develop coping plans • Provide education and utilize trauma-informed care practices • Refer to psychotherapy and/or psychiatry • Utilize motivational interviewing to increase motivation to change • Utilize teach-back method to assess understanding and catch misperceptions
Social	• Macrosystem: culture, social norms, economic system, political system, racism • Mesosystem: interactions between parties in the microsystem • Microsystem: family, school, peers, work, neighbors, medical providers	• Advocate and/or participate in policy change • Continued education. Practice cultural humility and continue to be self-reflective to catch bias in your care • Directly communicate with key microsystem parties (i.e., extended family members, school, specialty medical providers) • Encourage 504 or Individualized Education Program evaluation • Engage with social worker

or flare of a **chronic illness**, and about 7% of children experience at least one hospitalization in a 12-month period. Each of these encounter types represents an opportunity to build understanding of how children and families experience and cope with illness; from a well-defined, limited illness (e.g., streptococcal pharyngitis) to a complicated, chronic illness (e.g., asthma exacerbation in a child with multiple hospitalizations and significant family stress).

HELPING CAREGIVERS AND CHILDREN UNDERSTAND ILLNESSES

Health Belief Model

The **Health belief model** (HBM) was developed to understand the relationship between cognitions and behaviors surrounding health. This model can be used to understand how an individual's cognitions surrounding health impact health-related behaviors as well as how caregiver cognitions impact their child's health care. The relevant dimensions of the HBM include perceptions of susceptibility, severity, self-efficacy, and triggers for health-related behaviors. When conducting an evaluation with families, it can be helpful to identify both the child's and caregiver's perception of the child's susceptibility, or vulnerability, to illness as well as how severe or dangerous the illness is perceived. Self-efficacy can be defined as how confident the child or caregiver is that they can care for the illness on their own or complete the treatment as prescribed by a physician. Finally, triggers for health-related behaviors include internal triggers (i.e., previous experiences with illness, the symptoms of the condition) or external triggers (i.e., relatives, friends, healthcare providers, Internet, media) that cue the caregiver or child to pursue health care or other health-related behaviors.

Building aspects of the HBM into the evaluation of a child presenting with an acute or chronic illness can help identify caregiver and patient perspectives that may benefit from additional education, clarification, and/or intervention, particularly if there is an incongruency between the perceived and actual susceptibility and severity of illness and/or low self-efficacy. Some caregivers may view their child as more vulnerable to illness or that their condition is more severe and dangerous. Numerous factors could contribute to the development of this view, and commonly caregivers have experienced previous medical trauma and/or serious or life-threatening illness within the family. While the caregiver's intent is to protect their child from serious illness, inaccurate perceptions of child vulnerability may result in high healthcare utilization, excessive school absences, and may impact parenting resulting in insecure attachment, a lack of limit setting, and low expectations of their child. As a result, the child may internalize vulnerability and have high health anxiety, develop functional/somatic symptoms that reinforce caregiver misperceptions of health, avoid school, and have difficulties with social interactions. The pediatrician plays an extremely important role in supporting these families to regauge their perceptions of their child's health.

Communication With Caregivers

Pediatric clinicians can practice a form of preventive medicine to limit adverse psychosocial responses during the course of acute minor illnesses, chronic illness, and/or the discovery of benign, often transient physical findings. No matter the illness presentation, careful and clear communication with families is key to not only ensure proper understanding of the condition and treatment recommendations but also build a strong relational foundation. The *TEACHER* mnemonic is a useful technique to improve the quality of communication with children and their caregivers at the time of a visit (Table 25.2). Important components of communication include the primary differential diagnoses considered, testing planned, a summary of testing that has been completed to date and results, clear diagnosis if appropriate, treatment recommendations based on testing results, and clear communication regarding the level of risk based on all of these data. Caregivers may appreciate developing a concrete plan for responding to symptoms, which may include how to manage at home and school, what symptoms are considered an emergency/urgent/routine, access to on-call providers, and assurance for ongoing communication and reassessment. As much as possible, providing alternative methods for education,

TABLE 25.2 TEACHER—Method for Enhancing Communication With Pediatric Patients and Their Caregivers

T	Trust	Build trust and rapport with both caregiver(s) and the child by asking about their values, interests, and other nonmedical questions
E	Elicit	Elicit information from the caregiver(s) and child regarding concerns and the child's understanding of the reason for the visit
A	Agenda	Set an agenda early in the visit to help ensure that concerns are addressed
C	Control	Help the child feel control over the visit (e.g., knowing what will and will not happen) to help decrease fear and increase cooperation
H	Health plan	Establish a health plan with the child and caregiver(s) to meet the child's needs
E	Explain	Explain the health plan to the caregiver(s) and child in a way they can understand
R	Rehearse	Have the caregiver(s) and child rehearse the health plan as a way of assessing understanding; reinforce the caregiver(s) and child's jobs related to health care; explore any potential problems/barrier in the plan with the child and caregiver

From Bernzweig J, Pantell R, Lewis CC: Talking with children. In Parker S, Zuckerman B, editors: *Behavioral and developmental pediatrics*, New York, 1995, Little, Brown, p 7.

such as written materials, videos, and/or visuals, is recommended. Evaluating a caregiver's and patient's understanding of the diagnosis and treatment utilizing the teach-back method is a necessary step. All your hard work in providing education will be wasted if the family does not understand!

The discovery of benign, often transient physical findings, can be challenging to navigate as there can be a delicate balance between thorough education and the development excessive caregiver concern or unnecessary restrictions. Communication surrounding these benign or transient physical findings is crucial to keep a caregiver apprised of their child's medical findings, building a sense of trust with families, and to ensure an accurate understanding of the implications of the findings and recommendations. Common physical findings that require clear explanation to prevent a "nondisease" problem include a functional cardiac murmur, hyperbilirubinemia in infants, mild (physiological) adenopathy, tibial torsion, hydrocele, strawberry hemangioma, and umbilical hernia. For example, a benign functional cardiac murmur may be managed in several ways: (1) do not mention it because it is so frequently found and inconsequential; (2) tell the caregivers that their child "has a murmur coming from the heart that is called a functional murmur … It's not really important and we won't worry about it"; (3) explain to the caregivers that it is a sound heard when listening to a normal heart in a healthy child, does not reflect any cardiac problems, will disappear as the child grows, does not require any treatments or changes to the child's life, and if/how it will be monitored moving forward. Since the findings may be inconsequential for the child's health, it may be tempting to avoid informing the caregivers. A decision to withhold this information should be assessed carefully with the tenets of beneficence and nonmalfeasance at the forefront, balanced with the increased access to electronic medical records by families as well as the potential legal implications that could arise from withholding information. When in doubt, it is likely best to inform the caregivers verbally to support trust and an accurate understanding of the finding. The second explanation is vague and, for some vulnerable families, may predispose to "cardiac nondisease," a condition in which the caregivers leave the office uncertain of their child's cardiac status. Some caregivers may inappropriately restrict the child's activity or develop an inappropriate sense of vulnerability about the health of the child. The third explanation is preferred as it includes information about the specific finding, what the finding means for their child's health, any treatment or monitoring that will occur, why it is not a concerning finding, recommendations for the caregivers (i.e., no changes to the child's life), and alternative resources for information like written information, visuals, or videos. Offering opportunities to ask questions can support ease of mind. Finally, to evaluate the caregiver's understanding, utilize the teach-back method which may reveal misunderstanding or misconceptions that can be addressed. In follow-up visits, it can be helpful to check in families to assess their health beliefs, any activity restriction, and ensure ongoing understanding of any benign conditions.

Another common presentation that requires careful communication is hyperbilirubinemia in infants as it may appear serious or even life threatening to a caregiver but is characteristically benign and limited to the early neonatal period. Diagnostic and monitoring interventions (blood tests) and therapy (phototherapy accompanied by daily home nursing visits) are often overmedicated by clinicians, nurses, and other health personnel. In part, this is because hyperbilirubinemia can be associated with serious consequences in some circumstances. However, a pediatrician should be able to communicate the diagnosis and treatment of this condition to the caregivers in a manner that instills trust while maintaining/reinstating an exhausted caregiver's view of a healthy baby. It is most likely a benign condition that will resolve spontaneously or with a few days of phototherapy, will not recur, and will not have any lasting effect on the baby's growth and development. Without this kind of focused caregiver education, a common problem such as neonatal hyperbilirubinemia can induce in the new, likely exhausted, caregivers a lasting sense of vulnerability about the baby.

Communication With Children

Direct, transparent, accurate, and developmentally appropriate explanations during visits help children and caregivers understand and adapt to illness, medical evaluations, and treatment. Children tend to benefit from knowing what is happening with their body, what to expect in the evaluation and treatment, and what will be done to help them through anything difficult. If possible, having the child directly participate in the evaluation can provide deeper understanding of their perceptions, experiences, and coping style. It is key to provide transparent and accurate descriptions of the evaluation and treatment to children to manage expectations and instill/maintain trust in medical providers. Dishonesty ("the shot the nurse will give won't hurt you"), dismissing a child's experiences ("your belly really doesn't hurt that much"), separation from a caregiver during a procedure, and preoccupation with the disease (medical diagnosis) may increase the risk of medical trauma and result in adverse outcomes in children.

A Child's Understanding of Illness

Illness is a part of childhood. Acute illnesses occur frequently and are usually self-limited or responsive to medical therapy. During the first three years of life, most children experience between six and nine illnesses each year; most illnesses are respiratory or gastrointestinal infections. Between 4 and 10 years old, children average four to six illnesses annually. The high transmission rate throughout a family means that a family with two adults and two children will average 21 illnesses per year. A child's early experiences with these inevitable parts of childhood potentially shape several aspects of their development.

Every pediatric clinician who enters an examination room has one major objective: to get the diagnosis right and prescribe the appropriate treatment. This goal, coupled with empathy and the recognition that both child and caregiver are experiencing the stress of the illness (see Chapter 3), makes up the core components of pediatric practice. The next level of understanding is to ask the question, "What is the child's understanding of their symptoms and the reason they have been brought to the doctor?" The child may have limited understanding or misperceptions that should be addressed.

An understanding of a child's perspective on the acute illness visit is crucial for two reasons. First, it generates age-appropriate ways to communicate with children, a core pediatric value. Equally important is the clinician's recognition that *the experience of the office visit itself shapes the way a child learns and feels about their body, how their body works, how to verbalize and communicate physical symptoms, and what to expect through the healing process.* The cumulative experiences of illness management and experiences at the doctor's office contribute a child's coping with illness and subsequent adult perceptions of physical and psychological symptoms, response to illness, and perceptions of health care.

Perceptions About Illness Change With Cognitive Development

Children perceive the nature of their illness in a manner consistent with their cognitive level of development. The level of understanding of symptoms moves during childhood through a rapid developmental change from the magical responses ("You get sick because you eat too much candy") of preschool children to logic of early school-age children ("You get sick because you go out in the cold") to older school-age children, who are able to generalize symptoms and show some understanding of the role of a germ in causing disease, as well as beginning awareness of their contribution to the nature of the experience (Table 25.3).

As clinicians develop a better understanding of a child's internal response to an illness, they are in a better position to offer individualized targeted suggestions. In addition, this knowledge strengthens the therapeutic alliance with

TABLE 25.3   Growth in a Child's Understanding of Illness

Age (Years)	Understanding	Examples
4–6	Circular, magical, or global responses	"I got a boo-boo on my head because I didn't eat my soup!" (a child's reaction to a scalp laceration caused by falling and hitting his head on a table shortly after lunchtime, when his mother unsuccessfully encouraged him to eat tomato soup).
6–8	Concrete, rigid responses with a "parrot-like" quality; little comprehension by the child; enumeration of symptoms, actions, or situations associated with illness	"The cough is a bug that tickles my throat and makes me stay home and in bed. The bug can't play with my friends."
8–11	Increased generalization, with some indication of the child's contribution to the response; the quality of invariant causation remains	"I get these headaches sometimes because I fight with my sister and won't let her play with my things." When asked about his symptoms during a mild gastroenteritis episode, Sammy responded, "I got it because I ate some poison, just like last year when we all got sick at the restaurant."
11–13	Beginning use of an underlying principle; greater delineation of causal agents of illnesses	"Kids get sick when germs like a virus get into their body. It's the virus that makes us feel lousy, causes a fever and makes us want to sleep more."
Over 14	Organized description of mechanism(s) underlying illness and recovery; abstract principles	"Last year I had mono along with three of my friends. I know it's caused by a virus that makes you sleepy and not want to eat and zaps energy. But my friends got better quickly. I stayed out of school for a month. It seems that the mono virus was harder on my body and tougher to get rid of. My mom thinks it's because we've had a lot of stress in the family. She may be right because I know I get better quicker from a cold when things at home are cool."

Modified from Perrin EC, Gerrity PS: There's a demon in your belly: children's understanding of concepts regarding illness. *Pediatrics* 67:841, 1981.

children and their caregivers. Knowledge about frequently used coping strategies during an acute illness will bring some of these insights to the medical encounter. For example, it is important to understand that a child younger than 5 years often runs away from a clinician and hides behind or under an examination table. They may ask for a bandage or a kiss on a "boo-boo." These are direct coping mechanisms that reflect the child's magical thinking rather than the logical consequences of events. For a school-age child who may perceive a set of symptoms in concrete terms and may begin to show some understanding of causality, an astute clinician can make use of the new coping skills. Allowing the child to listen to their heart with a stethoscope, to ask questions about a medicine or an x-ray film, and encouraging them to talk about perceptions of the illness will give them an opportunity to learn about how their body works which can instill a sense of control, use age-appropriate coping skills, and enhance the therapeutic relationship. As always, ensuring that the child has an accurate understanding of the illness and treatment, as much as is developmentally appropriate, is key!

When Physical Symptoms Are Inconsistent With a Known Medical Condition

An early adolescent comes to the doctor with frequent physical symptoms such as headaches, abdominal pain, chest pain, back pain, sore throats, and/or neurological symptoms like weakness, loss of consciousness, and so on that are either mild and self-limited or cause significant pain, disability, and distress above what would be expected for a mild illness. Children frequently present with symptoms that are not consistent with a known medical condition. These situations are familiar to all pediatric clinicians. While these concerns come up frequently, a complicating factor in providing education to children and caregivers is the lack of a unified descriptive language amongst providers. Common terms include functional, somatic, psychosomatic, somatoform, amplified pain, medically unexplained, and/or mental health/stress related, amongst many others. Unfortunately, many of the terms used are stigmatizing and confusing to patients and families. As such, using the term **functional symptoms or disorder** is preferred as it describes a disorder of the body's communication pathways, rather than organic disease, and limits the emphasis on mental health.

There are numerous biopsychosocial factors (see Table 25.1) that may explain the adolescent's frequent doctor's visits with what appears to be functional symptoms. These encounters offer opportunities to explore how both the family and adolescent perceive and experience these physical symptoms as well as additional factors that may exacerbate symptoms. Biological factors that may contribute to functional symptoms include genetic predisposition to

functional symptoms and mental health concerns, sleep, nutrition, as well as differences in the patient's somatosensory cortex. A family history of functional symptoms may be difficult to prove, but it helps to explore whether other family members have similar symptoms to the patient or if there are frequent headaches, stomach aches, back pain, or other illnesses that do not have a clear medical etiology. Psychologically, there is a subset of patients who endorse premorbid depression and anxiety, and acute stressors may trigger or exacerbate functional symptoms. That said, there is no requirement for patients to have pre- or comorbid anxiety, depression, or trauma, and it is common that many patients with functional symptoms will not resonate with this psychological conceptualization of their symptoms. Rather than the presence of a comorbid mental health conditions, alexithymia (difficulty in identifying and communicating one's emotional experiences) and avoidant coping style are common for those with functional symptoms. Social and cultural factors to consider include the family's perspective of the child's overall health, how severe or dangerous the patient and family perceive the symptoms, and cultural norms and values surrounding both mental and physical health. In addition, consider the presence of additional social stressors such as racism and discrimination, bullying, school stressors (particularly high achieving, perfectionistic tendencies), romantic relationships, gender identity and social acceptance, and family relationships.

It is important to inform patients and families as soon as functional symptoms are being considered to avoid families feeling surprised or misled through the evaluation process. It can be helpful to describe that a holistic approach is being utilized to evaluate the patient's physical symptoms and that functional symptoms are on the differential in addition to a judicial medical workup. Normalization of functional symptoms can be helpful: every human experiences some degree of functional symptoms, it is the body's way of communicating with us. Evaluation of biopsychosocial factors that may contribute to the patient's physical symptoms may require a few follow-up visits to thoroughly investigate. Through the biopsychosocial evaluation, it is important to note *how* the patient and family discuss their physical symptoms and mental health such that similar language can be used when providing education regarding the functional nature of their symptoms.

If after completion of judicial and reassuring medical workup and evaluation of biopsychosocial factors that may be impacting symptoms, the patient's presentation is determined to be wholly or partially functional, it is necessary to inform the patient and their family of the conceptualization. This is a necessary and sometimes challenging step to interrupt the cycle and support the patient's healing. To begin this discussion, recap the medical evaluation that has been completed to date and the results of each test. It can be helpful for families to learn what conditions were on the differential, including functional symptoms, based on the patient's presentation. It is very important to note if and how the patient's symptoms are *inconsistent* with a known medical condition and that functional symptoms are *not* a diagnosis of exclusion. It is understandable that many families are concerned that a medical condition is being missed if functional symptoms are framed as a condition that is diagnosed after medical causes have been ruled out. Families may ask how you can rule out every medical condition and request further workup. Families may state concern that it is still not known what is causing the symptoms. Instead, framing the inconsistencies in the presentation as rule-in criteria can be reassuring to families as well as informing the families that it *is* known what is causing their symptoms, naming it directly, and identifying treatment options.

Common inconsistencies may include roaming pain symptoms, symptoms occurring at certain times of the day only, symptoms occurring in certain environments only, neurological symptoms that do not map to dermatomes, symptoms unresponsive to typical medication treatment, and symptoms more severe than would be expected based on the findings of the medical workup. Next, provide the family education on what functional symptoms are and how they are treated. It is important to stress that the physical symptoms the patient is experiencing are very real and not currently in the patient's control. To engage the family effectively and elicit a higher likelihood of buy-in, education should be based on the language that the family used to describe the patient's physical symptoms and mental health throughout the evaluation. Typically, families will fall in two camps: (1) biological basis with no to limited psychological contribution or (2) psychological basis with inclusion of the biological aspects of their symptoms. For the primarily biological conceptualization, determine if there was an illness that may have triggered the symptoms, like an injury or bacterial/viral illness. Then provide education about the nervous system and its primarily two functions: survival (fight, flight, freeze) and resting (rest and digest). The body automatically goes into survival mode when it experiences these scary physical symptoms. As such, when the patient had the injury or illness, their body automatically went into survival mode. Sometimes, the presence of physical symptoms increases the likelihood of more physical symptoms because the body is on guard and vigilant to the danger of illness or injury. While this is typically helpful and protective, the body can get "stuck" in survival mode and continue to send signals of symptoms even after the injury or illness has healed.

For families who resonate with the more psychological conceptualization, it can be helpful to emphasize a particular stressor or mental health concern reported by the patient and then normalize the physical response to such stressors (i.e., common to have heart racing, shortness of breath, and stomach pain with something very stressful). Then, connect the patient's stressors or mental health concern (anxiety, depression, etc.) to the nervous system as described above (i.e., anxiety activates survival mode).

It is next important to inform families that we know how to treat functional symptoms. Sometimes we find that knowing what the symptoms mean and that the body is safe can significantly reduce the symptoms and the patient may not need further treatment. Sometimes, patients do need extra support in rewiring communication between nervous system and the body, which can be supported by psychotherapy and/or physical/occupational therapy. Families who resonate with the biological conceptualization may benefit from extra explanation of psychotherapy as a way to rewire faulty communication between the nervous system and body that resulted in the patient getting stuck in survival mode. To "turn off" survival mode, psychotherapy teaches relaxation techniques, coping skills, and supports reframing of cognitions surrounding physical symptoms.

POSITIVE ASPECTS OF ACUTE ILLNESS

Parmelee has suggested that the multiple experiences with acute illness, a characteristic of everyone's childhood, guide the process of social competence. The manner and style of each family's response to an illness shape the child's sense of self, health beliefs, and their coping strategies. Children are often exposed to differing adult responses to acute illness symptoms which vary based on cultural views and responses to illness, environment (i.e., school, home), individual health beliefs, and the child's emotional response to symptoms. By practicing cultural humility—a lifelong practice of self-reflection, shifting power imbalances, openness, and curiosity—pediatricians can better understand the family's cultural values of illness and treatment which can then be integrated into their care plan. Children learn what it means to be sick, what rituals are involved in getting better, and that they will get well with time. A sense of the body, positive health beliefs, and what it means to be cared for by a caregiver are the positive aspects of an illness.

Clinicians can help caregivers achieve a balance between reasonable indulgence and maintaining a goal of recovery. It is a delicate balance that should encourage the healing process while the child learns about the value of being cared for by another individual. For many families, various healing rituals that are transferred through generations provide positive expectations that teach coping mechanisms. For example, some Native American people prefer to utilize herbs, manipulative therapies, community, and ceremonies to treat illness rather than medications or procedures prescribed by western medicine. It is important to note that there is incredible diversity within cultures and views of illness and healing cannot be assumed based upon belonging to a certain culture. As such, practicing cultural humility and being curious is the way to go.

CHRONIC ILLNESS

Primary care pediatric clinicians have considerably less experience with chronic illness or conditions than with acute illness in children. However, most pediatric practices are filled with one or more children with various chronic disorders managed by the pediatrician along with specialists. Caring for the psychosocial needs of children with chronic illness and their families can be guided effectively by a set of principles that simultaneously account for developmental considerations and the biology of the disease. A biopsychosocial approach to chronic illness does not require in-depth knowledge of a particular disorder's impact on a child. That said, it may be worthwhile to have a general understanding of the child's specific condition and/or connect with the social worker associated with the subspecialty team. Principles of managing a child with a chronic illness include:

- Availability to answer family questions
- Helping families set specific goals in areas related to the child's condition and its effects on daily activities
- Ensuring coordination of health and other services
- Monitoring care over time, including specific plans for follow-up
- Updating and monitoring family knowledge on a periodic basis
- Counseling regarding family responses to the condition
- Linking families with others who have children with similar chronic conditions

Certain characteristics are common to all chronic health conditions; they transcend the specific nature of the illness. For example, behavioral changes and mental health conditions occur twice as often in children with most chronic illnesses as in children without a chronic illness. Effects on caregivers' work schedules, job stability, relationships (sibling, caregivers), and family finances are common concerns regardless of the specific illness. In addition, social determinants of health play a significant role in not only severity and progression of chronic illness but also the family's adjustment to chronic illness. **Social determinants of health** include health literacy, socioeconomic status, insurance status, food insecurity, housing insecurity, caregiver employment, impact of illness on employment, social supports, zip code/neighborhood, and so on. Because time is a major constraint for all patient interactions, screening measures can be useful to expedite information gathering

in a standardized format (See Chapter 3 and Resource Appendix). Evaluation of social determinants of health can help elucidate if the family would benefit from a referral to a social worker to identify if there are additional resources or services that can help minimize barriers to healthcare access and/or maximize health-related behaviors.

Family-centered care, with a focus on therapeutic alliance, open communication, and comprehensive evaluation of the biopsychosocial factors of health, can support families in optimal understanding of their child's illness and its treatment as well as support identification of potential barriers to care and needed resources and services (see Table 25.1). Teaming with families can support productive problem solving surrounding their specific needs related to education, ability to adhere to treatment recommendations, reduce stigma, and identify concrete resource needs. In addition, coordination with subspecialty providers can ensure that all key players are on the same page to optimize the child's health care.

Although identification of caregiver concerns (the caregiver's agenda for the visit) is critical to all pediatric clinical encounters, it is especially important when working with a child who has a chronic disorder. Ask the caregiver and child to identify those things that they most want to see changed. Ask them to establish their care priorities. Encouraging them to identify three concerns often leads to the discovery of one that can be relatively easy to address. In addition to ensuring that concerns are addressed, these clinical encounters provide opportunities for recognition of successes to support self-efficacy. Successes can come in all shapes and sizes, such as making it to an appointment on time, securing additional services or resources, improvement in adherence, improvement in symptoms, getting good grades at school, developing a routine that works for the family, and so on.

MONITORING MENTAL HEALTH

There is a high prevalence of mental health concerns in pediatric patients with an estimated one in five meeting criteria for a diagnosable mental health concern, and rates are higher in children with chronic conditions such as asthma or diabetes. Pediatric clinicians are well positioned to detect behavioral and emotional problems in patients with chronic conditions, provide education to destigmatize mental health concerns and treatment, and refer to mental health providers. The use of screening tools can be a time-efficient way to longitudinally track behavioral and emotional functioning and identify which patients would benefit from additional evaluation and treatment (see Chapter 3 and Resource Appendix). The Pediatric Symptom Checklist (PSC-17) is a universal screener for behavioral and emotional problems with both caregiver and child forms that is available in two dozen languages. More condition/symptom-specific screeners are included in the Resource Appendix and include:

- ADHD: Vanderbilt ADHD Rating Scales or the Conners Fourth Edition (long, short, and ADHD index available)
- Anxiety: Screen for Child Anxiety Related Disorders (SCARED) or the Generalized Anxiety Disorder Scale-7 (GAD-7)
- Depression: Patient Health Questionnaire-9 Modified for Adolescents (PHQ-A)
- Behavior: Strengths and Difficulties Questionnaire (SDQ)
- Autism Spectrum Disorder: Modified Checklist for Autism in Toddlers, Revised (M-CHAT-R), Childhood Autism Spectrum (CAST), and the Autism Spectrum Quotient—Adolescent (AQ)
- Disordered Eating: Eating Attitudes Test (EAT-26)

PARTNERING TO IMPROVE TREATMENT ADHERENCE

When working with children or adolescents with chronic illness and their caregivers, it is not uncommon to find suboptimal adherence to a treatment after appropriate medications, advice, and education have been tried. This is particularly true for adolescents, as the requirements of caring for a chronic illness are at odds with developmentally appropriate focus on independence and separation from caregivers, increased influence of peers, and sense of invincibility. These situations are opportunities to reframe the nature of the problem and try some new approaches.

Motivational interviewing techniques can help identify the child and family's values and goals, understanding of their illness and treatment, what is going well in treatment, and barriers to optimal adherence. The goal of motivational interviewing is to provide education regarding treatment recommendations and rationale, elucidate the patient's and caregiver's health-related values, build awareness of incongruences between their values and behaviors, and support problem solving surrounding barriers to adherence. The first step to supporting optimal adherence is building a trusting relationship with the patient and family where the focus is assessing knowledge of medical condition and treatment recommendations, both the patient's and family's values, successes and barriers to optimal adherence, and the patient's and family's stage of change. The **transtheoretical model** (Table 25.4) supports evaluation of an individual's and/or family's stage of change and motivation to change behaviors. An important aspect of motivational interviewing is to accept the patient and family no matter their stage of change. Communication is key and motivational interviewing recommends the use of Open-ended questions, Affirmations/acceptance, Reflective listening, and Summaries (OARS acronym). Instead of challenging a patient/family who is not interested in changing, it can be more helpful to explore their values, paying close attention to incongruence between their stated values and behaviors as well as emphasizing change statements (Table 25.5). Change can take time and the most effective interventions are sparked from the patient's/family's values as well as their ideas to solve the problem. That said, when suboptimal adherence presents an acute danger to the child's life and health, it is necessary to be more direct in challenging a patient/family and may require the involvement of Children's Protective Services.

HOSPITALIZATION AND PROCEDURES

Hospitalization of a child involves removal of that child from a characteristically safe, nurturing, and predictable environment within the home to a place populated by strangers, to a crib or bed that is unfamiliar, to a place with walls and floors that are different from home colors and to sounds that are new and, at times, cacophonous. The child may see people in uniforms for the first time. Procedures, examinations, and treatments may be perceived as frighteningly invasive or traumatic. Any hospitalization, no matter how well managed, is stressful for the child. That stress can be a source of growth in experience and competence or can create additional illness complications and delay healing in its broadest sense.

Over the years, hospitals have improved the availability of resources and services that are designed specifically for the emotional needs and developmental capacities of children. Child life specialists are providers who are specially trained to provide developmentally appropriate education and preparation for procedures and treatments as well as support with coping through these experiences. In addition, many children's hospitals have additional resources to support coping and improve pleasurable opportunities in the hospital including art therapy, music therapy, patient technology, pet therapy, and schoolteachers. In addition, some hospitals have mental health providers, like social workers, psychologists, and psychiatrists.

Impact of Hospitalization

The impact of hospitalization is significant when viewed from the perspective of a sudden environmental change. A hospital environment brings predictable alterations to a child's relationships with family members, peers, school, and daily activities. Perhaps most significantly, going to the hospital means a loss of independence that is appropriate to the child's developmental level. Because the quest for independent activity and psychological

TABLE 25.4 Transtheoretical Model Stage Evaluation and Motivation Interviewing

Stage of Change	Stage Definition	Motivational Interviewing Interventions
Precontemplation	• No intention to change in the near future • Limited insight into the problem of the behavior	• Rapport and trust building • Utilize OARS (Open-ended questions, Affirmations/acceptance, Reflection, and Summaries) to: • Evaluate values and goals • Evaluate barriers, pros, and cons to change • Pay special attention to strength of resistance and sustain talk (see Table 25.5) • Gently highlight the discrepancies between values, goals, and behaviors
Contemplation	• Considering changing in the near future • Emerging insight into the problem of the behavior	• Explore and tolerate ambivalence using OARS • Pay special attention to "change talk" (see Table 25.5) and explore to help patient/family develop potential solutions
Preparation	• Recognition of the problem associated with the behavior • Motivation to change in the near future • Starting to plan how to change. May be taking small steps to change	• Pay special attention to "change talk" (see Table 25.5) • Clarify values and goals • Utilize OARS to help the patient/family develop concrete plans to make changes
Action	• Recently made changes to behavior • Intend to continue with behavior changes	• Affirm patient/family's ability to make changes • Encourage incremental changes as drastic changes are likely not realistic • Identify potential barriers and support patient/family in developing a plan for these situations
Maintenance	• Ongoing change to behavior	• Continue to support problem solving and developing plans
Relapse	• Individuals revert to old behaviors	• Normalize bumps in the road • Praise efforts to change and encourage patient/family to consider reengaging with change • Utilize barriers or triggers for relapse in future plans • Reevaluate and further develop coping plans

OARS, Open-ended questions, Affirmations/acceptance, Reflective listening, and Summaries.

autonomy begins at birth and is the energizing force that fuels development, most children are affected by the loss of independence when hospitalized. While many hospitals encourage and support caregiver presence at bedside, some family's circumstances and responsibilities prohibit their full attendance throughout hospitalization. This disruption may be very stressful, particularly for toddlers and younger children. In addition, children may be stripped of their usual patterns of coping with stress (e.g., withdrawing to the bedroom, a temper tantrum at dinnertime, asking for and receiving more nurturing time from caregivers). As such, it is common for children to experience distress and/or have a change in their behaviors during hospitalization.

Infant

When younger than 6 months, most infants seem to tolerate hospital experiences with minimal long-term behavioral or physiological reactions to separation experiences. Very young infants do distinguish caregivers and strangers in social interactions, so some transient change in behavior and responsiveness should be expected. The clinician will appreciate behavioral differences in the child when cared for by the caregiver rather than a nurse. An infant younger than 6 months has not reached the stage of perceiving themself as an independent being to the point that separation from a caregiver appears threatening. A young infant may show behavioral reactions (fussiness, inconsolability, sleep disturbances) or physiological reactions (vomiting, constipation,

TABLE 25.5 Motivational Interviewing: Resistance, Sustain, and Change Talk Definitions and Examples

Term/Acronym	Definition	Examples
Resistance Talk	Patient/family verbalizes that they are not willing/able to make a change.	Patient: "I am tired of people talking to me about my medications. I feel fine so what's the point." Clinician: "It's confusing why people keep asking you about your medications when you feel fine without them. What have you learned about why you have been prescribed those medications?"
Sustain Talk	Patient/family verbalizes reasons to not change.	Patient: "I have too much going on right now with school and sports. I don't think I can do anymore." Clinician: "It sounds overwhelming to think about doing anymore. What do you want to focus on right now?"
Change Talk	Patient/Family verbalizes interest in changing behaviors. Use DARN-CAT acronym to recognize and respond to change talk.	
DARN-CAT	Desire	Patient: "I [wish, want, hope, etc....] that I will just get used to it and taking my meds won't be so hard." Clinician: "I hear that you hope that taking your medications will get easier. If this wasn't a problem anymore, what would be different?"
	Ability	Patient: "I [would want to/can/could try] work on getting better at my meds." Clinician: "What change seems possible for you right now?"
	Reason	Patient: "[It's important because/It would help because] being sick holds me back." Clinician: "It sounds like taking your medications regularly is important to you. Being healthy will help you reach your goals. What is getting in the way? What steps could you take now?"
	Need	Patient: "I should do better. Something has to change with my medications ...." Clinician: "You want to make a change with your medications. What parts do you find the most challenging? What parts are you already doing well with?"
	Commitment	Patient: "I need to do better. I promise that I will work on taking my meds." Clinician: "I can hear that this is important to you, and you're committed to making some changes. Let's explore this more."
	Activation	Patient: "I am [going to/ready to] work on taking my meds" Clinician: "You sound ready to make some changes. Where were you thinking of starting?"
	Taking steps	Patient: "I am already taking my meds in the morning." Clinician: "That's great! You have already put in work to take your meds in the morning. What has been helpful to make this happen?"

poor weight gain, poor feeding) in response to a hospital experience. Young infants will begin to establish new relationships with sensitive, consistent caretakers and will build on these very quickly. Similarly, they will reestablish patterns of interactions with caregivers quickly after the separation, if it is brief. Alterations in sleep patterns and feeding may show the impact of hospitalization on the infant's schedule and state regulation. The more that stays the same for the infant—schedules, objects, and people—the less the stress.

Toddler

Toddlerhood tends to be one of the most challenging developmental stages to be hospitalized. Behavioral changes in a toddler are more dramatic and require a longer recovery phase. As they develop independence, the child has an accompanying awareness of the stress of disruptions to routine and potential separation from their caregivers. This response is particularly acute between the ages of 8 and 18 months. Language may play an important role in the toddler's reaction to hospitalization. Before the age of 18 months, the child's expressive and receptive language is limited; they may not understand why they need to stay in the hospital, why things are being done to them, what providers are saying to them, and they may be unable to verbally express their needs or wants. After the age of 18 months to 2 years, the acceleration of expressive and receptive language provides the toddler the equipment to interact with others in a more advanced form and therefore to understand, at least in part, some of the strange people and events around them and verbally communicate any wants or needs.

Toddlers also lack a sense of time, so they cannot appreciate a promise of going home soon or a prompt return by a caregiver. Temper tantrums, listlessness, refusal to eat, and sleep disturbances are characteristic responses of a typical toddler to a hospital setting. It is testimony to appropriate psychological growth. Regressive behavior in this situation should be seen as adaptive and appropriate because it allows for conservation of energy and a bid for help during this "crisis" situation. Regressive behavior usually subsides after hospitalization as long as medical trauma was minimal, any separation experience was not too intense or prolonged, and the attachment process was relatively secure before the hospitalization.

Preschooler

In contrast to the toddler's experience, a preschool child's response to hospitalization may call forth newly developed skills of imagination, verbal questioning, and magical thinking to understand and deal with the acute stresses of a strange environment. A 4- to 5-year-old can tolerate the absence of caregivers for a longer period because they now understand that "out of sight is not out of mind." Memory is better developed, and children at this age can use words to call up images, talk about planned events, and elicit conversations with hospital personnel. At the same time, magical thinking may produce distortions about causality, with associated fears, fantasies, and body distortions. Children at this age may feel personally responsible for their illness, that they did something wrong that caused their caregivers to bring them to the hospital or may make incorrect connections between events (i.e., eating causes worsening symptoms). Causal relationships may depend on the child's perception of the temporal or spatial placement of events. Linkage occurs automatically as the child generates their own hypotheses regarding events around them. These "explanatory models" may be resistant to change, no matter how many "facts" the caregiver or clinician provides.

School-Age Child

A hospitalized school-age child is often able to develop peer group friendships and attachments to nurses, physicians, and other personnel that may buffer the feelings arising from the disruption of hospitalization. Increasing verbal skills and the capacity to understand causality allow a school-age child to gain more mental control over the situation. They understand the basic causes of illness and the logic of treatment. Multidimensional causal models will be beyond their understanding. One thing causes a specific problem in a child's mind when they are in the concrete operational stage. However, the child may be able to exercise more options in their treatment and participate in their own care if these options are concrete and specific and make some sense to them, given their own understanding of the disease.

The hospital experience may become stressful for a school-age child because they may experience a lack of control which can result in a variety of emotional and behavioral responses. The concept of *locus of control* (a feeling of either internal or external control of events or an illness) may at times be useful in understanding and navigating a child through a stressful hospital experience. This approach provides the child greater clarity of what is happening and what the child can control and choices available. The loss of school relationships and fear of getting behind scholastically and socially may add to the distress for a child of this age.

Adolescent

As the child reaches adolescence, a primary developmental goal is independence and separation from their caregiver. A hospital experience, as well as the disease process, confronts the adolescent's identity and developmental goals directly. The loss of independence, coupled with an abrupt separation from peer groups and activities, may bring about psychological distress in a hospitalized teenager. The disease process, coupled with invasive hospital procedures, may distort the adolescent's concept of body image and disrupt future plans, real or imagined.

Developmental Regression

Children of all age groups can be expected to demonstrate a regression of some developmental milestones during and after a hospital experience. The intensity and duration of developmental regression are controlled by several determinants that have both preventive and therapeutic implications for the clinician:

- The child's developmental level with regard to social and language skills.
- Personality and temperament—what kind of child were they before hospitalization? The quality of the reaction to hospital experience will vary not only with the developmental level but also with the unique temperament of each child (see Chapter 2).
- Previous styles of coping with new situations.
- Characteristics of the illness—duration, acuteness, severity, invasive procedures, immobilization, isolation.
- Family's response to the illness—the behavioral reactions of close relatives may influence the child's behavior.
- Fears and fantasies—Ask the child, "What do you know about your illness?" or "Why are you in the hospital?" Observation of play or review of the child's drawings (see Chapter 4) or fantasies that are based on their own explanatory model of the illness.

In an attempt to lessen the adverse reactions of children to the hospital experience, pediatric professionals should not lose sight of the fact that *developmental regression symbolizes both a stress and a protective maneuver* to defend against the disruption of hospitalization and cope with the experience. In this sense, behavioral alterations in the hospital may be adaptive and represent a healthy response to the experience. For example, a toddler's mild-to-moderate protest is an appropriate adaptation to a strange new world that is inhabited by a new crib, an intravenous line, and numerous nurses and physicians. Preparing caregivers for these responses to hospitalization may help them understand their adaptive significance.

Measures to Help Children With Hospitalization and Procedures

Pediatric clinicians and other providers of health care for children may be advocates for their patients when hospitalization or a painful procedure is being considered by attending to the following issues:

- *Hospitalize children in a pediatric setting that is appropriately designed for children.* Colors and pictures on the walls should be child oriented. Toys in a playroom that provide flexibility of movement should be available. Encourage caregivers to engage with Child Life Specialists who are trained to provide coping support for illness and hospitalization as well as provide developmentally appropriate education of illness, cares, and procedures. During hospitalization, caregivers are encouraged to play with their child. Play is the "work" of childhood, and in this role, it provides children with an opportunity for symbolic expression of concerns and fantasies. The mere act of playing can be therapeutic.
- *Provide caregivers and the child with an age-appropriate explanation for the hospitalization.* Ensure accurate understanding by using the teach-back method with both the caregiver and the child (see Table 25.2).
- *For elective procedures (e.g., hernia repair, cardiac catheterization, myringotomy), provide the child with a description of the hospital setting and the procedures that will be encountered before anesthesia.* Hospital websites, children's books, coloring books, and medical toys may assist the child in preparing for the new experience. Some hospitals arrange tours through the children's facility to acquaint caregivers and children with the setting, uniforms, and routines before hospitalization. Many children's hospitals have comprehensive websites that can be used to prepare families for an admission.
- *Encourage caregivers to ask hospital staff for additional psychosocial support.* Children's hospitals tend to have many resources to support admitted children and often attempt to accommodate their needs as much as possible. For example, consistent nursing staffing can be beneficial to support feelings of attachment and trust. While it may not be 100% feasible to have consistent nursing support during an admission, caregivers can request this accommodation, and nursing leadership will often attempt to keep staffing as consistent as possible. In addition, caregivers can ask for Child Life Services (including music and art therapy) to provide procedure preparation, procedure support, and coping support. Many children's hospitals have psychologists, psychiatrists, or other mental healthcare providers should the child experience anxiety, changes to mood, or changes to behavior. Social workers are also available to support caregiver coping in addition to providing resources and logistical support.
- *Encourage family members to be present as much as possible.* The caregiver's presence in the hospital may assist the child in adaptation to the new setting by helping them master separation anxiety and self-control. Rooming-in may give caregivers the opportunity to assist in the care of the child. Caregiver participation in hospital care is beneficial to the well-being of children. This may include the caregiver reassuring and comforting the child during a poke, procedure, or induction of anesthesia as well as setting behavioral expectations.

- *Encourage the caregivers to maintain as much familiarity as possible.* Caregivers can bring a few familiar toys and books or a special comfort item (i.e., blanket, stuffed animal, etc.) as a way to lessen the effects of the separation. As much as possible, continue important routines like bedtime and morning routines. Set clear, simple limits and expectations on behavior as much as possible. Keep as many things as possible the same.

- *Encourage caregivers and providers to be truthful about procedures.* Caregivers can also remind hospital staff that transparency and accurate expectations are helpful for their child. Children are not helped by statements such as "It won't hurt," if it will. Mistrust builds anxiety. When painful procedures are planned, an explanation just before the procedure that "it will hurt for a moment" prepares a child older than 2 in an honest manner. Child Life Specialists can assist in providing developmentally appropriate education about procedures.

- *Encourage caregivers to advocate for **trauma-informed care** practices.* Hospitalization can create a power differential with medical providers holding more perceived power than caregivers and children. As such, caregivers may benefit from permission and encouragement to advocate for changes in providers' behaviors. Some common trauma-informed interventions that caregivers can ask for include the medical team rounding outside the child's room, communication preferences, request consolidation of cares, and asking providers to knock, introduce themselves, and inform the family what is planned for the visit (i.e., updates only, physical exam, vitals, medicine, pokes, dressing change, etc.). In addition, caregivers can ask providers to give realistic options for the child and age-appropriate opportunities for them to participate in their own care by making as many choices as possible.

- *Encourage caregivers to advocate for adequate pain control.* Pediatric clinicians must have knowledge about the need to improve recognition and management of pain in children. Untreated or undertreated pain has short- and long-term implications for children, caregivers, and healthcare providers including high acute distress, extended time required to complete procedures and allow for healing, medical and vicarious trauma, phobia, pain hypervigilance and sensitivity, and avoidance of health care.

  Medical management of pain. While adequate pain control is a priority for numerous inpatient providers, at times it can fall onto caregivers to communicate their child's pain level and response to treatment to the medical team. The pediatric clinician can support parents in navigating these situations by providing guidance on how to discuss pain concerns with the medical team. The Emergency Medical Services for Children Innovation & Improvement Center has developed toolkits, the Pediatric Education and Advocacy Kit (PEAK): Pain, to support both clinicians and families to achieve optimal pain control.

  Nonpharmacological pain management. In some pediatric centers, pain management has reached sophisticated levels in the form of hypnosis and other distraction-relaxation techniques, often provided by psychologists or Child Life Specialists. Relaxation techniques, self-talk, and distracting imagery can be combined to block out unpleasant sensations. Additional relaxation techniques include diaphragmatic breathing, progressive or passive muscle relaxation, guided imagery, and grounding techniques. The use of biofeedback combines relaxation techniques and distraction, while enabling real-time feedback about the body's response to these interventions. Distraction reduces pain by redirecting the child's attention away from the painful stimulus and toward a pleasant experience. During a painful procedure, children can be distracted by virtual reality, TV, video games, blowing bubbles, hand holding, whistling, singing, storytelling, puppets, and visual or auditory engagement with toys. Unpleasant procedures experienced by infants can be modified by rocking, singing, sucking, and even playing peek-a-boo.

- *Develop coping plans.* When a child is faced with a known painful or distressing care or procedure, having a coping plan already developed can be helpful to increase predictability, reduce distress, and instill some sense of control. Communication preferences of both the caregiver and child should be included in a coping plans, such as how the need for the care or procedure is communicated to the child, the timing of communication (i.e., 1 hour before, 1 day before, as soon as possible), and the level of communication the child wants during the care or procedure (i.e., step-by-step narrative, informing prior to starting only, counting to three for pokes). It is important to identify support persons (caregiver, Child Life Specialist, etc.) for the care of procedure and how the child would like support (holding hand, sitting on lap, verbal reassurance, supporting relaxation techniques, etc.). Including comfort or distracting items in the coping plan can be helpful to avoid scrambling to find something at the last moment. Common items for pokes include topical analgesia (e.g., a eutectic mixture of lidocaine and prilocaine), the use of Buzzy (a device that vibrates which can detract from the poke sensation), or the use of a shot blocker. Finally, sometimes children may have severe anxiety related to

> ### ⚠ HEADS UP–ILLNESS
>
> - Be mindful of the child's/caregiver's perception of the experience of being ill (Health Beliefs) and its congruence with the medical formulation of the problem. Incongruencies require additional education and intervention.
> - Careful consideration of the biopsychosocial framework surrounding benign or self-limited medical problems combined with careful communication and anticipatory guidance is necessary to prevent caregivers from perceiving the condition as serious, which may result in activity restrictions or perceptions of a vulnerable child. Examples include a benign cardiac murmur, uncomplicated neonatal jaundice, or an umbilical hernia.
> - Frequently ask, "Have I considered that the experience of this office visit is shaping the way this child learns about their body, physical symptoms, and illness as well as the process of healing?" Asking the question is the initial step in changing communication techniques and procedures to enhance social competency and self-esteem.
> - Recognize the child who is brought to your office frequently for minor functional or behavioral concerns. When a medical assessment consistently rules out physical illness or symptoms are inconsistent with a known medical condition, it is an opportunity to explore biopsychosocial factors that may contribute to the child's presentation.
> - When adherence to a therapeutic recommendation is suboptimal, reevaluate the caregiver's and patient's conceptualization of the problem, priorities, values, and stage of change. Utilize motivational interviewing techniques to support alignment between values and behaviors. Children's Protective Services may need to be considered if there are acute concerns for the patient's health or life.
> - Behavioral changes and mental health conditions occur twice as often in children with most chronic illnesses. Screening for depression, anxiety, and behavioral concerns can be a time-efficient to monitor for these concerns in addition to incorporating a biopsychosocial framework into evaluations.
> - A hospital experience is a major psychosocial shift in the experience of all children and adolescents. Clinicians who are aware of the developmental significance of this experience at different stages in development are prepared to provide education and anticipatory guidance while helping the caregivers and hospital staff understand and ameliorate difficult behavior and regressions.
> - Regressions in development and/or behavior during an illness are common, often temporary, and necessary to support coping.
> - Cognitive and behavioral strategies, as well as the use of safe pain-relieving medications, should be considered during routine office procedures, hospitalizations, or outpatient procedures.

cares or procedures and may benefit from an anxiolytic either prescribed directly by the medical team or through a psychiatry consultation.

The desired outcomes for a hospitalized child include healing as quickly and completely as possible, be provided support in line with their biopsychosocial needs, and they are given the opportunity to grow from the experience. The clinician's role is to understand and support the child's developmental work while caring for the child's physical illness. The clinician should monitor the environment to ensure that it is providing the appropriate support. The caregivers should be provided with expectations for their child's physical and psychological recovery. They should hopefully emerge from the experience of their child's hospitalization as better caregivers, as better observers of their child's physical and mental health, as better participants in the healing process, and with an enhanced sense of competency as guardians of their child's health. The child's physician must support these processes through knowledge and sensitivity.

RECOMMENDED RESOURCES

Resources for children to understand and cope with their illness or hospitalization are available in the Resources Appendix.

For Caregivers

A different dream for my child: Meditations for parents of critically or chronically ill children by Jolene Philo.

Afraid of the doctor: Every parent's guide to preventing and managing medical trauma by Meghan Marsac, PhD, & Melissa Hogan, JD.

When your child has a chronic medical illness: A guide for the parenting journey by Frank Sileo, PhD, & Carol Potter, MFT.

When your child is sick: A guide to navigating the practical and emotional challenges of caring for a child who is very ill by Joanna Breyer.

When your child hurts: Effective strategies to comfort, reduce stress, and break the cycle of chronic pain by Rachel Coakley, PhD.

Your child in the hospital: A practical guide for parents by Nancy Keene & Rachel Prentice.

For Clinicians

Agency for Clinical Innovation: Pain management network. http://www.aci.health.nsw.gov.au/chronic-pain/painbytes

Emergency Medical Services for Children Innovation and Improvement Center: *Pediatric Education and Advocacy Kit (PEAK): pain.* https://emscimprovement.center/education-and-resources/peak/peak-pediatric-pain/

Michigan Medicine: *Trauma-informed care with adolescents.* https://www.michiganmedicine.org/trauma-informed-careadolescent-patients

The Center for Pediatric Traumatic Stress: *The Health Care toolbox, pediatric medical traumatic stress.* https://www.health-caretoolbox.org/

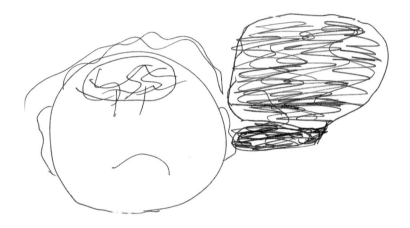

A migraine headache

A 12-year-old boy was asked to draw a picture of his (migraine) headache. The picture tells a great deal about the illness experience. By BL.

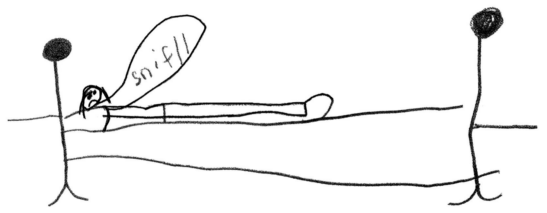

A girl draws a picture of what it is like to be sick with a cold. The bed seems confining and her expression is very sad. These "cinema noir" pictures are typical of children with acute illness. By Louise Dixon, age 7.

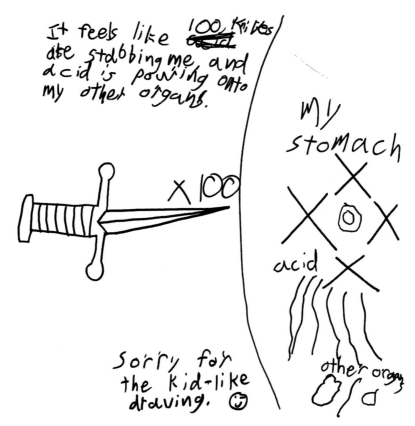

A 12-year-old boy with severe abdominal pain illustrates it in this drawing. He has multiple psycho-social stressors.

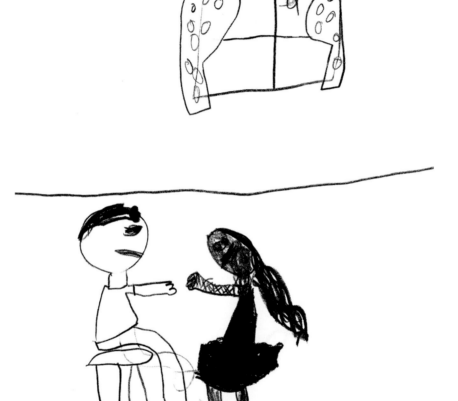

A girl shows a doctor applying an arm cast. The doctor is drawn only in outline, whereas the patient is drawn in color with more details. Detail and color often signal importance, and the patient is clearly the center here. By Louise Dixon, age 7.

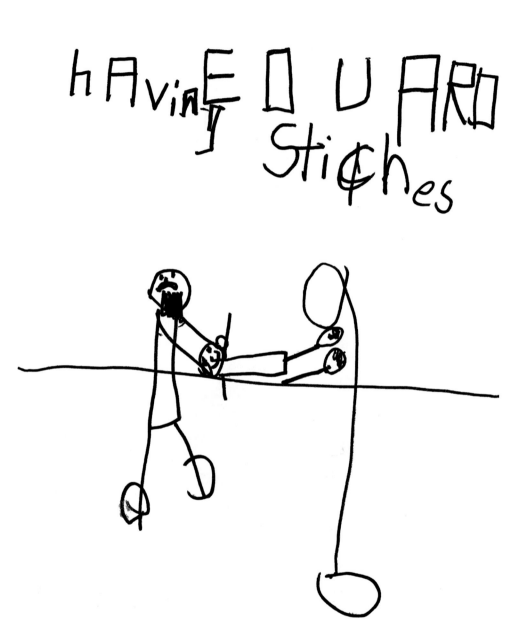

"Having stitches." A boy, age 6, shows his doctor fixing him up. The nurse is less well drawn and is faceless. The lack of hands and disconnected leg might suggest a sense of losing control or of powerlessness in the situation.

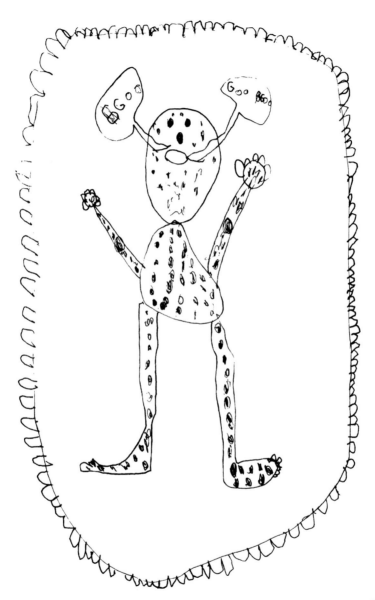

A boy, age 7, draws his baby brother with chickenpox on a blanket, perhaps as a wall of safety.

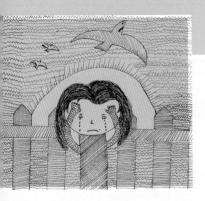

26

Stressful Events: Separation, Loss, Violence, and Death

Destiny G. Tolliver

This chapter describes child exposure to violence and trauma and children's emotional responses to the significant loss events that touch their lives, including their responses to death, family disruption, and other stressors.

KEYWORDS

- Children and trauma
- Children's understanding of death
- Grief reactions
- Suicide
- Sibling loss
- Divorce and separation
- Parental loss
- Child exposure to violence
- Catastrophic events

Small losses are an inevitable part of the landscape of childhood. Examples are the first time infants are aware of their parent's momentary absence, a toddler's struggle with separation at bedtime, and a preschooler's brave leap from a safe, known environment to the bigger world of a school. With each small, predictable, and manageable loss comes an opportunity for growth, and in each successful resolution and adaptation to loss comes increased coping skills and a greater sense of self.

In contrast to the losses we expect as part of the progress of normal development, exposure to traumatic events such as death of a loved one, violence close to home, and terrorism near or far presents a true crisis to a child. The clinician can help by seeing these crises through a child's eyes and then mobilizing support for the child as needed. A risk will then become an opportunity for growth.

This chapter focuses on the conceptual assumptions, interventions, and insights that will help clinicians provide monitoring and assistance to bereaved children and their families. Age-specific stressors of childhood are discussed in the context of loss and grieving in order to guide support by a clinician. We provide an overview of adverse childhood experiences (ACEs) and then discuss developmental responses associated with the death of a close family member to provide a framework for how a child experiences losses in general. These fundamental concepts should inform the clinician how a child might experience other losses.

CHILDREN AND TRAUMA

Children in the United States are exposed to traumatic violence and loss in epidemic proportions. Each day in the United States, seven children are murdered, 52 children are wounded or killed by guns, and 87 children are arrested for violent crimes. Children are also often witnesses to violence in their homes and communities. Additionally, there has been increasing attention to a wide variety of ACEs, which are associated with negative physical and mental health outcomes in childhood and through adulthood. ACEs include abuse, neglect, household adversity, caregiver mental illness, caregiver substance use, family separation, and community violence. Due to interpersonal and structural forms of oppression (including racism, xenophobia, homophobia, transphobia, and ableism), which lead to concentrated individual and community disadvantage, children who are marginalized by race, immigration status, sexual or gender

Original chapter by Maria Trozzi and Suzanne D. Dixon.

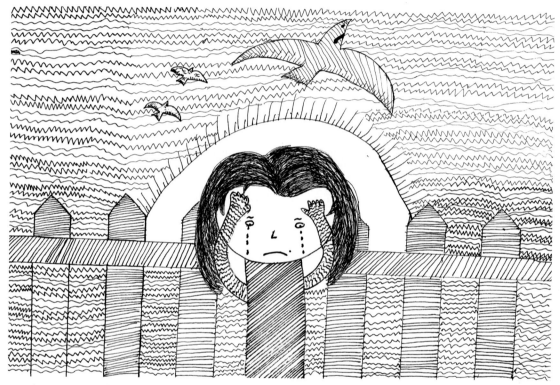

A teen uses simple geometrical shapes to convey a sense of hope (as well as sorrow). By Sherey Harris, age 18.

identity, or disability are at increased risk of experiencing ACEs. For example, racism can lead to interpersonal trauma including bullying, microaggressions, or hate crimes, in addition to structural traumatic experiences such as living in disinvested communities, criminal legal system involvement, and child welfare system involvement. Additionally, trauma is commonly an intergenerational phenomenon, meaning that children who experience ACEs often have caregivers who themselves have been traumatized. A caregiver's experience of trauma may impact their ability to support a child during traumatic events, and clinicians should incorporate a two-generation approach to caring for families impacted by trauma and loss.

CHILDREN'S UNDERSTANDING OF LOSS AND DEATH: DEVELOPMENTAL PERSPECTIVE

> *A simple child*
> *That lightly draws its breath*
> *And feels its life in every limb*
> *What should it know of death?*
>
> *– Wordsworth*

For adults, death is a disruption in their usual "steady state" and results in a sense of disequilibrium. **Children's understanding of death** is different, however. For children, death can represent a developmental interference that results in a suspension of their ongoing cognitive and emotional growth. It is this "stall factor" that must be taken into account for children at different developmental stages. The goal of clinical intervention with children is to get them "unstuck," to help them get through, over, under, or around a temporary barrier to their normal and healthy forward movement. The clinician should view the child's ability to cope with a significant trauma, loss, or death in relation to specific factors (Box 26.1).

BOX 26.1 Individual Factors that Influence Ability to Cope with Loss

- The child's ability to make sense of the death from the perspective of his own developmental level
- The child's history of loss and death
- Repeated and/or multiple losses that diminish capacity to cope
- The child's normal ability to cope with change, temperament, and situational stress

---

DEVELOPMENTAL FRAMEWORK

Much of our understanding about how children perceive loss is derived from Piaget's theories about children's cognitive development (see Chapter 2). This framework is a helpful starting point in assessing a child's reaction to the death of a loved one. Remember, however, that children regress under stress such as a major loss, and changes in the age and stage boundaries to more "basic" responses may be seen in such circumstances. These changes in response to death are meant as broad guidelines only and are presented in Table 26.1.

Infants (0–2 Years)

Before age 3, infants and toddlers are thought to have no cognitive conceptualization of death. Its effect on them is linked to what is lost, to the relationship with a significant other, and to the consistency that is or is not part of their life. It seems indisputable that infants and toddlers react strongly to the loss of a meaningful person and show their **grief reactions** in alterations in behavior. However, what is controversial is whether the very youngest child is capable of mourning without a mature understanding of the meaning of the loss. Behavioral change indicative of internal stress is expected when an infant loses a significant care provider. Consistency in care, attentiveness, and emotional responsiveness is needed for the infant to continue to thrive. These are essential elements that are lost to an infant who loses a primary care provider.

A significant loss in an infant may be expressed as irritability, whining, loss of self-care abilities, withdrawal, increases in aggression, poor feeding, and sleep disturbances.

The following suggestions may be useful in the case of loss of a parental figure:

- If the deceased was the infant's primary caregiver, identify a permanent surrogate caregiver as soon as possible. Do not divide the job or delay in this designation if at all possible. Consistency is key to coping.
- Learn the deceased caregiver's routines; keep the same as much as possible.
- Provide a consistent, nurturing, and dependable environment.
- Be prepared for regression in behavior and developmental competency. This regression may even have a delayed onset.

Preschooler (3–5 Years)

Preschoolers have a concept of death, but they view it as temporary or reversible, as going someplace else or

TABLE 26.1   Children's Understanding of Death at Different Ages

Age	Understanding
Infants 0–2 years	Have no cognitive understanding of death. Death is the same as a significant separation Respond to changes in routine, caregivers, and emotional chaos in family situation Experience separation anxiety, irritability, and regression
Preschoolers (3–5 years)	Death is temporary, reversible, living under different circumstances Literal thinking about causes Link seemingly unrelated factors to the death (transductive reasoning) Use magical thinking to explain death
School age (6–8 years)	Death is final, irreversible, but not universal See death as a person or spirit that catches you Death "catches" the elderly, disabled, klutzes May be contagious Concerned with safety, predictability Need for details
Preadolescents (9–12 years)	Adult understanding: death is final, irreversible, universal Disconnect between thinking and emotions Understand the biological aspects of death Interested in rituals, roles, ceremonies Understand causality: may feel guilty about contributing to it Intellectualize death: thoughts more available than feelings
Adolescents (13–18 years)	Adult understanding: death is final, irreversible, universal Engage in high-risk activities (challenge own mortality) Understand existential implications of death Reject adult rituals and support May see some aspects of stigma

as changing in a reversible way. Children this age want and expect to continue a relationship with their deceased loved one through prayers, writing, or engaging in one-sided conversations. They think the person is coming back. Children who place the deceased loved one in heaven want to visit, call, or write to them. Their thinking tends to be egocentric, that the death was caused by or was linked to their own actions, or that the cause is magical. They often attribute faulty thinking to death, define associations based on their own rule structure, and make spurious associations.

Preschoolers need simple, straightforward explanations of death, and what it means in concrete forms. "Grandpa died. His body totally stopped working." Many preschoolers will need help to operationally define death by answering specific questions: "Can he eat? Can he sleep? Does he still dream? Does he go to the bathroom? Will he breathe under the ground? Can he hear me in heaven? Does he need his wheelchair still?" Be particularly careful to respond with concrete, simple explanations to these kinds of queries. Avoid euphemisms like "lost," "sleeping," "passed," "with the angels." At best, they confuse young children. At worst, they may scare them.

In explaining death to their young children, adults often jump immediately to their own spiritual beliefs. Although this can be comforting and, in general, should be part of the process, it may also be confusing. For instance, preschool children are perplexed by how the body and spirit can simultaneously be in the grave and in heaven. Although religious beliefs can be shared with young children, they usually require some explanation and many opportunities to bring up the child's specific questions, no matter how concrete or even disturbing they may be to the adults.

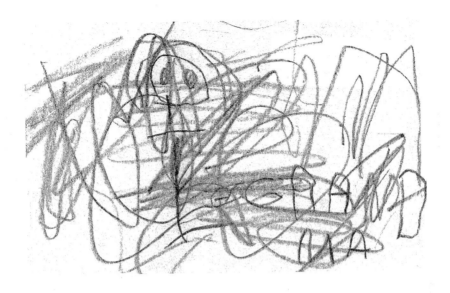

A 4-year-old girl draws her grandmother in the year after her death. The figure is simple compared with the writing beside it. It is orange but scribbled all over with gray. By Louise Dixon, age 4.

School Age (6–8 Years)

Children of school age understand death to be final and irreversible, but *not universal*. They know that people who die stay dead, but they do not think that they themselves will die. Death is often personalized, perceived as a character who can grab you at any unsuspected time, a dangerous, and wily presence. Children may come up with explanations, such as how fast they can run, to allow them to distance and defend themselves from death. However, unlike younger children, a death presents a child this age with the challenge of questioning their own and others' safety. "Is life still safe?" becomes an overriding question. An ongoing sense of impending disaster or unpredictable happenings exists unless the safety issue is addressed. Disruption of one's own life is also seen as a threat to safety. So again, reassurance of continuity and consistency adds to a sense of safety.

Predictability, that is, what will be the same versus what will be different because of this death, is an inescapable concern confronting a school-age child. The child needs direct, simple answers to what changes will happen that will affect their life. The child may ask after a sibling's death, "Will I have my own room now? Can I have their toys?" Although adults may initially view these questions as egotistical and completely unfeeling, the child is really asking

how the world will change fundamentally because of this death. Both the specifics and the general concern should be answered directly with support and assurance.

Other typical concerns prompted by a parent's death are illustrated by comments such as the following: "If my friend's mom died, are you (i.e., the parent) going to die also? Who will take care of me? Am I safe? Will I be safe?" Parents, particularly those in single-parent households, should face these important questions directly and seriously. It would *not* be useful to respond, "Don't worry about that" or "I'm too healthy to die." Remind the child that *everyone* dies someday, but that unlike their friend's mom, most people live to be very, very, very old. "If I were to die, your Aunt is prepared to care for you until you are grown up." Children are generally satisfied with that response, and it teaches them that you can talk about death, thus opening the door for more questions and voiced concerns.

Although discussing the details of a death (e.g., What happens to the body? Was there blood? What did it look like?) is difficult for adults, most school-age children have a need for some details about these events to help them feel more in control of the overwhelming event by learning the specifics. What seems to be morbid curiosity to an adult is really the way for a child to get a handle on an incomprehensible situation. The emotional response will come later.

Adults in the child's life have an opportunity to face these questions with them, and by doing this, they are telling their child that they can face stressful life events together. In contrast, refusing to discuss issues or to give flip answers sends the wrong message. "If it's unmentionable, it's unmanageable." Children are left with uncertainty, fear, and no place to go to get their questions answered and their needs met. Emotional coping comes out of the knowledge base at this age, so first the facts, then the hugs.

Preadolescents (9–11 Years)

Preadolescents have an adult understanding of death: it is final, irreversible, and universal. Most youngsters this age understand that everyone dies someday, even them, and that it is forever. This new awareness may actually heighten anxiety for youngsters this age as the result of an increased sense of vulnerability at this stage. They may view death as a punishment for bad behavior as they begin to explore moral development at this age. They are able to understand the biological aspects of death, such as what happens if the heart has a blockage or what effect a brain tumor has on life function. Physical causability is usually understood at this age, at least as final cause of death. In addition, children this age can understand the concept of specific and possible multiple causes and effects. That leads them to wonder about what part, if any, they may have played that contributed to a death. They may feel guilty in ways that they may not even understand; adults need to help them process such complicated ideas and emotions.

Preadolescents are fascinated with the religious and cultural rituals that surround death and display a curiosity about topics such as cremation, burial, embalming, and the afterlife. Adults in their lives may find these questions disarming, particularly if they are without any coherent emotional display or if posed at inappropriate times. However, if approached in a straightforward way, youngsters are reminded that they can trust adults to give them useful information about "difficult to talk about" topics.

Many preadolescents respond without a display of emotion or may even be sarcastic when faced with a loved one's death. They intellectualize death because their thoughts are often more available to them than their feelings. This may bewilder and concern adults who think that their typically sensitive and caring 11-year-old has been replaced with an insensitive person, when in reality

it just takes longer for children at this age to identify and let out feelings.

Even adolescents continue to use magical thinking in their formulations of death, in ways that may be less obvious but still have profound effects on young people. At any age, magical thinking should be uncovered and challenged. Simply ask the question, "What made your (mother, father, friend, pet) die? Why do you think they died?" Offer a simple statement of your own beliefs around the issue. And then wait. The child or adolescent has been given fuel to reconstruct his thinking and a supportive place to discuss it. The clinician may respond, "Many young people have ideas like that—it's a way of saying we cared. But wishes do not make things happen. Bad thoughts can't harm people."

A preadolescent is dependent on the adults in their life to make life feel safe, especially in times of crisis such as death. This may be very hard at this age because much behavior is as confusing as the thoughts and emotions of the child. Parents and other support people should remember to do the following:

- Be authentic. Children pick up platitudes, gloss-overs, and ambivalence like radar.
- Verbalize that, in spite of your grief, you are still able to care for them. Help them feel that they are safe and that their lives will go on.
- Give them repeated opportunities to discuss the death, but do not push too hard. It will take weeks to months to get at feelings. Provide openings and then wait.
- Talk about your own grief and how your feelings influence your own behavior. Provide a prototype of how to behave at a loss.

Children can face intensely difficult emotional times if the adults in their life continue to make them feel safe throughout. By explaining their own emotions and continuing to care for their children in spite of their feelings, adults can model how grief and its intense emotions can be faced with the adults in their lives.

Adolescents (12–18 Years)

This period brings in several new cognitive abilities, emotional processes, and developmental gains that have an impact on the experience of death.

- Adolescents are actively engaged in the normal developmental task of separation from the significant adults in their lives. A close death, such as the death of a parent or sibling, can derail this intense separation-individuation process and make the maturational process scary and overwhelming.
- Adolescents often engage in high-risk behavior, almost as though they need to "flirt with death." They are

fascinated with death but may be overwhelmed when it intrudes closely on their lives. This is hard for them to admit.

- Paradoxically, adolescents intellectually have an adult's understanding of death, but they behave as though they themselves were immortal. Many adolescents during this period will face the death of a peer, and it shatters all their fantasies of immortality. The intellectualization cover that is typical at this age may make it harder to get at such a devastating developmental and emotional experience. Peer loss is a huge event.
- Adolescents are capable of understanding the existential implications of death as they gain the ability to think abstractly. However, they may not have fully formed their understanding at this level before confronting death. So these abstractions for the reasons, consequences, and meaning of death may not be available to them on a personal level.
- Adolescents are interested in exploring society's attitudes about life and death. They will monitor how their immediate circle of family and friends, as well as the broader society, responds to, explains, and grieves a death. They look to others to help make sense of these overwhelming events while seeming to ignore the usual conventions or to challenge beliefs.

Although teens often reject traditional adult rituals surrounding death and create their own with the help of their peers, they do need adults in their life to help them sort out the often colliding feelings of sadness, anger, disbelief, and isolation. Adults may feel rejected when attempting to provide emotional support at this age. However, just their continued presence and availability during the crisis are therapeutic. Adults must interpret this distancing as developmentally appropriate and respect it while remaining available for reassurance and support.

Parental Death at Different Developmental Stages

The loss of a parent has long-term consequences, no matter when it occurs. For infants younger than 2 who lose parents, there is a risk of attachment disorders and serious emotional, cognitive, and developmental problems unless someone steps in quickly. For preschoolers, a variety of somatic complaints, anxiety symptoms, clinginess, and aggressive behavior would be typical. They may be overly responsible to take care of the surviving parent or blame themselves for the parent's death. This may take time to resolve or may linger as anxiety, depression, or separation phobias.

Middle childhood parental loss may deal a blow to self-esteem and set up a child for short- and long-term emotional problems. Academic achievement and friendships are at risk, and they may even have a fear of being stigmatized by peers. The key here is the mental health of the surviving parent. An overly adult demeanor may mean the child feels too much responsibility. Difficulties with relationships may persist into adulthood.

Children older than 12 may become anxious, have long-term difficulty with trust, and may feel alienated from peers. They may harbor guilt about past behavior and are prone to a variety of complex emotional problems into adulthood. Help from outside as well as inside the family is usually needed.

SPECIAL CASE OF SUICIDE

Adolescent **suicide** is becoming an increasingly frequent tragedy. Statistics reveal that every day in this country, many youth between the ages of 13 and 25 will attempt suicide, and many will die by suicide. Why do so many adolescents attempt to kill themselves? Why, if they have an adult understanding of death, can they see "ending their lives" as an option? Unfortunately, adolescents are often unable to look beyond the act itself and fail to fully comprehend that the consequences of death are final and irreversible.

Adults who care for, teach, and live with adolescents must help them face the stark reality of the act of suicide through clear discussion with them whenever a suicide is in news or happens in their school or neighborhood. Conversation should emphasize facts such as the following:
- Suicide is killing yourself.
- People who die by suicide do not know how to get help to solve problems.
- You do not come back.
- It will not glorify your memory.
- It is a permanent solution to a temporary problem.
- Adolescents need to look for help with problem solving.
- No problem is solved by suicide.

CHILDREN'S GRIEF REACTIONS—SPECIAL CHARACTERISTICS

Children of all ages have grief responses that are different from those of adults. Their behavior must be understood as indicating grief so that appropriate support can be provided.

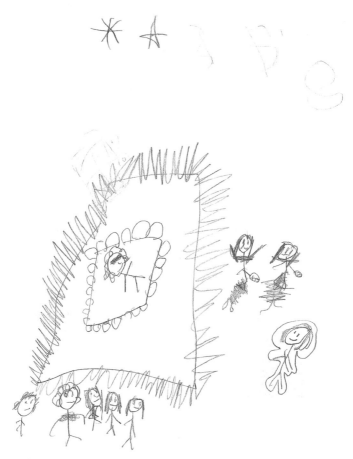

A 5-year-old shows her grandmother's burial. The coffin, on wheels, is placed in the grassy grave. Her grandmother is visible in the drawing, but her eyes are masked. The family is gathered at the bottom of the page. To the side, we see Jesus and two angels, dancing, soon to be joined by grandma. By Dori Dedmon, age 6.

- **Children grieve in spurts.** Children fluctuate between expressions of anger, sadness, anxiety, and confusion and then, in a moment, resumption of their normal behavior. They do not continuously show overt signs of grieving. This leads some to believe that children do not recognize the loss or understand its implications and therefore do not grieve appropriately. The behavior is adaptive, however, because children have a limited capacity to tolerate emotional pain and will pull away from it cognitively and emotionally when it all becomes too much for them. Adults might mistrust the child's intermittent display of intense feelings and see them as disingenuous. Children, even very young children, experience intensely painful responses that adults must understand within a developmental framework.

- **Children grieve longer than adults, contrary to popular thinking.** They *re-grieve* the loss over and over again at each new stage in development as they change their perspective on themselves and the world around them and make more mature meaning of the significance of the past loss. The grief process recurs over and over.

- **Childhood grief is manifested in qualitatively different ways.** Adults often think the child is not grieving after a loss because the emotions and behavior do not match the sad demeanor we expect. However, there may be marked changes in the child's behavior. Difficulty concentrating, heightened sibling squabbles, inappropriate and aggressive behavior, moodiness, withdrawal, disorganization, and temper tantrums are symptoms of grieving in childhood. Because of differences in cognitive ability and temperament, children are apt to use more primitive defense mechanisms than adults do, particularly denial and regression. Common psychosomatic symptoms include headaches, stomachaches, bowel and bladder difficulties, and sleep disturbances. The clinician can interpret such behavior as manifestations of grief for baffled families and school personnel.

MONITORING THE GRIEF PROCESS

A prolonged duration or intensity of these normal behavioral responses and symptoms may indicate the need for clinical intervention, whereas brief periods of turmoil are usually evidence of expected grief work. Chronic depression or hostility, longing to join the deceased, persistent fear or panic, and chronic loss of appetite or ability to sleep indicate the need for professional referral. For a school-age child, regular communication with the teacher regarding the child's classroom behavior is recommended because this should show gradual normalization after a brief period of disruption. Especially during the first several months after a loss, caring adults can help the grieving child significantly by providing a stable environment and well-defined behavioral boundaries, but doing so with empathy. Well-intentioned teachers who become more permissive do not serve the grieving child, particularly because the school environment is often the only place that feels the same for the child. Similarly at home, the same level of expectation, routine and pattern is more supportive than a more permissive or lenient approach. A significant adult who is physically and emotionally available to the child over time is essential to recovery. Six months to a year is a reasonable time frame for resolution of acute grief reactions. A longer duration or lack of progress in resolution will require a mental health referral.

CHALLENGES TO SUCCESSFUL GRIEVING

For a child to grieve a loss, they must perceive the world to be safe and "back to normal." Often, one loss leads to secondary losses that may, in effect, have a more profound influence on a child's sense of loss. For example, when a parent dies and the family must move or there is a financial downturn, it may be these events that complicate and prolong the grief process. A deceased parent may be fantasized as away on a trip, but the immediacy of moving, leaving friends, changing schools, and so forth goes beyond the child's ability to use denial as a coping strategy. Especially during the first few months following a loss within the family unit, family dynamics are apt to change because of explosive emotions, significant depression, financial stress, and new schedules. This is all part of the predictable "grief"

landscape that a clinician must consider in seeing the stresses from the child's point of view.

Certain other factors can significantly derail the child's mourning process and require clinical intervention:

- The inability of the significant adult in the child's life to mourn. Stony silence can be devastating to a child's sense of safety. There has to be emotional space in which to mourn.
- The significant adult's inability to tolerate the child's expression of grief. A "stiff upper lip" is not to be encouraged.
- Forced hypermaturity of the child; requirement to exemplify adult behavior, such as to take care of siblings and prepare meals.
- Overwhelming secondary losses or a history of unresolved losses.
- Ambivalence toward the deceased person or confusion about details of the death.
- Inability to make meaning of the loss, lack of ability to accept the finality of the loss, fantasy ideas beyond a few weeks.

RITUALS AROUND DEATH

Clinicians must view a child's conception of death and grief reaction in religious and cultural contexts that are determined by the child's family and tradition.

Most bereavement specialists agree that it is of assistance to children to attend funerals and other rituals associated with the death of a loved one. However, an adult, not necessarily an immediate family member but a familiar and supportive person, should prepare the child for the experience directly and without euphemisms, accompany the child, and be available to answer questions. A child should be told what their role will be and that they can leave if needed (this rarely happens). For a child to benefit from this experience, they must be old enough to make sense of the event and be assured of the adult for direct support. Keeping a child separate from the family and community during this time is usually more harmful to a child older than 4 than inclusion. Abandonment at a time of family upheaval can be stressful for a young child. Their fantasies about the death and the funeral are more scary than anything that will happen in reality. Participation in all or part of the grieving ritual is to be supported in the vast majority of cases. If given support, children will leave if it gets overwhelming.

SPECIAL ISSUES IN LOSS

Pet Loss

Few, if any, children will grow up without facing the painful experience of the death of their pet. Some parents, in an effort to shield their children from the pain, mistakenly disallow

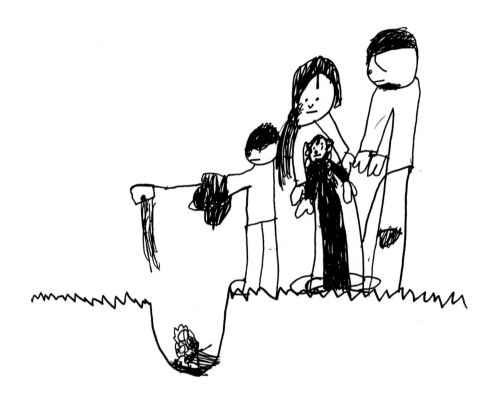

This picture depicts the burial of a child's grandfather. Each family member places dirt in the grave. The artist draws her brother doing this. By E. O., a girl aged 7.

the child the opportunity to face the grief that is a necessary byproduct of affection and connection to their beloved pet. The unexpected and hidden aspect of the event makes it difficult for a child to profit from this learning opportunity.

In fact, the death of a pet provides a rich opportunity for a youngster to strengthen coping skills and learn how to face losses. The family can grieve together, naming the feelings and recognizing and respecting each family member's individual way of dealing with feelings. Finally, the family can engage in the rituals involved in saying goodbye. Parents and other caring adults serve their children by not trivializing or denying their feelings of grief but, at the same time, by not being overwhelmed by them or exaggerating them. Simple, clear, and short rituals and discussions are best.

Sibling Loss

The death of a sibling presents an enormous challenge to the surviving child. They have weathered the death of a contemporary whose loss will continue to be felt throughout their life. The surviving sibling has also lost their parents as they knew them because the complicated mourning process that parents face in this circumstance is intense and prolonged. Marital conflict, depression, guilt, social isolation, and possible resentment of the surviving children may exacerbate parents' grief and further inhibit their ability to be emotionally available to their surviving children. To gain affection and ease their parents' pain, the surviving child may attempt to "replace" a deceased sibling, thereby compromising the youngster's own identity development. Some children will hold on to their grief until they see parental grief resolve and feel safer revealing their own feelings. An explosion of emotion may occur weeks to months down the line. This often confuses and angers parents. Too often, the tendency to idealize the dead child also makes it difficult for the surviving siblings to deal with their own ambivalent feelings (e.g., unresolved sibling rivalry) or with anger at the deceased or at their parents (e.g., for not preventing the death or for seeming to care more about the deceased child). Finally, a survivor's guilt is commonly felt by the surviving sibling and must be challenged. Many times, brief counseling is needed to explore these issues, separate from any group family therapy. Sibling survivor groups may be an additional help. This issue will need to be revisited over time.

Parental Loss

It is not clear exactly how many children experience the death of a parent, but estimates are about 5% to 8%, and about three-fourths of these deaths are anticipated. Additionally, during the COVID-19 pandemic, an estimated 10.5 million children experienced the loss of a caregiver (and 7.5 million experienced COVID-19-associated orphanhood) as of May 2022. In the United States, there was a higher rate of caregiver death among children who are Black, Hispanic, or Indigenous. The ramifications of this high rate and disproportionate burden of caregiver and extended family member deaths will be seen over the coming years.

The death of a parent affects the child's development profoundly in the short and long term. All such children are depressed or dysphoric at 3 months after a parent's death, and 20% have continuing serious problems at 1 year. Anticipate that about a third of such children will have behavioral problems that require mental health referral. In addition to the child's developmental age at the time of death (see earlier), the next most important consideration is the emotional availability of the surviving parent or other supportive adult. Children can do their necessary grief work only if and when life feels safe again, and sometimes that is delayed if a lot of family disruption takes place. The acute grieving period, usually 2 to 3 years, is a time of adjustment because each family member feels a real need to be understood and has the least capacity to give understanding.

Children may idealize and overidentify with the deceased parent while distorting their view of the remaining parent. They are particularly concerned about any perceived vulnerability of the remaining parent. Depending on the cause of death, safety or health issues may become exaggerated. A common concern for the surviving parent is whether a young child will remember the deceased parent. Looking at family photos and videos and storytelling are not universally welcomed by the children, who may fear the surviving parent's strong display of emotion. Letting children take it in at their own pace is the best way to handle this. The health and adjustment of the surviving parent are key to the child's ability to cope. When a child faces a life-threatening illness or injury, a new crisis must be faced by the child, family, and clinician. Although family members are all grieving the same person, that person had a unique relationship with each of them.

The Dying Child

Before the 1970s, most professionals used a protective approach regarding disclosure of information to a dying child. Today, most researchers and clinicians agree that an open approach with disclosure about diagnosis, treatment, and prognosis promotes coping skills and adaptive behavior for most children and families. In a recent study, none of the parents who talked to their dying child about death expressed any regrets; in contrast, 27% of parents who did not talk with their child expressed regret. Children should be given information that allows them to understand the illness and treatment. The child may vacillate between denial and acceptance of the situation. With some people, the child may practice mutual pretense, with both parties ignoring the illness, whereas with others, the child may be open about the seriousness of the illness and their own

---

BOX 26.2   Factors to Consider Before Discussing Death With a Dying Child

- Parents' **philosophical stance** on death. What are their religious and cultural views about life, death, and the afterlife? These should be supported but within a developmental framework.
- Parents' **emotional stance** on death. Is either parent in denial about death as an eventuality? Is either parent likely to be stoic or hyperemotional?
- Child's **age, experience, and level of development**.
- Family's **coping strategies**. What history of crisis or illness can predict its ability to cope with this illness? What are the other stressors a family is facing?
- Child's **perception of participation or control**. Does the child require detailed information about procedures or treatment? Can she look at "the big picture"?

---

fears and fantasies of impending death. Listening to the child can mitigate a sense of isolation. Spinetta suggests five factors that should be considered by caregivers before discussing the illness or death with a dying child (Box 26.2).

A child's understanding of death will depend on their developmental stage (see earlier). Most children with a prolonged illness will actually advance in their understanding of death as they face it. Some children in middle childhood will acquire a very adult notion of death and dying. A few may regress. The clinician should regularly pose open-ended questions to allow the child to reveal their understanding of the circumstances and have a place to express concerns and worries.

Today, a dying child is often actively involved with the treatment team. Because many children will die at home, the parents play a much more active role in treatment as well. When curative therapy has been augmented or replaced by palliative care, the treatment team should take special care to not abandon the child or family, because this will compound the loss. The primary care clinician's role is central to this support by identifying the needs of the child and the treatment choices and assisting with decision-making. In this way, the primary care clinician's work is complementary to that of a specialist caring for the child. The natural tendency is to withdraw from the child and family because most clinicians feel defeated by death and helpless to do anything. That's the wrong thing to do—it makes the loss for the child and family even worse.

GETTING HELP

When a child is facing their own death or the death of someone close, the primary clinician should be not only a source of personal support but also a source of community resource information. Developmentally appropriate grief groups are outstanding supports for children and the parent or parents who bring them. Children can be helped to express their grief through individual and group play, artwork (see the artwork in this chapter), journaling, and sharing time. Selected books and videos can be particularly helpful to a bereaved child. The Good Grief Program at Boston Medical Center offers an annotated bibliography that catalogs books by the type of loss and the reading level (see "Recommended Reading").

CHILDREN AND VIOLENCE

What is the effect on children who live with trauma and violence in their world? Lenore Terr defined childhood psychological **trauma** as "the mental result of one blow or a series of blows, rendering the young person temporarily helpless and breaking past ordinary coping and defensive operations." Violence, in particular, is an important form of trauma that is increasingly experienced or witnessed by children. The media have brought school violence home to every household in America. Interpersonal violence, also referred to as "domestic" violence, occurs in rural and urban areas without regard to class or ethnicity. A study of 6-year-old children by Schuler and Nair indicated that 43% of these young children had seen a beating, 13% saw a knife threat, and 7% saw an actual stabbing or shooting. Young children are deeply affected by witnessing violence, particularly when the perpetrator or victim is a family member.

The child's reaction to violence, and the trauma experienced, will depend on a number of factors, including age and developmental stage, previous exposure to violence, whether the perpetrator or the victim is known, and whether the violence is a single incident or is chronic. Children exposed to violence have an increased level of aggression, are more anxious, and have higher rates of delinquency and social problems. Children are usually more affected than adults suspect, and most communicate their fear and uncertainty about their lives through behavior rather than language.

The following are clinical clues that a child or adolescent may have witnessed overwhelming violence:

- Hypervigilance, jumpiness
- Hyperactivity, frantic activity
- Nightmares
- Separation anxiety, clinginess
- Risk-taking behavior
- Withdrawal, isolation
- Emotional numbing

Posttraumatic stress disorder (PTSD) develops in a significant percentage of children who experience violence (Box 26.3). Studies of the etiology of PTSD in children have shown that witnessing interpersonal violence is

BOX 26.3   Posttraumatic Stress Disorder

Diagnostic Criteria
Posttraumatic Stress Disorder in Individuals Older
Than 6 Years

Note: The following criteria apply to adults, adolescents, and children older than 6 years. For children 6 years and younger, see corresponding criteria below.

A. Exposure to actual or threatened death, serious injury, or sexual violence in one (or more) of the following ways:
1. Directly experiencing the traumatic event(s).
2. Witnessing, in person, the event(s) as it occurred to others.
3. Learning that the traumatic event(s) occurred to a close family member or close friend. In cases of actual or threatened death of a family member or friend, the event(s) must have been violent or accidental.
4. Experiencing repeated or extreme exposure to aversive details of the traumatic event(s) (e.g., first responders collecting human remains; police officers repeatedly exposed to details of child abuse).
   Note: Criterion A4 does not apply to exposure through electronic media, television, movies, or pictures, unless this exposure is work related.

B. Presence of one (or more) of the following intrusion symptoms associated with the traumatic event(s), beginning after the traumatic event(s) occurred:
1. Recurrent, involuntary, and intrusive distressing memories of the traumatic event(s).
   Note: In children older than 6 years, repetitive play may occur in which themes or aspects of the traumatic event(s) are expressed.
2. Recurrent distressing dreams in which the content and/or effect of the dream are related to the traumatic event(s).
   Note: In children, there may be frightening dreams without recognizable content.
3. Dissociative reactions (e.g., flashbacks) in which the individual feels or acts as if the traumatic event(s) were recurring. (Such reactions may occur on a continuum, with the most extreme expression being a complete loss of awareness of present surroundings.)
   Note: In children, trauma-specific reenactment may occur in play.
4. Intense or prolonged psychological distress at exposure to internal or external cues that symbolize or resemble an aspect of the traumatic event(s).
5. Marked physiological reactions to internal or external cues that symbolize or resemble an aspect of the traumatic event(s).

C. Persistent avoidance or stimuli associated with the traumatic event(s), beginning after the traumatic event(s) occurred, as evidenced by one or both of the following:
1. Avoidance of or efforts to avoid distressing memories, thoughts, or feelings about or closely associated with the traumatic event(s).
2. Avoidance of or efforts to avoid external reminders (people, places, conversations, activities, objects, situations) that arouse distressing memories, thoughts, or feelings about or closely associated with the traumatic event(s).

D. Negative alterations in cognitions and mood associated with the traumatic event(s), beginning or worsening after the traumatic event(s) occurred, as evidenced by two (or more) of the following:
1. Inability to remember an important aspect of the traumatic event(s) (typically due to dissociative amnesia and not due to other factors, such as head injury, alcohol, or drugs).
2. Persistent and exaggerated negative beliefs or expectations about oneself, others, or the world (e.g., "I am bad," "No one can be trusted," "The world is completely dangerous," "My whole nervous system is permanently ruined").
3. Persistent, distorted cognitions about the cause or consequences of the traumatic event(s) that lead the individual to blame himself/herself or others.
4. Persistent negative emotional state (e.g., fear, horror, anger, guilt, or shame).
5. Markedly diminished interest or participation in significant activities.
6. Feelings of detachment or estrangement from others.
7. Persistent inability to experience positive emotions (e.g., inability to experience happiness, satisfaction, or loving feelings).

E. Marked alterations in arousal and reactivity associated with the traumatic event(s), beginning or worsening after the traumatic event(s) occurred, as evidenced by two (or more) of the following:
1. Irritable behavior and angry outbursts (with little or no provocation) typically expressed as verbal or physical aggression toward people or objects.
2. Reckless or self-destructive behavior.
3. Hypervigilance.
4. Exaggerated startle response.
5. Problems with concentration.
6. Sleep disturbance (e.g., difficulty falling or staying asleep or restless sleep).

(Continued)

BOX 26.3 Posttraumatic Stress Disorder—cont'd

F. Duration of the disturbance (Criteria B, C, D, and E) is more than 1 month.

G. The disturbance causes clinically significant distress or impairment in social, occupational, or other important areas of functioning.

H. The disturbance is not attributable to the physiological effects of a substance (e.g., medication, alcohol) or another medical condition.

Specify whether:

With dissociative symptoms: The individual's symptoms meet the criteria for posttraumatic stress disorder, and in addition, in response to the stressor, the individual experiences persistent or recurrent symptoms of either of the following:

1. **Depersonalization**: Persistent or recurrent experiences of feeling detached from, and as if one were an outside observer of, one's mental processes or body (e.g., feeling as though one were in a dream, feeling a sense of unreality of self or body or of time moving slowly).

2. **Derealization**: Persistent or recurrent experiences of the unreality of surroundings (e.g., the world around the individual is experienced as unreal, dreamlike, distant, or distorted).

   Note: To use this subtype, the dissociative symptoms must not be attributable to the physiological effects of a substance (e.g., blackouts, behavior during alcohol intoxication) or another medical condition (e.g., complex partial seizures).

Specify if:

With delayed expression: If the full diagnostic criteria are not met until at least 6 months after the event (although the onset and expression of some symptoms may be immediate).

Posttraumatic Stress Syndrome in Children 6 Years and Younger

A. In children 6 years and younger, exposure to actual or threatened death, serious injury, or sexual violence in one (or more) of the following ways:

1. Directly experiencing the traumatic event(s).

2. Witnessing, in person, the event(s) as it occurred to others, especially primary caregivers.

3. Learning that the traumatic event(s) occurred to a parent or caregiving figure.

B. Presence of one (or more) of the following intrusion symptoms associated with the traumatic event(s), beginning after the traumatic event(s) occurred:

1. Recurrent, involuntary, and intrusive distressing memories of the traumatic event(s).

   Note: Spontaneous and intrusive memories may not necessarily appear distressing and may be expressed as play reenactment.

2. Recurrent distressing dreams in which the content and/or effect of the dream are related to the traumatic event(s).

   Note: It may not be possible to ascertain that the frightening content is related to the traumatic event.

3. Dissociative reactions (e.g., flashbacks) in which the child feels or acts as if the traumatic event(s) were recurring. (Such reactions may occur on continuum, with the most extreme expression being a complete loss of awareness of present surroundings.) Such trauma-specific reenactment may occur in play.

4. Intense or prolonged psychological distress at exposure to internal or external cues that symbolize or resemble an aspect of the traumatic event(s).

5. Marked physiological reactions to reminders of the traumatic event(s).

C. One (or more) of the following symptoms, representing either persistent avoidance of stimuli associated with the traumatic event(s) or negative alterations in cognitions and mood associated with the traumatic event(s), must be present, beginning after the event(s) or worsening after the event(s):

Persistent Avoidance of Stimuli

1. Avoidance of or efforts to avoid activities, places, or physical reminders that arouse recollections of the traumatic event(s).

2. Avoidance of or efforts to avoid people, conversations, or interpersonal situations that arouse recollections of the traumatic event(s).

Negative Alterations in Cognitions

3. Substantially increased frequency of negative emotional states (e.g., fear, guilt, sadness, shame, confusion).

4. Markedly diminished interest or participation in significant activities, including constriction of play.

5. Socially withdrawn behavior.

6. Persistent reduction in the expression of positive emotions.

D. Alterations in arousal and reactivity associated with the traumatic event(s), beginning or worsening after the traumatic event(s) occurred, as evidenced by two (or more) of the following:

1. Irritable behavior and angry outbursts (with little or no provocation) typically expressed as verbal or physical aggression toward people or objects (including extreme temper tantrums).

2. Hypervigilance.

3. Exaggerated startle response.

4. Problems with concentration.

5. Sleep disturbance (e.g., difficulty falling or staying asleep or restless sleep).

E. The duration of the disturbance is more than 1 month.
F. The disturbance causes clinically significant distress or impairment in relationships with parents, siblings, peers, or other caregivers or with school behavior.
G. The disturbance is not attributable to the physiological effects of a substance (e.g., medication or alcohol) or another medical condition.

Specify whether:

With dissociative symptoms: The individual's symptoms meet the criteria for posttraumatic stress disorder, and the individual experiences persistent or recurrent symptoms of either of the following:

1. **Depersonalization**: Persistent or recurrent experiences of feeling detached from, and as if one were an outside observer of, one's mental processes or body (e.g., feeling as though one were in a dream, feeling a sense of unreality of self or body or of time moving slowly).
2. **Derealization**: Persistent or recurrent experiences of unreality of surroundings (e.g., the world around the individual is experienced as unreal, dreamlike, distant, or distorted).

Note: To use this subtype, the dissociative symptoms must not be attributable to the physiological effects of a substance (e.g., blackouts) or another medical condition (e.g., complex partial seizures).

Specify if:

With delayed expression: If the full diagnostic criteria are not met until at least 6 months after the event (although the onset and expression of some symptoms may be immediate).

as traumatic as being the victim of sexual abuse. Clinical experience suggests that PTSD can be a chronic problem and a source of ongoing problems in school, relationships, and emotional development. One of the unmistakable symptoms of chronic exposure to violence is the child's foreshortened view of the future. They cannot imagine next year's vacation or what they will be when they grow up.

Because the scars carried by children who are chronically exposed to violence are invisible, and because their immediate caregivers may also be victims or perpetrators, it is incumbent on the clinician to recognize symptoms and ask questions that can lead to intervention. Think about PTSD when evaluating a child with behavior or learning problems who has witnessed a violent event any time in the past.

Asking about violence takes little time, does not require special expertise, and demonstrates concern. The following are indications that a referral to a community resource such as a mental health specialist, a community organization or support group, or the department of social services should be made:

- Symptoms have persisted for more than 6 months. Behavioral change with distress lasting less than 3 months is labeled adjustment disorder, but it should be gradually improving across that time.
- The trauma was particularly violent or involved the death or departure from the home of a parent or primary caretaker.
- Continuing revisualization of the violent event.
- The child's caretakers are unable to empathize with or support the child.

PTSD requires a mental health referral, with other agencies involved as indicated to ensure child safety. About

BOX 26.4   Factors that Influence A Child's Ability to Cope with Serious Trauma or Violence

Enhanced Risk
- Predisposition to anxiety and/or depression in self or in a family
- Preexisting family and school problems
- Preexisting developmental and/or physical disabilities
- No stable family member as a support
- Poor economic security
- Moving, immigration, cultural, or family isolation

Protective Factors
- Higher intellectual abilities
- Enhanced language skills
- Special talents, abilities
- School success. Other experience with success and mastery
- Participation in outside activities, for example, scouting, sports, church groups, special camps
- Physical and emotional availability of an adult support person

20% to 30% of child survivors of serious trauma will need extended mental health care. It is unclear why PTSD does not develop in some children who are exposed to chronic violence. However, resiliency factors such as the presence of a strong role model and activities that promote competence and self-esteem (Box 26.4) remind us that an understanding, nurturing parent, a dedicated coach, or a member of

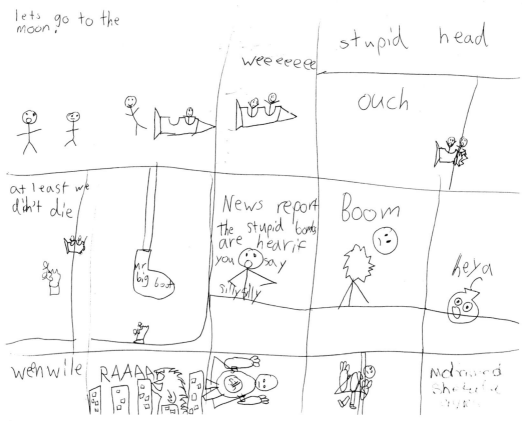

An 8-year-old boy describes his drawing as a space journey that starts and is interrupted by a crash. A news report is embedded in his story; a bomb knocks the head off the reporter. The story continues with more bombs directed at tall city buildings and a disembodied person who has crashed into a pole. By Mohammed Shetula.

the clergy who works with youth can positively change the child's view of himself. Some children who have weathered severe violence with apparent good resolve may suffer from symptoms years later. The clinician may have to probe the past to identify the source of current emotional, social, or behavioral complaints.

WHEN VIOLENCE OCCURS AT HOME

Children who experience violence within the home are at even greater risk than those who see it in the community. Estimates indicate that as many as 10% of youngsters witness such violence. The children in such homes are at serious risk of being physically harmed themselves, but they are also likely to have anxiety, depression, and enhanced aggressive behavior. Over the long term, they are at increased risk for anxiety and depression, poor school performance, and substance use. Behavior problems of both the internalizing and externalizing types are seen in a large proportion of children 6 to 18 years old who have witnessed interpersonal violence.

Child health care clinicians commonly have variable knowledge about, or screening practices for, interpersonal violence among families in their practices. This can be remedied by routinely asking at health encounters whether a parent feels or has felt at risk. A referral to a community resource should be available. A high level of suspicion for interpersonal violence as a possible cause of childhood behavioral concerns needs to be part of the clinician's thinking. It can be accomplished during a clinical interview or through a psychosocial parent questionnaire that includes an assessment of interpersonal violence (see Kemper and Kelleher, 1996, in "References").

WHEN CATASTROPHE STRIKES

Many children may face the threat of disasters such as hurricanes or earthquakes, which are increasing threats as climate change progresses, the widespread threat of gun violence in homes, communities, and schools (Box 26.5), and the fears and insecurities that accompany news of war and terrorism around the world. The feelings experienced by children, even very young children, include anxiety, confusion, fear, irritability, and depression. Very young children may suffer symptoms of stress such as crying and whining, repressive behavior, separation anxiety and fear of being alone, sleep disorders, illness, changes in normal patterns of behavior, aggression, and fear.

Why some children in a family appear to be resilient and others suffer permanent psychological scars in the wake of an overwhelming event is a subject of much inquiry. However, experts all agree what resilience is *not*. It is not rare; most

---

> ### BOX 26.5   School Shootings And Drills
>
> In 2022 there were 51 school shootings resulting in injury or death. School shootings are traumatic events that, in addition to the risk of injury or death for a particular child in the moment, can also directly lead to the loss of peers and trusted adults, with resulting grief, as discussed in this chapter. Additionally, the rise in school shootings has also led to an increased use of active shooter drills in schools. Such drills have a risk of traumatizing students, families, and staff and can have a negative effect on youth emotional health. There are mixed data on their effectiveness. For places where these drills are being implemented, various groups including Everytown for Gun Safety Support Fund, the American Federation of Teachers, and the National Education Association recommend avoiding drills that simulate actual incidents, notifying parents, students, and teachers in advance, developing developmentally appropriate content in collaboration with staff and mental health specialists, and working to combine drills with support systems that support student well-being. Clinicians can discuss perceptions around active shooter drills with families and advocate for developmentally appropriate and evidence-based practices.

children have the capacity to be resilient. Second, people are not born resilient. Resilience is developed.

What, then, are the strategies that parents can use when children are facing threats that may be imminent or threats that are more nebulous? The following strategies are important for helping toddlers and young children manage the stress of exposure to man-made and natural disasters: Clinicians should be aware of these strategies to assist if the occasion warrants it.

- **Infants and children** younger than 6 years rely exclusively on the emotional competence of their primary caregiver. How a parent communicates about escaping to safety from a disaster, the emotional tone that is set, and the age-appropriate explanations about what will happen in the next few minutes or hours will determine the child's reaction. Communicate in a clear, calm voice, hold the child close physically when possible, and reassure the child that you, the adult, are in charge and will make everything all right.
- Exposure to the media should be avoided since very young children have no capacity to distinguish real-time action from the replay displays of destruction. There is no sense of distance or time in the presentations of these images at a young age.

- **Elementary-aged children** will understand the life event or threat not just from their primary caregiver's perspective but also from that of their peers and other adults. They worry about the safety of their limited world of home, neighborhood, and school. It is critical to assure these children that you are in charge, that you will do your best to keep them safe, and that other helping adults, such as neighbors, paramedics, and mayors, will do their best to keep everyone safe as well.
- **Preadolescents** view themselves as members of a more complex world; they are part of a family, a community of school and sports, a religious and an ethnic group, and a citizen of a town, a state, and a nation. They have the capacity to worry in times of threat about their immediate safety, as well as how the event or threat will change their future.
- **Adolescents** are caught in the middle between understandable feelings of terror and their own imposed pressure to be mature in the face of a threat. They rely on the adults in their lives to make them feel safe and yet may want to participate in creating safety nets for others. They may be philosophical and/or political in their attempts to make sense of the event.

In summary, for children of any age, adults whom they know and trust will provide the most safety and security in times of crisis and stress. Adults should never promise anything that they cannot control, but they should reassure children that they are doing everything to make them safe and secure. They should explain action plans, a crisis response, and immediate future events, all with confidence and competence. For older children who may want to watch and listen to the media, parents should join them so that they can respond to any concerns. They should preserve whatever routines can be maintained in their children's lives, such as bedtime rituals. They should anticipate the symptoms of stress in their children and be available to comfort them.

RECOMMENDED READING

American Academy of Pediatrics, George Cohen (lead author). Helping children and families deal with divorce and separation. *Pediatrics.* 2002;110:1019–1023.

Books and videos on loss for children and adolescents: an annotated bibliography. The Good Grief Program, One Boston Medical Center Place, 1996, Boston.

Galeo S, Ahera J, Resnick H, et al. Psychological sequelae of the September 11 terrorist attacks in NYC. *N Engl J Med.* 2002;346:982–987.

Lamberg L. In the wake of tragedy: studies track psychological response to mass violence. *JAMA.* 2003;291:587–589.

Sourkes B. *Armfuls of time: the psychological experience of the child with a life-threatening illness.* Pittsburgh: University of Pittsburgh Press; 1995.

Stein MT, Heyneman EK, Stern EJ. Recurrent nightmares, aggressive doll play, separation anxiety and witnessing domestic violence in a nine year old girl. *J Dev Behav Pediatr.* 2004;25:419–422.

Swick S, Dechant E, Jellinek M. Children of victims of September 11th: a perspective on the emotional and developmental challenges they face and how to help meet them. *J Dev Behav Pediatr.* 2002;23:378–384.

Tanner JL. Parental separation and divorce: can we provide an ounce of prevention? *Pediatrics.* 2002;110:1007–1009.

Terr L: *Too Scared to Cry.* New York, Basic Books, 1990.

Walman vander, Molen JW. Violence and suffering in television news: toward a broader conception of harmful television content in children. *Pediatrics.* 2004;113:1771–1775. (See this whole issue to read about this topic in more detail.).

Winston F, Kassam-Adams N, Garcia-Espana F, et al. Screening for risk of persistent posttraumatic stress in injured children and their parents. *JAMA.* 2003;290:643–649.

Kemper KJ, Kelleher KJ, Rationale for family psychosocial screening. *Ambul Child Health.* 1996;1(4):311–324.

Resources for Children and Families

Grollman EA. *Talking about death: a dialogue between parents and the child.* Boston: Beacon Press; 1990.

Mundy M. *Sad isn't bad: a good grief guidebook for kids dealing with loss.* St Meinrad, IN: Abby Press; 1998.

The Dougy Center for Grieving Children: *35 ways to help a grieving child*, Portland, The Dougy Center for Grieving Children.

Grieving Children, 1999. www.dougy.org. See Good Grief Program (above), Boston Medical Center, for a complete bibliography.

<https://everytownresearch.org/issue/child-teen-safety/>

<https://www.ojjdp.gov/ojstatbb/crime/qa05101.asp>

Zullig KJ. Active shooter drills: a closer look at next steps. *J Adolesc Health.* 2020;67(4):465–466. https://doi.org/10.1016/j.jadohealth.2020.07.028.

Moore-Petinak N, Waselewski M, Patterson BA, Chang T. Active shooter drills in the United States: a national study of youth experiences and perceptions. *J Adolesc Health.* 2020;67(4):509–513. https://doi.org/10.1016/j.jadohealth.2020.06.015.

Duffee J, Szilagyi M, Forkey H, et al. Trauma-informed care in child health systems. *Pediatrics.* 2021;148(2): e2021052579.

Hillis SD, Blenkinsop A, Villaveces A, et al. COVID-19–associated orphanhood and caregiver death in the United States. *Pediatrics.* 2021;148(6): e2021053760.

Hillis S, N'konzi JN, Msemburi W, et al. Orphanhood and caregiver loss among children based on new global excess COVID-19 death estimates. *JAMA Pediatr.* 2022;176(11):1145–1148. https://doi.org/10.1001/jamapediatrics.2022.3157.

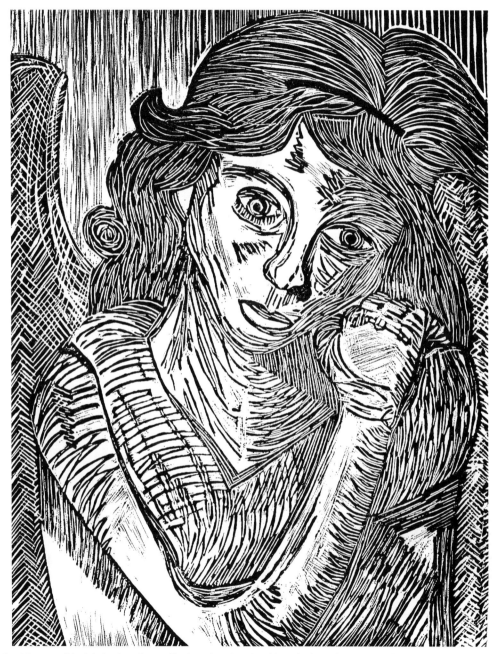

An 18-year-old girl depicts herself after the death of her father. A woodcut by Loni Blankenship, age 18.

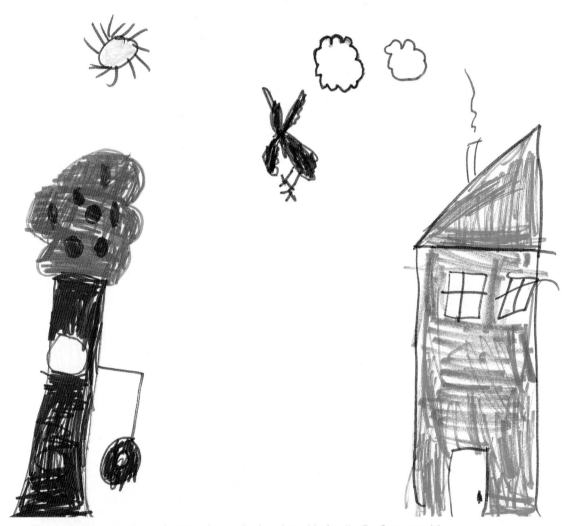

This boy draws an empty house when asked to draw his family. By Cameron M.

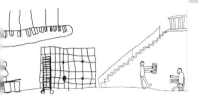

27

Resources for Families: An Annotated Bibliography

Caroline J. Kistin and Jenny S. Radesky

> *Listen to the MUSTN'TS, child, Listen to the DON'TS Listen to the SHOULDN'TS The IMPOSSIBLES, the WONT'S Listen to the NEVER HAVES Then listen close to me—Anything can happen, child, ANYTHING can be.*
>
> **—Where the Sidewalk Ends by Shel Silverstein**

Resources about parenting, health, and child development can be a helpful supplement to other supports and referrals made by primary care clinicians. However, since the advent of the internet and the explosion of books by parenting experts, it can be a lot for caregivers to navigate. By knowing several good books and reliable websites, child health clinicians can help families find good information that suits their individual learning style. This is even more important now that caregivers are offered a vast amount of information—much of it low quality or even misinformation—online and through social media.

This collection of resources begins with the "Classics"—books about child development and parenting that may have been written decades ago but have stood the test of time and continue to offer important insights to parents. These books are also great for clinicians in training and are good to know about in case caregivers ask about them. For family resources about specific health or behavior topics—such as prematurity (Chapter 7) or autism spectrum disorder (Chapter 14)—please refer to the respective chapters on these topics.

We then list here several dozen books for children that may be helpful for teaching them about topics like emotions, their bodies, or coping with illness. Books are incredible health literacy tools for young people. As we discuss throughout this textbook, young children learn through storytelling— they are magical thinkers who build parasocial relationships with characters and learn by watching them. Older children and adolescents also appreciate learning by watching characters navigate difficult situations; for

teens, seeing a challenging topic played out through a book or graphic novel is often more approachable than being taught about it directly by an adult.

Finally, we provide a list of web-based resources that are trusted and comprehensive and can be a go-to source of handouts and information.

BOOK FOR PARENTS-CHILD DEVELOPMENT CLASSICS

Brazelton TB: *Touchpoints: your child's emotional and behavioral development: birth-3: the essential reference for the early years*, New York, 2006, HarperCollins. An easy-to-read reference book in which parents' questions and concerns about their child's behavior, development, and feelings are anticipated and answered in chronological (part I) as well as problem (part II) form.

Brazelton TB, Sparrow JD: *Touchpoints 3-6*, Cambridge, 2002, Perseus Publishing. An extension of Dr. Brazelton's original book, *Touchpoints*, that now extends the age from 3 to 6 years. There are few books on typical development and behavior in preschool children for parents and clinicians. This one fills the gap.

Fraiberg S: *The magic years*, New York, 1959, Charles Scribner's Sons, (updated 1996). Now a child development classic. Child psychoanalyst Fraiberg discusses early psychological development (birth to 6 years) as though the reader were experiencing the child's inner world. More theoretical than many books in this list, it discusses typical developmental problems and their management—but is easy to read.

Previous edition chapter by Martin T. Stein and Suzanne D. Dixon.

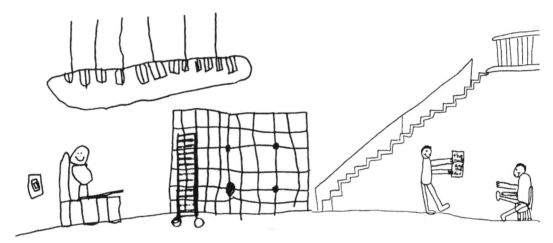

"Reading together." Left illustration by Ben Stein, age 5. Right illustration by Josh Stein, age 8.

Gopnik A, Meltzoff AN, Kuhl PK: *The scientist in the crib: what early learning tell us about the mind*, 2001, Perennial. Written by three pioneer researchers in infant cognitive science, a journey through the discoveries about how much babies and young children know, how available they are to learn, and how much parents teach them during everyday activities. Among the best reviews of contemporary early development research for parents and clinicians—and easy to read.

Brazelton TB, Sparrow JD: *Calming your fussy baby* (2003); *Discipline* (2003); *Sleep* (2003); *Toilet training* (2004), Cambridge, Da Capo Press. Short monographs written in a comforting style for parents as they experience typical fluctuations in development.

Faber A, Mazlish E: *Siblings without rivalry*, New York, 1987, Avon Books, (updated 2012). This book offers practical guidelines supplemented with the views and experiences of parents in a parenting workshop. Thought-provoking ideas for role-playing. Helpful comic strips and reminder strips on how to handle different situations make this book a good source for parents and professionals.

Ferber R: *Solve your child's sleep problems*, New York, 1985, Simon & Schuster, (updated 2006). Clear explanations of the developmental basis of sleep disturbances in a family context. Specific, sensible suggestions for solving problems from sleep rhythm disturbances to enuresis. Has been the subject of criticism for the approach of "Ferberizing" and crying it out, but worth knowing for pediatric clinicians.

Green RW: *The explosive child: a new approach for understanding and parenting easily frustrated, chronically inflexible children*, ed 6, New York, 2021, HarperCollins. From an experienced child psychologist who offers specific approaches for parents of children with defiance, oppositionality, and meltdowns. Offers practical ways to reduce hostility and antagonism between child and parent with an emphasis on communication and collaborative problem solving.

Greenspan S: *The challenging child*, New York, 1996, Addison-Wesley. A valuable book for motivated parents of "difficult" children that gives insight into the child while offering child-rearing guidelines. Dr. Greenspan describes five personality patterns and devotes a chapter to each (sensitive child, self-absorbed child, defiant child, inattentive child, active-aggressive child). A nice neutral chapter of environmental and dietary influences on children's behavior is also included.

Phelan T: *1-2-3 Magic: effective discipline for children 2-12 years*, ed 6, 2016, Parent Magic. A straightforward behavioral method of discipline that uses counting to help parents stop unwanted behavior and start wanted behavior without arguing, yelling, or spanking. Easy-to-follow steps for a motivated parent.

Parenting Teenagers

Pashe P, Greydanus D, eds: *Caring for your teenager*, New York, 2003, Bantam Books (for American Academy of Pediatrics). The third of a three-book series developed by the American Academy of Pediatrics. Well-written and easy-to-use comprehensive guide for parents of 12- to 21-year-olds. Practical advice on everything from typical development to nutrition to school failure to family conflicts. Straightforward coverage of sexuality, substance use, sexually transmitted infections, reproductive health, and eating disorders. Reader-friendly format and illustrations make it informative for all parents.

Child and Health Care

Eisenberg A, Murkoff HE, Hathaway SE: *What to expect the first year*, ed 3, New York, 2014, Workman Publishing. Comprehensive and practical guide to newborn and infant care. Format is easy to read with chapters that identify issues at monthly stages. Useful sections on nutrition, language development, and safety.

Leach P: *Your baby and child: from birth to age 5*, revised ed, New York, 1997, Alfred A Knopf. Developmental psychologist Penelope Leach has written an encyclopedia for parents of children from birth to 5 years. Leach uses an approach to everyday care and common behavioral issues that is based on development of the child and the family. Subtitles within the chapter, many excellent drawings and pictures, and a comprehensive index with definitions facilitate reading this book and make it accessible to most parents.

Spock B, Needlman R: *Dr. Spock's baby and child care*, ed 10, New York, 2018, Pocket Books (soft-cover), EP Dutton (hardcover). This eighth edition of Dr. Spock's classic guide to parenting and child rearing is a compilation of information on child development, parenting skills, and common medical conditions. Dr. Spock's advice on parenting (captured in the book's opening statement, "Trust yourself. You know more than you think.") has engaged parents for multiple generations.

Weisbluth M: *Healthy sleep habits, happy child*, ed 4, New York, 2015, Ballantine Books. A popular parent guide to understanding natural sleep cycles, ways to promote restful sleep, and problems related to sleep. Emphasis on individual temperaments. Some parents feel this book sets expectations a bit high.

Barkley R: *Taking charge of ADHD*, ed 4, New York, 2020, Guilford Press. A well-organized guide of suggestions for helping children with attention-deficit/hyperactivity disorder (ADHD). Practical lists of suggestions and charts. The text can get a bit technical, but the advice given is good.

Hallowell E, Ratey J: *Driven to distraction*, New York, 1994, Touchstone (updated 2011). A best-selling book that any parents who think they or their children have ADHD probably will have read. The authors use stories from their patients to demonstrate the different forms of ADHD. It offers sound advice on how to identify ADHD and what to do about it.

Serious Illness and Death

Kübler-Ross E: *On children and death*, reprint ed, New York, 1997, Scribner. From the person who gave the classic descriptions of the grieving process, this book explains children's understanding of death and how to assist in the process.

Trozzi M: *Talking with children about loss: words, strategies, and wisdom to help children cope with death, divorce, and other difficult times*, New York, 1999, Putnam. Intended for parents and professionals, this book gently leads the reader through the most difficult terrain: how to help your child deal with the painful feelings of significant loss in a way that actually enhances healthy psychological development. This easy-to-read book uses many examples: facing the death of a family member or a pet, divorce, chronic illness, and welcoming a new sibling with special needs, as well as the inevitable losses and changes that all children face. Practical suggestions for management and intervention are included. Good for parents, teachers, and other professionals who care for children facing the death of themselves or family members.

Feeding

Brazelton TB, Sparrow JD: *Feeding*, Cambridge, 2004, Da Capo Press. Feeding patterns from the newborn to the 5-year-old are described in the context of developmental abilities and family expectations, with a discussion of common feeding problems and solutions.

Satter E: *How to get your kid to eat—but not too much*, Palo Alto, 1987, Bull. This practical resource shows parents how to help children develop healthy eating behavior. It also discusses childhood distortions about eating and feeding that may be precursors to eating disorders in later life.

Satter E: *Child of mine: feeding with love and good sense*, ed 3, Palo Alto, 2000, Bull. This nutritional guidebook offers information on the developmental and social aspects of feeding from infancy through adolescence. Types of behavior that encourage the formation of healthy eating

patterns are reviewed, and technical nutrition information is translated into practical and basic concepts.

BOOKS FOR CHILDREN

Emotions

Huebner D: *What to do when you worry too much: a kid's guide to overcoming anxiety*, 2021, American Psychological Association.—Great workbook for parents and school-aged children.

Modd D: *Shelley the hyperactive turtle*, 2006, Woodbine House.—Shelley the turtle explains that receiving an ADHD diagnosis is not so scary.

Carlson N: *This morning Sam went to Mars*, 2013, Free Spirit Publishing.—Sam's mind is always wandering. He meets with a doctor to learn about ways to focus.

Esham B: *Mrs. Gorski, I think I have the wiggle fidgets*, 2008, Mainstream Connections Publishing.—David's teacher is always frustrated with David's impulsivity. He learns some techniques to help. [Best for older readers]

Nelson-Schmidt M: *Jonathan James and the whatif monster*, 2012, Kane Miller EDC Publishing.—Jonathan James is always asking "what if" about his fears, but he starts asking "what if those things don't happen."

Henkes K: *Wemberly worried*, 2000, Greenwillow Books.—Wemberly worries and worries, and she learns to face her fears as she starts school.

Green A: *The monster in the bubble*, 2009, Monsters in my Head, LLC.—Monster likes everything to be the same, and he is scared of taking risks.

Green A: *Don't feed the worry bug*, 2011, Monsters in my Head, LLC.—Wince the monster of worry decides not to feed his worry bug anymore.

McCloud C: *Have you filled a bucket today?*, 2006, Nelson Pub and Marketing LLC.—This book uses the analogy of a bucket to discuss self-esteem and building others up with our words and actions.

Carlson N: *Henry and the bully*, 2010, Viking Books for Young Readers.—Henry the mouse learns how to deal with a bully.

Cook J: *Bully B.E.A.N.S.*, 2009, National Center for Youth Issues.—A creative approach to standing up to bullies! Julia Cook has several books about behavior that help build children's insight into things like personal space and impulsive talking.

Peters A: *The color thief: a family's story of depression*, 2015, Albert Whitman & Company.—A young boy describes the course of his father's depression as a world that loses colors.

Sterling C: *Some bunny to talk to: a story about going to therapy*, 2014, Magination Press.—Bunny realizes therapy is not so scary after all.

Llenas A: *The color monster: a story about emotions*, 2018, Little, Brown Books for Young Readers.—Color Monster needs help sorting out his emotions.

Becker S: *Even superheroes have bad days*, 2016, Union Square Kids.—Superheroes consider using their powers against others when having a bad day, but they realize real superheroes use their powers for good.

Wright L: *I can handle it!*, 2017, Laurie Wright.—Sebastien is trying to learn how to handle frustration. Great book for kids struggling with transitions and frustration tolerance.

Dewney A: *Llama llama mad at mama*, 2010, Scholastic.—Llama and mama go shopping, and llama learns from the tantrum he throws. [Best for younger readers]

Manning J: *Millie fierce*, 2012, Philomel Books.—Millie struggles with controlling her anger and impulsive behavior, and she learns an important lesson.

Greenwood E: *My mixed emotions*, 2018, DK Children.—An explanation of all the emotions and some practical steps and examples of how to handle them. [Best for older readers]

Green A: *The very frustrated monster*, 2012, Monsters in my Head.—Monster is having a bad day, but he learns to reframe his troubles.

Cain J: *The way I feel*, 2000, AmazonUS/INDPB.—A young girl uses pictures and descriptions of the many emotions she experiences. [Best for younger readers]

Willey K: *Breathe like a bear: 30 mindful moments for kids to feel calm and focused anywhere*, 2017, Rodale Kids.—30 examples of mindfulness exercises.

Autism

Rudolph S: *All my stripes: a story for children with autism*, 2015, Magination Press.—Zane the zebra struggles with feeling different because of his autism, but his mama reminds him of all of his unique skills and talents.

Larson EM: *I am utterly unique: celebrating the strengths of children with Asperger syndrome and high functioning autism*, 2006, AAPC Publishing.—An alphabet book highlighting the amazing skills of children with autism. [Best for older readers]

Pain and Coping

Miles B: *Imagine a rainbow: a child's guide for soothing pain*, 2006, Magination Press.

Zoffness R: *The chronic pain and illness workbook for teens: CBT and mindfulness-based practices to turn the volume down on pain*, 2019, Instant Help.

Cuthbert T: *Be the boss of your pain: self-care for kids*, 2007, Free Spirit Publishing.

Viorst J: *Alexander and the terrible, horrible, no good, very bad day*, 1972, Atheneum Books for Young Readers.

Rogers F: *Going to the hospital*, 1988, Puffin.

Hautzig D: *A visit to the Sesame Street hospital*, 1985, Random House Books for Young Readers.

Bourgeois P: *Franklin goes to the hospital*, 2000, Scholastic.

Palacio RJ: *Wonder*, 2012, Alfred A. Knopf.

Developmental and Situational Conflicts

Berenstain S, Berenstain J: *First time books: the berenstain bears: go to the doctor; go to visit the dentist; moving day; and the sitter; get in a fight; trouble with friends; trouble with money; and the messy room; learn about strangers; and too much TV; and too much junk food; go out for the team; and mama's new job; forget their manners; and the truth; get stage fright; trouble at school; in the dark; and the bad habit*, New York, 1981–1997, Random House. Inexpensive picture books that highlight some stressful experiences. Written for older toddlers and preschoolers in a pleasant and reassuring manner.

Berger T: *I have feelings*, New York, 1977, Human Sciences Press. Nice, reflective book for kindergarten through sixth grade. An example of several books that help children to reflect on themselves through another child's eyes.

Cole J, Degan B: *The magic school bus: inside the human body*, New York, 1990, Scholastic. For ages 6 to 9 years. The Magic School Bus series is great for teaching children about science and nature.

BOOKS FOR TEENAGERS

Mental Health

Quinn P, Stern J: *Putting on the brakes: young people's guide to understanding attention deficit hyperactivity disorder*, revised ed, New York, 2001, Magination Press. A book written for 8- to 13-year-olds that uses wonderful analogies to explain what ADHD is and how to address the problems that it presents. Practical and straightforward.

Galanti R: *Anxiety relief for teens: essential CBT skills and mindfulness practices to overcome anxiety and stress*, 2020, Zeitgeist Young Adult.

Van Djik S: *Don't let your emotions run your life for teens: dialectical behavior therapy skills for helping you manage mood swings, control angry outbursts, and get along with others*, 2021, Instant Help.

Health and Puberty/Sexuality

McCoy K, Wibbelsman C: *The teenage body book*, revised ed, New York, 1999, Perigee Books. This book is based on questions commonly asked by teenagers concerning their bodies and bodily changes. The authors are a former editor of *Teen Magazine* and a physician who specializes in adolescent medicine. The authors cover a wide range of topics, including normal physical development and birth control. Case vignettes and examples of letters from teens are used to illustrate various problems. Detailed line drawings are plentiful and excellent. This book is more appropriate for those in mid to late adolescence; it may be too sophisticated for younger adolescents.

Harris RH, Emberley M: *It's perfectly normal: changing bodies, growing up, sex and sexual health*, Cambridge, 1994, Candlewick Press. A wonderful book for preteens and their parents. Informative, easy to read, accurate, and unbiased. Nice cartoons and illustrations.

Harris RH, Emberley M: *It's so amazing! A book about eggs, sperm, birth, babies, and families*, Cambridge, 1999, Candlewick Press. Similar format written for younger children (kindergarten through fourth grade).

Maderas L: *What's happening to my body? A book for girls: a growing-up guide for parents and daughters*, ed 3, New York, 2000, New Market Press and *What's happening to my body? A book for boys: a growing-up guide for parents and sons*, ed 3, New York, 2000, New Market Press. Excellent comprehensive books to be read with preadolescents. The new edition has information on AIDS and sexually transmitted diseases.

INTERNET RESOURCES

The internet democratized access to information about medical conditions and their treatment, meaning that anyone with a computer or smartphone can look up symptoms, treatment guidelines, and a range of health recommendations from great to deceptive. Research shows that parents and teens regularly search online for health information—especially around topics that they may not feel comfortable asking about—so it is crucial to help them sort the good from the bad.

These days, child health clinicians should expect that families will have already searched for answers to their pressing questions about child health and development before attending the health care visit. This presents an opportunity to validate the drive to take charge of their health, to ask about what they have learned so far, and to listen closely to their additional questions, concerns, or uncertainties. Help families not only by providing links to trusted websites that they can return to again and again but also by having conversations that support their literacy about health information online. This includes:

- *Who is writing the material and what's their agenda?* In addition to the name of the author(s) the site should provide the background and credentials of the contributors. Help families look for qualified professionals with specific education and training in the issues on which they write. Some social media influencers can sound convincing but also have products to sell or an agenda to grow their own personal "brand."
- *Is it a nonprofit, or is there sponsorship from a company?* Help parents look for information from hospitals and professional societies, and help them recognize when health claims or products are being promoted by someone who is being paid, so therefore may not be as trustworthy.
- *Look for the date of the material.* Lots of current health topics are frequently changing, so online sites need to be updated and reviewed frequently.
- *Check multiple sources to verify information.* Misinformation is unfortunately rampant online and can sound too good to be true. Artificial intelligence programs can even generate believable health misinformation. Therefore encourage caregivers and teens to check multiple sites and sources to check that advice and information are consistent across them.

RELIABLE WEB RESOURCES

http://www.babycenter.com—This site focuses largely on pregnancy and the first year. Many features on this site change daily, including polls, news, games, and the largest baby name reference available. Monitored chat, questions and answers, and lots of special features. Well written and reviewed.

www.healthychildren.org—The AAP site for parents contains evidence-based articles on a wide range of topics written by pediatricians.

www.kidshealth.org—A great site for parents and youth from the Nemours Foundation.

https://www.aacap.org/AACAP/Families_Youth/Resource_Centers/AACAP/Families_and_Youth/Resource_Centers/Home—The American Academy of Child and Adolescent Psychiatry developed Facts for Families to provide concise and up-to-date information on psychological issues that affect children, teenagers, and their families. Each statement is available in multiple languages.

https://www.mottchildren.org/your-child—Resources for parents from developmental and behavioral and general pediatricians at the University of Michigan. Well-researched, accessible, and in-depth information on a range of topics with links to other information, organizations, and support groups.

https://www.aap.org/socialmedia—Resources from the AAP Center of Excellence on Social Media and Youth Mental Health, relevant to parents of young children to teens. Contains evidence-based answers to parents' questions and links to resources about health relationships with media.

https://parentandteen.com/—Center for Parent-Teen Communication. Provides practical information about how to talk about challenging topics and allow more emotional connection.

https://www.zerotothree.org/resources/—Resources for families, as well as clinicians and policymakers, focused on evidence-based parenting practices that support child development in the first 3 years of life.

https://www.samhsa.gov/talk-they-hear-you/parent-resources—This website, from the Substance Abuse and Mental Health Services Administration, includes resources for parents about how to talk to youth about substance use.

https://livesinthebalance.org/—Website from Ross Greene (author of *The Explosive Child*) that advocates and provides resources for developmentally sensitive school supports and avoiding punitive discipline and expulsion. Provides resources on identifying children's lagging skills and how to address them.

https://www.thetrevorproject.org/—Comprehensive resources on sexual orientation, gender identity, mental health, and community resources that can be useful for caregivers and youth.

http://www.pflag.org—Resources for parents, caregivers, friends of LGBTQ+ children include how to support youth wellness.

https://developingchild.harvard.edu/resources/—Evidence-based resources from the Harvard Center on the Developing Child about child development, as well as the community programs and policies that support child and family wellness.

https://childmind.org/resources/—The family resource center has online parenting guides and informational materials on learning disabilities, mental health conditions, diagnoses including autism, ADHD, and anxiety, and other resources.

https://reachoutandread.org/what-we-do/resources-2/—The Reach Out and Read online resources for families include early literacy guides and book recommendations, as expected, but also helpful links for caregivers to information on stress relief, healthy routines, and family wellness.

https://www.commonsensemedia.org/—Information for caregivers on parenting practices, child development, social media use, cellphones, and many other topics that can be searched by both child age and content focus.

https://www.pbs.org/parents—Resources include ideas about activities families can do together to support child's socioemotional development. Information can be looked up by child age or by topic area.

www.nctsn.org/—The National Child Traumatic Stress Network has online resources on child and family trauma, as well as trauma-based and trauma-focused care.

https://www.uclahealth.org/marc/mindful-meditations—UCLA Mindful Awareness Research Center: Website with free guided meditations to help with anxiety, worries, and difficult physical sensations.

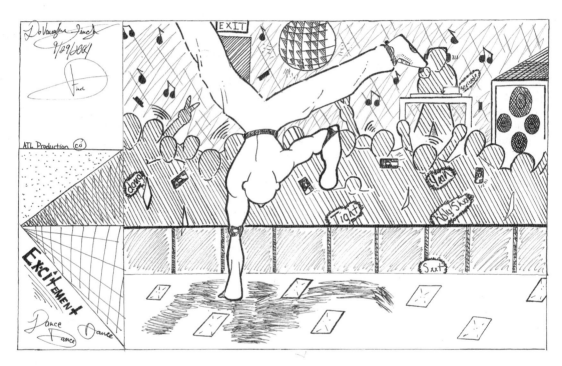

Illustration By DeVaughn Finch, age 18.

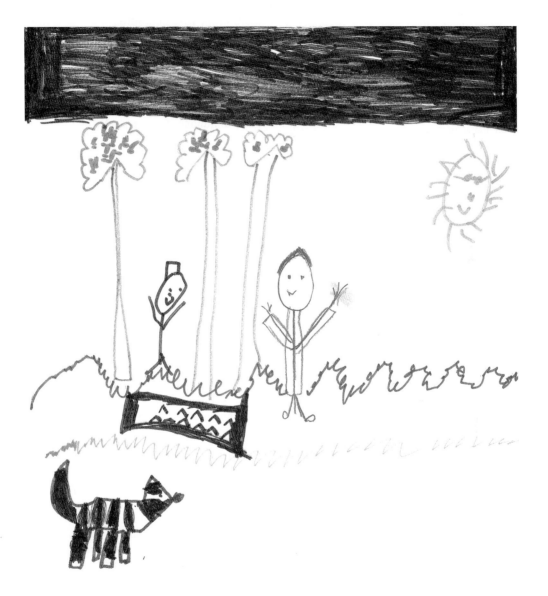

Pets are very important to children and frequently appear in drawings, often not the least or last but central to the action. A 6-year-old boy shows himself with his dad and his dog. The dog crossed the stream and is off on his own. By T.M.M.

Section I: Screening Checklists as Aids to Interview

The clinical interview, at its best, forms the foundation for a therapeutic relationship with child and parents. To supplement the interview and conduct developmental and mental health surveillance, the American Academy of Pediatrics recommends using standardized screening checklists at specific well-child encounters and whenever concerns are raised. Most of the tests below have been evaluated for validity, reliability, and predictive value. However, a screening test is not diagnostic. Rather, it suggests a problem that must then be evaluated further through a comprehensive and focused interview by a primary care clinician. Referral for a developmental assessment or a mental health consultation may follow, depending on the clinician's interpretation of the screening test and clinical interview.

Rating scales for behavioral conditions (e.g., depression) cannot take the place of a careful clinical interview, which helps identify the contributors and possible solutions unique to each patient. Rating scales, however, are often helpful in the assessment of severity of symptoms and monitoring progress over time. They also help prevent omissions that may occur during an interview alone and may provide potential educational value as a parent or older child answers questions that raise a concern that may not have been considered previously. They may help parents become better observers of their child's developmental changes and behavior.

When a screening test is used, it is important for the clinician to interpret the results for the child and family and to build their health literacy and self-understanding. Especially within a trusted clinician-parent and clinician-child relationship, discussing sensitive screening results or social determinants of health can help a family feel more understood, more engaged, and more willing to take next steps. (In contrast, if positive screening test results are brushed over, this could contribute to families feeling more vulnerable and less engaged.) Screening for developmental, behavioral, and mental conditions and/or social determinants of health should always be done with current knowledge about available referral sources in the community—so that, if a concern is identified, it can be acted on.

REFERENCES

Council on Children With Disabilities; Section on Developmental Behavioral Pediatrics; Bright Futures Steering Committee; Medical Home Initiatives for Children With Special Needs Project Advisory Committee: Identifying infants and young children with developmental disorders in the medical home: an algorithm for developmental surveillance and screening, *Pediatrics* 118(1):405–420, 2006.

Dworkin PH, Garg A: Considering approaches to screening for social determinants of health, *Pediatrics* 144(4):e20192395, 2019.

Sokol R, Austin A, Chandler C, et al: Screening children for social determinants of health: a systematic review, *Pediatrics* 144(4):e20191622, 2019.

Section II: Developmental and Behavioral Screening Test Examples

Perinatal Mental Health

The Edinburgh Postnatal Depression Scale (see page 424) is a 10-item scale that is used to screen for antenatal and postpartum depression. It is usually administered approximately 6 to 12 weeks postpartum.

Early Childhood Development

Table A1 shows selected early and middle childhood development scales that are commonly used in primary care practice, their psychometric properties, and what domains they cover. This appendix shows examples of the Ages and Stages Questionnaire (note its appearance, with illustrations to help aid parents in understanding different developmental skills), the Parents' Evaluation of Developmental Status (PEDS) and Modified Checklist for Autism in Toddlers, Revised Edition (M-CHAT-R) questionnaires. The Denver II is also shown; although this instrument is rarely administered in primary clinics currently due to being a provider-administered test that requires training, materials, and extra time, its visual representation of progression of developmental skills across early childhood is helpful for learners.

Behavioral and Mental Health Screening

As noted in several chapters of this book (Chapters 21, 22, and 25), screening for behavioral and mental health problems is recommended when concerns arise and at annual well-child exams for tweens and teens. Examples of commonly used instruments include:

- Beck Depression Inventory-II is a 21-item self-report scale that has a substantial body of research and is validated to measure the severity of depression symptoms in children and adults ages 13 and over. It has a low reading level (average grade level 3.6), so is easy to implement with adolescents.
- Children's Depression Inventory, Second Edition screens for cognitive, affective, and behavioral signs of depression in children ages 7 to 17. It has a second-grade reading level and comes as a long form (27 items) and short form (10 items).
- Strengths and Difficulties Questionnaire is a free 25-item measure that assesses behaviors, emotions, and relationships in children ages 4 to 17 years. It is often used as a research tool but can be used as a screening tool for emotional symptoms, conduct problems, hyperactivity/inattention, and peer relationship problems.
- Screen for Child Anxiety Related Emotional Disorders (SCARED) is a free 41-item scale that is administered to children ages 8 to 18 years and their parents. It can

TABLE A1 Standardized Parent-Completed Developmental-Behavioral Screening Instruments in Early and Middle Childhood

Tool, Source, and Languages Available	Age Range	Description	No. of Items and Scoring	Accuracy	Completion Time
Ages and Stages Questionnaire (ASQ) https://agesandstages.com English, Spanish, French, and Arabic, Vietnamese, and Chinese; other languages available on website	4–60 months	Series of 1 9 age-specific questionnaires screening communication, gross motor, fine motor, problem-solving, and personal adaptive skills. Features clear drawings and simple directions help parents report on children's skills.	30 items Pass/fail score for each domain	Normed on 2008 children from diverse ethnic and socioeconomic backgrounds, including Spanish speaking; sensitivity: 0.70–0.90 (moderate to high); specificity: 0.76–0.91 (moderate to high)	10–15 min
Survey of Well-being of Young Children (SWYC) https://www.tuftsmedicine.org/medical-professionals-trainees/academic-departments/department-pediatrics/survey-well-being-young-children/age-specific-forms	2–60 months	Depending on the child's age, the form includes either three or four components: (1) cognitive, language and motor development; (2) social-emotional development; (3) family risk factors, including parental depression, discord, substance abuse, and hunger; and for children between 15 months and 36 months (4) autism.	Approx. 40 items; varies by age Scoring guide provides thresholds for concern by age	Has been compared to the ASQ and CBCL	10–5 min
Parents' Evaluations of Developmental Status (PEDS) www.pedstest.com English, Spanish, Vietnamese, Arabic, Swahili, Indonesian, Chinese, Taiwanese, French, Somali, Portuguese, Malaysian, Thai, and Laotian versions available	Birth to 8 years	Ten questions eliciting parents' concerns. Can be administered in waiting rooms or by interview in Spanish and English. Determines when to refer, provide a second screen, counsel, reassure or carefully monitor development, behavior and academic progress. single response form used for all ages; may be useful as a surveillance tool.	10 items, Identifies levels of risk for various kinds of emotional and developmental problems and delays Risk categorization; provides algorithm to guide need for referral, additional screening, or continued surveillance	Standardized with 771 children from diverse ethnic and socioeconomic backgrounds, including Spanish speaking; sensitivity: 0.74–0.79 (moderate); specificity: 0.70–0.80 (moderate)	2–10 min

Continued

TABLE A1   Standardized Parent-Completed Developmental-Behavioral Screening Instruments in Early and Middle Childhood—cont'd

Tool, Source, and Languages Available	Age Range	Description	No. of Items and Scoring	Accuracy	Completion Time
Modified Checklist for Autism in Toddlers (M-CHAT) English, Spanish, Turkish, Chinese, and Japanese versions available www.firstsigns.com	16–48 months	Parent-completed questionnaire designed to identify children at risk of autism from the general population.	23 items Risk categorization (pass/fail)	Standardization sample included 1293 children screened, 58 evaluated, and 39 diagnosed with an autistic spectrum disorder; validated using ADI-R, ADOS-G, CARS, DSM-IV; sensitivity: 0.85–0.87 (moderate); specificity: 0.93–0.99 (high)	5–10 min
Pervasive Developmental Disorders Screening Test-II (PDDST-II), Stage 1-Primary Care Screener	12–48 months	Parent-completed questionnaire designed to identify children at risk of autism from the general population.	22 Risk categorization (pass/fail)	Validated using extensive multimethod diagnostic evaluations on 681 children at risk of autistic spectrum disorders and 256 children with mild-to-moderate other developmental disorders; no sensitivity/specificity data reported for screening of an unselected sample; sensitivity: 0.85–0.92 (moderate to high); specificity: 0.71–0.91 (moderate to high)	10–15 min to complete; 5 min to score

	Age	Description	Scoring	Validation	Time
Social Communication Questionnaire (SCQ) (formerly Autism Screening Questionnaire-ASQ) English and Spanish versions www.wpspublish.com	≥4 years	Parent-completed questionnaire; designed to identify children at risk of autistic spectrum disorders from the general population; based on items in the ADI-R.	40 Risk categorization (pass/fail)	Validated using the ADI-R and DSM-IV on 200 subjects (160 with pervasive developmental disorder, 40 without pervasive developmental disorder); for use in children with mental age of at least 2 years and chronologic age ≥4 years; available in two forms: lifetime and current; sensitivity: 0.85 (moderate); specificity: 0.75 (moderate)	5–10 min
Pediatric Symptom Checklist	4–16 years	Thirty-five short statements of problem behavior, including both externalizing (conduct) and internalizing (depression, anxiety, adjustment, etc.). Ratings of never, sometimes or often are assigned a value of 0, 1, and 2, and scores above cutoffs indicate when referrals are needed.	Single refer/nonrefer score	All but one study showed high sensitivity (80%–95%) but somewhat scattered specificity (68%–100%)	About 7 min

ADI-R, Autism Diagnostic Interview—Revised; *DSM-IV*, Diagnostic and Statistical Manual of Mental Disorders—Fourth Edition.
Modified with permission from Glascoe FP: *Collaborating with parents.* Nashville, Tennessee, Ellsworth & Vandermeer, 1998. Additional information from Council on Children With Disabilities; Section on Developmental Behavioral Pediatrics; Bright Futures Steering Committee; Medical Home Initiatives for Children With Special Needs Project Advisory Committee: Identifying infants and young children with developmental disorders in the medical home: an algorithm for developmental surveillance and screening, *Pediatrics* 118 (1):405–420, 2006.

be used to follow the severity of anxiety symptoms over time. The SCARED questionnaire generates scores for general anxiety, panic/somatic symptoms, separation anxiety, social phobia, and school phobia.

- Pediatric Symptom Checklist (PSC) is a 35-item free tool that assesses inattention, hyperactivity/impulsivity, school problems, somatic symptoms, mood symptoms, and disruptive behavior symptoms. It is validated for ages 11 and older.
- Patient Health Questionnaire (see Chapter 21) is a free 9-item tool validated for ages 12 to 18 years to screen for mental health symptoms.
- Generalized Anxiety Disorder 7-item scale is a free questionnaire used to screen for anxiety in children aged 11 years and older.

Attention Deficit/Hyperactivity Disorder and Learning Problems (see Chapter 19)

- NICHQ Vanderbilt Assessment Scale screens for attention deficit/hyperactivity disorder (ADHD) in children aged 6 to 12 years. It is a 55-item scale with versions for parents and teachers and generates scores for inattentive, hyperactive/impulsive, oppositional-defiant, conduct, and anxiety-depression symptoms. The teacher respondent form also indicates concerns for learning disabilities.
- Conners Scale (Fourth edition) for ADHD has two forms: one for early childhood (ages 2–6 years) and one for children/teens (6–18 years). This scale can be used by primary care providers and subspecialists and generates scores in domains, including executive functioning, learning problems, peer problems, and atypical behaviors.

Edinburgh Postnatal Depression Scale

Please read each group of statements carefully and then circle the one in each group that describes the way you have been feeling during the past week.

1   I have been able to laugh and see the funny side of things
   0 as much as I always could
   1 not quite so much now
   2 definitely not so much now
   3 not at all
2   I have looked forward with enjoyment to things
   0 as much as I ever did
   1 rather less than I used to
   2 definitely less than I used to
   3 hardly at all
3   I have blamed myself unnecessarily when things went wrong
   3 yes, most of the time
   2 yes, some of the time
   1 not very often
   0 no, never
4   I have been anxious or worried for no good reason
   0 no, not at all
   1 hardly ever
   2 yes, sometimes
   3 yes, very often
5   I have felt scared or panicky for no very good reason
   3 yes, quite a lot
   2 yes, sometimes
   1 no, not much
   0 no, not at all

6   Things have been getting on top of me
   3 yes, most of the time I haven't been able to cope at all
   2 yes, sometimes I haven't been coping as well as usual
   1 no, most of the time I have coped quite well
   0 no, I have been coping as well as ever
7   I have been so unhappy that I have had difficulty sleeping
   3 yes, most of the time
   2 yes, sometimes
   1 not very often
   0 no, not at all
8   I have felt sad or miserable
   3 yes, most of the time
   2 yes, quite often
   1 not very often
   0 no, not at all
9   I have been so unhappy that I have been crying
   3 yes, most of the time
   2 yes, quite often
   1 only occasionally
   0 no, never
10   The thought of harming myself has occurred to me
   3 yes, quite often
   2 sometimes
   1 hardly ever
   0 never

PEDIATRIC SYMPTOM CHECKLIST

Please mark under the heading that best fits your child:

	Never	Sometimes	Often
1. Complains of aches or pains	☐	☐	☐
2. Spends more time alone	☐	☐	☐
3. Tires easily, little energy	☐	☐	☐
4. Fidgety, unable to sit still	☐	☐	☐
5. Has trouble with a teacher	☐	☐	☐
6. Less interested in school	☐	☐	☐
7. Acts as if driven by a motor	☐	☐	☐
8. Daydreams too much	☐	☐	☐
9. Distracted easily	☐	☐	☐
10. Is afraid of new situations	☐	☐	☐
11. Feels sad, unhappy	☐	☐	☐
12. Is irritable, angry	☐	☐	☐
13. Feels hopeless	☐	☐	☐
14. Has trouble concentrating	☐	☐	☐
15. Less interest in friends	☐	☐	☐
16. Fights with other children	☐	☐	☐
17. Absent from school	☐	☐	☐
18. School grades dropping	☐	☐	☐
19. Is down on him or herself	☐	☐	☐
20. Visits doctor with doctor finding nothing wrong	☐	☐	☐
21. Has trouble sleeping	☐	☐	☐
22. Worries a lot	☐	☐	☐
23. Wants to be with you more than before	☐	☐	☐
24. Feels he or she is bad	☐	☐	☐
25. Takes unnecessary risks	☐	☐	☐
26. Gets hurt frequently	☐	☐	☐
27. Seems to be having less fun	☐	☐	☐
28. Acts younger than children his or her age	☐	☐	☐
29. Does not listen to rules	☐	☐	☐
30. Does not show feelings	☐	☐	☐
31. Does not understand other people's feelings	☐	☐	☐
32. Teases others	☐	☐	☐
33. Blames others for his or her troubles	☐	☐	☐
34. Takes things that do not belong to him or her	☐	☐	☐
35. Refuses to share	☐	☐	☐

© 1998 Michael Jellinek, M.D., Massachusetts General Hospital (reprinted with permission from the author)

Procedures and Scoring Criteria for the Pediatric Symptoms Checklist

- For children 4 and 5 years of age, responses to items 5, 6, 17, and 18 are not counted due to their emphasis on school issues, which may not be relevant.
- The value of 0 is assigned to "never," 1 to "sometimes," and 2 to "often." Add these values to obtain a score for the entire test.
- The presence of significant behavioral or emotional difficulties is suggested when children ages 4 to 5 years receive 24 or more points, and when children ages 6 to 16 years receive 28 or more points.
- To determine what kinds of mental health problems are present, determine the three factor scores on the PSC:

PSC Attention Subscale consists of these five items:

4. Fidgety, unable to sit still
7. Acts as if driven by motor
8. Daydreams too much
9. Distracted easily
14. Has trouble concentrating

Children who receive 7 or more points on these five items need a workup for ADHD. The American Academy of Pediatrics recently revised its recommendations on how to diagnose ADHD, and the article is in the May 2000 issue of *Pediatrics*—a must read.

PSC Internalizing Subscale consists of these five items:

11. Feels sad
13. Feels hopeless
19. Is down on self
22. Worries a lot
27. Seems to have less fun

It is a screen for depression and anxiety. Children who receive 5 or more points on these five items need to be referred for counseling and may eventually need to be considered for antidepressives, anxiolytics, etc.

PSC Externalizing Subscale consists of these seven items:

16. Fights with other children
29. Does not listen to rules
31. Does not understand other's feelings
32. Teases others
33. Blames others for his troubles
34. Takes things that do not belong to them
35. Refuses to share

It is a screen for conduct disorder, oppositional-defiant disorder, rage disorder, etc. Children who receive 7 or more points on these seven items need behavioral intervention.

PSC Developmental/Academic Screening (33)

If a child fails the whole test, the child should be referred for an academic/developmental assessment. Children with mental health problems almost invariably have academic problems, and children with developmental or academic problems are at high risk of mental health problems.

Parents whose children pass the PSC but endorse numerous items should benefit from in-office counseling. If this has been tried and not found to be successful, such families should be referred for such services as parent training classes and behavioral intervention programs.

Those with academic failure and difficulties (whose parents endorse items about poor school performance, absence from school, etc.), whether or not the PSC is passed, should be referred for intellectual and educational testing.

A short form of the Pediatric Symptom Checklist is available in Gardner W, et al: The PSC-17: a brief pediatric symptom checklist for psychosocial problem subscales: a report from PROS and ASPN, *Ambul Child Health* 5:225–236, 1999.

M-CHAT (THE MODIFIED CHECKLIST FOR AUTISM IN TODDLERS), REVISED (16–30 MONTHS OF AGE)

Please answer these questions about your child. Keep in mind how your child *usually* behaves. If you have seen your child do the behavior a few times, but he or she does not usually do it, then please answer **no**. Please circle **yes** or **no** for every question.

1.	If you point at something across the room, does your child look at it? (for example, if you point at a toy or an animal, does your child look at the toy or animal?)	Yes	No
2.	Have you ever wondered if your child might be deaf?	Yes	No
3.	Does your child play pretend or make-believe? (For example, pretend to drink from an empty cup, pretend to talk on a phone, or pretend to feed a doll or stuffed animal?)	Yes	No
4.	Does your child like climbing on things? (for example, furniture, playground equipment, or stairs)	Yes	No
5.	Does your child make unusual finger movements near his/her eyes? (for example, does your child wiggle his or her fingers close to his or her eyes?)	Yes	No
6.	Does your child point with one finger to ask for something or to get help? (for example, pointing to a snack or toy that is out of reach)	Yes	No
7.	Does your child point with one finger to show you something interesting?	Yes	No
8.	Is your child interested in other children? (for example, does your child watch other children, smile at them, or go to them?)	Yes	No

9.	Does your child show you things by bringing them to you or holding them up for you to see – not to get help, but just to share? (for example, showing you a flower, a stuffed animal, or a toy truck)	Yes	No
10.	Does your child respond when you call his or her name? (for example, does he or she look up, talk or babble, or stop what he or she is doing when you call his or her name?)	Yes	No
11.	When you smile at your child, does he or she smile back at you?	Yes	No
12.	Does your child get upset by everyday noises? (for example, does your child scream or cry to noise such as a vacuum cleaner or loud music?)	Yes	No
13.	Does your child walk?	Yes	No
14.	Does your child look you in the eye when you are talking to him or her, playing with him or her, dressing him or her?	Yes	No
15.	Does your child try to copy what you do? (for example, wave bye-bye, clap, or make a funny noise when you do)	Yes	No
16.	If you turn your head to look at something, does your child look around to see what you are looking at?	Yes	No
17.	Does your child try to get you to watch him or her? (for example, does your child look at you for praise, or say "look" or "watch me"?)	Yes	No
18.	Does your child understand when you tell him or her to do something? (for example, if you don't point, can your child understand "put the book on the chair" or "bring me the blanket"?)	Yes	No
19.	If something new happens, does your child look at your face to see how you feel about it? (for example, if he or she hears a strange or funny noise, or sees a new toy, will he or she look at your face?)	Yes	No
20.	Does your child like movement activities? (for example, being swung or bounced on your knee).	Yes	No

Scoring the Modified Checklist for Autism in Toddlers, Revised (M-CHAT-R)

For most items, YES is a typical response, and NO is an at-risk response. However, items 2, 5, and 12 are reverse scored, meaning that NO is a typical response and YES is an at-risk response. To score the M-CHAT-R, add up the number of at-risk responses and follow the algorithm below:

- **Total Score 0–2**: The score is LOW risk. No Follow-up is needed. Child has screened negative. Rescreen at 24 months if the child is younger than 2 years old (or after 3 months has elapsed), and refer as needed if developmental surveillance or other tools suggest risk for autism spectrum disorder.
- **Total Score 3–7**: The score is MODERATE risk. Administer the M-CHAT-R Follow-up items that correspond to the at-risk responses. Only those items which were scored at risk need to be completed. If two or more items continue to be at-risk, refer the child immediately for (1) early intervention and (2) diagnostic evaluation.
- **Total Score: 8–20**: The score is HIGH risk. It is not necessary to complete the M-CHAT-R Follow-up at this time. Bypass Follow-up, and refer immediately for (1) early intervention and (2) diagnostic evaluation.

Section III: Social Determinants of Health Screening

Screening for social determinants of health, including material hardship, exposure to violence, and other stressors that influence child well-being has become more common over the past decade. Several screening tools are shown in Table A2, but research continues to examine the best ways to implement these tools and follow up to ensure that families access appropriate resources. Experts in this field stress that screening for social determinants of health should be strengths based and family centered, involving shared decision-making and respect for family autonomy in terms of what resources they want help with. Rather than being a "screen-and-refer" model, these tools should open opportunities for discussions about family circumstances and be embedded within a comprehensive, integrated process that facilitates connections to known community resources that address families' priorities and needs.

TABLE A2 Screening Tools for Social Determinants of Health (SDOH) Available for Use in Pediatric Ambulatory Settings

Screening Tool	Time to complete (min)	SDOH Domains Assessed	Available Languages	Appropriate for Low-Literacy Populations	Validity and/or Reliability Assessed
SEEK PSQ	3–4	Food insufficiency Health-related needs Parental intimate partner violence, depression, stress, drug or alcohol problems Tobacco use in the home Gun in the home	English; Spanish	Not reported	Yes
iScreen	10	Food insufficiency Housing instability Financial problems Need for health/disability benefits Child care/education needs/after-school care Health insurance needs Child behavioral health concerns Tobacco exposure Transportation difficulties Neighborhood safety Immigration concerns Household concerns about violence, drugs/alcohol, incarceration of a household member, problems with child support or custody	English; Spanish	Yes	No
ASK Tool	Not reported	Food insufficiency Housing instability Difficulty paying bills, parental employment, need for legal aid Child care needs Child violence and bullying exposure, physical or sexual abuse Parental mental illness or substance abuse Child separation from caregiver Safe adult in child's life	English; Spanish	Not reported	No
WE CARE Screening Instrument	4–5	Food insufficiency Housing instability Difficulty paying bills Parental employment/education Lack of child care Household intimate partner violence, alcohol, and drug use Parental depressive symptoms	English; Spanish	Yes	Yes

TABLE A2   Screening Tools for Social Determinants of Health (SDOH) Available for Use in Pediatric Ambulatory Settings—cont'd

Screening Tool	Time to complete (min)	SDOH Domains Assessed	Available Languages	Appropriate for Low-Literacy Populations	Validity and/or Reliability Assessed
FAMNEEDS	Not reported	Food insufficiency Housing instability Difficulty paying bills/meeting basic needs Employment/education, need for benefits, legal aid Need for child/elder care Help needed in getting health insurance Transportation problems Health literacy Parental social support, experience of discrimination Parental experience of violence Parental depressive symptoms Parental tobacco/alcohol/drug use	English; Spanish; Haitian Creole; Urdu; Punjabi; Hindi; Arabic	Not reported	No
Child ACE Tool	5	Parental Education Parental marital status Suspected child maltreatment Intimate partner violence in the household Mental illness in the household Substance abuse in the household Household member is incarcerated	English; Spanish	Not reported	No
Health-Related Social Problems Screener	20	Food insufficiency Housing instability Difficulty paying bills Use of income support programs Parental employment Household income Parent and child health insurance status, barriers to health care No regular healthcare provider Parental intimate partner violence victimization	English; Spanish	Yes	No

ASK, Addressing Social Key Questions for Health; *FAMNEEDS*, Family Needs Screening Program; *NR*, not reported.
Adapted from Sokol R, Austin A, Chandler C, et al: Screening children for Social Determinants of Health: a systematic review, *Pediatrics* 144 (4):e20191622, 2019.

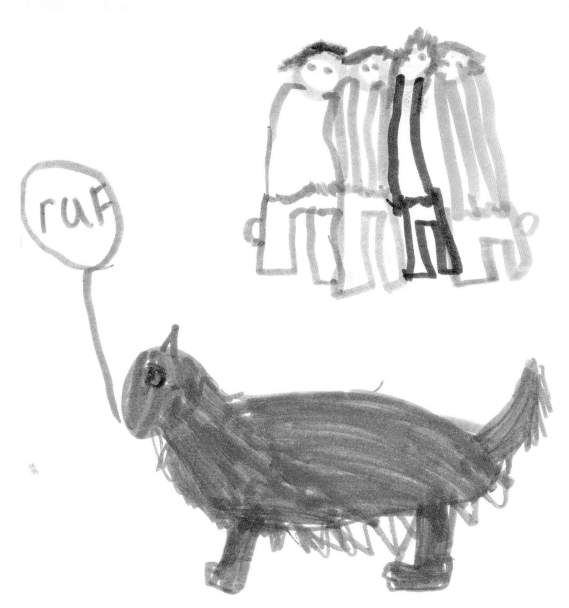

And finally, the tail wags. By a boy, age 5.

Note: Page numbers followed by *f* indicate figures, *t* indicate tables, and *b* indicate boxes